PRACTICAL
Dermatopathology

Content Strategist: Belinda Kuhn
Content Development Specialists: Sven Pinczewski, Joanne Scott
Editorial Assistant: Trinity Hutton
Project Manager: Maggie Johnson
Design: Stewart Larking
Marketing Manager (UK/USA): Carla Holloway

SECOND EDITION

PRACTICAL
Dermatopathology

Ronald P Rapini MD

Josey Professor and Chairman
Department of Dermatology
Professor of Pathology
University of Texas Medical School
and MD Anderson Cancer Center
Houston, TX, USA

ELSEVIER
SAUNDERS

Edinburgh, London, New York, Oxford, Philadelphia, St Louis, Sydney, Toronto 2012

For additional online content visit
www.expertconsult.com

Expert | CONSULT

Saunders is an imprint of Elsevier Inc.

ISBN-13: 978 0323 06658 7
E-book ISBN: 978 1 4557 3800 7

British Library Cataloguing in Publication Data
A catalogue record for this book is available from the British Library

Library of Congress Cataloging in Publication Data
A catalog record for this book is available from the Library of Congress

Rapini, Ronald P.
Practical dermatopathology. – 2nd ed.
1. Skin – Diseases – Diagnosis.
I. Title
616.5'07 – dc22

Printed in China
Last digit is the print number: 9 8 7 6 5 4 3

Contents

Preface

The first edition of this book was a complete overhaul of a similar book I co-authored in 1988, published as *Atlas of Dermatopathology.* A practical approach to skin biopsies is presented to supplement existing textbooks of dermatopathology. I hope that the lists of differential diagnoses for clinical and pathologic changes found in Chapter 1 will serve as a starting point in the evaluation of a skin biopsy. The first edition was compact enough for residents to carry around, and even experienced dermatopathologists sometimes kept a copy near the microscope for a quick list of differential diagnoses. Since many have complained about a very worn-out copy of the first edition, we have embarked upon a second edition, deciding to keep the size compact. Adding clinical photographs would have made the book too thick, so we are providing these along with additional histologic photographs on a website instead. I have listed the important clinical and histologic features and variations for both common and unusual diseases, italicizing the most characteristic features. I have tried to distill the most important facts into this text. To be concise, I have omitted discussion of normal skin histology, electron microscopy, hair, nails, oral mucosa, disease pathogenesis, and treatment. Of course, knowledge of the pathogenesis is critical in understanding skin disease, and detailed correlation between the clinical and pathologic features is very important in making a specific diagnosis. The reader can readily find this information in some of the major textbooks listed at the end of this book, most of which give many references. I have not given extensive references because of space considerations, and because most physicians now have ready access to computerized literature searching for contemporary references. Essentially this is a book that aids in making a diagnosis. Making a correct diagnosis is of utmost importance, because the treatment can then be found in a variety of sources. The physician without a specific diagnosis is doomed to treat patients by trial and error.

The book has been organized so that one can quickly look up a disease or a pathologic feature and immediately find the important criteria and a differential diagnosis. Pure pathologists will complain that rashes in Chapters 2 and 3 are organized by their clinical morphology instead of by histology. They would prefer to have chapters on lichenoid, perivascular, and spongiotic dermatitis instead. But they can find that kind of thinking in Sections 1.72, 1.109, and 1.132. There is no perfect way to organize diseases in this kind of text, and this book reflects the perspective of an author who is both a clinician and a histopathologist. Organization strictly by etiology or clinical features provides the reader with no starting point in evaluating a biopsy with a specific pathologic change. Textbooks organized by pathologic changes often end up discussing a given disease in multiple fragmented locations throughout the book, because most inflammatory diseases present with variable histologic patterns.

I must alert the reader to additional pitfalls in the use of this book. In my efforts to publish "classic" examples of each disease, the reader may be confused when examining a lesion showing only some of the typical features. There is no substitute for experience in dealing with all of the numerous variations that may occur (experientia docet). Uncommon presentations of common diseases are common. There is not enough space to publish both low- and high-power photomicrographs of all conditions, otherwise, several expensive volumes would be needed to adequately cover the gamut of skin diseases. This is not meant to minimize the importance of scanning microscopy. Skin lesions evolve through time, and it has not been possible for any author to illustrate the incipient or non-diagnostic stages of all of these skin diseases in a single volume. The reader should realize that the lists found in Chapter 1 and elsewhere in the book purposely do not include every possibility, although they are reasonably complete. My bias toward being a "lumper" may be apparent, so that many conditions considered by "splitters" to be separate entities are often grouped together as "Variations" under some other heading. I appreciated comments from readers of inevitable errors or omissions found in the first edition, and I solicit additional feedback on this newest version.

Ronald P Rapini, MD
2012

Acknowledgements

Richard Zuehlke MD organized some of the ideas used in Chapter 1, which were presented in his *Syllabus of Dermatologic Histopathology*, the fourth edition of which was published by Westwood Pharmaceuticals in 1982. That guide updated lists of differentials prepared by Victor I Spear MD in 1962 at University of Michigan, crediting the 1954 book *Systematized Histopathology* by Drs Walter R Nickel and James H Lockwood. Loren Golitz MD provided me with valuable fellowship training in dermatopathology and served as a role model educator and collector of slides for teaching purposes.

I thank many other faculty, colleagues (and residents and students!) who have taught me over the years. Special thanks to recent dermatopathology fellows Darren Whittemore DO, Valencia Thomas MD, Kimara Whisenant MD, and Scott Bangert MD for help with some of the new second edition photos.

I cannot list all of those individuals who have shared their cases or provided slides for my teaching collection. They are too numerous to mention individually.

Ronald P Rapini, MD

Dedication

To Mary Jo, my love, who tolerates (most of the time) the competing affection I feel for academic work.

To Joann and Vince Rapini, my parents, who laid the foundation for my life.

To Brianna and Sarina, my children, in whom I hope to have instilled the drive to do something meaningful while being considerate of others.

CHAPTER 1

Clinical and Pathologic Findings with Differential Diagnostic Lists

The differential diagnostic lists that follow in this chapter serve as a starting point for evaluation of an unknown skin biopsy. Such lists have some advantages over algorithms because they provide multiple pathways for getting back on track toward the correct diagnosis. By contrast, some algorithms provide fatal forks in the road that, if selected incorrectly, might lead the pathologist toward a misdiagnosis based upon too much emphasis upon one criterion. Instead, it is best to consider multiple criteria in concert.

A. Overview of clinical findings

The most important clinical questions are *location* of lesions (arms, head, legs, etc.), *symptoms* (pruritus, pain, etc.), *duration* (acute or chronic), *arrangement* of lesions (solitary, generalized, annular, linear, etc.), *morphology* (macules, papules, plaques, vesicles, etc.), and *color* (red, blue, brown, black, white, yellow, etc.). The smart pathologist will not read out a skin biopsy of an inflammatory condition without calling for clinical information. Some pseudomalignancies are distinguished from bona fide malignancies mainly by clinical differences (1.118). The difference between a lichenoid keratosis and lichen planus, which may be nearly identical histologically, for example, primarily rests upon the former being a solitary papule and the latter being a rash with more than one lesion.

B. Overview of pathologic findings

Pathologists organize most of the histologic findings of skin lesions according to *epidermal* changes, *dermal* changes, *adipose* changes (panniculitis, if inflammatory), *patterns* or arrangements of inflammatory or neoplastic cells, and specific *types of cells* found. *Architecture* of skin lesions (arrangements of cells) is considered along with cytologic changes such as atypia. *Cytologic atypia* (hyperchromatism, pleomorphism, prominent nucleoli, increased nuclear to cytoplasmic ratio, and abnormal mitoses) is subjective, and the precise quantification of atypia into mild, moderate or severe is in the eye of the beholder to some extent. Atypia is often used as evidence of malignancy, but it must be considered along with clinical findings and the lesion architecture. Dermatopathologists with a background in clinical dermatology tend to emphasize the clinical information and cellular architecture over the cytologic features. Those with a pathology background often stress cytology at the expense of clinical features and architecture. If the histologic findings do not fit the clinical situation, then the disparity must be rectified!

The *art of pathology* is to be dogmatic about the diagnosis as often as possible, while not being afraid to hedge and give a differential diagnosis when the diagnosis is uncertain.[156,158] The correct diagnosis sometimes must be expressed as a list of probabilities, and the helpful pathologist should list the possibilities in the order of likelihood. Pathologists may be subcategorized into home-run hitters and hedgers. The *home-run hitters* try to "force" a diagnosis, and give only one most likely diagnosis. They are either very, very correct, and look very smart, or else they strike out and miss the diagnosis completely. This can be dangerous. For example, they might diagnose a lesion as a definite Spitz nevus, which subsequently is found to be a melanoma when it metastasizes. Most Spitz nevi can be diagnosed with relative certainty, but there are always those difficult cases for which all the experts can have their opinions, using the best of criteria, but for which there remains an element of uncertainty. Simple histology has its limits in predicting biologic behavior.

Hedger pathologists, by contrast, seldom make a specific diagnosis, and instead often give a long differential diagnostic list, even to the point of listing histologic possibilities that are ridiculous from a clinical standpoint. They rarely strike out, but they are sometimes not very helpful, and are not appreciated by clinicians. Frequently these pathologists might add the comment to the report that "clinical correlation is recommended", feeling that this will relieve them from having to do any correlation themselves. They dream of the clinician doing the correlation, based upon the pathologist's microscopic description. Unfortunately, some of the clinicians are in no better position to do the correlation either, so then this type of report becomes worthless. Someone simply has to take the responsibility for making sense of it all and doing the correlation, and simply punting this duty back and forth between the clinicians and the pathologists does no good. Sometimes they actually may need to speak to one another. The lack of clinical correlation is one of the biggest problems seen frequently in dermatopathology, probably more commonly than errors of fact. Wise pathologists avoid the two extremes of the home-run hitter and the hedger.

1. Epidermal changes

Acantholysis (1.2)
Atrophy of epidermis (1.9)
Dyskeratosis (1.27)
Follicular plugging (1.47)
Horn cysts (1.59)
Hypergranulosis (1.60)
Hyperplasia of epidermis (1.61)
Hypogranulosis (1.63)
Liquefaction degeneration of basal layer (1.64)

DOI: 10.1016/B978-0-323-06658-7.00001-4

Necrotic keratinocytes (1.86)
Papillomatosis (1.102)
Parakeratosis (1.104)
Pseudoepitheliomatous (pseudocarcinomatous) hyperplasia (1.116)
Spongiosis (1.132)
Squamous eddies, keratin pearls, and squamatization (1.134)
Transepidermal elimination (1.140)
Vacuolization of keratinocytes (1.144)

2.   Dermal changes

Atrophy of dermis (1.8)
Black deposits (1.12)
Blue amorphous material (1.15)
Brown deposits (1.17)
Calcification (1.19)
Edema of dermis (1.30)
Elastic tissue changes (1.31)
Eosinophilic pink amorphous material (1.35)
Hemosiderin (1.58)
Melanin incontinence (1.79)
Mucin and myxomatous changes (1.83)
Scars, sclerosis, fibrosis (1.125)
Thrombi (1.137)

3.   Cell types

Basaloid cells (1.11)
Clear or pale cells (1.22)
Eosinophils (1.36)
Epithelioid cells (1.38)
Extravasated erythrocytes (1.40)
Foam cells (1.46)
Granulomas (1.51)
Lymphocytes and histiocytes (1.76)
Mast cells (1.78)
Multinucleated giant cells (1.84)
Neutrophils (1.89)
Plasma cells (1.111)
Small cells ("oat cells") (1.130)
Spindle cells (1.131)

4.   Patterns of inflammation and neoplastic proliferation

Epidermotropism and pagetoid proliferation (1.37)
Folliculitis (1.47)
Grenz zone (1.53)
Interface dermatitis (1.64)
Interstitial dermatitis (1.65)
Lichenoid dermatitis (1.72)
Nodular and diffuse dermatitis (1.91)
Panniculitis (1.101)
Perivascular dermatitis, superficial (1.109)
Perivascular dermatitis, superficial and deep (1.109)
Single filing of cells (1.128)
Vasculitis (1.145)

C. Differential diagnostic lists
1.1 Abdomen lesions

(see also Umbilicus lesions 1.143, Trunk lesions 1.141)
Accessory nipple (29.12)
Cutaneous endometriosis (29.9)
Dysplastic nevus (20.5)
Melanocytic nevus (20.5)
Omphalomesenteric duct remnant (29.11)
Pemphigoid gestationis (6.3)
Pruritic urticarial plaques of pregnancy (3.6)
Seborrheic keratosis (18.2)
Striae (27.2)

1.2 Acantholysis

Acantholysis is the loss of cohesion between keratinocytes as a result of dissolution of intercellular connections, sometimes resulting in an intraepidermal vesicle. Acanthocyte is an old name for keratinocyte, and means "prickle cell", referring to the desmosomal spines that normally connect the cells. The process differs from spongiosis (1.9) in that acantholytic keratinocytes tend to be rounded rather than elongated, the desmosomal spines appear destroyed rather than stretched, and exocytosis of lymphocytes into the epidermis is usually absent. Dyscohesive melanocytes in melanoma (20.11) may resemble acantholysis (20.11), but in this situation the term acantholysis is not used (call it "dyscohesion").

Actinic keratosis (sometimes) (18.8)
Darter's disease (11.3)
Familial dyskeratotic comedones (10.1)
Hailey–Hailey disease (5.5)
Herpes virus infection (14.2)
Impetigo (occasionally) (12.2)
Incidental finding or artifact
Pemphigus (all varieties, 5.4)
Pityriasis rubra pilaris (2.10, rarely)
Squamous cell carcinoma (sometimes) (18.11)
Staphylococcal scalded skin syndrome (12.2)
Transient acantholytic dermatosis (Grover's disease) (5.6)
Warty dyskeratoma (18.7)

Acanthosis (see Hyperplasia of epidermis, 1.61)
1.3 Acneiform lesions

This is a clinical group of conditions characterized by erythematous papules, pustules, and/or comedones, resembling acne (pilosebaceous unit inflammation). See also Follicular eruptions (1.47), Neutrophil eruptions (1.89), and Comedones (1.24).

Acne variants (10.1)
Arthropod bites (15.7)
Bowel bypass syndrome (4.1)
Candidiasis (13.4)
Dermatitis herpetiformis (6.5)
Drug-induced acneiform eruptions (3.5)
Folliculitis (10.2)
Grover's disease (5.6)
Impetigo (12.1)
Miliaria (10.6)
Perioral dermatitis (10.1)

Pustular vasculitis (4.1)
Pyoderma faciale (10.1)
Varicella (14.2)

1.4 Alopecia

Alopecia is hair loss.[55,58] It is commonly subdivided into scarring and non-scarring. Some pathology laboratories prefer to section punch biopsies of alopecia both horizontally and vertically, to maximize the view of more follicles. This author is not a fan of horizontal scalp biopsy sections, but nevertheless they are popular. Vertical scalp biopsies perform comparably to horizontal ones.[113a]

A. Non-scarring alopecia

Alopecia areata (10.9)
Androgenetic alopecia (10.12)
Drug-induced alopecia (3.5)
Genodermatoses: Ectodermal dysplasia (11.2), Progeria (9.6), Rothmund–Thomson syndrome (11.5), etc.
Hair shaft disorders (most are not covered in this book): trichorrhexis nodosa, monilithrix, trichorrhexis invaginata (11.1), pili annulati, pili torti, trichothiodystrophy, mechanical trauma, etc.
Lipedematous alopecia (10.13)
Psoriasis, severe (2.8)
Seborrheic dermatitis, severe (2.1)
Syphilis, secondary (12.13)
Telogen effluvium (10.14)
Temporal arteritis
Thyroid disease
Traction alopecia (can scar if severe, 10.11)
Trichotillosis (10.11)

B. Scarring alopecia

Acne keloidalis nuchae (10.2)
Alopecia mucinosa (10.8)
Alopecia neoplastica (secondary to neoplasm, especially metastatic, on the scalp, Chapter 28)
Aplasia cutis congenita (17.4)
Burns (6.7)
Folliculitis (10.2)
Herpes zoster (14.2)
Lichen planopilaris (2.11)
Lupus erythematosus (17.6)
Nevus sebaceus (21.2)
Pemphigoid, cicatricial (6.2)
Pseudopelade of Brocq (10.10)
Radiodermatitis (9.2)
Scleroderma and morphea (9.3)
Tinea capitis (13.1)
Trauma (10.11)

1.5 Annular lesions

These lesions form clinical rings. Similar terms are gyrate and circinate. See also Serpiginous (1.127), Linear (1.73), and Reticulated (1.123).

A. Annular reactive erythemas (many are reactions to infections, drugs, or other)

Cutis marmarata (3.10)
Erythema ab igne (3.9)
Erythema annulare centrifugum (3.3)
Erythema chronicum migrans (12.14, Lyme disease, also in infectious group)
Erythema gyratum repens (3.4)
Erythema marginatum (3.1, rheumatic fever, also in infectious group)
Erythema multiforme (3.2)
Livedo reticularis (3.10)
Necrolytic migratory erythema (3.2)
Urticaria (3.1)

B. Annular infections

Chromomycosis, rarely annular (13.10)
Hansen's disease (12.12)
Impetigo (12.1)
Lupus vulgaris (12.10)
Syphilis, more annular on the face in black skin (12.13)
Tinea (13.1)
Warts, especially recurring after cryotherapy (14.1)

C. Non-infectious annular granulomas

Granuloma annulare and actinic granuloma (7.1)
Sarcoidosis (7.5)

D. Annular eczematous and papulosquamous diseases

Eczema, especially nummular (2.1)
Erythrokeratodermia variabilis (11.1)
Ichthyosis linearis circumflexa (11.1)
Lichen planus (2.11)
Pityriasis rosea (2.4)
Psoriasis (2.8)
Reiter's disease (circinate balanitis, 2.8)
Seborrheic dermatitis (2.1)

E. Annular vesiculopustules

Chronic bullous disease of childhood (6.4)
Linear IgA bullous dermatosis (6.4)
Pemphigus (5.4)
Subcorneal pustular dermatosis (2.8)

F. Annular neoplastic diseases

Basal cell carcinoma (18.14)
Desmoplastic trichoepithelioma (22.2)
Mycosis fungoides (24.1)
Sebaceous hyperplasia (21.1)
Targetoid hemosiderotic hemangioma (25.2)

G. Miscellaneous annular lesions

Elastosis perforans serpiginosa (9.13)
Lupus erythematosus (especially subacute cutaneous lupus erythematosus, 17.6)
Porokeratosis (18.4)
Purpura annularis telangiectodes (Majocchi's disease) (4.8)

1.6 Arm lesions (includes forearms)

(see also Hand lesions 1.56, Leg lesions 1.67)

A. Common

Actinic keratosis (18.8)
Arthropod bites (15.7)
Basal cell carcinoma (18.14)
Contact dermatitis (2.2)
Eczema (2.1)
Erythema multiforme (3.2)
Granuloma annulare (3.1)
Keratosis pilaris (10.5)
Lentigo simplex (20.3) and solar lentigo (20.4)
Lichen planus (2.11)
Melanocytic nevus (20.5)
Psoriasis (especially elbows, 2.8)
Solar purpura (4.15)
Squamous cell carcinoma (18.11)
Trauma

B. Uncommon

Atypical mycobacteria (12.11)
Epidermal nevus (18.1)
Idiopathic guttate hypomelanosis (17.10)
Lichen striatus (2.5)
Lupus erythematosus (17.6)
Pseudoxanthoma elasticum (axilla, antecubital, 9.8)
Sporotrichosis (13.11)

1.7 Arthritis and skin disease

Drug eruption (3.5)
Gonococcemia (12.18)
Gout (8.5)
Loefgren's syndrome (7.5)
Lupus erythematosus (17.6)
Lyme disease (12.14)
Multicentric reticulohistiocytosis (7.8)
Psoriasis (2.8)
Pyoderma gangrenosum (4.12)
Reiter's disease (2.8)
Relapsing polychondritis (17.8)
Rheumatic fever (12.2)
Rheumatoid arthritis (3.7, 4.1, 7.3)
Sepsis and subacute bacterial endocarditis (4.1)
Sweet's syndrome (3.7)
Vasculitis (4.1)
Viral infections (Chapter 14)
Yersiniosis (1.7)

1.8 Atrophy of the dermis

Dermal atrophy is a decreased thickness of the dermis. In most of these diseases, the epidermis is also atrophic (1.9). In some of them, the dermis is not actually thin, but adipose tissue is deposited higher up in the dermis than usual, or the fat clinically appears herniated, due to lack of dermal support, even though the dermis is not actually thin. Panniculitis (Chapter 16) can also produce the appearance of dermal atrophy, although the atrophy is primarily in the adipose.

Acrodermatitis chronica atrophicans (12.14)
Aging skin (9.1)
Anetoderma (9.11)
Aplasia cutis congenita
Atrophoderma of Pasini and Pierini (9.4)
Corticosteroids (especially injected)
Focal dermal hypoplasia (Goltz syndrome, 11.8)
Morphea (9.4)
Nevus lipomatosus (29.1)
Piezogenic pedal papules (29.1)
Scars (27.2)

1.9 Atrophy of the epidermis

Epidermal atrophy is a decreased thickness of the epidermis, particularly the spinous layer.

Acrodermatitis chronica atrophicans (12.14)
Actinic keratosis, atrophic (18.8)
Aging, sun-damaged, or radiation-damaged skin (9.1, 9.2)
Anetoderma (9.11)
Aplasia cutis congenita (17.4)
Atrophie blanche (4.13)
Atrophoderma (9.4)
Corticosteroids (especially topical)
Degos disease (4.10)
Dermatomyositis (17.7)
Graft-versus-host disease, chronic (17.3)
Lichen planus, atrophic (usually acanthotic) (2.11)
Lichen sclerosus (9.5)
Lupus erythematosus (17.6, always consider when extreme atrophy)
Necrobiosis lipoidica (7.2)
Neoplasms in the dermis will often cause epidermal atrophy
Poikiloderma atrophicans vasculare (24.1)
Poikiloderma congenitale (11.5)
Porokeratosis (18.4, central portion sometimes)
Progeria (Werner's syndrome) (9.6)
Scar (27.2)
Striae (27.2)

1.10 Axilla lesions

Acanthosis nigricans (18.5)
Acrochordons (27.4)
Axillary granular parakeratosis (1.27)
Candidiasis (13.4)
Chromhidrosis
Contact dermatitis (2.2)
Cystic hygroma (25.10)
Erythrasma (12.5)
Fibrous hamartoma of infancy (27.9)
Fox–Fordyce disease (10.7)
Hailey–Hailey disease (5.5)
Hidradenitis suppurativa (10.1)
Hyperhidrosis
Intertrigo (2.2)
Inverse psoriasis (2.8)
Neurofibromatosis (axillary freckling)
Pemphigus vegetans (5.4)

Pseudoxanthoma elasticum (9.8)
Scabies (15.9)
Seborrheic dermatitis (2.1)
Trichomycosis axillaris (12.5)

1.11 Basaloid cells

Basaloid cells are tumor cells that resemble basal cells of the epidermis (compare with small cells, 1.130). They have a dark oval nucleus and very little cytoplasm.

Basal cell carcinoma (18.14)
Seborrheic keratosis (18.2)
Ameloblastoma (18.14)
Cloacogenic carcinoma (18.14)
Sebaceous tumors (especially sebaceous adenoma, sebaceous epithelioma, and sebaceous carcinoma, Chapter 21)
Follicular tumors (especially trichoepithelioma and pilomatricoma, Chapter 22)
Sweat gland tumors (Chapter 23)

1.12 Black deposits (histologic)

(compare with Brown deposits 1.17)

Amalgam tattoo (7.6)
Argyria (8.18)
Foreign bodies (7.6)
Mercury (7.6)
Tattoos (7.6)

1.13 Black clinical lesions

(see also Blue 1.14, Brown 1.18)

Angiokeratoma (25.2)
Angiosarcoma (25.7)
Black dermatographism (7.6)
Blue nevus (20.8)
Calciphylaxis (8.15)
Comedo, open (1.24)
Coumarin necrosis (4.18)
Deep fungus infection (Chapter 13)
Disseminated intravascular coagulation (4.14)
Ecthyma gangrenosum (12.17)
Eschar
Foreign body or exogenous substance (7.6)
Gangrene
Lentigo simplex (20.3), solar lentigo (20.4)
Melanoma (20.11)
Meningococcemia (12.19)
Purpura (1.120)
Terra firma dermatosis[126] (dirt on the skin)
Vascular neoplasms (Chapter 25)
Venous lake (25.2)

Blister (see Vesicles, 1.147)

1.14 Blue clinical lesions

(see also Brown 1.18, Gray 1.54, and Black 1.13)

A. Blue skin

Argyria (3.5)
Blue nevus (20.8)
Cyanosis and methemoglobinemia

Cysts (Chapter 19, sometimes)
Dermal and subcutaneous nodules (various)
Drugs (3.5, especially chlorpromazine, antimalarials, amiodarone, clofazimine, minocycline)
Erythema dyschromicum perstans (3.11)
Foreign body or tattoo (7.6)
Hidrocystoma (19.11)
Maculae ceruleae (15.7, pediculosis)
Melanocytic nevus (20.5)
Melanoma (20.11)
Mongolian spot (20.10)
Nevus of Ota, Nevus of Ito (20.9)
Ochronosis (8.16)
Purpura (1.120)
Vascular neoplasms (Chapter 25)

B. Blue nails

Argyria (3.5)
Aspergillus infection (13.13)
Cyanosis
Drugs (3.5, tetracycline)
Heavy metal poisoning (mercury, copper)
Hemorrhage (1.121, old)
Pseudomonas infection (12.17)
Wilson's disease

C. Blue sclera[135]

Anemia, iron deficiency
Corticosteroid therapy
Ehlers–Danlos syndrome (9.9)
Marfan syndrome (9.9)
Minocycline
Myasthenia gravis
Nevus of Ota (20.9)
Ochronosis (8.16)
Osteogenesis imperfecta (9.9)
Pseudoxanthoma elasticum
Thinning of the sclera revealing retina

1.15 Blue material (H&E stain)

Bacteria and some fungi (Chapters 12 and 13)
Calcium (1.19)
Foreign materials (7.6)
Hematoxylin precipitate
Keratohyaline granules (1.63)
Mucin (light blue, 1.83)
Nuclei and nuclear dust (4.1)
Solar elastosis (light blue, 9.1) or radiodermatitis (light blue to pink, 9.2)

1.16 Bone changes and skin lesions

Buschke–Ollendorff syndrome (27.6, osteopoikilosis)
Conradi–Hunerman syndrome (11.1, chondrodysplasia punctata)
Ehlers–Danlos syndrome (9.9, hypermobile joints)
Epidermal nevus syndrome (18.1)
Epidermolysis bullosa dystrophica (6.6)
Goltz syndrome (11.8, osteopathia striata)

Incontinentia pigmenti (11.6)
Klippel–Trenaunay–Weber syndrome (25.1, bony hypertrophy)
Langerhans cell histiocytosis (24.18, osteolytic lesions)
Leishmaniasis (15.1, bony erosion)
Linear scleroderma (9.3, bony involvement)
Maffucci syndrome (25.1, dyschondroplasia)
Marfan syndrome (9.9, tall, pectus excavatum, arachnodactyly)
McCune–Albright's syndrome (20.2, polyostotic fibrous dysplasia)
Mycetoma (13.14, erosion and deformity)
Nail–patella syndrome (triangular lunulae, iliac horns, renal failure)
Neoplasms (osteolytic lesions)
Neurofibromatosis (26.1, many bony changes)
Nevoid basal cell carcinoma syndrome (18.14, cysts, hypertelorism, frontal bossing, bifid ribs)
Nevus sebaceus syndrome (21.2)
North American blastomycosis (13.8, infection)
Osteogenesis imperfecta (9.9, brittle bones)
Pachydermoperiostosis (9.7, periosteal proliferation)
Rhinoscleroma (12.9)
Rhinosporidiosis (13.15)
Scrofuloderma (abscess, 12.10)
Syphilis, congenital (12.13, dactylitis, epiphysitis, osteoperiostitis, saddle nose, Higoumenakis sign, saber shins)
T-cell leukemia-lymphoma (24.3, osteolytic lesions)
Xanthoma disseminatum (7.13, osteolytic lesions)

1.17 Brown deposits (histologic)

Dematiacious fungi (13.3, 13.10, 13.16)
Foreign bodies (7.6)
Formalin pigment (acid formaldehyde hematin).[108] This is a brown precipitate resulting from hemoglobin in formalin with a pH below 6. It is a common artifact, especially in areas of red blood cells
Gout (8.5)
Hemosiderin (1.58)
Melanin (1.79)
Monsel's solution (7.6, ferrous subsulfate, used for hemostasis)
Ochronosis (8.16)
Oxalosis (yellow–brown, 8.15)

1.18 Brown clinical lesions (hyperpigmentation)

(see also Black 1.13, Blue 1.14)
Acanthosis nigricans (18.5)
Accessory nipple (29.12)
Albright's syndrome (20.2)
Cronkhite–Canada syndrome (1.49)
Dermatofibroma (27.1)
Dermatosis papulosa nigra (18.2)
Dowling–Degos disease (17.10)
Drugs (3.5, phenothiazines, meclorethamine, psoralen, arsenic, etc.)
Dyskeratosis congenita (11.4)

Endocrinopathies (17.10, Addison's disease, Cushing's disease, etc.)
Erythema ab igne (3.9)
Erythema dyschromicum perstans (2.15)
Fixed drug eruption (3.5)
Goltz syndrome (11.8)
Granuloma faciale (4.2)
Hemochromatosis (8.17)
Incontinentia pigmenti (11.6)
Laugier–Hunziker syndrome (17.10)
Leopard syndrome (20.3)
Liver and kidney disease (1.75, 1.66)
Macular amyloidosis (8.40)
Melanocytic neoplasms (Chapter 20)
Melasma (17.10)
Ochronosis (8.16)
Pellagra (2.1)
Phytophotodermatitis (1.110)
Pigmented adnexal neoplasms (Chapters 22 and 23)
Pigmented basal cell carcinoma (18.14)
POEMS syndrome (24.12)
Post-inflammatory hyperpigmentation (17.10)
Riehl's melanosis (17.10)
Seborrheic keratosis (18.2)
Stasis dermatitis (2.1)
Terra firma dermatosis[126] (dirt on the skin)
Tinea nigra (13.3)
Tinea versicolor (13.2)
Transient neonatal pustular melanosis (5.2)
Urticaria pigmentosa (24.17)

1.19 Calcification

Calcium salts appear as dark blue to purple, brittle deposits on H&E stain (shatter into shards like peanut brittle candy that has been cut by a butter knife). Sometimes instead it has the appearance of bluish granular material. Calcium salts can be stained with alizarin red (more specific) or von Kossa stains (black). Eosinophilic laminated *psammoma bodies* (1.35) will sometimes calcify, and are seen in meningioma, papillary thyroid carcinoma, and ovarian carcinoma. *Schauman bodies* are round, blue, calcified, laminated inclusions in multinucleated macrophages, usually seen with sarcoidosis (7.5), but also seen with other granulomas (1.51). *Calcareous bodies* (purplish oval calcified concretions) are seen with cysticercosis (15.3) and other parasites.

Acrodermatitis chronica atrophicans (12.14)
Basal cell carcinoma (18.14)
Calcifying aponeurotic fibroma (27.16)
Calciphylaxis (8.15)
Cysts (especially pilar) (19.2)
Dermatomyositis (17.7)
"Dystrophic" calcification (8.15)
Foreign bodies, trauma, and injection sites (7.6)
Gout (8.5)
"Metastatic" calcification (8.15)
Osteoma cutis (29.8)
Panniculitis (Chapter 16, especially pancreatic fat necrosis, lupus profundus, and subcutaneous fat necrosis of the newborn)
Perforating calcific elastosis (9.8)

Peyronie's disease (27.15)
Pilomatricoma (22.3)
Proliferating trichilemmal cyst (22.4)
Pseudoxanthoma elasticum (9.8)
Subepidermal calcified nodule (8.15)
Scleroderma (9.3, especially CREST syndrome)
Trichoepithelioma (22.2)

1.20 Cheilitis (inflammation of the lip)

(see also Lip lesions 1.74)
Acrodermatitis enteropathica (17.1)
Actinic cheilitis (18.8)
Candidiasis (13.4)
Cheilitis granulomatosis (7.7)
Contact dermatitis (2.2)
Drugs (retinoids, etc.) (3.5)
Erythema multiforme (3.2)
Herpes simplex (14.2)
Lip licking (2.2)
Sarcoidosis (7.5)
Squamous cell carcinoma (18.11)
Verruca plana (14.1)
Xerotic eczema (2.1)

1.21 Chord-like lesions

(see also Linear lesions 1.73)
Mondor's disease (4.16)
Sclerosing lymphangitis of penis (4.16)
Superficial thrombophlebitis (16.7)
Trauma
Trousseau's syndrome (4.16)

1.22 Clear or pale cell neoplasms

(see also Vacuolization of keratinocytes 1.144, Pale epidermis 1.99)
The cells of these neoplasms appear similar to foam cells (1.46), but the cytoplasm is more uniformly pale or clear rather than bubbly. The paleness is usually due to the removal of a substance from the cytoplasm during processing, generally glycogen, mucin, or lipid.
Adipose tumors (Chapter 29)
Balloon cell nevus and balloon cell melanoma (20.5 and 20.11)
Clear cell acanthoma (18.6)
Clear cell basal cell carcinoma (18.14)
Clear cell hidradenoma (23.9)
Clear cell sarcoma (20.11)
Clear cell syringoma (23.7)
Eccrine carcinoma (23.13)
Hidroacanthoma simplex (23.10)
Metastatic renal cell carcinoma (28.4)
Pagetoid diseases (1.37)
PEComa (27.21)
Pilomatricoma (shadow cells, 22.3)
Sebaceous gland tumors (Chapter 21)
Squamous cell carcinoma (18.11)
Trichilemmoma (22.5)

1.23 Clefts (histologic)

"Cleft" is used here to mean an empty space. It may have previously contained fluid, crystals, lipid, or some other material that was removed during processing of the tissue, but in some cases it is simply an artifact. We have excluded vesicles and bullae, vascular spaces, and spaces in which there is some evidence of materials within them.
Actinic keratosis (18.8): occasional separation at dermal/epidermal junction ("Freudenthal's lacunae")
Amyloidosis (8.4) and Colloid milium (8.2): fissured clefts within hyalinized material
Basal cell carcinoma (18.14): prominent retraction of tumor from surrounding stroma ("stromal retraction")
Cholesterol clefts: oblong-shaped clefts
Cysts (19.1): clefts around loose keratin flakes
Darier's disease (11.3) and warty dyskeratoma (18.7): suprabasal lacunae
Gout (8.5): needle-shaped clefts within gouty deposits
Lichen planus (2.11): occasional cleft between dermal/epidermal junction due to liquefaction degeneration ("Max Josef space")
Paraffinoma (7.6): Swiss cheese holes in dermis
Scleredema (8.12) and sclerotic fibroma (27.1): clefts between collagen bundles
Spitz nevus (20.6): prominent clefts around melanocytic nests
Subcutaneous fat necrosis and sclerema neonatorum (16.4 and 16.5): small needle-shaped clefts in the subcutaneous fat

1.24 Comedones (singular is comedo)

Acne variants (10.1)
Dilated pore of Winer (22.1)
Familial dyskeratotic comedones (10.1)
Favre–Racouchot syndrome and actinic damage (9.1)
Nevus comedonicus (18.1)
Trichofolliculoma (22.1)
Trichostasis spinulosa (22.1)

1.25 Cystic lesions

A cyst is a closed cavity or localized sac containing fluid or some fluctuant material, often lined by epithelium. Unlined cysts are sometimes called pseudocysts. The horn pseudocysts of seborrheic keratosis are called pseudocysts because they are really invaginations of a papillomatous epidermis. Most of the *"true"* lined cysts are in Chapter 19. Others are listed here.
Abscess (12.1)
Auricular pseudocyst (19.13)
Conventional cysts (Chapter 19)
Digital mucous cyst (8.9)
Focal mucinosis (8.11)
Follicular neoplasms (especially pilomatricoma, Chapter 22)
Ganglion cyst (8.9)
Hemangioma (25.1)
Lymphangioma (25.10)
Mucocele (8.10)
Pilonidal cyst (10.1)

Sweat gland neoplasms (especially solid-cystic hidradenoma, Chapter 23)

1.26 Diabetes mellitus and skin disease

Acanthosis nigricans (18.5)
Bullosis diabeticorum (6.9)
Candidiasis (13.4)
Diabetic dermopathy (pigmented macules of shins, 17.10)
Granuloma annulare, disseminated (7.1)
Hemachromatosis (8.17)
Leg ulcers (1.142)
Lipodystrophy (16.11)
Necrobiosis lipoidica diabeticorum (7.2)
Perforating dermatosis, acquired (9.12)
Progeria (9.6)
Scleredema diabeticorum (8.12)
Xanthomas (7.9)

1.27 Dyskeratosis

(see Fig. 1.27A–C)
Dyskeratotic cells are abnormally or prematurely cornified individual keratinocytes in the epidermis that stain intensely pink with the H&E stain. A small remnant of a basophilic nucleus may be present. Similar pink blobs have been called *colloid bodies, cytoid bodies, hyaline bodies, Kamino bodies* (in Spitz nevus) or *Civatte bodies* when they are present in the deep epidermis or superficial dermis. Colloid bodies generally occur in diseases in which there is interface dermatitis and liquefaction degeneration of the basal layer (1.64), and may actually represent altered collagen or basement membrane, fibrin, and immunoglobulin, as well as degenerated keratinocytes. *Caterpillar bodies* are linear dyskeratotic cells, colloid bodies or degenerated basement membrane material found on the roof of a blister of porphyria cutanea tarda (8.1), resembling a caterpillar. *Corps ronds* and *grains* are acantholytic dyskeratotic cells. Corps ronds have a round nucleus, often with a perinuclear halo, while grains have a more oval, grain-like nucleus. There has been considerable confusion regarding the distinction between dyskeratotic, *apoptotic*, and necrotic keratinocytes. All appear intensely pink with the H&E stain. They may be impossible to distinguish with routine staining, or they may all represent the same thing. For example, in graft-versus-host disease, some authors refer to these cells as dyskeratotic, while others say that they are necrotic. Hence, there is some duplication between these two lists of diseases (see Necrotic keratinocytes, 1.87).

Acrodermatitis enteropathica (17.1)
Arthropod bites (15.7)

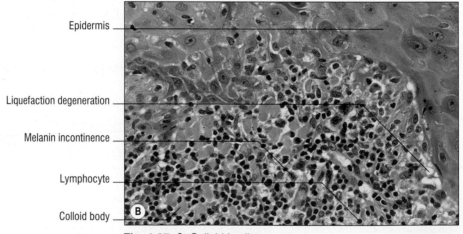

Epidermis

Liquefaction degeneration

Melanin incontinence

Lymphocyte

Colloid body

Fig. 1.27 A Colloid bodies.

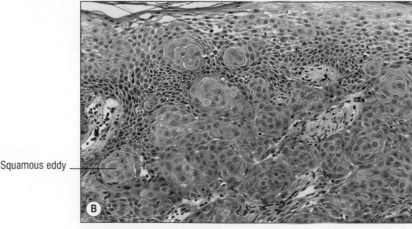

Squamous eddy

Fig. 1.27 B Squamous eddies in an irritated seborrheic keratosis may be considered a form of dyskeratosis.

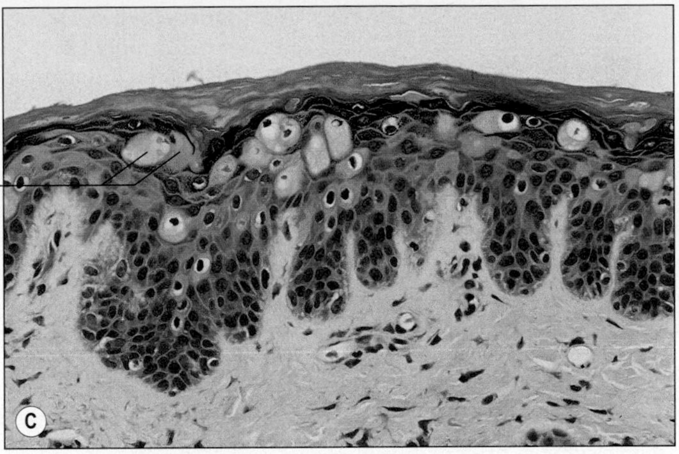

Fig. 1.27 C Pagetoid dyskeratosis.

Darter's disease (11.3)
Familial dyskeratotic comedones (10.1)
Graft-versus-host disease (17.3)
Grover's disease (5.6)
Hailey–Hailey disease (5.5)
Herpes virus infections (14.2)
Incontinentia pigmenti (verrucous second stage) (11.6)
Lichen planus (2.11)
Lichen sclerosus (9.5)
Lichen striatus (2.5)
Lupus erythematosus (17.6)
Many epithelial neoplasms, especially malignant and
    irritated benign epidermal tumors (Chapter 18) and
    irritated benign and malignant adnexal tumors
    (Chapters 21 through 23)
Orf and milker's nodules (14.5)
Pagetoid dyskeratosis:[164] a peculiar incidental finding of
    dyskeratosis in pale keratinocytes with orthokeratosis,
    of uncertain significance (1.37)
Porokeratosis (18.4)
Spitz nevus (Kamino bodies) (20.6)
Viral warts (14.1)
Warty dyskeratoma (18.7)

1.28 Ear lesions

Acanthoma fissuratum (2.3)
Accessory tragus (29.10)
Actinic keratosis (18.8)
Atypical fibroxanthoma (27.12)
Auricular pseudocyst (19.13)
Basal cell carcinoma (18.14)
Calcinosis (8.15)
Chondrodermatitis nodularis helicis (17.9)
Epidermoid cyst (19.1)
Keloid (27.2)
Lentigo maligna (20.11)
Lupus erythematosus (17.6)
Lupus pernio (7.5)
Ochronosis (8.16)
Relapsing polychondritis (17.8)
Seborrheic dermatitis (2.1)
Solar lentigo (20.4)

Squamous cell carcinoma (18.11)
Venous lake (25.2)
Weathering nodules (9.1)

1.29 Eczematous diseases

(see also Papulosquamous 1.103)
Eczematous diseases are those characterized by scaling and
erythema, and often spongiosis and parakeratosis, suggesting epidermal changes. Papulosquamous diseases are often
lumped together with eczematous diseases, but the "splitters" consider papulosquamous lesions to be more hyperkeratotic, thicker and more heaped-up, and more sharply
demarcated than eczematous lesions. Further discussion of
eczema appears in Section 2.1. Most of the diseases that might
be called eczematous appear in Chapter 2, but others that
may exhibit similar clinical morphology are listed here.

Acrodermatitis enteropathica (17.1)
Darier's disease (11.3)
Desquamation post-erythema in viral exanthems,
    Kawasaki's disease, sunburn, scarlet fever, and drug
    eruptions
Drug eruptions (most are not eczematous, 3.5)
Eczematous and papulosquamous diseases (Chapter 2)
Exfoliative erythroderma (1.39)
Follicular mucinosis (10.8)
Ichthyosis (11.1)
Immunodeficiencies (especially Wiscott–Aldrich
    syndrome, X-linked agammaglobulinemia, 2.1)
Inborn errors of metabolism (especially phenylketonuria,
    Hurler's syndrome, Hunter's syndrome, 2.1, 8.14)
Langerhans cell histiocytosis (purpuric, seborrheic
    dermatitis-like, 24.18)
Mycosis fungoides (24.1)
Onchocerciasis (15.5)
Scabies (15.9)
Tinea (13.1)

1.30 Edema of the dermis

Dermal edema produces paleness in the dermis by the accumulation of interstitial fluid. Paleness in the dermis can also
be due to mucin accumulation (1.83). Edema in the epidermis
is called spongiosis (1.132).

Acute eczema (2.1)
Arthropod bites (15.7)
Burns (6.7)
Cellulitis and erysipelas (12.3)
Contact dermatitis (2.2)
Erythema multiforme (3.2)
Fixed drug eruption (3.5)
Lichen sclerosus (9.5)
Lymphedema
Polymorphous light eruption (17.5)
Sweet's syndrome (3.7)
Urticaria (3.1)
Vasculitis (4.1)
Vesiculobullous diseases (1.147, especially pemphigoid, herpes gestationis, bullous mastocytosis, bullous lupus erythematosus, dermatitis herpetiformis)

1.31 Elastic tissue changes

Elastic tissue changes may not be apparent with the H&E stain. An index of suspicion is necessary so that special stains, such as the Verhoeff–van Gieson stain may be done.

Acrokeratoelastoidosis (2.15)
Actinic granuloma (7.1)
Anetoderma (macular atrophy) (9.11)
Blepharochalasis (9.10)
Connective tissue nevus (27.6)
Cutis laxa (9.10)
Elastofibroma (27.6)
Elastosis perforans serpiginosa (9.13)
Erythema ab igne (3.9)
Mid-dermal elastolysis (9.15)
Pseudoxanthoma elasticum (9.8)
Perforating calcific elastosis (9.8)
Scars and keloids (27.2)
Solar elastosis (9.1)
Striae distensae (27.2)

1.32 Elbow lesions

Calcinosis cutis (8.15)
Dermatitis herpetiformis (6.5)
Epidermolysis bullosa (6.6)
Frictional lichenoid dermatosis (2.3)
Granuloma annulare (7.1)
Lichen simplex chronicus and prurigo nodularis (2.3)
Lipoid proteinosis (8.3)
Psoriasis (2.8)
Rheumatoid nodule (7.3)
Tuberous xanthoma (7.9)

1.33 Encapsulated or sharply circumscribed neoplasms

The following neoplasms have a tendency to be sharply circumscribed or encapsulated in the dermis or the subcutaneous fat, without an obvious connection to the epidermis.

Angioleiomyoma (29.6)
Giant cell tumor of tendon sheath (27.9)
Lipomas (29.2)
Neurilemmoma (26.2)

Neurofibroma (26.1)
Pilomatricoma (22.3)
Solitary glomus tumors (25.5)
Sweat gland tumors (Chapter 23): hidradenoma papilliferum, cylindroma, nodular hidradenoma, eccrine spiradenoma

1.34 Eosinophilia in blood with skin disease

Angiolymphoid hyperplasia with eosinophilia (25.4)
Atopic dermatitis (2.1)
Churg–Strauss syndrome (4.5)
Coccidioidomycosis (13.6)
Drug eruptions (3.5)
Eosinophilia–myalgia syndrome (3.5)
Eosinophilic fasciitis (9.3)
Hypereosinophilic syndrome (24.16)
Internal malignancy
Mycosis fungoides (24.1)
Parasitosis (internal or in skin, Chapter 15)
Pemphigoid (6.1)
Urticaria (3.1)

1.35 Eosinophilic pink amorphous material (H&E stain)

Eosinophilic material appears in these diseases (usually in the dermis). The terms *hyaline* or hyalinized are often used to refer to homogenized pink material in general. Hyaline is generally periodic acid-Schiff (PAS)-positive and diastase resistant. The term *sclerosis* (1.125) is used for hyalinized collagen with decreased fibroblasts. *Psammoma bodies* are laminated, hyalinized, or calcified structures that may be found with meningioma (26.6), melanocytic nevus (20.5), thyroid carcinoma, or psammomatous melanotic Schwannoma (26.2).

Amyloidosis (8.4)
Ancient melanocytic nevus (20.5)
Colloid (hyaline) bodies (1.27)
Colloid milium (8.2)
Corticosteroid material
Eosinophilic cellulitis (flame figures) (3.8)
Fibrin and thrombi (1.137)
Fibrous proliferations (scar, keloid, fibromatosis) (1.125, Chapter 27)
Gout (see Section 8.5)
Granuloma with caseation (1.51)
Juvenile hyaline fibromatosis (8.3)
Kamino bodies (1.27)
Lichen sclerosus (9.5)
Lipoid proteinosis (8.3)
Necrobiosis lipoidica (7.2)
Necrosis (1.86, 1.87)
Porphyria (especially erythropoietic protoporphyria, 8.1)
Radiodermatitis, chronic (9.2)
Rheumatoid nodule (7.3)
Russell bodies (1.111)
Scleroderma (9.3)
Sweat gland tumors (especially cylindroma, eccrine spiradenoma, and nodular hidradenoma) (Chapter 23)

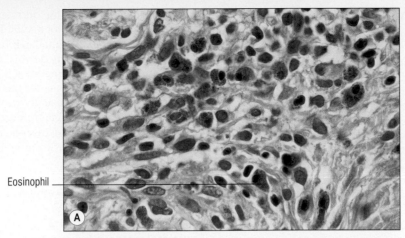

Eosinophil

Fig. 1.36 A Eosinophils.

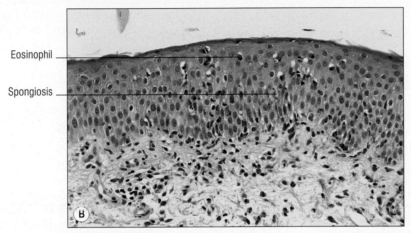

Eosinophil

Spongiosis

Fig. 1.36 B Eosinophilic spongiosis.

Vasculitis (especially hyalinizing segmental vasculitis, in which vessel walls become hyalinized) (Chapter 4)

1.36 Eosinophils in skin

(see Fig. 1.36A,B)
Eosinophils have a bilobed nucleus (fewer lobes than neutrophils), and prominent eosinophilic granules in the cytoplasm. The presence of eosinophils in the skin can be non-specific, but the following conditions should be considered if eosinophils are easy to find. Some diseases, such as lupus erythematosus, usually do not have eosinophils at all.

A. Eosinophils in the epidermis (eosinophilic spongiosis)

Allergic contact dermatitis (2.2)
Arthropod bites (15.7)
Eosinophilic pustular folliculitis (10.2)
Erythema toxicum neonatorum (5.3)
Incontinentia pigmenti (11.6)
Pemphigus and pemphigoid (5.4 and 6.1)

B. Eosinophils in the dermis

Angiolymphoid hyperplasia with eosinophilia (25.4)
Arthropod bites and parasitic infestations (Chapter 15)
Coccidioidomycosis and occasionally other deep fungi (13.6)

Contact dermatitis (2.2)
Dermatitis herpetiformis (6.5)
Dermatophytosis (sometimes, 13.1)
Drug eruptions (3.5)
Eczema (especially atopic dermatitis) (2.1)
Eosinophilic cellulitis (Well's syndrome) (3.8)
Eosinophilic pustular folliculitis (10.2)
EPPER (eosinophilic polymorphic pruritic eruption associated with radiotherapy, 9.2)
Erythema multiforme (sometimes) (3.2)
Granuloma annulare (sometimes, 7.1)
Granuloma faciale (4.2)
Hodgkin's lymphoma (24.15)
Hypereosinophilic syndrome
Juvenile xanthogranuloma (7.10)
Langerhans cell histiocytosis (24.18)
Mycosis fungoides (24.1)
Pemphigoid gestationis (6.3)
Pemphigus (5.4) and *pemphigoid* (6.1)
Pruritic urticarial papules and plaques of pregnancy (PUPPP) (3.6)
Urticaria (3.1)
Urticaria pigmentosa (24.17)
Urticarial vasculitis (4.1), eosinophilic vasculitis (4.1), and Churg–Strauss vasculitis (4.5)

1.37 Epidermotropism and pagetoid cells

(see also Clear cell neoplasms 1.22)

Epidermotropism refers to migration of malignant cells into the epidermis, usually without significant spongiosis. *Exocytosis* refers to the migration of cells (usually lymphocytes, neutrophils, or eosinophils) into the epidermis, usually in association with spongiosis (1.132), and usually used for benign conditions. *Pagetoid cells* are cells in the epidermis, often pale or atypical, resembling Paget's disease. Pagetoid cells may or may not arrive in the epidermis by means of epidermotropism. *Pagetoid melanocytes* (Chapter 20) are best known in melanoma, but are also seen in benign melanocytic neoplasms such as Spitz nevus, pigmented spindle cell nevus, congenital nevus in neonates, recurrent nevus, and acral nevus. Care must be taken not to mistake melanocytes in *tangentially sectioned epidermis* for pagetoid cells,[160] nor to mistake common *artifactual vacuoles* around keratinocytes for pagetoid cells (1.144).

   Paget's disease: pale cells with adenocarcinoma staining features. Carcinoembryonic antigen (CEA), EMA, CK-7, CK-8, usually positive. Mucin in cytoplasm is often positive with mucicarmine, Alcian blue, colloidal iron, and PAS with and without diastase. Basal cells are often compressed and uninvolved. No dyskeratosis

   Bowen's disease (squamous cell carcinoma in situ, 18.10): pale keratinocytes may be present which contain glycogen (PAS positive, diastase labile) with frequent dyskeratosis (1.27). Full-thickness atypia often involves basal cells also. High molecular weight keratin positive. Mucin stains, CEA, EMA, CK-7, CK-8 and low molecular weight keratin negative. However, cases have been published with exceptions, such as positive staining for CK-7 and EMA. Usually no pagetoid cells in the stratum corneum, which sometimes occurs with Paget's disease and melanoma

Borst–Jadassohn phenomenon: discrete clones of basaloid, squamatized, or pale keratinocytes in the epidermis that appear different than their neighbors. This can be benign or malignant. It is mainly seen with *irritated seborrheic keratosis* (18.2) or Bowen's disease (18.10), and rarely with hidroacanthoma simplex (a form of eccrine poroma limited to the epidermis, 23.10).

   Melanoma (20.11): S-100 (very sensitive, but not specific), HMB-45 and MART-1 (both very specific, but not sensitive) stains positive. Fontana melanin stain is also positive, but is less useful because keratinocytes may contain melanin transferred from melanocytes. Melanosomes by electron microscopy

   Mycosis fungoides (24.1): malignant T-lymphocytes (sometimes cerebriform) in spaces called Pautrier microabscesses. Stains such as CD45 (leukocyte common antigen, used for screening), CD4 (T-helper cells), and CD3 (pan-T cells) usually positive

Lymphomatoid papulosis (24.5): CD30 positive large atypical lymphocytes, and most smaller ones in the epidermis stain with T-cell markers

Langerhans cell histiocytosis (24.18): malignant Langerhans cells, often kidney-shaped nuclei, CDla or S-100 positive

Sebaceous carcinoma (21.5): oil red-O stain positive (need frozen section). Sometimes Bowenoid changes (oil red-O negative carcinoma) in the epidermis coexist with sebaceous carcinoma in the dermis. EMA positivity is useful if frozen section not available

Merkel cell tumor (26.7): small cell tumor (1.130) is almost always present also in the dermis, in addition to the epidermotropic cells. Sometimes Bowen's disease can coexist, or the small cells enter the epidermis. Merkel cell carcinoma cells are usually positive for CK20 (perinuclear dot pattern) and neuron-specific enolase

Clear cell acanthoma (18.6): discrete clone of pale keratinocytes in a psoriasiform epidermis, positive for glycogen and keratin

Hidroacanthoma simplex (23.10): this is an eccrine poroma with Borst–Jadassohn features, and sweat ducts are present

Pagetoid dyskeratosis[164] (1.27)

Epidermotropic adnexal carcinoma (23.13): rare

Epidermotropic metastatic carcinoma or melanoma: very rare. Usually carcinoma or melanoma cells within the epidermis imply that a neoplasm is primary, but in this case metastatic melanocytes or epithelial cells actually infiltrate the epidermis. This usually can only be diagnosed with certainty when more than one lesion is present, making it more apparent that the lesions are metastatic.

1.38 Epithelioid cells

Epithelioid cells are defined as cells that resemble (-oid) epithelial cells (keratinocytes). They have large oval, pale, vesicular nuclei and abundant eosinophilic cytoplasm. The term "epithelioid cell" confuses neophytes because it is most often used to describe large monocyte-derived macrophages (histiocytes, 1.76) that often form granulomas, but is also used to describe many tumor cells that have a similar appearance. Sometimes immunostaining may be needed to identify the type of epithelioid cell. Vimentin will stain all of these (all mesenchymal lesions) except most examples of squamous cell carcinoma (an epithelial neoplasm). SCC stains with cytokeratin cocktail, while epithelioid sarcoma stains with both vimentin and cytokeratin. True histiocytes found in granulomas, atypical fibroxanthoma, and malignant fibrous histiocytoma usually stain with CD68 or alpha-1 antitrypsin. S-100 protein stains melanocytic neoplasms and Langerhans cell histiocytosis. CD la stains only the Langerhans cell histiocytosis. CD31, CD34, and Ulex stain most vascular neoplasms with proliferating endothelial cells (see Chapter 30).

A. Most common

   Granulomas (1.51)
   Melanoma (20.11)
   Spitz nevus (spindle and epithelioid cell nevus, 20.6)
   Squamous cell carcinoma (18.11)

B. Uncommon

   Angiolymphoid hyperplasia with eosinophilia ("histiocytoid" hemangioma, 25.4)
   Atypical fibroxanthoma (27.12)
   Epithelioid angiosarcoma (25.7)
   Epithelioid sarcoma (27.14)
   Langerhans cell histiocytosis (24.18)
   Malignant fibrous histiocytoma (27.11)

Erythema (see red)

1.39 Exfoliative erythroderma

This is a term used by clinicians for *generalized scaling and erythema* over an extensive part of the body. It is important to try to determine one of the causes in the following list. The histology depends on which of these is the underlying etiology.

Contact dermatitis (2.2)
Crusted "Norwegian" scabies (15.9)
Darier's disease (11.3)
Dermatomyositis (17.7)
Drug eruption (3.5)
Eczema (2.1)
Graft-versus-host disease (17.3)
Ichthyosis variants (11.1)
Idiopathic erythroderma (common)
Immunodeficiencies, especially Wiskott–Aldrich syndrome (2.1), Omenn syndrome (2.1)
Mycosis fungoides (especially *Sezary syndrome)* (24.1)
Onchocerciasis (15.5)
Pemphigus foliaceus (5.4)
Pityriasis rubra pilaris (2.10)
Post-erythema stage of viral exanthems (Chapter 14)
Psoriasis (2.8)
Scarlet fever (12.2)
Staphylococcal scalded skin syndrome (12.2)

1.40 Extravasated erythrocytes (red blood cells)

(see also Purpura 1.120)

A. In the epidermis

Mucha-Habermann disease (2.14) is by far the most common, although erythrocytes may enter the epidermis occasionally in other diseases.

B. In the dermis

Amyloidosis (8.4)
Cellulitis (12.3)
Gonococcemia (12.18)
Herpes virus infections (14.2)
Langerhans cell histiocytosis (24.18)
Meningococcemia (12.19)
Pityriasis lichenoides (2.14)
Pityriasis rosea (sometimes) (2.4)
Stasis dermatitis (2.1)
Vascular neoplasms (Chapter 25)
Vasculitis and purpuric diseases (Chapter 4)

1.41 Eye and skin lesions

(see also Eyebrow 1.42, Eyelid 1.43, Blue sclera 1.14)
Albinism (11.9, nystagmus)
Ataxia telangiectasia (11.2, bulbar telangiectasia)
Atopic dermatitis (2.1, cataracts)
Behçet's syndrome (4.11, uveitis)
Cat scratch disease (12.15, Parinaud's oculoglandular syndrome)
Congenital syphilis (12.13, interstitial keratitis)

Cytomegalovirus (14.9, retinitis)
Hansen's disease (12.12, iritis)
Herpes virus infections (14.2, keratitis, iritis)
Ichthyosis (11.1, mostly corneal changes)
Incontinentia pigmenti (11.6, rarely blindness, strabismus)
Juvenile xanthogranuloma (7.10, xanthogranulomas, glaucoma, iritis)
Kawasaki's disease (14.10, conjunctivitis)
Loefgren's syndrome (7.5, iritis)
Neurofibromatosis (26.1, Lisch nodules of iris)
Pretibial myxedema (8.7, exophthalmos)
Pseudoxanthoma elasticum (9.8, angioid streaks, retinal hemorrhages, blindness)
Reiter's disease (2.8, conjunctivitis, iritis)
Relapsing polychondritis (17.8, ocular inflammation)
Rothmund–Thompson syndrome (11.5, cataracts)
Sarcoidosis (7.5, iritis)
Sturge–Weber syndrome (25.1, glaucoma)
Toxoplasmosis (15.15, chorioretinitis)
Tuberous sclerosis (27.3, several complications)
Vogt–Koyanagi–Harada syndrome (17.2, uveitis)

1.42 Eyebrow lesions

(see also Madarosis 1.77)
Alopecia areata (10.9)
Dermoid cyst (1.42)
Porphyria (especially EP and PCT, 8.1): hypertrichosis
Seborrheic dermatitis (2.1): scale and erythema
Ulerythema ophryogenes (10.5): follicular plugging and scale

1.43 Eyelid lesions

(see also Madarosis 1.77)
Acne rosacea (10.1)
Acrochordon (27.4)
Amyloidosis (8.4)
Angioedema (3.1)
Anthrax (12.4)
Ascher's syndrome (7.7)
Atopic dermatitis (2.1)
Basal cell carcinoma (18.14)
Cat scratch disease (12.15)
Cellulitis, orbital (12.3)
Chagas disease (Romana's sign, 15.14)
Chalazion and sty (10.1)
Cicatricial pemphigoid (6.1)
Contact dermatitis (2.2)
Dacryocystitis
Dermatomyositis (heliotrope, 17.6)
Herpes simplex (14.2)
Hidrocystoma (19.11)
Kawasaki syndrome (conjunctivitis, 14.10)
Lipoid proteinosis (8.3)
Measles (conjunctivitis, 14.7)
Milia (19.1)
Molluscum contagiosum (14.4)
Myxedema (8.6)
Necrobiotic xanthogranuloma (7.11)
Pediculosis (phthirus pubis on eyelashes, 15.7)

Reiter's syndrome (conjunctivitis, 2.8)
Sebaceous carcinoma (4.5)
Seborrheic dermatitis (2.1)
Seborrheic keratosis (18.2)
Stevens–Johnson syndrome (3.2)
Syringoma (23.7)
Thyroid disease
Trichinosis
Vitiligo (17.2)
Xanthelasma (7.9)

1.44 Face lesions
(see also Nose 1.95, Eyelid 1.43, Eyebrow 1.42)

A. Common
Acne (10.1)
Actinic keratosis (18.8)
Atopic dermatitis (especially infants, 2.1)
Basal cell carcinoma (18.14)
Contact dermatitis (2.2)
Demodicosis (15.8)
Dermatosis papulosa nigra
Dilated pore of Winer (22.1)
Epidermoid cyst (19.1)
Follicular neoplasms (most, Chapter 22)
Herpes simplex and varicella zoster (14.2)
Impetigo (12.1)
Lentigo maligna (20.11)
Lentigo, solar (20.4)
Lupus erythematosus (17.6)
Melanocytic nevus (20.5)
Melasma (17.10)
Nevus sebaceus (21.2)
Photocontact dermatitis (2.2)
Photodermatitis (1.110)
Photodrug reaction (3.5)
Pityriasis alba (2.6)
Port wine stain (25.1)
Pseudofolliculitis barbae (10.2)
Sebaceous hyperplasia (21.1)
Seborrheic dermatitis (2.1)
Seborrheic keratosis (18.2)
Spider hemangiomas (1.136)
Squamous cell carcinoma (18.11)
Verruca plana (14.1)

B. Uncommon
Angiolymphoid hyperplasia with eosinophilia (25.4)
Angiosarcoma (25.7)
Atypical fibroxanthoma (27.12)
Chronic actinic dermatitis (2.2)
Eosinophilic folliculitis (10.2)
Erysipelas (12.3)
Fifth disease (14.7)
Follicular mucinosis (10.8)
Gianotti–Crosti syndrome (14.11)
Granuloma faciale
Leishmaniasis (15.1)
Lepromatous leprosy (12.12)
Lupus vulgaris (12.10)

Lymphocytoma cutis (24.14)
Nevus of Ota (20.9)
Palisaded encapsulated neuroma (26.8)
Pemphigus erythematosus (5.4)
Polymorphous light eruption (17.5)
Sarcoidosis (7.5)
Sebaceous neoplasms, most (Chapter 21)
Solar urticaria (3.1)
Subepidermal calcified nodule (8.15)
Tinea facei (13.1)
Warty dyskeratoma (18.7)

1.45 Fever with rash
(see also Morbilliform 1.81)

A. Bacterial diseases (many in Chapter 12)
B. Fungal diseases (many in Chapter 13)
C. Viral diseases (many in Chapter 14)
D. Rheumatologic diseases
Dermatomyositis (17.7)
Lupus erythematosus (17.6)
Still's disease

E. Other reactive conditions
Drug eruption (3.5)
Leukemia, lymphoma (Chapter 24)
Loefgren's syndrome (7.5)
Pustular psoriasis (2.8)
Sweet's syndrome (3.7)
Weber–Christian disease (16.2)

Fibrosis (see Scars)
Finger lesions (see Hands)
1.46 Foam cells

Foam cells (foamy cells) have a bubbly (foamy) cytoplasm. Most are macrophages (1.76) that have phagocytized lipid material, but some are cells of another derivation that have a similar multivacuolated cytoplasm. Compare with clear cells (1.22). *Touton giant cells* (1.84) are macrophage-derived multinucleated cells that contain lipid. A wreath of nuclei encircles a smooth pink cytoplasm, and a foamy cytoplasm is present outside the wreath. Touton giant cells are mainly seen in juvenile xanthogranuloma, but can occasionally be seen in other xanthomatous conditions as well.
Atypical fibroxanthoma (27.12)
Atypical mycobacteria and rarely other bacterial infections (Chapter 12)
Balloon cell nevus and balloon cell melanoma (20.5 and 20.11)
Dermatofibroma (uncommonly, 27.1)
Fox–Fordyce disease (10.7)
Granular cell tumor (more granular than foamy, 24.18)
Hibernoma (29.4)
Juvenile xanthogranuloma (7.10)
Langerhans cell histiocytosis (24.18)
Leprosy (lepromatous) (12.12)
Liposarcoma (29.5)
Malakoplakia (12.21)

Necrobiotic xanthogranuloma (7.11)
Panniculitis (any type may exhibit foam cells if there is damage to adipose, but foam cells are most characteristic of Weber–Christian disease, Chapter 16)
Pneumocytosis (15.12)
Rhino scleroma (12.9)
Sebaceous gland tumors (Chapter 21)
Verruciform xanthoma (7.12)
Xanthoma disseminatum and other histiocytosis variants (7.13)
Xanthomas (7.9)

1.47 Follicular plugging and follicular eruptions

Follicular plugging is hyperkeratosis within hair follicles (usually in the infundibulum). In some of these conditions, there is adnexocentric inflammation around follicles or other adnexal structures such as sweat glands. A few of these just appear to be follicular on a clinical basis, such as some of the transepidermal elimination diseases.

Acne variants (10.1)
Atopic dermatitis (2.1)
Darier's disease (keratosis follicularis) (11.3)
Eczema with follicular accentuation (2.1)
Follicular mucinosis (10.8)
Folliculitis variants (10.2)
Fox–Fordyce disease (10.7)
Graft-versus-host disease (follicular type) (17.3)
Hidradenitis suppurativa (10.2)
Ichthyosis vulgaris (11.1)
Keratosis pilaris (10.5)
Kyrle's disease (9.12)
Lichen planopilaris (2.11)
Lichen sclerosus (9.5)
Lichen simplex chronicus (2.3)
Lichen spinulosus (10.5)
Lupus erythematosus (17.6)
Miliaria (actually is sweat duct occlusion, 10.6)
Mycosis fungoides, follicular variant (24.1)
Perforating folliculitis (10.3)
Pityriasis rubra pilaris (2.10)
Prurigo nodularis (2.3)
Scurvy and phrynoderma (4.17)
Seborrheic dermatitis (2.1)
Transepidermal elimination diseases (1.140)
Trichostasis spinulosa (10.4)

1.48 Foot lesions

(see also Hands 1.56, and also Palm and sole 1.100)
Acral lentiginous melanoma (20.11)
Acral pseudolymphomatous angiokeratoma (24.14)
Atherosclerotic ulcers
Buerger's disease (4.19)
Chilblains (3.12)
Clear cell sarcoma (20.11)
Contact dermatitis (2.2)
Eczema (2.1)
Epidermolysis bullosa (6.6)
Foreign body granuloma (7.6)
Kaposi sarcoma (25.9)

Larval migrans (15.6)
Lichen planus (2.11)
Mycetoma (13.14)
Purpuric glove and sock syndrome (14.7)
Stasis dermatitis and ulcers (2.1, 16.9)
Tinea pedis (13.1)
Tungiasis (15.11)

1.49 Gastrointestinal tract and skin

A. Neoplasms of intestinal tract
Arsenical keratoses (keratoses, especially of palms and soles, GI carcinoma, 18.9)
Cowden's disease (trichilemmomas, GI polyps or malignancy, 22.5)
Cronkite–Canada syndrome (hyperpigmentation, alopecia, GI polyps, enteropathy, 17.10)
Dermatomyositis (rash, internal malignancy, 17.7)
Extramammary Paget's disease (Paget's disease on skin, GI carcinoma, 18.13)
Gardner's syndrome (cutaneous cysts, lipomas, desmoid tumors, GI adenomatous polyps, often malignant, 19.1)
Kaposi sarcoma (vascular skin lesions, GI vascular lesions, 25.9)
Leser–Trelat syndrome (rapid onset of seborrheic keratoses, GI carcinoma, 18.2)
Muir–Torre syndrome (sebaceous neoplasms, keratoacanthoma, GI carcinoma, 21.3)
Necrolytic migratory erythema (rash, glucagonoma, 3.2)
Neurofibromatosis (neurofibromas, café-au-lait macules, GI polyps, 26.1)
Pancreatic fat necrosis (panniculitis, pancreatitis or pancreatic carcinoma, 16.8)
Peutz–Jegher's syndrome (lentigines of lips, small intestinal polyps with malignant potential, 20.3)
Tylosis (palmar–plantar keratoderma, esophageal carcinoma, 2.15)

B. Bleeding or pain of intestinal tract
Blue rubber bleb nevus syndrome (25.1)
Degos disease (infarction and bleeding, 4.10)
Ehlers–Danlos syndrome (9.9)
Epidermolysis bullosa (6.6)
Hemangiomatosis (25.1)
Kaposi sarcoma (25.9)
Osler–Weber–Rendu syndrome (1.136)
Pseudoxanthoma elasticum (9.8)
Vasculitis (especially Henoch–Schoenlein purpura, 4.1)

C. Diarrhea or inflammatory bowel disease
Acrodermatitis enteropathica (17.1)
Aphthous stomatitis (17.11)
Bowel bypass syndrome (4.1)
Carcinoid (28.5)
Crohn's disease of the skin (7.7)
Cronkhite–Canada syndrome (17.10)
Dermatitis herpetiformis (gluten sensitive enteropathy often asymptomatic, 6.5)
Erythema nodosum (16.1)
Graft-versus-host disease (17.3)
Mastocytosis (24.17)

Pyoderma gangrenosum (4.12)
Pyoderma vegetans (4.12)
Pyostomatitis vegetans (4.12)
Reiter's disease (2.8)
Scleroderma (malabsorption, diarrhea, 9.3)
Sweet's syndrome (3.7)
Typhoid fever (12.2)
Yersiniosis (12.23)

D. Miscellaneous

Omphalomesenteric duct remnant (29.11)

1.50 Gingival lesions

(see also Mouth 1.82)

Addison's disease (melanosis, 17.10)
Amalgam tattoo (pigment, 7.6)
Ameloblastoma (tumor, 18.14)
Cowden's disease (22.5)
Drug-induced hyperplasia (phenytoin, nifedipine, cyclosporine, etc., 3.5)
Gingivitis due to infection or irritation
Juvenile hyaline fibromatosis (hyperplasia, 8.3)
Kaposi sarcoma (tumor, 25.9)
Leukemia, lymphoma (bleeding, Chapter 24)
Leukoplakia, traumatic or premalignant (1.71)
Lipoid proteinosis (hyperplasia, 8.3)
Melanoma (tumor, 20.11)
Mucosal pemphigoid (ulcers, 6.2)
Papillon–Lefevre syndrome (periodontitis, 2.15)
Paraneoplastic pemphigus (ulcers, 5.4)
Pemphigus vulgaris (ulcers, 5.4)
Racial pigmentation
Scurvy (bleeding, 4.17)

1.51 Granulomas

A granuloma is an aggregate of monocyte-derived histiocytes (macrophages, 1.76), sometimes mixed with other inflammatory cells. Large histiocytes in a granuloma are often called epithelioid cells (1.38). These epithelioid cells may fuse to form multinucleated giant cells. It is important to stress that such multinucleated giant cells do not have to be present to meet the criteria for a granuloma. Non-infectious granulomas are mainly covered in Chapter 7, and infectious ones are covered in Chapters 12, 13, and 15. The subcategories of granulomas listed below are not always accurate. For example, granuloma annulare may not palisade (it often has mainly just interstitial lymphocytes and histiocytes), tuberculosis or syphilis may not caseate, and granulomas in sarcoidosis may be surrounded by considerable lymphocytic inflammation.

Evaluation of granulomas should include polarization to look for foreign bodies and special stains for infectious organisms. Such stains include the tissue Gram stain for bacteria (Brown–Brenn), fungal stains (PAS = periodic acid-Schiff, and GMS = Gomori's methenamine silver), acid-fast bacterial stains (Ziehl–Neelsen, auramine, or Fite), spirochete stain (Warthin–Starry), or stains for leishmania (Giemsa).

1. The most common granulomas in skin by far

Foreign body granulomas (re-excision sites, exogenous and endogenous materials such as uric acid in gout, hair, keratin)

Ruptured cysts or follicles ("pimples": acne, folliculitis, hidradenitis, see Chapters 10 and 19)

2. Infectious diseases

Usually, infectious granulomas will have plasma cells or neutrophils. If no plasma cells or neutrophils are present, then a granuloma is unlikely to be infectious. The presence of plasma cells or neutrophils does not mean that it is likely to be infectious, however, because common ruptured cysts and follicles can also have neutrophils or plasma cells.

Deep fungal infections (Chapter 13)
Leishmaniasis (15.1)
Mycobacterial infections (tuberculosis, atypical acid-fast bacillus infection, leprosy (12.10, 12.11, 12.12))
Syphilis and yaws (12.13)
Tularemia (12.6)

3. Palisading granulomas

Palisading granulomas surround a central focus of degenerated connective tissue ("necrobiosis", a word that is difficult to define, see under caseating below), mucin accumulation, or fibrin. The first three are the classic common members of this group.

Granuloma annulare (7.1)
Necrobiosis lipoidica (7.2)
Rheumatoid nodule (7.3)
Calcifying aponeurotic fibroma (27.16)
Caseating granulomas (below, may appear to palisade)
Cat scratch disease (12.15)
Churg–Strauss syndrome (4.5)
Collagen-implant granuloma (from injected collagen)
Epithelioid sarcoma (27.14)
Foreign body granulomas (7.6)
Necrobiotic xanthogranuloma (7.11)
Rheumatic fever nodule (12.2)
Wegener's granulomatosis (4.6)

4. Caseating granulomas

These develop necrosis in the center of the granulomas. When prominent, it grossly resembles cheese (hence, "caseation"). Caseating granulomas may resemble the palisading granulomas, but the necrosis is greater than the "necrobiosis" seen in some palisading granulomas. "Necrobiosis" is sometimes defined as "mild necrosis" of connective tissue.

Atypical mycobacteria (12.11)
Erythema induratum (16.6)
Granulomatous rosacea (10.1)
Leishmaniasis (15.1)
Local beryllium granuloma (not systemic berylliosis, 7.6)
Tertiary syphilis (12.13)
Tuberculosis (12.10)
Tularemia (12.6)

5. Linear granulomas

Leprosy (granulomas follow nerves, 12.12)

6. Tuberculoid granulomas

These diseases form well-demarcated nodules called tubercles. They are said to be "naked" tuberculoid granulomas if there are relatively few lymphocytes around the tubercles (especially common in sarcoidosis).

Beryllium and zirconium granulomas (7.6)
Leprosy (TT and BT, 12.12)
Sarcoidosis (7.5)
Syphilis (late secondary, tertiary, 12.13)
Tuberculosis (most forms, 12.10)

7. Uncommon or "other" granulomas

Actinic granuloma (7.4)
Cheilitis granulomatosa (7.7)
Crohn's disease (7.7)
Foam cell diseases (1.46)
Granulomatous lymphoma: lymphomatoid
    granulomatosis (24.1), granulomatous T-cell lymphoma
    (24.6), granulomatous slack skin (24.6)
Granulomatous panniculitis (Chapter 16)
Granulomatous vasculitis: Churg–Strauss
    granulomatosis (4.5), Wegener's granulomatosis (4.6),
    temporal arteritis, interstitial granulomatous
    dermatitis (7.1), and lymphomatoid granulomatosis
    (24.1)
Halogenodermas (3.5)
Lichen nitidus (2.12)
Panniculitis (Chapter 16)
Reticulohistiocytosis (7.8)

1.52 Green lesions

Chloroma (usually more blue–gray, 24.16)
Pseudomonas infection (12.3, 12.17)
Tattoo (mostly potassium dichromate, 7.6)

1.53 Grenz zone

A Grenz zone is a narrow band of sparing between the epidermis and a dense infiltrate in the dermis (from the German word for boundary).
Acrodermatitis chronica atrophicans (12.15)
B-cell lymphoma and leukemia (usually) (24.1 and 24.16)
Granuloma faciale (4.2)
Lepromatous leprosy (12.12)
Pseudolymphoma (24.14)

1.54 Grey lesions

(see also Blue 1.14)
Argyria (8.18)
Chloroma (24.16)
Drugs (3.5, antimalarials, amiodarone, phenothiazine, etc.)
Erythema dyschromicum perstans (3.11)
Heavy metal toxicity (gold, bismuth, etc.)
Mongolian spot (20.10)
Nevus of Ota and Ito (20.9)
Riehl's melanosis (17.10)

1.55 Groin lesions

(see also Penis 1.107, Vulva 1.149)
Acrochordons (27.4)
Candidiasis (13.4)
Condyloma acuminatum (14.1)
Erythrasma (12.5)
Granuloma inguinale (12.8)
Herpes simplex (14.2)

Hidradenitis suppurativa (10.1)
Intertrigo (2.2)
Lichen sclerosus (9.5)
Malakoplakia (12.21)
Molluscum contagiosum (14.4)
Paget's disease (18.13)
Pediculosis pubis (15.7)
Pemphigus vegetans (5.4)
Psoriasis (2.8)
Scabies (15.9)
Seborrheic dermatitis (2.2)
Tinea cruris (13.1)

1.56 Hand and finger lesions

(see also Palm and sole lesions 1.100)

A. Common

Acral melanocytic nevus (20.5)
Actinic keratosis (18.8)
Burn (6.7)
Callus and corn (2.3)
Contact dermatitis (2.2)
Digital mucous cyst (8.9)
Eczema (2.1)
Epidermoid cyst (19.1)
Erythema multiforme (3.2)
Foreign body granuloma
Friction blisters (5.7)
Granuloma annulare (7.1)
Keratoacanthoma (18.12)
Paronychia (infection around the nail, usually due to
    Staphylococcus 12.3, or *Candida* 13.4)
Psoriasis (2.8)
Pyogenic granuloma (25.3)
Raynaud's phenomenon
Scabies (especially fingerwebs, 15.9)
Solar lentigo (20.4)
Squamous cell carcinoma (18.11)
Tinea manuum (13.1)
Verruca vulgaris (14.1)
Vitiligo (17.2)

B. Uncommon

Acquired digital fibrokeratoma (27.5)
Acral pseudolymphomatous angiokeratoma (24.14)
Acrodermatitis continua (2.8)
Acrokeratoelastoidosis (2.15)
Acrokeratosis verruciformis (18.3)
Acropustulosis of infancy (5.1)
Aggressive digital adenoma and adenocarcinoma (23.13)
Angiokeratoma (25.2)
Anthrax (12.4)
Atypical mycobacterial infection (12.11)
Bazex disease (1.105)
Blistering distal dactylitis (12.3)
Calcifying aponeurotic fibroma
Colloid milium (8.2)
Dermatomyositis (Gottron's papules, 17.7)
Epidermolysis bullosa (6.6)

Erysipeloid (12.3)
Erythema elevatum diutinum (4.3)
Erythermalgia (3.13)
Flegel's disease (2.7)
Giant cell tumor of tendon sheath (27.9)
Hand–foot–mouth disease (14.6)
Hereditary hemorrhagic telangiectasia (1.136)
Herpetic whitlow (14.2)
Id reaction (2.1)
Infantile digital fibromatosis (27.7)
Keratoderma (2.15)
Knuckle pad (27.15)
Lichen planus (2.11)
Lupus erythematosus (17.6)
Orf and milker's nodule (14.5)
Periungual fibromas (27.3)
Porphyria cutanea tarda (8.1)
Purpuric glove and sock syndrome (14.7)
Reticulohistiocytosis (7.8)
Rheumatoid nodule (7.3)
Scleroderma (9.3)
Septic vasculitis (gonococcemia 12.18, subacute bacterial endocarditis 4.1, etc.)
Sporotrichosis (13.11)
Supernumerary digit (27.5)
Sweet's syndrome (3.7)
Tularemia (12.6)

1.57 Heart and skin lesions

Amyloidosis (8.4, cardiomyopathy)
Behçet's syndrome (4.11, pericarditis)
Carney's complex (20.3, atrial myxoma)
Cutis laxa (9.10, aortic dilatation)
Degos disease (4.10, pericarditis)
Dermatomyositis (17.7, conduction defects)
Ehlers–Danlos syndrome (9.9, aortic dilatation)
Emboli (4.16, septic, cholesterol)
Exfoliative erythroderma (1.39, high output failure)
Fabry's disease (25.2, cardiomyopathy)
Hemochromatosis (8.17, heart failure)
Infectious diseases (Chapters 12 and 13, numerous)
Kawasaki's disease (14.10, aneurysm)
Leopard syndrome (20.3, EKG abnormalities, pulmonic stenosis)
Lupus erythematosus (17.6, endocarditis, heart block)
Lyme disease (12.14, myocarditis)
Multicentric reticulohistiocytosis (7.8, pericarditis)
Myxedema (8.6, dilatation cardiomegaly, pericardial effusion)
Progeria (9.6, atherosclerosis)
Pseudoxanthoma elasticum (9.8, aortic aneurysm)
Reiter's disease (2.8, pericarditis)
Relapsing polychondritis (17.8, valvular disease)
Rheumatic fever (12.2, carditis)
Sarcoidosis (7.5, conduction defects)
Scleroderma (9.3, pericarditis)
Tuberous sclerosis (27.3, rhabdomyomas)
Vasculitis (4.1, coronary arteritis)

Viral diseases (especially Coxsackie, mononucleosis)
Xanthomas (7.9, coronary artery disease)

1.58 Hemosiderin

Hemosiderin is a brown iron-containing pigment usually derived from the disintegration of extravasated red blood cells (1.40). It tends to be golden brown, more refractile, and more clumped than melanin (1.79), but the distinction can be difficult at times, requiring special melanin stains or iron stains. Hemosiderin is often phagocytized by macrophages called hemosiderophages (1.76). Consider other brown pigments (1.17) and other clinical conditions with a brown color (1.18).

Dermatofibroma (27.1)
Erythema ab igne (3.9)
Giant cell tumor of tendon sheath (27.9)
Granuloma faciale (4.2)
Hemochromatosis (8.17)
Monsel's solution (used for hemostasis, iron pigment similar to hemosiderin, 7.6)
Pityriasis lichenoides (2.14)
Purpura pigmentosa chronica (4.8)
Stasis dermatitis (2.1)
Vascular neoplasms (Chapter 25)
Vasculitis (Chapter 4)

1.59 Horn cysts

A horn cyst is an island of keratin within an epithelial proliferation. A granular layer is sometimes present. A *horn pseudocyst* appears identical to a horn cyst, but actually represents an invagination of a papillomatous stratum corneum. Often this connection to the surface cannot be seen unless serial sections are obtained. Horn cysts are often used as evidence of follicular differentiation in basaloid neoplasms. See Chapter 19 for a discussion of dermal and subcutaneous cysts.

Seborrheic keratosis (18.12)
Keratotic basal cell carcinoma (18.14)
Melanocytic nevi (occasionally, 20.5)
Trichoepithelioma and trichoadenoma (22.2)
Nodular hidradenoma (occasionally) (23.9)
Microcystic adnexal carcinoma (23.13)

Hyalinization (see Eosinophilic material)

1.60 Hypergranulosis

Hypergranulosis is a thickened granular layer, almost always accompanied by hyperkeratosis. Because nearly any hyperkeratotic lesion may occasionally show hypergranulosis, it has limited usefulness in differential diagnosis.

Acrokeratosis verruciformis (18.3)
Epidermal nevus (18.1)
Epidermolytic hyperkeratosis (11.1)
Hyperkeratotic seborrheic keratosis and stucco keratosis (18.2)
Lichen planus (2.11)
Lichen simplex chronicus and prurigo nodularis (2.3)
Molluscum contagiosum (14.4)
Normal acral skin
Pemphigus foliaceus and erythematosus (5.4)
Verruca vulgaris (14.1)

Hyperkeratosis (see Hyperplasia of epidermis, 1.61)

1.61 Hyperplasia of epidermis

(see also Psoriasiform hyperplasia 1.119, Pseudoepitheliomatous hyperplasia 1.116)

Hyperplasia means an increase in the thickness of a tissue, usually through an increase in the number of cells. It differs from neoplasia by its theoretical capability of a return to a normal condition, whereas neoplasia implies uncontrolled, progressive growth that usually does not regress. A *collarette* of epithelium is defined as epithelium at the edge of a lesion, sometimes part of hyperplastic adnexal structures, which tend to bow inwardly and clutch alterations of the dermis. Examples of lesions that often have collarettes include lichen nitidus (2.12), verruca vulgaris (14.1), Spitz nevus (20.2), angiokeratoma circumscriptum (25.2), pyogenic granuloma (25.3), and lymphangioma circumscriptum (25.10). *Hyperkeratosis* is a thickened stratum corneum. *Orthokeratosis* is hyperkeratosis without parakeratosis. It can be thickened in the normal basket-weave manner, or it can become very dense (*compact hyperkeratosis*). *Acanthosis* is a thickened Malpighian (spinous) layer. Hyperkeratosis and acanthosis usually occur together in epidermal hyperplasia. There are exceptions; lichen sclerosus, for example, often has hyperkeratosis with spinous layer atrophy. Epithelium, particularly hyperplastic epidermis, is said to be squamotized (squamatized) when it is more pale and glassy, with the basal cells having more pink cytoplasm than usual. It is important to realize that there is considerable regional variation in what is normal, so that the thicker epidermis of acral areas such as the palms or soles, which normally have a compact stratum corneum, should not be mistaken for pathologic hyperkeratosis or acanthosis. True hyperkeratosis and acanthosis are often accompanied by parakeratosis (1.104). Hyperkeratosis and acanthosis are non-specific findings common to many diseases, especially chronic ones. Only some of the more important ones are listed.

Acquired digital fibrokeratoma (27.5)

Angiokeratoma (25.2)

Atypical mycobacterial infections (12.11)

Chronic cutaneous lupus erythematosus (17.6)

Chronic radiodermatitis (9.2)

Corn or callus (2.3)

Crusted "Norwegian" scabies (15.9)

Cutaneous horn (hornu cutaneum): a clinical term referring to a massive horn-like growth due to hyperkeratosis. It is most commonly due to actinic keratosis, squamous cell carcinoma, verruca vulgaris, or seborrheic keratosis

Darier's disease (11.3)

Deep fungal infections (Chapter 13)

Dermatofibroma (27.1)

Diseases with papillomatosis (1.4)

Diseases with pseudoepitheliomatous hyperplasia (1.2)

Eczema and papulosquamous diseases in Chapter 2

Epidermal neoplasms (most of those in Chapter 18 technically have neoplasia rather than hyperplasia)

Halogenodermas (3.5)

Ichthyosis (11.1)

Lichen sclerosus (9.5)

Normal acral skin

Reactive perforating collagenosis (9.14)

Tuberculosis verrucosa cutis (12.10)

1.62 Hypertrichosis

Becker's nevus (20.3)

Drug induced (3.5, cyclosporine, minoxidil, androgens, etc.)

Familial hypertrichosis

Fawn tail

Hirsutism

Hypertrichosis lanuginosa (1.105)

Melanocytic nevus (especially congenital, 20.5)

Mucopolysaccharidoses (8.14)

Porphyria (8.1)

Smooth muscle hamartoma (29.6)

Hyperpigmentation (see Brown)

1.63 Hypogranulosis

Hypogranulosis is a decreased thickness of the granular layer. Because it may occur in any condition where there is parakeratosis (sometimes indicating a faster epidermal turnover time with less time to develop a granular layer), the finding of hypogranulosis has limited diagnostic importance except in ichthyosis vulgaris.

Acrodermatitis enteropathica (17.1)

Beneath parakeratosis, especially psoriasis (2.8) and cornoid lamellae of porokeratosis (18.4)

Ichthyosis vulgaris (11.1)

Necrolytic migratory erythema (3.2)

Normal mucous membranes

Pellagra (8.19)

Pityriasis lichenoides (2.14)

Pityriasis rotunda

Hypopigmentation (see White, 1.150)

Induration (see Scars, Sclerosis, Fibrosis, 1.125)

1.64 Interface dermatitis, basal layer liquefaction degeneration, vacuolar alteration, hydropic degeneration

Interface dermatitis is dermatitis in which there is a degenerative change at the dermal–epidermal junction, with inflammation (mostly lymphocytes) mostly at the interface between the epidermis and dermis. *Liquefaction degeneration*, *vacuolar alteration*, and *hydropic degeneration* are three synonyms for this degenerative change that occurs at the basal layer. Liquefaction degeneration was the preferred term until Ackerman and his trainees started popularizing his term vacuolar alteration, so most books use the latter term because of his strong influence. Tiny vacuolar spaces appear at the dermal–epidermal junction, often leaving the junction indistinct. This may result in formation of a subepidermal blister. The term lichenoid dermatitis (1.72) overlaps with interface dermatitis, but "lichenoid" is used when there is a prominent band-like inflammatory infiltrate. Some authorities divide interface dermatitis into the *lichenoid type*, and the *vacuolar type*, the latter having a less impressive inflammatory infiltrate.

Bloom's syndrome (11.5)
Dermatomyositis (17.7)
Erythema dyschromicum perstans (3.11)
Erythema multiforme (3.2)
Graft-versus-host disease (17.3)
Interface dermatitis of HIV infection (14.12)
Lichen nitidus (2.12)
Lichen planus (2.11)
Lichen sclerosus (9.5)
Lichenoid and fixed drug eruptions (3.5)
Lichenoid keratosis (18.8)
Lupus erythematosus (17.6)
Lymphomatoid papulosis (24.5)
Mucha–Habermann disease (2.14)
Mycosis fungoides (24.1)
Poikiloderma atrophicans vasculare (17.4)
Radiodermatitis (9.2)
Rothmund–Thomson syndrome (11.5)
Secondary syphilis (sometimes, 12.13)
Some viral exanthems (14.7)

1.65 Interstitial dermatitis

This is defined as the unimpressive presence of inflammatory cells scattered in the spaces between collagen bundles in the dermis, as opposed to the more common perivascular dermatitis (1.109). It is not as dense as nodular and diffuse dermatitis (1.91) or lichenoid dermatitis (1.72). Of course, many of these other patterns may have a few interstitial inflammatory cells, but the list here primarily includes those where interstitial inflammation is the major finding.

Cellulitis (12.3)
Erythema marginatum (3.1 and 12.2)
Granuloma annulare (7.1)
Interstitial drug reaction (3.5)
Interstitial mycosis fungoides (24.1)
Sweet's syndrome (3.7, usually more diffuse)
Urticaria (3.1)
Well's syndrome (3.8, usually more diffuse)

Intertriginous eruptions (see Axilla 1.10 or Groin 1.55)

1.66 Kidney and the skin

Amyloidosis (8.4, deposition)
Birt–Hogg–Dube syndrome (22.6, renal cell carcinoma)
Bullous disease of hemodialysis (8.1, pseudoporphyria)
Cryoglobulinemia (4.9, glomerulonephritis)
Diabetic skin lesions (1.26, nephropathy)
Fabry's disease (25.2, renal failure)
Gout (8.5, nephrolithiasis)
Impetigo (12.2, nephritis)
Kyrle's disease (9.12, renal failure)
Lupus erythematosus (17.6, nephritis)
Myeloma (24.12, Bence Jones proteinuria)
Nail–patella syndrome (triangular lunulae, iliac horns, renal failure)
Nephrogenic fibrosing dermopathy (8.20)
Pruritus without rash (1.115)

Pseudoxanthoma elasticum (9.8, hypertension, renal artery involvement)
Renal cell carcinoma (28.4)
Sarcoidosis (7.5, calcium stones)
Scarlet fever (12.2, nephritis)
Scleroderma (9.3, renal failure)
Tuberous sclerosis (27.3, angiomyolipomas)
Vasculitis (many types, Chapter 4)

1.67 Leg lesions (includes thigh)

(see also Foot lesions 1.67)

A. Common

Actinic keratosis (lower leg, 18.8)
Arthropod bites (15.7)
Dermatofibroma (27.1)
Eczema (2.1)
Folliculitis (10.2)
Lichen simplex chronicus (2.3)
Panniculitis (all types, 1.101 and Chapter 16)
Psoriasis (2.8)
Purpura pigmentosa chronica (4.8)
Stasis dermatitis and ulcers (2.1)
Stucco keratosis (18.2)
Vasculitis (Chapter 4)
Verruca vulgaris and plana (14.1)

B. Uncommon

Atrophie blanche (4.13)
Clear cell acanthoma (18.6)
Diabetic dermopathy (17.10)
Disseminated superficial actinic porokeratosis (18.4)
Epidermal nevus (18.1)
Incontinentia pigmenti (11.6)
Kaposi sarcoma (25.9)
Kyrle's disease (9.12)
Lichen amyloidosus (8.4)
Lichen planus, hypertrophic (2.11)
Lichen striatus (2.5)
Livedo reticularis (3.10)
Necrobiosis lipoidica (7.2)
Pretibial myxedema (8.7)

1.68 Leonine facies

Carcinoid (28.5)
Chronic actinic dermatitis
Cutis verticis gyrata
Leishmaniasis (15.1)
Leprosy (12.12)
Lipoid proteinosis (8.3)
Lymphoma, leukemia (Chapter 24)
Multicentric reticulohistiocytosis (7.8)
Multiple keratoacanthoma syndrome (18.12)
Mycosis fungoides (24.1)
Progressive nodular histiocytoma (7.13)
Sarcoidosis (7.5)
Scleromyxedema (8.8)

1.69 Leukocytosis and skin disease

Infections (numerous, mostly Chapter 12)
Leukemia (24.16)
Psoriasis, pustular (2.8)
Pyoderma gangrenosum (4.12)
Sezary syndrome (24.1)
Sweet's syndrome (3.7)
Systemic corticosteroid therapy

1.70 Leukopenia and skin disease

Acquired immunodeficiency syndrome (14.12)
Drug induced (3.5)
Infections, severe (Chapters 12 and 14)
Leukemia, lymphoma (Chapter 24)
Lupus erythematosus (17.6)
Viral diseases (Chapter 14)

1.71 Leukoplakia

(see also Mouth lesions 1.82, Tongue lesions 1.139, Palate lesions 1.98)
Leukoplakia is defined as any white plaque in the mouth (occasionally the term has been applied to other mucous membranes). The term is confusing because some authors use it to be synonymous with only the premalignant form, or sometimes it is defined as any white plaque other than candidiasis.

Candidiasis (thrush, 13.4)
Hairy leukoplakia (14.8)
Lichen planus (2.11)
Premalignant leukoplakia (18.8)
Squamous cell carcinoma (18.11)
Trauma (reactive hyperplasia, buccal bite line, etc.)
Verrucous carcinoma (oral florid papillomatosis, 18.11)
Warts (human papillomavirus, especially condyloma acuminatum and Heck's disease, 14.1)
White sponge nevus (17.11)

1.72 Lichenoid dermatitis

(see Fig. 1.72)
Lichenoid is *defined by the pathologist as a band-like infiltrate* of inflammatory cells in the superficial dermis, parallel to the epidermis. Liquefaction degeneration of the basal layer (interface dermatitis, 1.64), colloid bodies (1.27), and melanin incontinence (1.79) frequently occur together. The band of inflammatory cells is usually mostly lymphocytes, except there may be plasma cells (syphilis, mucous membranes, Zoon's balanitis), or eosinophils (lichenoid drug reaction).

The *clinician defines lichenoid differently* to mean papules or plaques resembling lichen (symbiotic growth of algae and fungi) stuck on the skin. Some diseases that are lichenoid clinically are not lichenoid histologically (e.g., lichen simplex chronicus and lichen spinulosus). Lichen planus is both clinically lichenoid and pathologically lichenoid. Many of the diseases listed below that are histologically lichenoid are not clinically lichenoid. If it is a rash, usually it is lichen planus, lupus erythematosus, or drug eruption. If a solitary papule, then lichenoid keratosis.

Flegel's disease (2.7)
Graft-versus-host disease, chronic (17.3)
Keratosis lichenoides chronica (2.13)

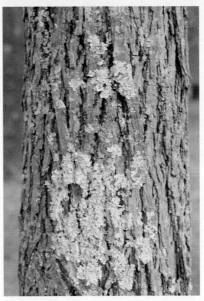

Fig. 1.72 Lichen on a tree (for those who work too hard to enjoy the woods).

Langerhans cell histiocytosis (24.18)
Lichen planus (2.11)
Lichen sclerosus (9.5)
Lichen striatus (sometimes) (2.5)
Lichenoid drug eruption (3.5)
Lichenoid keratosis (18.8)
Lichenoid pigmentary purpura (4.8)
Lupus erythematosus (17.6)
Mycosis fungoides (24.1)
Pityriasis lichenoides (2.14)
Poikiloderma atrophicans vasculare (17.4)
Some neoplasms (Chapters 18 and 20)
(Bowen's disease, melanoma, Spitz nevus, halo nevus, superficial basal cell carcinoma, etc.) The neoplastic cells may be hiding in the band-like infiltrate
Syphilis, lichenoid secondary (12.13)
Zoon's balanitis (2.11)

1.73 Linear lesions

(see also Annular lesions 1.5, Chord-like lesions 1.21, Serpiginous lesions 1.127)
These lesions tend to appear in a straight-line configuration. When injury to the skin (such as a scratch) reproduces new lesions, the process is called the *Koebner phenomenon* or Koebnerization, and often this is linear.

Basal cell carcinoma (uncommon linear variant, 18.14)
Bites and stings (such as Portuguese man-of-war, 15.7)
Contact dermatitis (especially to plants, 2.2)
Darier's disease, linear variant (11.3)
Epidermal nevus (18.1)
Goltz syndrome (11.8)
Incontinentia pigmenti (11.6)
Kyrle's disease (9.12)
Lichen nitidus (2.12)
Lichen planus (2.11)
Lichen striatus (2.5)
Linea alba, linea nigra

Molluscum contagiosum (14.4)
Nevus sebaceus (21.2)
Phytophotodermatitis (2.2)
Pigmentary demarcation lines such as Futcher's lines
Porokeratosis, linear variant (18.4)
Psoriasis (2.8)
Reactive perforating collagenosis (9.14)
Scleroderma and morphea, linear variant (9.3)
Self-induced and factitial lesions
Sporotrichoid lesions (1.133)
Striae (27.2)
Sweat gland neoplasms (rare variants such as eccrine poroma and eccrine spiradenoma, Chapter 23)
Thrombophlebitis, lymphangitis (16.7)
Trichoepitheliomas (rare linear variant, 22.2)
Verruca vulgaris and *verruca plana* (14.1)

1.74 Lip lesions

(see also Mouth lesions 1.82)

A. Common

Actinic cheilitis (18.8)
Candidiasis (13.4)
Contact cheilitis (2.2)
Erythema multiforme (3.2)
Fordyce spots (21.1)
Herpes simplex (14.2)
Labial lentigo (20.3)
Lip licking dermatitis (2.2)
Mucocele (8.10)
Perleche (2.2)
Premalignant leukoplakia (18.8)
Pyogenic granuloma (25.3)
Retinoid cheilitis (3.5)
Squamous cell carcinoma (18.11)
Venous lake (25.2)
Verruca vulgaris (14.1)
Vitiligo (17.2)

B. Uncommon

Addison's disease (17.10)
Angioedema (3.1)
Ascher's syndrome (7.7)
Cheilitis glandularis (7.7)
Cheilitis granulomatosis of Melkersson Rosenthal syndrome (7.7)
Collagen injection granulomas (7.6)
CREST syndrome (9.3)
Heck's disease (14.1)
Laugier–Hunziker syndrome (20.4)
Microcystic adnexal carcinoma (23.13)
Mucosal neuroma (26.3)
Osler–Weber–Rendu syndrome (1.136)
Pemphigus vulgaris (5.4)
Peutz–Jegher's syndrome (20.4)
Pilar sheath acanthoma (22.1)
Plasma cell cheilitis (2.11)
Sarcoidosis (7.5)
Secondary syphilis (12.13)

Liquefaction degeneration of basal layer (see interface dermatitis, 1.64)

1.75 Liver and skin disease

Amyloidosis (8.4)
Drug eruptions (3.5)
Gaucher's disease (hyperpigmentation)
Graft-versus-host disease (17.3)
Hemachromatosis (8.17)
Infectious hepatitis (14.7) and other viruses in Chapter 14
Lymphoma (Chapter 24)
Metastatic cancer (Chapter 28)
Porphyria (8.1)
Primary biliary cirrhosis (pruritus, xanthomas)
Pruritus without rash (1.115)
Sarcoidosis (7.5)
Spider angiomas (25.1)
Syphilis (12.13)
Terry's nails (1.85)
Wilson's disease (1.14, blue lunulae)
Xanthomas (7.9)

1.76 Lymphocytes and histiocytes

Mononuclear (*lymphohistiocytic*) infiltrates in the dermis are very common; therefore, we provide no list of diseases for this finding. It is useful to think of almost all inflammatory skin diseases as lymphohistiocytic, leaving us only to learn the exceptions! The term *mononuclear cell* refers to lymphocytes and histiocytes, even though there are obviously many types of cells that possess one (mono) nucleus. The equally unfortunate term *round cell* is also a synonym for mononuclear cell. Mononuclear cells are to be distinguished from neutrophils and eosinophils, which have segmented nuclei. The term "*histiocyte*" has been criticized as being confusing because it has been used for a diversity of cells found within the dermis that are now known to be heterogeneous by today's more sophisticated methods. In old-time pathology a histiocyte was a phagocytic cell (macrophage) in the reticuloendothelial system that differed from a lymphocyte by having a larger, paler nucleus and more abundant cytoplasm. A macrophage that has phagocytized melanin is called a *melanophage* (1.79), and one that has consumed hemosiderin is called a hemosiderophage or *siderophage* (1.58). Those that have eaten lipid material are called *lipophages*, and are one form of foam cells (1.46).

In almost all instances in this book, the term "histiocyte" is used for a monocyte-derived macrophage. Histiocytes appear epithelioid (1.38) and therefore some other cells that look epithelioid have been erroneously called "histiocytes", or said to be "*histiocytoid*". For example, histiocytoid hemangioma is a synonym for angiolymphoid hyperplasia (25.4), in which endothelial cells lining blood vessels resemble histiocytes. Most examples of "histiocytic lymphoma" in the old terminology actually represent B-lymphocyte malignancies. The proliferating cells in histiocytosis X (24.18) and congenital self-healing reticulohistiocytosis (24.18) are really Langerhans cells. The proliferating cells of regressing atypical histiocytosis (lymphomatoid papulosis, 24.5) are actually T-lymphocytes, and neoplastic T cells in cytophagic histiocytic panniculitis (24.1) are merely accompanied by reactive histiocytes that have phagocytized erythrocytes and leukocytes.

Lymphocytes are predominant in most rashes, and as the predominant reacting inflammatory cells for most neoplasms, so it is impossible to provide a list of disorders that have lymphocytes. It is important to stress that lymphohistiocytic inflammation in a skin disease does not indicate that a condition is chronic, contrary to common teachings in pathology courses that neutrophils are *"acute" inflammatory cells* and lymphocytes and histiocytes are *"chronic" cells*. Many acute conditions (e.g., allergic contact dermatitis, erythema multiforme) are primarily lymphocytic, while some chronic conditions (e.g., psoriasis) may attract many neutrophils. Since most lymphohistiocytic infiltrates are predominantly lymphocytic, this book will simply state that the infiltrate is lymphocytic. If histiocytes become a significant component of the infiltrate, then the differential diagnosis of granulomas (1.51) usually applies.

Macules (flat lesions without elevation, see under appropriate color)

Maculopapular (see Morbilliform)

1.77 Madarosis

Madarosis is loss of the eyelashes or eyebrows.
Alopecia areata (10.9)
Anhidrotic ectodermal dysplasia (11.2)
Atopic dermatitis (Hertoghe's sign, 2.1)
Ectodermal dysplasia (11.2)
Erythroderma (1.39)
Familial eyebrow hypoplasia
Hypothyroidism (1.138)
Leprosy lepromatous (12.12)
Monilithrix (1.4)
Pilitorti (1.4)
Progeria (9.6)
Rothmund–Thomson syndrome (11.5)
Secondary syphilis (12.13)
Self-induced or factitial plucking (10.11)
Ulerythema ophryogenes (10.5)

1.78 Mast cells

(see Fig. 1.78)
Mast cells are easily recognized when they have the typical "fried egg" appearance (round nucleus centrally placed within amphophilic cytoplasm). They are more difficult to recognize when they resemble lymphocytes or spindled fibroblasts. An index of suspicion is needed so that special stains such as the Giemsa, toluidine blue, or chloroacetate esterase can be done if needed. Do not mistake mast cells for plasma cells (1.111). Mast cells are present in small numbers in normal skin. As a rough guideline, more than six mast cells per high-powered field is probably an increased number.
Mucinous areas (1.23)
Neural tumors (Chapter 26)
Urticaria (3.1)
Urticaria pigmentosa and mastocytosis (11.10)

1.79 Melanin incontinence

Melanin incontinence (pigmentary incontinence) is the presence of melanin in the superficial dermis, due to the loss of melanin from damaged cells of the basal layer. In contrast, the presence of melanin deep in the dermis usually means it is being synthesized there by a melanocytic neoplasm (Chapter 20), many of which are pigmented whether they are superficial or deep. Some *pigmented neoplasms* contain melanocytes capable of synthesizing melanin, such as pigmented BCC (18.14), pigmented Bowen's disease (18.10), pigmented cysts (Chapter 19), pigmented follicular tumors (Chapter 22), pigmented sweat gland tumors (Chapter 23), pigmented neurofibroma (26.1), melanotic Schwannoma (26.2), and pigmented DFSP (27.10). Damage to the basal layer in interface dermatitis often results in melanin incontinence. Melanin in the dermis is often phagocytized by macrophages that are then called *melanophages* (1.76).
Any inflammatory disease in darkly pigmented skin
Erythema dyschromicum perstans (3.11)
Incontinentia pigmenti (third stage, 11.6)
Interface dermatitis (1.64)
Macular and lichen amyloidosis (8.4)
Melanocytic neoplasms (Chapter 20)
Post-inflammatory hyperpigmentation (17.10)

1.80 Monoclonal gammopathy or paraproteinemia

Monoclonal gammopathy[125] of uncertain significance occurs in 1% of the normal population over 50 years old, and in 3% over age 70. Only about 11% of those patients eventually develop multiple myeloma.

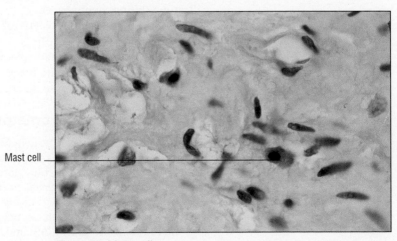

Mast cell

Fig. 1.78 Mast cells.

Amyloidosis (8.4)
Cryoglobulinemia (4.9)
Dermatitis herpetiformis (6.5)
Erythema elevatum diutinum (4.3)
Lichen myxedematosus (8.8)
Lymphoma (Chapter 24)
Multiple myeloma (24.12)
Mycosis fungoides (24.1)
Necrobiotic xanthogranuloma (7.11)
Normolipemic plane xanthoma (7.9)
POEMS syndrome (24.12)
Pyoderma gangrenosum (4.12)
Scleredema of Buschke (8.12)
Scleromyxedema (8.8)
Subcorneal pustular dermatosis (2.8)
Waldenström's macroglobulinemia (4.9)

1.81 Morbilliform (exanthematous, maculopapular, scarlatiniform) eruptions

These diseases present as generalized small 2–5 mm erythematous macules and/or papules, especially on the trunk, usually with little or no scale except in the later desquamative stages. Some would argue about the differences between these terms (scarlatiniform being rougher like sandpaper) but all four terms listed above are roughly synonyms. The term maculopapular is frequently misused non-specifically for any rash. Many of these diseases are accompanied by fever (1.45).

A. Bacterial

Corynebacterium hemolyticum infection (12.2)
Listeriosis
Lyme disease (12.14)
Rheumatic fever (12.2)
Scarlet fever (12.2)
Secondary syphilis (12.13)
Toxic shock syndrome (12.2)

B. Viral

Adenovirus (14.7)
Arbovirus infection (including dengue, 14.7)
Echovirus (14.7)
Fifth disease (14.7)
Gianotti–Crosti syndrome (14.11)
Hepatitis B
Human immunodeficiency virus disease (14.12)
Kawasaki disease (14.10)
Mononucleosis (14.8)
Roseola (14.7)
Rubella (14.7)
Rubeola (14.7)

C. Other infections

Rocky Mountain spotted fever (14.13)
Toxoplasmosis
Typhus (14.13)

D. Non-infectious

Drug eruption (3.5)
Follicular eruptions (1.47)

Graft-versus-host disease (17.3)
Leukemia (24.16)
Purpuric eruptions (1.120)
Reactive erythemas (Chapter 3)
Red papular eruptions (1.122)
Still's disease and juvenile rheumatoid arthritis
Transfusion reaction and serum sickness

1.82 Mouth lesions

(see also Gingiva 1.50, Lips 1.74, Palate 1.98, Tongue 1.139)
Ameloblastoma (nodule, 18.14)
Aphthous ulcers (ulcers, 17.11)
Behçet's syndrome (ulcers, 4.11)
Burns (ulcers, 6.7)
Candidiasis (leukoplakia, 13.4)
Condyloma acuminatum (verrucous papules, 14.1)
Contact stomatitis (leukoplakia, erythema, 2.2)
Cowden's syndrome (fibromas, 22.5)
Darier's disease (cobblestoned leukoplakia, 11.3)
Drug-induced stomatitis (chemotherapy, etc., 3.5)
Dyskeratosis congenita (premalignant leukoplakia, 11.4)
Epidermolysis bullosa (blisters, ulcers, 6.6)
Erythema multiforme (ulcers, 3.2)
Fibroma (27.1)
Hand–foot–mouth disease (vesicles, 14.6)
Heck's disease (papules, 14.1)
Herpangina (ulcers, 14.6)
Herpes virus (vesicles, ulcers, 14.2)
Histoplasmosis (ulcers, 13.9)
Leukoplakia, premalignant (white plaque, 1.71)
Leukoplakia, traumatic (white plaque, 1.71)
Lichen planus (reticulated plaques, erosions, 2.11)
Lupus erythematosus (ulcers, 17.6)
Measles (Koplik spots, 14.7)
Mucosal neuroma (multiple papules, 26.3)
Mucosal pemphigoid (vesicles, ulcers, 6.2)
Pachyonychia congenita (leukoplakia, 9.15)
Pemphigus (vesicles, ulcers, 5.4)
Pyostomatitis vegetans (pustules, 17.11)
Reiter's disease (erosions, 2.8)
Squamous cell carcinoma (nodules, plaques, 18.11)
Stevens–Johnson syndrome (ulcers, 3.2)
Syphilis, mucous patch (leukoplakia, 12.13)
Trauma (biting, dentures, etc.)
Tuberculosis cutis orificialis (12.10)
Verruca vulgaris (papules, 14.1)
Verruciform xanthoma (white plaque, 7.12)
Verrucous carcinoma (white plaque, 18.11)
White sponge nevus (white plaque, 17.11)

1.83 Mucin and myxomatous changes

Dermal mucin contains acid mucopolysaccharide and stains pale blue, smudgy, thread-like or granular on H&E staining. It can be stained with Alcian blue, toluidine blue, or colloidal iron stains (Chapter 30). *Sialomucin* (the product of salivary glands) and other *epithelial mucins* often contain neutral mucopolysaccharide as well as acid mucopolysaccharide, and therefore stain with PAS and mucicarmine, as well as with Alcian blue, toluidine blue, and colloidal iron.

Myxomatous refers to the presence of abundant mucin, a term usually used when H&E staining shows a pale, washed-out area because much of the mucin is lost during processing. Such paleness can be confused with edema (1.30).

Basal cell carcinoma (18.14)
Degos disease (4.10)
Dermatomyositis (17.7)
Digital mucous cyst (8.9)
Eosinophilia myalgia syndrome (3.5)
Familial myxovascular fibromas (27.3)
Fibrous tumors (Chapter 27)
Focal mucinosis of the skin (8.11)
Follicular mucinosis (10.8)
Granuloma annulare (7.1)
Lichen myxedematosus and scleromyxedema (8.8)
Lupus erythematosus (17.6)
Metastatic adenocarcinoma (28.2)
Mucocele (8.10)
Mucopolysaccharidoses (8.14)
Myxedema (especially pretibial) (8.6, 8.7)
Myxoid liposarcoma (29.5)
Myxoma (27.17)
Nephrogenic fibrosing dermopathy (8.19)
Neural tumors, most (Chapter 26)
Pachydermoperiostosis (9.7)
Reticular erythematous mucinosis (8.13)
Scleredema (8.12)
Spindle cell lipoma (29.2)
Sweat gland carcinoma (especially mucinous carcinoma) (23.13)
Young scars and keloids (27.2)

1.84 Multinucleated giant cells

1. Macrophage-derived giant cells (1.76)

Langhans giant cells (not to be confused with Langerhans cells, 24.18) have a ring of nuclei at the cell periphery. *Foreign body giant cells* have nuclei that are haphazardly distributed through the cytoplasm, and are seen in many diseases besides foreign body granulomas. The distinction between these two kinds of cells is not very important, since either kind can be found in a wide variety of disorders. *Touton giant cells are* foamy and are discussed in Section 1.46.

Granulomatous diseases (1.51)

2. Melanocytic giant cells are more common in benign lesions than malignant

Melanocytic nevus (20.5)
Melanoma (less commonly, and then are atypical) (20.11)
Spitz nevus (20.6)

3. Epithelial giant cells are derived from keratinocytes

Herpes virus infections (14.2)
Miscellaneous diseases can rarely have multinucleated keratinocytes for no apparent reason

4. Endothelial giant cells

Cytomegalovirus infection (these giant cells are rarely seen in the skin, 14.9)

5. Giant cells in other neoplasms

Fibrohistiocytic proliferations (dermatofibroma, giant cell tumor of tendon sheath, atypical fibroxanthoma, and malignant fibrous histiocytoma, Chapter 27)
Hodgkin's lymphoma (Reed–Sternberg cells, 24.15)
Pleomorphic lipoma (floret giant cells, 29.2)

1.85 Nail lesions[59]

A. Associated with skin disease

Alopecia areata (hammered brass pits, 10.9)
Contact dermatitis (dystrophy, 2.2)
Darier's disease (longitudinal ridges, triangular distal wedges, 11.3)
Dyskeratosis congenita (dystrophy, 11.4)
Ectodermal dysplasia, anhidrotic (dystrophy, 11.2)
Eczema adjacent to nail plate (dystrophy, 2.1)
Epidermolysis bullosa (absence or dystrophy, 6.6)
Lichen planus (longitudinal ridges, pterygium, 2.11)
Pachyonychia congenita (thick nails, keratoderma, leukoplakia, 9.15)
Pityriasis rubra pilaris (dystrophy 2.10)
Psoriasis (pits, onycholysis, dystrophy, 2.8)
Reiter's disease (dystrophy, 2.8)

B. Associated with systemic disease

Beau's lines (transverse ridge from illness)
Clubbing (pulmonary and cardiac disease)
Koilonychia (spoon nails from iron deficiency or genetic)
Lindsay's half and half nails (white proximal nail, kidney disease)
Mee's lines (white transverse bands, arsenic)
Muehrcke's nails (narrow transverse white bands, hypoalbuminemia)
Nail–patella syndrome (triangular lunula)
Terry's nails (total white nail except distal 1.2 mm, liver disease)
Yellow nail syndrome (pulmonary disease)

C. Primary nail diseases

Anonychia (lack of nails, usually congenital)
Candidiasis (white dystrophy, 13.4)
Glomus tumor (pain, erythema, 25.5)
Habit tic deformity (transverse or midline longitudinal ridges from picking at cuticle)
Median canaliform dystrophy (longitudinal midline fir tree splitting)
Melanocytic nevus (pigmented streak, 20.5)
Melanoma (pigmented streak, 20.11)
Melanonychia striata (pigmented streak, 20.3)
Nail–patella syndrome (triangular lunulae)
Onychauxis (thick nails, trauma, etc.)
Onychogryphosis (ram's horn nail)
Onycholysis (separation of nail plate due to trauma, drugs, psoriasis, etc.)
Onychomadesis (nail shedding beginning proximally)
Onychomycosis (white thickening, onycholysis, fungus, 13.1)
Onychophagia (nail biting)

Onychoschizia (splitting distal edge, thyroid disease)

Onychotillomania (compulsive picking at nails)

Paronychia (infection around nail, 12.3)

Squamous cell carcinoma (dystrophy, 18.11)

Twenty-nail dystrophy (idiopathic dystrophy with childhood onset)

Unguium incarnatus (ingrown nail)

Verruca, periungual (dystrophy, 14.1)

Verrucous carcinoma (dystrophy, 18.11)

1.86 Neck lesions

Acanthosis nigricans (18.5)

Acrochordon (27.4)

Actinic keratosis (18.8)

Basal cell carcinoma (18.14)

Contact dermatitis (2.2)

Cysts (especially epidermoid, branchial cleft, thyroglossal, Chapter 19)

Eczema (2.1)

Elastosis perforans serpiginosa (9.13)

Hibernoma (29.4)

Kimura's disease (25.4)

Mid-dermal elastolysis (9.15)

Pilomatricoma (22.3)

Pleomorphic lipoma (29.2)

Poikiloderma of Civatte (17.10)

Pseudofolliculitis barbae (10.2)

Pseudoxanthoma elasticum (9.8)

Spindle cell lipoma (29.2)

Squamous cell carcinoma (18.11)

Tinea (14.1)

1.87 Necrotic keratinocytes, necrotic epidermis, apoptosis

Necrosis refers to cell death with subsequent degeneration. Because necrotic keratinocytes are brightly eosinophilic ("dead reds"), they can be difficult to distinguish from *dyskeratotic keratinocytes* (1.27). In fact, dyskeratosis may actually be necrosis in most cases. An in-vogue term, *apoptosis*,[121] may be impossible to distinguish from necrosis with routine H&E staining, and the distinction has been actively debated. Apoptosis has been defined as a special type of necrosis that is active, as opposed to passive necrosis, and it also has been called programmed cell death. In graft-versus-host disease, a necrotic keratinocyte with an adjacent lymphocyte is sometimes called "satellitosis" or "*satellite cell necrosis*".

Burns (6.7)

Erythema multiforme and its variants (toxic epidermal necrolysis and Stevens–Johnson syndrome) (3.2)

Glucagonoma syndrome (3.2)

Graft-versus-host disease (17.3)

Herpes, papilloma, Coxsackie, and other viral infections (Chapter 14)

Hypoxemia, pressure (6.8)

Numerous neoplasms, especially *malignant epidermal tumors* (Chapter 18) and malignant adnexal tumors (Chapters 21 through 23)

Photodermatitis (1.110)

Pityriasis lichenoides (2.14)

Radiodermatitis (9.2)

Rowell syndrome (17.6)

Severe bite reactions (15.7)

Severe cellulitis (12.3)

Severe contact dermatitis (2.2)

Severe vasculitis, emboli, infarction, or coagulopathy (Chapter 4)

Some drug eruptions (*fixed drug eruption* (3.5), warfarin necrosis)

Syphilis (rare "lues maligna," 12.13)

1.88 Necrotic dermis
(see also Eosinophilic material 1.35, Scars, sclerosis, and fibrosis 1.125)

Amebiasis (15.13)

Deep fungal infections (especially opportunistic, Chapter 13)

Degos disease (4.10)

Ecthyma gangrenosum (12.20)

Hydroa vacciniforme (17.5)

Hypoxia (pressure necrosis, decubiti, etc.)

Necrotizing fasciitis (12.3)

Protothe`cosis (15.2)

Thrombotic and embolic diseases (1.137, 4.16)

Toxoplasmosis (15.15)

1.89 Neutrophils
(see Fig. 1.89)

Neutrophils usually have more than two segmentations of the nucleus, while eosinophils (1.36) have two or less. Both neutrophils and eosinophils can have a brightly eosinophilic cytoplasm, but with H&E staining it is more granular in eosinophils. Whenever there are many neutrophils, fragmentation of nuclei (*nuclear dust, karyorrhexis, leuko-cytoclasis*) is common, and this is not specific for leukocytoclastic vasculitis (4.1).

A. Neutrophilic microabscesses or pustules in the epidermis (especially in the stratum corneum or superficial spinous layer)

1. Three most common (usually subcorneal)

Impetigo (includes "impetiginization" = secondary infection of other dermatoses, especially of eczemas, 12.1)

Psoriasis (and related entities) (2.8)

Superficial fungal infections (dermatophytosis and candidiasis) (Chapter 13)

2. Other diseases with neutrophils in the epidermis (often pustules clinically)

Acne and folliculitis (Chapter 10)

Acropustulosis of infancy (5.1)

Atypical mycobacterial infections (12.11)

Clear cell acanthoma (18.6)

Deep fungal infections (Chapter 13)

Gonococcemia (12.18)

Halogenodermas (3.5)

Mucha–Habermann disease (2.14)

Necrolytic migratory erythema (3.2)

Neonatal pustular melanosis (5.2)

Pemphigus erythematosus or foliaceus (sometimes) (5.4)

Pustular vasculitis (4.1)

Pyoderma gangrenosum (4.12)

Pyogenic granuloma (25.3)

Scabies (15.9)

Some arthropod bites or stings (such as fire ants) (15.7)

Syphilis and yaws (some types, 12.13)

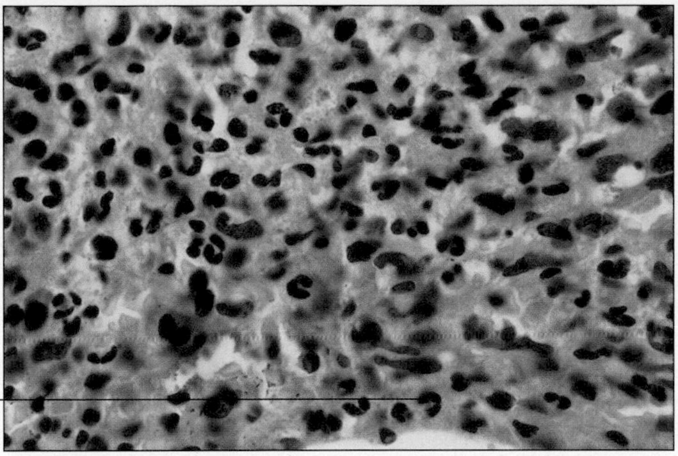

Fig. 1.89 Neutrophils.

B. Neutrophils in the dermis (in some of these, neutrophils may be found in the epidermis also)

1. *Subepidermal blistering diseases*
    Bullous lupus erythematosus (17.6)
    Bullous pemphigoid (sometimes, 6.1)
    Dermatitis herpetiformis (6.5)
    Epidermolysis bullosa acquisita (sometimes)
    Linear IgA bullous dermatosis and chronic dermatosis of childhood (6.4)
2. *Neutrophilic dermatosis group*
    Behçet's syndrome (4.11)
    Bowel bypass syndrome (4.1)
    Pyoderma gangrenosum (4.12)
    Rheumatoid neutrophilic dermatitis (3.7)
    Sweet's syndrome (3.7)
3. *Infectious diseases (Chapters 12 and 13)*
    Consider sepsis, cellulitis, abscess, deep fungus infection, bacterial infection; consider special stains for organisms such as CMS, PAS, Gram, AFB.
4. *Ruptured cysts or follicles (Chapters 10 and 19)*
5. *Leukocytoclastic vasculitis (4.1)*
6. *Erythema elevatum diutinum (4.3)*
7. *Granuloma faciale (4.2)*
8. *Ulcerations (1.142)*
9. *Areas of necrosis tend to attract neutrophils (1.86, 1.87)*
10. *Neutrophilic eccrine hidradenitis (10.15)*
11. *Urticaria (3.1)*

1.90 Nipple lesions

Accessory nipple (29.12)
Contact dermatitis (2.2)
Neurofibroma (26.1)
Nevoid hyperkeratosis
Paget's disease (18.13)
Papillary adenoma (23.5)
Sebaceous hyperplasia (Montgomery's tubercles, 21.1)

1.91 Nodular and diffuse dermatitis

These diseases produce a dense infiltrate of cells in the dermis, either arranged into nodules or diffusely throughout the dermis.

Cellulitis and many infectious diseases (12.3)
Eosinophilic cellulitis (Well's syndrome) (3.8)
Erythema elevatum diutinum (4.3)
Granuloma faciale (4.2)
Granulomatous diseases (1.51)
Leukemia (24.16)
Lupus erythematosus (sometimes, 17.6)
Lymphoma (24.10)
Mastocytosis (24.17)
Plasmacytoma (myeloma) (24.12)
Polymorphous light eruption (sometimes, 17.5)
Pseudolymphoma (24.14)
Sweet's syndrome (3.7)
Undifferentiated metastatic carcinoma (Chapter 28)

1.92 Nodules (clinical, in general)

A. Many neoplasms and cysts

B. Granulomas (1.51)

C. Reactive

Arthropod bite (15.7)
Fibrous proliferations (Chapter 27)
Lymphocytoma cutis (24.14)
Panniculitis (Chapter 16)
Sweet's syndrome (3.7)
Vasculitis (Chapter 4)

D. Follicular

Acne, nodulocystic (10.1)
Folliculitis decalvans (10.2)
Hidradenitis suppurativa (10.1)

E. Depositions

Calcinosis cutis (8.15)
Gout (8.5)
Osteoma cutis (29.8)
Xanthomas (7.9)

F. Infections

Atypical mycobacterial infection (12.11)
Deep fungal infections (Chapter 13)
Furuncle, bacterial (12.1)

Inflamed molluscum (14.4)
Majocchi's granuloma (13.1)
Nodular scabies (15.9)
Orf and milker's nodule (14.5)
Parasitic infestation (Chapter 15)

G. Juxta-articular nodules (near joints)

Calcinosis cutis (8.15)
Gout (8.5)
Granuloma annulare (7.1)
Multicentric reticulohistiocytosis (7.8)
Osteoarthritis (Heberden's node)
Osteochondroma
Rheumatic fever nodule (12.12)
Rheumatoid nodule and rheumatoid joint destruction (7.3)
Synovial cyst (8.9)
Xanthomas, tuberous (7.9)

1.93 Nodules in children (clinical)

The first four listed possibilities are predominant common considerations.

Arthropod bite (15.7)
Juvenile xanthogranuloma (7.10)
Mastocytoma (24.17)
Spitz nevus (20.6)
Accessory tragus (29.10)
Acute lymphoblastic leukemia (24.16)
Cysts (dermoid, branchial cleft, etc., Chapter 19)
Fibromatosis (27.15)
Hemangioma and vascular malformation (25.1)
Infantile digital fibromatosis (27.7)
Inflamed molluscum contagiosum (14.4)
Langerhans cell histiocytosis (24.18)
Metastatic retinoblastoma, neuroblastoma (28.5)
Nasal glioma (26.5)
Pilomatricoma (22.3)
Pseudorheumatoid nodule (7.1)
Pyogenic granuloma (25.3)
Scabies, nodular (15.9)
Supernumerary digit (27.5)

1.94 Normal-appearing skin (histologic)

The following diseases should be considered when initial examination of routine sections appears to show no abnormality. Besides subtle findings that are easy to miss, the "best special stain in dermatopathology" (deeper levels cut into the block) may be helpful in many cases.

A. Epidermal abnormality

Ichthyosis (11.1)
Interface dermatitis (1.64, subtle liquefaction degeneration of the basal layer without much inflammation, especially Graft-versus-host disease 17.3, or Dermatomyositis 17.7)
Parapsoriasis (2.9)
Porokeratosis (18.40): look for cornoid lamella
Tinea and *Candida* (13.1): get special stains

B. Pigmentary abnormality

Vitiligo and other diseases with hyperpigmentation or hypopigmentation (17.2)

C. Adnexal abnormality

Alopecia, etc. (Chapter 10)

D. Dermal abnormality

Connective tissue alteration: scleroderma, connective tissue nevus, atrophoderma, anetoderma, cutis laxa, etc. (Chapter 9)
Foreign material: argyria, hemochromatosis, tattoo, macular amyloidosis (Chapter 8)
Mucin deposition: myxedema, scleredema, etc. (1.83)
Subtle interstitial dermatitis (1.65)
Subtle neoplasms: blue nevus, metastasis in lymphatics, fibrous neoplasm
Subtle perivascular dermatitis (1.109)
Urticaria (3.1) and telangiectasia macularis eruptiva perstans (24.17)

1.95 Nose lesions

Acanthoma fissuratum (2.3)
Actinic keratosis (18.8)
Angiofibroma (fibrous papule, 27.3)
Basal cell carcinoma (18.14)
Leishmaniasis (15.1)
Lupus erythematosus (17.6)
Lupus pernio (7.5)
Melanocytic *nevus* (20.5)
Microcystic adnexal carcinoma (23.13)
Nasal glioma (26.5)
Pagetoid cells (see Epidermotropism 1.37)
Relapsing polychondritis (17.8)
Rhinoscleroma (12.9)
Rhinosporidiosis (13.15)
Rosacea (10.1)
Sebaceous hyperplasia (21.1)
Trichoepithelioma (22.2)

1.96 Painful nodules

Some of these are often remembered using mnemonics such as ENGLAND, GLENDA, ANGEL, BENGAL, or LENDANEGG.

Eccrine spiradenoma (23.11)
Neurilemmoma (26.2)
Glomus tumor (25.5)
Leiomyoma (29.6)
Angiolipoma (29.2)
Neuroma (26.3)
Dercum's disease (adiposis dolorosa, 29.2)
Arthropod bite or sting (15.7)
Blue rubber bleb nevus (25.1)
Chondrodermatitis nodularis helicis (17.9)
Cutaneous endometriosis (29.9)
Dermatofibroma (sometimes, 27.1)
Erythema nodosum (16.1)
Erythema nodosum leprosum (12.12)
Osier's nodes (4.1)
Panniculitis (Chapter 16)

Sweet's syndrome (3.7)
Vasculitis (1.145)

1.97 Pain or paresthesia without skin lesions

Delusions of parasitosis
Herpes zoster (14.2)
Neurodermatitis (2.1)
Neuropathy
Notalgia paresthetica
Polycythemia rubra vera
Porphyria (8.1)
Systemic disease (kidney, liver)

1.98 Palate lesions

(see also Mouth)
Candidiasis (13.4)
Herpangina (14.6)
Kaposi sarcoma (25.9)
Lymphoma ("lethal midline granuloma," 24.6)
Necrotizing sialometaplasia (17.11)
Squamous cell carcinoma (18.11)
Syphilis (perforation of palate, 12.13)
Viral disorders (rubella, mononucleosis, parvovirus, etc., 14.7, 14.8)

1.99 Pale epidermis

(see also Vacuolization of epidermis 1.144, Clear cell neoplasms 1.22, Pagetoid cells 1.37)
Acrodermatitis enteropathica (17.1)
Hartnup's disease (2.1)
Necrolytic migratory erythema (3.2)
Pellagra (8.19)
Psoriasis (2.8)
Radiodermatitis (9.2)
Syphilis (2.13)

1.100 Palm and sole lesions

(see also Hands and fingers 1.56, Foot 1.48)
Acral lentiginous melanoma (20.11)
Acral melanocytic nevus (20.5)
Acropustulosis of infancy (5.1)
Arsenical keratosis (18.9)
Callus and corn (2.3)
Contact dermatitis (2.2)
CREST syndrome (telangiectasias, 9.3)
Darier's disease (pits, 11.3)
Drug eruptions (3.5)
Eccrine poroma (23.10)
Ectodermal dysplasia (11.2)
Eczema (2.1)
Epidermolysis bullosa (especially Weber–Cockayne type, 6.6)
Erythema multiforme (3.2)
Erythermalgia (3.13)
Fibromatosis (27.15)
Friction blister (5.7)
Graft-versus-host disease (17.3)
Hand–foot–mouth disease (14.6)

Id reaction (2.1)
Juvenile plantar dermatosis (2.2)
Kawasaki's disease (14.10)
Keratoderma (2.15)
Keratosis punctata (2.15)
Measles, atypical (14.7)
Nevoid basal cell carcinoma syndrome (pits, 18.14)
Osler–Weber–Rendu syndrome (1.136)
Pachyonychia congenita (1.82)
Palmar erythema (liver disease, connective tissue disease, pregnancy, estrogens)
Piezogenic pedal papules
Pityriasis rubra pilaris (2.10)
Psoriasis (2.8)
Reiter's disease (2.8)
Rocky Mountain spotted fever (14.13)
Scabies, crusted "Norwegian" (15.9)
Syphilis, secondary (12.13)
Talon noir (black heel, traumatic intracorneal hemorrhage)
Tinea nigra (13.3)
Tinea pedis, tinea manuum (13.1)
Tripe palms (18.5)
Verruca vulgaris and plantaris (14.1)
Xanthoma (eruptive, planar, 7.9)

1.101 Panniculitis

Alpha-1 antitrypsin deficiency (16.10)
Calciphylaxis (8.15)
Cold panniculitis (16.3)
Eosinophilic panniculitis
Erythema induratum (16.6)
Erythema nodosum (16.1)
Factitial panniculitis
Foreign body granuloma (7.6)
Infection-related panniculitis (bacterial, fungal, parasitic, Chapters 12, 13, 15, 16)
Leukemic panniculitis (24.16)
Lipodystrophy (16.11)
Lipomembranous panniculitis (16.9)
Lupus panniculitis (17.6)
Lymphoma, subcutaneous (Chapter 24)
Pancreatic fat necrosis (16.8)
Polyarteritis nodosa (4.4)
Post-corticosteroid injection panniculitis
Rheumatoid nodule (7.3)
Sarcoidosis (7.5)
Sclerema neonatorum (16.4)
Scleroderma (9.3)
Subcutaneous fat necrosis of the newborn (16.5)
Superficial thrombophlebitis (16.7)
Weber–Christian disease (16.2)

1.102 Papillomatosis

(see also Verrucous 1.146)
Papillomatosis is an irregular undulation of the epidermal surface. The first four diseases listed below are by far the most common. Sometimes these four cannot be distinguished by routine H&E sections, and are signed out without

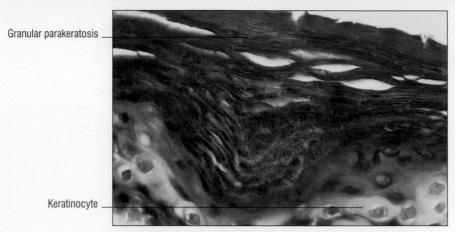

Granular parakeratosis

Keratinocyte

Fig. 1.104 Granular parakeratosis.

commitment as "benign keratosis", "papilloma", or "fibroepithelial papilloma".

A. The most common

Acrochordon (27.4)
Actinic keratosis (18.8)
Seborrheic keratosis (18.2)
Verruca vulgaris (14.1)

B. Others

Acanthosis nigricans (18.5)
Acrokeratosis verruciformis (18.3)
Darier's disease (11.3)
Epidermal nevus (18.1)
Lipoid proteinosis (8.3)
Nevus sebaceus (21.2)
Orf and milker's nodule (14.5)
Papules (see under location or specific color)
Some melanocytic nevi (20.5)
Squamous cell carcinoma, sometimes (18.11)
Syringocystadenoma papilliferum (23.3)
Tuberculosis verrucosa cutis (12.10)

1.103 Papulosquamous diseases

(see also Eczematous diseases 1.29)
These are lesions with thick scale, erythema, and sharp demarcation. Nearly all of them are listed in Chapter 2, but some others with that clinical appearance are listed here.
Diseases in Chapter 2
Basal cell carcinoma, superficial type (18.14)
Bowen's disease (18.10)
Epidermal nevus (18.1)
Fungal infections (Chapter 13)
Ichthyosis (11.1)
Lupus erythematosus, discoid (17.6)
Mycosis fungoides (24.1)
Nevus sebaceus (21.2)
Porokeratosis (18.4)
Scabies, crusted "Norwegian" (15.9)
Seborrheic keratosis, irritated (18.2)
Squamous cell carcinoma (18.11)
Syphilis, secondary (12.13)
Tinea (13.1)

Tuberculosis verrucosa cutis (12.10)
Verruca vulgaris (14.1)

1.104 Parakeratosis

(see Fig. 1.104)
Parakeratosis refers to pyknotic keratinocyte nuclei within the stratum corneum, where nuclei are not normally present. It is common to many diseases where there are *changes within the epidermis*, and is often accompanied by hyperkeratosis (1.61), hypogranulosis (1.63), and acanthosis (1.61). Most parakeratotic diseases are *scaly*, a clinical finding that again implies epidermal pathology. Scale is especially common to eczematous (1.29) and papulosquamous diseases (1.103). Parakeratosis is a very non-specific change, but several patterns of parakeratosis may be helpful clues in differential diagnosis.

A. Alternating parakeratosis

Parakeratosis (often over dysplasia) alternates with orthokeratosis, with orthokeratosis most prevalent over adnexa that are spared by the dysplasia. There may be a bluish and pinkish alternating appearance of the stratum corneum.
Actinic keratosis (18.8)

B. Columns of parakeratosis

Columns of parakeratosis, which may be impressive.
Porokeratosis (18.4, cornoid lamellae)
Verruca vulgaris (14.1)

C. Confluent parakeratosis

Extensive parakeratosis, tends to involve broad areas of stratum corneum.
Bowen's disease (18.10)
Psoriasis (2.8)

D. Focal parakeratosis: small foci of parakeratosis

Guttate psoriasis (2.8, with mounds of neutrophils in stratum corneum)
Most of the "eczemas" (2.1)
Parapsoriasis (2.9)
Pityriasis lichenoides (2.14)
Pityriasis rosea (2.4)

E. Sputtering, checkerboard, and shoulder parakeratosis

Parakeratosis seems to start and stop in a sputtering or checkerboard patchwork manner and is present at the edges over plugged follicles.

Pityriasis rubra pilaris (2.10)

F. Mounds of parakeratosis with neutrophils

Psoriasis (2.8, especially guttate)

G. Sandwich parakeratosis

Parakeratosis over orthokeratosis over the granular layer, resembles layers of a sandwich.

Tinea (13.1)

H. Axillary granular parakeratosis[140]

Axillary granular parakeratosis is a peculiar pattern of hundreds of granules in the stratum corneum thought to be a reaction to deodorant in the axilla.

1.105 Paraneoplastic syndromes

Paraneoplastic syndromes are dermatoses in which the skin lesions have a parallel course along with and associated with systemic malignancy. Cure of the malignancy might cause a resolution of the cutaneous lesions. Also included here are some genodermatoses associated with systemic neoplasms, which arguably are not truly paraneoplastic.

Acanthosis nigricans (abdominal adenocarcinoma, 18.5)

Acquired ichthyosis (lymphoma, 11.1)

Amyloidosis (myeloma, 8.4)

Arsenical keratosis (GI adenocarcinoma, 18.9)

Ataxia–telangiectasia (lymphoma, 11.12)

Bazex syndrome (acrokeratosis paraneoplastica, aerodigestive tract carcinoma, 2.15)

Birt–Hogg–Dube syndrome (renal cell carcinoma, 22.6)

Bloom's syndrome (variety of neoplasms, 11.10)

Carcinoid (flushing, pancreatic or GI neoplasm, 28.5)

Cowden's disease (breast and thyroid cancer, 22.5)

Cronkhite–Canada syndrome (GI malignancy, 17.10)

Cryoglobulinemia (Waldenström's macroglobulinemia, myeloma, 4.9)

Dermatitis herpetiformis (lymphoma, 6.5)

Dermatomyositis (various malignancies in 25% of adults, 17.7)

Dyskeratosis congenita (various tumors, 11.4)

Erythema gyratum repens (lung cancer, 3.4)

Erythromelalgia (myeloproliferative malignancy, 3.13)

Exfoliative erythroderma (mainly lymphoma, 1.39)

Fat necrosis (pancreatic carcinoma, 16.8)

Follicular mucinosis (mycosis fungoides, 10.8)

Gardner's syndrome (cysts, lipomas, GI adenocarcinoma, 19.1)

Granuloma annulare, systemic type (myeloproliferative disorders, 7.1)

Herpes zoster (usually no malignancy, 14.2)

Howell–Evans keratoderma (esophageal carcinoma, 2.15)

Hyperpigmentation, generalized (melanoma, 1.18)

Hypertrichosis lanuginosa acquisita (lung and colorectal carcinoma)

Leser–Trelat sign (eruptive SKs with adenocarcinoma, 18.2)

Muir–Torre syndrome (sebaceous neoplasms, keratoacanthomas, GI carcinoma, 21.3)

Multicentric reticulohistiocytosis (30% risk of malignancy various cancers, 7.8)

Multiple endocrine neoplasia type 1 (Wermer syndrome) (angiofibromas, parathyroid, pancreatic, pituitary tumors, 27.3)

Multiple endocrine neoplasia type 2a (Sipple syndrome) (pruritic hyperpigmentation and hyperkeratosis of the back, pheochromocytoma, thyroid carcinoma)

Multiple endocrine neoplasia type 2b (mucosal neuromas, thyroid carcinoma, 26.3)

Multiple keratoacanthoma syndrome (GI carcinoma, 18.12)

Necrolytic migratory erythema (glucagonoma, 3.2)

Neurofibromatosis (malignant Schwannoma, 26.9)

Paraneoplastic pemphigus (myeloproliferative malignancy, 5.4)

Progeria (variety of malignancies, 9.6)

Pruritus without rash (various malignancies, especially myeloproliferative, 1.115)

Pyoderma gangrenosum (leukemia, 3.7)

Rothmund–Thomson syndrome (osteogenic sarcoma, 11.5)

Stewart–Treves syndrome (mastectomy, lymphedema, angiosarcoma, 25.7)

Superficial thrombophlebitis (various malignancies, 16.7)

Sweet's syndrome (leukemia, 3.7)

Tripe palm (acanthosis palmaris, lung and GI carcinoma, 18.5)

Trousseau's syndrome (phlebitis with neoplasm, 4.16)

1.106 Pedunculated lesions

These lesions protrude from a narrow stalk.

Accessory nipple (29.12)

Accessory tragus (29.10)

Acquired digital fibrokeratoma (27.5)

Acrochordon (27.4)

Condyloma acuminatum (14.1)

Congenital wattle (29.10)

Cutaneous horn (1.61)

Fibroma of the mouth (27.1)

Melanocytic nevus (some, 20.5)

Neurofibroma (26.1)

Nevus lipomatosus (29.1)

Omphalomesenteric duct polyp (29.11)

Pedunculated melanoma (rare, 20.11)

Pyogenic granuloma (25.3)

Rhinosporidiosis (13.15)

Seborrheic keratosis (some, 18.2)

Supernumerary digit (27.5)

Yaws (12.13)

1.107 Penis lesions

Balanitis xerotica obliterans (9.5)

Behçet's syndrome (4.11)

Bowen's disease (erythroplasia of Queyrat, 18.10)

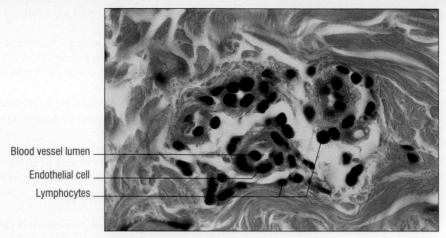

Fig. 1.109 Perivascular lymphocytes.

Bowenoid papulosis (18.10)
Candidiasis (13.4)
Chancroid (12.7)
Condyloma acuminatum (14.1)
Condyloma lata (12.13)
Contact dermatitis (2.2)
Fixed drug eruption (3.5)
Granuloma inguinale (12.8)
Herpes simplex (14.2)
Lentigo simplex (2.8)
Lichen nitidus (2.12)
Lichen planus (2.11)
Lymphogranuloma venereum (14.14)
Median raphe cyst (19.12)
Molluscum contagiosum (14.4)
Pearly penile papules (27.3)
Peyronie's disease (27.15)
Psoriasis (2.8)
Reiter's disease (circinate balanitis, 2.8)
Scabies (15.9)
Sclerosing lipogranuloma (7.6)
Sclerosing lymphangitis (4.16)
Squamous cell carcinoma (18.11)
Syphilis, primary (12.13)
Verrucous carcinoma (Buschke–Lowenstein tumor, 18.11)
Vitiligo (17.2)
Zoon's balanitis (2.11)

1.108 Perianal lesions

Amebiasis (15.13)
Candidiasis (13.4)
Carcinoma (18.11)
Cellulitis, perianal streptococcal (12.3)
Cloacogenic carcinoma (18.14)
Condyloma acuminatum (14.1)
Condyloma lata (12.13)
Contact dermatitis (2.2)
Crohn's disease (7.7)
Cytomegalovirus infection (usually ulcers, 14.9)
Fissures
Granuloma inguinale (12.8)
Hemorrhoids

Herpes simplex (14.2)
Hidradenoma papilliferum (23.2)
Lichen sclerosus (9.5)
Lymphogranuloma venereum (14.14)
Malakoplakia (12.21)
Paget's disease, extramammary (18.13)
Pilonidal sinus (10.1)
Pinworms
Pruritus ani
Psoriasis (2.8)
Schistosomiasis (1.108)

1.109 Perivascular dermatitis

(see Fig. 1.109)
Numerous "rashes" belong here. This term is used when the dermal inflammatory cells (mostly lymphocytic, 1.76) are mainly around blood vessels. This is by far the *most common pattern* of inflammation in the dermis, because inflammatory cells initially come out of the blood vessels. It is useful to think of almost all inflammatory skin diseases as showing perivascular dermatitis, leaving the pathologist to remember only the exceptions. Most books subdivide perivascular dermatitis into "superficial" and "superficial and deep" subtypes. This splitting is far less helpful toward making a specific diagnosis than is the clinical correlation, and the concomitant search for other findings, such as epidermal changes and inflammatory cell types. Other patterns, such as lichenoid (1.72) and nodular (1.91), may show areas of perivascular dermatitis, but when those patterns are found, the correct differential diagnosis is generally found under those headings rather than under perivascular dermatitis. Splitting of categories into hybrids such as perivascular with interstitial dermatitis (1.65), perivascular and interface (1.64), perivascular with spongiotic (1.132), and perivascular with psoriasiform (1.119) is of limited practical help.

A. Perivascular dermatitis, superficial

Eczema (2.1)
Morbilliform eruptions (1.81, especially viral eruptions 14.7, and drug eruptions 3.5)
Purpura pigmentosa chronica (4.8)
Some erythemas (Chapter 3), especially erythema multiforme (3.2)

B. Perivascular dermatitis, superficial and deep

Arthropod assaults (15.7)
Erythemas (Chapter 3), especially gyrate erythemas such as erythema annulare centrifugum
Eythema chronicum migrans (12.14)
Lupus erythematosus (17.6, also periadnexal)
Polymorphous light eruption (17.5)
Syphilis, secondary (12.13)

1.110 Photodermatitis

(see also Face 1.44)
The following eruptions are aggravated by exposure to sunlight.

Actinic keratosis (18.8)
Actinic reticuloid (2.2)
Bloom's syndrome (11.10)
Chronic actinic dermatitis (2.2)
Cockayne's syndrome (11.10)
Darier's disease (11.3)
Dermatomyositis (17.7)
Hartnup's disease (2.1)
Herpes simplex (14.2)
Hydroa aestivale (17.5)
Hydroa vacciniforme (17.5)
Lupus erythematosus (17.6)
Pellagra (2.1)
Persistent light reactor (2.2)
Photocontact dermatitis (2.2)
Photodrug reaction (3.5)
Polymorphous light eruption (17.5)
Porphyrias (8.1)
Rothmund–Thomson syndrome (11.5)
Solar urticaria (3.1)
Sunburn (6.7)
Xeroderma pigmentosa (11.11)

1.111 Plasma cells

(see Fig. 1.111A,B)
Plasma cells have eccentric (pushed to one side), "clock-face" dotted nuclei, amphophilic (purplish) cytoplasm that stains somewhat with both the eosin and hematoxylin dyes, and a pale perinuclear Golgi zone known as a hof. Mast cells may resemble plasma cells, because they also have an amphophilic cytoplasm, but mast cells (1.78) have a more solid chromatin

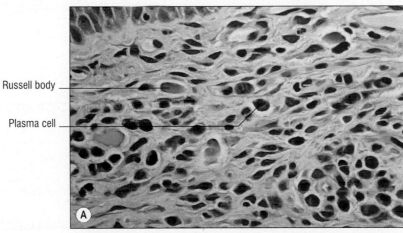

Russell body
Plasma cell

Fig. 1.111 **A** Plasma cells with Russell bodies.

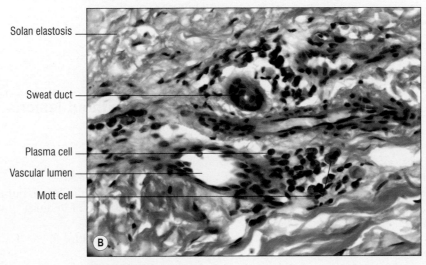

Solan elastosis
Sweat duct
Plasma cell
Vascular lumen
Mott cell

Fig. 1.111 **B** Mott cells.

pattern within a central nucleus, and sometimes the mast cell cytoplasm appears more granular, especially with stains such as Giemsa. There are three forms of "constipation" in very active plasma cells which may occur in any of the diseases on this list. *Russell bodies* are intensely eosinophilic unilocular PAS-positive bodies that form in the cytoplasm, particularly prevalent in rhinoscleroma, for example. *Mott cells* are plasma cells containing multilocular eosinophilic cytoplasmic inclusions resembling scybala or rabbit pellet stools. *Dutcher bodies* are eosinophilic inclusions in the nucleus, instead of the cytoplasm, mostly seen in blood smears.

A. Inflammatory diseases

Mucous membranes and skin near mucous membranes and the scalp will frequently contain numerous plasma cells, regardless of the pathologic process.

Amyloidosis (sometimes, 8.4)

Chronic folliculitis (acne, folliculitis decalvans, hidradenitis, etc.) (10.1 and 10.2)

Infectious diseases (especially syphilis, yaws, pinta, Lyme disease, rhinoscleroma, leishmaniasis, granuloma inguinale, chancroid, HIV virus, deep fungal infections)

Lupus erythematosus (sometimes a few plasma cells, 17.6)

Necrobiosis lipoidica (7.2)

Plasmacytosis mucosae, Zoon's balanitis, plasma cell vulvitis (2.11)

Rosai–Dorfman disease (7.17)

Scleroderma and morphea (sometimes) (9.3)

B. Neoplasms

Actinic keratosis, squamous cell carcinoma (18.8, 18.11)

Kaposi sarcoma (sparse plasma cells, 25.9)

Lymphocytoma cutis (24.14)

Lymphoma (especially B-cell, 24.10)

Plasmacytoma and multiple myeloma (24.12)

Syringocystadenoma papilliferum (23.3)

1.112 Poikiloderma

Poikiloderma is the combination of atrophy of the epidermis (1.9), telangiectasia (1.136), hyperpigmentation (1.18), and hypopigmentation (1.150), giving the skin a *mottled appearance*. If the skin has a red or discolored net-like appearance, also consider reticulated lesions (1.123).

Arsenic toxicity (18.9)

Bloom's syndrome (11.10)

Cockayne's syndrome (11.10)

Corticosteroid topical overuse

Dermatomyositis (17.7)

Dyskeratosis congenita (11.4)

Erythema ab igne (3.9)

Goltz syndrome (11.8)

Graft-versus-host disease (17.3)

Hereditary sclerosing poikiloderma

Kindler's syndrome (congenital poikiloderma and epidermolysis bullosa)

Lupus erythematosus (17.6)

Mycosis fungoides (24.1)

Photodamaged skin (*dermatoheliosis*) (9.1)

Poikiloderma atrophicans vasculare (24.1)

Poikiloderma congenitale (11.5)

Poikiloderma of Civatte (17.10)

Post-inflammatory pigmentary alteration (17.10)

Radiodermatitis (9.2)

Weary's syndrome (hereditary acrokeratotic poikiloderma)

Xeroderma pigmentosum (11.11)

1.113 Pregnancy rashes

Atopic eruption of pregnancy (formerly prurigo gestationis of Besnier) (3.6)

Folliculitis of pregnancy (10.2)

Impetigo herpetiformis (2.8)

Papular dermatitis of Spangler (questionable entity, 3.6)

Pemphigoid gestationis (6.3)

Perforating calcific elastosis (9.8)

Pruritic urticarial papules and plaques of pregnancy (PUPPP, 3.6)

Pruritus gravidarum (itch without rash, 1.75)

1.114 Pruritus with skin lesions

Pruritus is the most misspelled word in dermatology (it is –us, not an –itis, a suffix used for inflammation of anything). Any skin lesion can itch, but some of the itchiest are in this list.

Amyloidosis (macular and lichen types, 8.4)

Arthropod bites (15.7)

Contact dermatitis (2.2)

Delusions of parasitosis (Ekbom's syndrome) and Morgellon's disease (15.9)

Dermatitis herpetiformis (6.5)

Drug eruptions (3.5)

Eczema (2.1)

Exfoliative erythroderma (1.39)

Kyrle's disease (9.12)

Lichen planus (2.11)

Lichen sclerosus (9.5)

Lichen simplex chronicus and prurigo nodularis (2.3)

Mastocytosis (24.17)

Mycosis fungoides (24.1)

Pruritic urticarial papules and plaques of pregnancy (PUPPP, 3.6)

Pruritus ani

Scabies (15.9)

Urticaria (3.1)

Varicella (14.2)

1.115 Pruritus without lesions

AIDS (14.12)

Aquagenic pruritus

Brachioradial pruritus

Central nervous system disease

Diabetes mellitus (1.26, often listed, but probably not a real increased incidence of itching)

Drug allergy (3.5)

Hereditary localized pruritus

Hyperparathyroidism

Internal malignancy

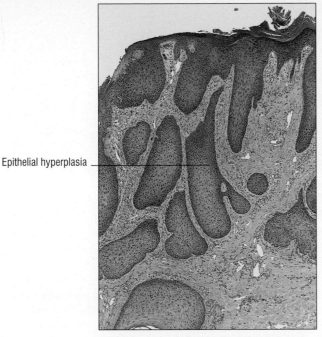

Fig. 1.116 A Pseudocarcinomatous hyperplasia.

Epithelial hyperplasia

Acanthosis

Blood vessel

Eosinophilic sweat duct

B

Fig. 1.116 B Sweat duct metaplasia producing a pseudocarcinomatous appearance.

Iron deficiency
Kidney disease
Liver disease
Myeloproliferative disorders (Chapter 24)
Neuropathy
Notalgia paresthetica
Occult xerosis (2.1)
Polycythemia rubra vera
Pruritus gravidarum
Psychological disorders
Scabies (15.9)
Systemic parasitosis
Thyroid disease (1.138)

1.116 Pseudoepitheliomatous (pseudocarcinomatous) hyperplasia

(PEH, see also Hyperplasia of epidermis 1.61)
(see Fig. 1.116A,B)
PEH is extreme epidermal proliferation that may simulate well-differentiated squamous cell carcinoma. It may be extremely difficult to distinguish from carcinoma, and is mainly differentiated by clinical findings or the discovery of some reason for its presence.
   Atypical mycobacterial infection (12.11)
   Borders of ulcers and healing wounds (particularly previous biopsy sites and areas of trauma, pyoderma gangrenosum, stasis ulcer, scrofuloderma, and granuloma inguinale)
   Chronic arthropod bite (15.7)
   Condyloma acuminatum (14.1)
   Deep fungal infections (Chapter 13)
   Granular cell tumor (26.4)
   Halogenoderma (3.5)
   Hypertrophic lichen planus (2.11)
   Keratoacanthoma (18.12)

Lichen simplex chronicus (2.1)
Orf and milker's nodule (14.5)
Pemphigus vegetans (5.4)
Prurigo nodularis (2.3)
Syringosquamous metaplasia (3.5)
Tuberculosis verrucosa cutis (12.10
Verrucous lupus erythematosus (17.6)

1.117 Pseudoepitheliomatous hyperplasia with intraepithelial microabscesses of neutrophils

Atypical mycobacterial infection (12.11)
Deep fungus infection (Chapter 13)
Halogenoderma (3.5)
Keratoacanthoma (18.12)
Pemphigus vegetans (5.4)
Pyoderma gangrenosum (4.12)
Pyoderma vegetans (4.12)
Tuberculosis verrucosa cutis (12.10)

1.118 Pseudomalignancies

Most of the following conditions are considered to be benign, but may simulate a malignancy. Others traditionally included in this list are now actually considered malignant some or all of the time (e.g., keratoacanthoma, proliferating trichilemmal cyst, lymphomatoid papulosis, and atypical fibroxanthoma)!
   Acral melanocytic nevus (20.5)
   Actinic reticuloid (24.1)
   Ancient melanocytic nevus (20.5)
   Angiolymphoid hyperplasia with eosinophilia (25.40)
   Bowenoid papulosis (18.10, behaves like condyloma acuminatum, but may be carcinoma in situ)
   Condyloma acuminatum after podophyllin treatment (14.1)

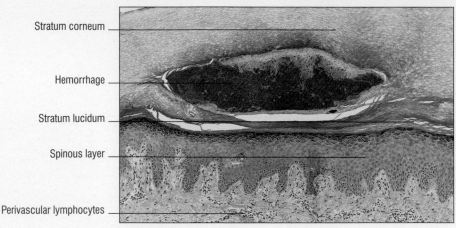

Fig. 1.120 Talon noir (black heel), hemorrhage in the stratum corneum from trauma.

Labels (from top to bottom): Stratum corneum, Hemorrhage, Stratum lucidum, Spinous layer, Perivascular lymphocytes

Diseases with pseudocarcinomatous hyperplasia (1.116)
Halo nevus (20.5)
Intravascular papillary endothelial hyperplasia (25.8)
Irritated seborrheic keratosis or verruca vulgaris (18.2 and 14.1)
Keratoacanthoma (18.12, most are probably squamous cell carcinoma)
Kikuchi's syndrome (14.8)
Lymphocytoma cutis (24.14)
Lymphomatoid papulosis (24.5, probably already is low-grade lymphoma with good prognosis)
Necrotizing sialometaplasia (17.11)
Nodular fasciitis (pseudosarcomatous fasciitis) (27.8)
Pigmented spindle cell nevus (20.6)
Pleomorphic fibroma (27.4)
Pleomorphic lipoma (29.2)
Proliferating trichilemmal cyst (22.4, some are actually squamous cell carcinoma)
Recurrent or irritated melanocytic nevus (20.5)
Spitz nevus (20.6)
Spongiotic simulants of mycosis fungoides (1.132)
Sweat gland neoplasms (Chapter 23, may simulate metastatic adenocarcinoma)
Targetoid hemosiderotic hemangioma (25.1)
Trichoepithelioma (22.2)

1.119 Psorlasiform hyperplasia

(see also Hyperplasia of epidermis 1.61)
These diseases usually have regular acanthosis resembling psoriasis. The rete ridges tend to be clubbed and about the same length, instead of irregular acanthosis with pointed rete ridges as in lichen simplex and in the majority of the diseases listed under Hyperplasia of epidermis. Parakeratosis is often confluent (1.104), and some of these conditions will also have neutrophils in the stratum corneum (1.88).
   Bowen's disease (18.10, not really hyperplasia, since it is squamous cell carcinoma in situ, look for atypia)
   Chronic eczema (2.1): often more irregular acanthosis
   Clear cell acanthoma (18.6)
   Mycosis fungoides (24.1): look for atypical epidermotropism

Pellagra, acrodermatitis enteropathica, and necrolytic migratory erythema may sometimes be somewhat psoriasiform (but rete ridges are usually not so elongated)
Pityriasis rubra pilaris (2.10)
Psoriasis and Reiter's syndrome (2.8): look for neutrophils in mounds
Secondary syphilis and pinta (12.13): look for plasma cells

1.120 Purpura

(clinical, see also Extravasated erythrocytes 1.40)
(see Fig. 1.120)
   Amyloidosis (8.4)
   Bacterial endocarditis (4.1)
   Coagulopathies (4.14)
   Coumarin necrosis (4.18)
   Cryoglobulinemia (4.9)
   Drug eruption (3.5)
   Gardner–Diamond syndrome
   Gonococcemia (12.18)
   Hematoma
   Henoch–Schoenlein purpura (4.1)
   Herpes zoster (14.2)
   Idiopathic thrombocytopenic purpura (4.14)
   Langerhans cell histiocytosis
   Meningococcemia (12.19)
   Mucha–Habermann disease (2.14)
   Plague (12.23)
   Purpura fulminans (disseminated intravascular coagulopathy (DIC), 4.14)
   Purpura pigmentosa chronica (4.8)
   Purpuric glove and sock syndrome (14.7)
   Relapsing fever (12.14)
   Rickettsial infections (14.13)
   Scurvy (4.17)
   Septic vasculitis (4.1)
   Solar purpura (4.15)
   Stasis dermatitis (2.1)
   Talon noir (black heel)
   Thrombocytopenia (4.14)

Trauma
Vascular neoplasms (Chapter 25)
Vasculitis (Chapter 4)
Waldenström's hyperglobulinemic purpura (4.9)

Pustules (see Neutrophils 1.89)

1.121 Red lesions (erythematous lesions)

Most inflammatory conditions are red; therefore, the list of possibilities for red lesions is too long to be very useful. For scaly red lesions, see Eczematous 1.29 and Papulosquamous 1.103. Erythemas without scale are found in Chapter 3. See Nodules 1.92, many of which are red. Many neoplasms are red, especially vascular ones. Malignancies are often red because of the inflammatory response. *Salmon red* (orange red) color is often seen with pityriasis rubra pilaris and mycosis fungoides.

1.122 Red papules, multiple

(see also Morbilliform 1.81)
  Acne (10.1)
  Arthropod bites (15.7)
  Drug eruptions (3.5)
  Eruptive xanthomas
  Erythema multiforme (3.2)
  Folliculitis (10.2)
  Gianotti–Crosti syndrome (14.11)
  Granuloma annulare (7.1)
  Guttate psoriasis (2.8)
  Lymphomatoid papulosis (24.5)
  Miliaria (10.6)
  Pityriasis lichenoides (2.14)
  Pityriasis rosea (2.4)
  Scabies (15.9)
  Urticaria (3.1)
  Viral exanthems (14.7)

1.123 Reticulated lesions

(see also Annular 1.5, Linear 1.73, Serpiginous 1.127, and Poikiloderma 1.112)
Reticulated lesions have a net-like pattern.
  Cholesterol emboli (4.16)
  Confluent and reticulated papillomatosis (18.5)
  Cutis marmarata (3.10)
  Dowling–Degos disease (reticulated anomaly of the flexures)
  Dyskeratosis congenita (11.4)
  Erythema ab igne (3.9)
  Erythema infectiosum (Fifth disease, 14.7)
  Lichen planus (2.11)
  Livedo reticularis (3.10)
  Livedoid vasculitis (4.13)
  Lupus erythematosus (17.6)
  Mycosis fungoides (24.1)
  Reticular erythematous mucinosis syndrome (8.13)

Scaling (see Eczematous, 1.29)

1.124 Scalp lesions

  Alopecia (1.4)
  Angiolymphoid hyperplasia with eosinophilia (25.4)

Angiosarcoma (25.7)
Aplasia cutis congenita (17.4)
Cicatricial pemphigoid (6.2)
Contact dermatitis (2.2)
Cylindroma (23.4)
Folliculitis (10.2)
Lupus erythematosus (17.6)
Melanocytic nevus (20.5)
Meningioma (26.6)
Metastatic neoplasm (Chapter 28)
Nevus sebaceus (21.2)
Pilar cyst (19.2)
Proliferating trichilemmal cyst (22.4)
Prurigo nodularis (2.3)
Psoriasis (2.8)
Seborrheic dermatitis (2.1)
Seborrheic keratosis (18.2)
Syringocystadenoma papilliferum (23.3)
Tinea capitis (13.1)

1.125 Scars, sclerosis, and fibrosis

The following diseases have induration, sometimes due to *sclerosis* (increased collagen with decreased numbers of fibroblasts), or *fibrosis* (increased collagen with increased numbers of fibroblasts). *Desmoplasia* or desmoplastic stroma is a densely collagenous stroma associated with a neoplasm.
  Acrodermatitis chronica atrophicans (12.14)
  Acrosclerosis
  Amyloidosis (8.4)
  Ataxia–telangiectasia (11.2)
  Carcinoma en cuirasse (28.3)
  Chemical exposure (polyvinyl chloride, etc.)
  Cockayne syndrome (11.10)
  Desmoplastic melanoma (20.11)
  Drugs (bleomycin, pentazocine, etc., 3.5)
  Eosinophilia–myalgia syndrome (3.5)
  Eosinophilic fasciitis (9.3)
  Fibrohistiocytic proliferations and neoplasms (Chapter 27)
  Foreign bodies and drug injection sites (7.6)
  Graft-versus-host disease (chronic, 17.3)
  Hurler's syndrome (8.14)
  Hypodermitis sclerodermiformis (lipodermatosclerosis, 16.9)
  Keloids (27.2)
  Lichen sclerosus (9.5)
  Lipodystrophy (16.11)
  Lymphedema
  Microcystic adnexal carcinoma (23.13)
  Morphea (9.3)
  Nephrogenic fibrosing dermopathy (8.19)
  Pachydermoperiostosis (9.7)
  Panniculitis (Chapter 16)
  Paraneoplastic syndrome (1.105)
  POEMS syndrome (24.12)
  Porphyria cutanea tarda and erythropoietic porphyria (8.1)
  Pretibial myxedema (8.7)
  Progeria (9.6)
  Radiodermatitis (9.2)
  Scar (27.2)

Scleredema (8.12)
Scleroderma (9.3)
Scleromyxedema (8.8)
Vibration exposure (jack hammer, chainsaw, etc.)

1.126 Scrotum lesions

Angiokeratoma of Fordyce (25.2)
Bowen's disease (18.10)
Calcinosis scroti (8.15)
Candidiasis (13.4)
Condyloma acuminatum (14.1)
Contact dermatitis (2.2)
Elephantiasis nostras
Epidermoid cyst (19.1)
Herpes simplex (14.2)
Leiomyoma (29.6)
Lichen simplex chronicus (2.3)
Paget's disease (18.13)
Pediculosis pubis (15.7)
Sclerosing lipogranuloma (7.6)

1.127 Serpiginous lesions

(see also Annular 1.5, Linear 1.73, Reticulated 1.123)
These lesions have a snake-like appearance.
Coelenterate stings (jellyfish, etc.)
Epidermal nevus (18.1)
Erythema gyratum repens (3.4)
Erythrokeratodermia variabilis (11.1)
Hypomelanosis of Ito (11.7)
Ichthyosis hystrix (11.1)
Incontinentia pigmenti, third stage (11.6)
Larval migrans (15.6)
Lupus erythematosus (subacute cutaneous, 17.6)

1.128 Single filing of cells

Single filing ("Indian filing", not politically correct) is the extension of single rows of cells between collagen bundles.
Congenital melanocytic nevus (20.5)
Glomus cell tumor (25.5)
Granuloma annulare (7.1)
Lymphoma and leukemia (24.10 and 24.16)
Metastatic carcinoma, especially breast (Chapter 28)
Pseudolymphoma (occasionally) (24.14)

1.129 Skin-colored papules or nodules

Skin-colored refers to the color of the patient's normal skin. The term "flesh-colored" is often used, but it is less accurate because the skin of darker races is technically not flesh in color, as in Caucasians.
Acrochordon (27.4)
Connective tissue nevus (27.6)
Neurofibroma (26.1)
Nevus, intradermal (20.5)
Subcutaneous nodules (1.135)
Syringoma (23.7)
Trichoepithelioma (22.2)
Verruca plana (14.1)

1.130 Small cell ("oat cell") neoplasms

Small cell tumors are made up of cells with uniform, round, dark vesicular nuclei and very little cytoplasm. They resemble basaloid tumor cells but are more rounded, less cohesive, and are unrelated to keratinocytes. Often, immunostaining (28.5), electron microscopy, or clinical information is needed to distinguish these.
Lymphoma or leukemia (Chapter 24)
Metastatic anaplastic carcinoma (Chapter 28)
Metastatic visceral neuroendocrine carcinoma, metastatic carcinoid (28.5)
Metastatic neuroblastoma, retinoblastoma, Ewing's sarcoma, and rhabdomyosarcoma (all usually in children, all very rare in skin, 28.5)
Metastatic small cell carcinoma of the lung (28.5)
Merkel cell carcinoma (26.7)
Metastatic small cell melanoma (20.11, rare)
Metastatic small cell (basaloid) eccrine carcinoma (23.13, very rare)

1.131 Spindle cell neoplasms

These are neoplasms made up of elongated spindled cells. The first three (fibrous, muscle, and nerve) create a common differential diagnostic problem. Immunostains may be needed. Vimentin will stain almost all of these (all mesenchymal neoplasms). Most examples of squamous cell carcinoma (an epithelial neoplasm) are vimentin negative, and cytokeratin cocktail positive, but spindle cell squamous cell carcinoma may stain with both vimentin and cytokeratin. Desmin, muscle-specific actin, and smooth muscle actin identify the smooth muscle neoplasms. S-100 protein stains the neural and melanocytic neoplasms. CD31, CD34, and Ulex stain most vascular neoplasms with proliferating endothelial cells (see Chapter 30).
Fibrous proliferations (most, Chapter 27)
Melanocytic neoplasms: blue nevus, spindle and epithelioid cell nevus, nevus of Ota, nevus of Ito, Mongolian spot, melanoma, desmoplastic nevus (Chapter 20)
Neural neoplasms (most, Chapter 26)
Smooth muscle neoplasms: leiomyoma, leiomyosarcoma (29.6 and 29.7)
Spindle cell lipoma (29.2)
Squamous cell carcinoma (sometimes, 18.11)
Vascular tumors: hemangiopericytoma (25.6) and Kaposi sarcoma (25.9)

1.132 Spongiosis

Spongiosis is mainly intercellular edema between keratinocytes in the epidermis. The edema may cause keratinocytes to become elongated and stretched, eventually producing spongiotic intraepidermal vesicles (1.147). Spongiosis is nearly always accompanied by exocytosis (migration into the epidermis) of lymphocytes, and sometimes of neutrophils or eosinophils. Spongiosis should not be confused with keratinocyte vacuolization by other mechanisms (1.144), acantholysis (1.2), or with Pautrier microabscess formation (24.1). Spongiosis is the hallmark of eczema, although it may not be present in all stages. It also commonly appears non-specifically in many rashes and irritated neoplasms.
Arthropod bites (15.7)
Contact dermatitis (2.2)

Eczema (2.1)
Eosinophilic spongiosis (1.36, eosinophils in epidermis with spongiosis)
Erythema multiforme (3.2)
Gianotti–Crosti syndrome (2.7)
Herpes gestationis (6.3)
Id reaction (2.1)
Irritated seborrheic keratosis (18.2)
Lichen striatus (2.5)
Miliaria (10.6)
Mucha–Habermann disease (2.14)
Pityriasis alba (2.6)
Pityriasis rosea (2.4)
Spongiform pustules (1.89, neutrophils in epidermis with spongiosis)
Tinea and candidiasis (13.1)

1.133 Sporotrichoid lesions

(lymphocutaneous syndrome, nodular lymphangitis, see also Linear lesions, 1.73)
Nodules appear in a linear pattern, often following the course of lymphatics. Sometimes the mnemonic SLANT has been used to remember them.
Sporotrichosis (13.11)
Leishmaniasis (15.1)
Atypical mycobacterial infection (12.11)
Nocardiosis (12.17)
Tularemia (12.6)
Furunculosis (12.1)

1.134 Squamous eddies, keratin pearls, and squamatization

A *squamous eddy* is a concentric whorled appearance of keratinocytes, showing gradually increasing keratinization towards the center. A *keratin* or *horn pearl* is similar, but the keratinization is more abrupt and complete in the center. Cornification is not as abrupt and complete as in a *horn cyst* (1.59), however. Keratohyaline granules are sparse or absent in squamous eddies or pearls but may be present in some horn cysts. *Dyskeratosis* (1.27), which exhibits brightly pink eosinophilia similar to the keratinization in a horn pearl, differs by involving single keratinocytes. *Squamatization* means that the epithelium is more eosinophilic than usual, because of more keratinization or dyskeratosis, and is usually also hyperplastic.
Discoid lupus erythematosus (17.6)
Diseases with pseudoepitheliomatous hyperplasia (1.116)
Hypertrophic lichen planus (2.11)
Irritated seborrheic keratosis (18.2)
Irritated verruca vulgaris (14.1)
Keratoacanthoma (18.12)
Other irritated epithelial tumors, occasionally (Chapter 18)
Proliferating trichilemmal cyst (22.4)
Squamous cell carcinoma (18.11)

1.135 Subcutaneous nodules

A. Neoplasms

Adnexal neoplasms (Chapters 22 and 23, especially pilomatricoma, hidradenoma, spiradenoma, and chondroid syringoma)
Cysts (Chapter 19)

Fibrous proliferations (Chapter 27, especially benign fibrous histiocytoma, malignant fibrous histiocytoma, nodular fasciitis)
Metastatic neoplasms (Chapter 28)
Miscellaneous neoplasms (Chapter 29, especially angioleiomyoma, *lipoma*, liposarcoma)
Neural neoplasms (Chapter 26, especially neurofibroma, neurilemmoma, malignant peripheral nerve sheath tumor)
Vascular neoplasms (Chapter 25, especially intravascular papillary endothelial hyperplasia, angiolymphoid hyperplasia with eosinophilia)

B. Granulomas

Foreign body granuloma (7.6)
Pheohyphomycosis and hyalohyphomycosis (13.17, 13.18)
Rheumatoid nodule (7.3)
Sarcoidosis (7.5)
Subcutaneous granuloma annulare (7.1)

C. Miscellaneous

Calcinosis cutis (8.15)
Gouty tophus (8.5)
Osteoma cutis (29.8)
Panniculitis (Chapter 16)

1.136 Telangiectasia

(see also Poikiloderma 1.112)
Angiokeratoma corporis diffuse (25.2)
Ataxia–telangiectasia (11.12)
Bloom's syndrome (11.10)
Carcinoid syndrome (28.5)
Corticosteroid overuse
CREST syndrome (9.3)
Dermatomyositis (17.7)
Dyskeratosis congenita (11.4)
Essential telangiectasia
Goltz syndrome (11.8)
Livedo reticularis (3.10)
Liver disease
Lupus erythematosus (17.6)
Osler–Weber–Rendu syndrome
Photodamaged skin (dermatoheliosis, 9.1)
Pregnancy or estrogen therapy
Radiodermatitis (9.2)
Rosacea (10.1)
Telangiectasia macularis eruptiva perstans (24.17)
Unilateral nevoid telangiectasia
Xeroderma pigmentosum (11.11)

1.137 Thrombi

Angiolipoma (29.2)
Coagulopathies (thrombotic thrombocytopenic purpura, disseminated intravascular coagulation, 4.14)
Degos disease (4.10)
Dysproteinemia (especially cryoglobulinemia and macroglobulinemia, 4.9)
Echthyma gangrenosum (12.20)

Emboli (4.16)
Intravascular lymphoma (24.13)
Lupus anticoagulant syndrome (7.6)
Opportunistic deep fungal infections (Chapter 13)
Thrombophlebitis (16.7)
Trousseau's syndrome (4.16)
Vascular neoplasms (Chapter 25)
Vasculitis (Chapter 4)
Warfarin-induced necrosis (4.18)

1.138 Thyroid disease and the skin

Alopecia areata (thyroiditis, 10.9)
Ascher's syndrome (thyroid, lip, eyelid enlargement, 7.7)
Cowden's disease (thyroid carcinoma, 22.5)
Erythema ab igne (hypothyroid, 3.9)
Multiple endocrine neoplasia type 2a (Sipple syndrome) (pruritic hyperpigmentation and hyperkeratosis of the back, pheochromocytoma, thyroid carcinoma)
Multiple endocrine neoplasia type 2b (mucosal neuromas, pheochromocytoma, thyroid carcinoma, 26.3)
Myxedema (pretibial type 8.7, Graves disease, or generalized hypothyroid myxedema 8.8)
Onychoschizia (nail splitting, thyroid disease in general)
Telogen effluvium (hyper- or hypothyroidism)
Vitiligo (thyroiditis, 17.2)

1.139 Tongue lesions

Amyloidosis (macroglossia, 8.4)
Aphthous ulcer (17.11)
Black hairy tongue
Candidiasis (13.4)
Condyloma acuminatum (14.1)
Fibroma (27.1)
Geographic tongue (2.8)
Granular cell tumor (26.4)
Hairy leukoplakia (14.8)
Hemangioma (25.1)
Kawasaki's syndrome (strawberry tongue, 14.10)
Leukoplakia, benign and premalignant (1.71)
Lichen planus (2.11)
Lingua plicata (scrotal tongue, Melkersson–Rosenthal syndrome, 7.7)
Median rhomboid glossitis (13.4)
Osler–Weber–Rendu syndrome Reiter's syndrome (2.8)
Scarlet fever (strawberry tongue, 12.2)
Squamous cell carcinoma (18.11)
Syphilis, secondary (mucous patch, 12.13)
Vitamin deficiencies

1.140 Transepidermal elimination (perforating diseases)

In this group of diseases, some substance (commonly elastic tissue, collagen, or foreign material) is being eliminated through the epidermis. Since this sometimes results in a channel through the epidermis, this group of diseases has been called the "perforating disorders". The first four diseases are the original members of this group, but perforating folliculitis might not vary sufficiently from any folliculitis in which the follicles have ruptured. Some authors have expanded the concept greatly and would add many more diseases to the partial list provided here.

Elastosis perforans serpiginosa (9.13)
Kyrle's disease (9.12)
Perforating folliculitis (10.3)
Reactive perforating collagenosis (9.14)
Perforating granuloma annulare (7.1) and necrobiosis lipoidica (7.2)
Perforating pseudoxanthoma elasticum (9.8)
Periumbilical perforating calcific elastosis (9.8)
Transepidermal elimination of foreign bodies or endogenous substances (gout, calcium, cartilage, etc.)

1.141 Trunk lesions

A. Common

Acne (10.1)
Basal cell carcinoma (18.14)
Drug eruption (3.5)
Dysplastic nevus (20.7)
Epidermoid cyst (19.1)
Hemangioma, cherry (25.1)
Herpes zoster (14.2)
Keloid (27.2)
Lipoma (29.2)
Melanocytic nevus (20.5)
Melanoma (20.11)
Morphea (9.3)
Pityriasis rosea (2.4)
Psoriasis (2.8)
Seborrheic keratosis (18.2)
Tinea corporis (13.1)
Tinea versicolor (13.2)
Varicella zoster (14.2)
Viral exanthems (14.7)

B. Uncommon

Atrophoderma (9.4)
Becker's nevus (20.3)
Confluent and reticulated papillomatosis (18.5)
Darier's disease (11.3)
Dermatofibrosarcoma protuberans (27.10)
Dermatomyositis (17.7)
Erythema ab igne (3.9)
Erythema annulare centrifugum (3.3)
Grover's disease (5.6)
Hypomelanosis of Ito (11.7)
Macular amyloidosis (8.4)
Mycosis fungoides (24.1)
Nevus of Ito (20.9)
Reticular erythematous mucinosis (8.13)
Scleredema (8.12)
Secondary syphilis (12.13)

1.142 Ulcers

A. Neoplasms

Angiosarcoma (25.7)
Atypical fibroxanthoma (27.12)
Basal cell carcinoma (18.14)

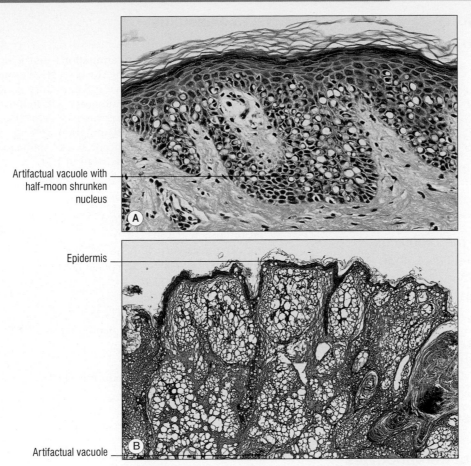

Artifactual vacuole with half-moon shrunken nucleus — A

Epidermis

Artifactual vacuole — B

Fig. 1.144 A Tissue processing artifact. **B** Freezing artifact.

Melanoma (20.11)
Metastatic neoplasm (Chapter 28)
Squamous cell carcinoma (18.11)

B. Vasculopathies

Atherosclerosis
Behçet's syndrome (4.11)
Buerger's disease (thromboangiitis obliterans, 4.19)
Cryoglobulinemia and other coagulopathies (4.9, 4.14)
Necrobiosis lipoidica (7.2)
Pressure ulcer (decubitus, 6.8)
Pyoderma gangrenosum (4.12)
Raynaud's disease
Sickle cell disease
Stasis (2.1)

C. Infections

Actinomycosis (12.16)
Amebiasis (15.13)
Anthrax (12.4)
Atypical mycobacterial infection (12.11)
Chancroid (12.7)
Deep fungus infections (Chapter 13)
Ecthyma (*Staphylococcus*, *Streptococcus*, 12.1)

Ecthyma gangrenosum (12.20)
Granuloma inguinale (12.8)
Herpes simplex (14.2)
Leishmaniasis (15.1)
Mycetoma (13.14)
Nocardiosis (12.17)
Scrofuloderma (12.10)
Syphilis (12.13)
Tularemia (12.6)

D. Neurological conditions

Neurotrophic ulcer
Notalgia paresthetica

E. Miscellaneous

Aphthous ulcers (17.11)
Aplasia cutis congenita (17.4)
Bites (15.7)
Burns, cold injury (6.7)
Panniculitis (Chapter 16)
Post-bullous disease (1.147)
Radiodermatitis (9.2)
Scleroderma and morphea (9.3)
Trauma, factitial

1.143 Umbilicus lesions

(see also Trunk lesions 1.141)

A. Solitary lesions

Endometriosis (29.9)
Fibrous umbilical polyp
Metastatic adenocarcinoma (Sister Mary Joseph nodule, 28.2)
Omphalomesenteric duct remnant (29.11)
Pyogenic granuloma (25.3)
Umbilical hernia

B. Eruptions that favor the umbilicus

Chronic bullous disease of childhood (6.4)
Pemphigoid gestationis (6.3)
Perforating calcific elastosis (9.8)
Psoriasis (2.8)
Scabies (15.9)
Seborrheic dermatitis (2.1)
Typhoid fever rose spots (12.2)
Vitiligo (17.2)

Vacuolar alteration (see Interface dermatitis, 1.64)

1.144 Vacuolization of keratinocytes

(see Fig. 1.144)

Intracellular or extracellular clear spaces may cause keratinocytes to appear vacuolated. This should not be confused with *pagetoid cells* (1.37), or *spongiosis* (1.132, which is mostly intercellular edema between keratinocytes). Liquefaction degeneration of the basal layer is discussed in Section 1.64. See also *clear cell neoplasms* (1.22) and pale epidermis (1.99).

Tissue processing artifact: this is by far the most common cause of vacuoles within keratinocytes, causing the nucleus to shrink away from the cytoplasm.
Freezing artifact
Radiodermatitis (9.2)
Epidermolytic hyperkeratosis (11.1)
Mucous membranes usually have a vacuolated appearance.
Papillomavirus infection (14.1) vacuolization (koilocytosis) occurs around the pyknotic (raisin-like) nuclei in the upper spinous layer, often in association with hypergranulosis
Other viral infections (Chapter 14), especially orf and milker's nodule, may occasionally have keratinocyte vacuolization, but usually it is not as prominent as in papillomavirus infections. Keratinocytes in herpes virus infections, for example, are more likely to be ballooned (enlarged with a pale nucleus and pale cytoplasm) rather than vacuolated
Bowen's disease, arsenical keratosis, and squamous cell carcinoma (Chapter 18) occasionally have keratinocyte vacuoles in addition to dysplasia and dyskeratosis
Refsum's disease (11.1)

1.145 Vasculitis

(see Chapter 4)

Vasculitis literally means inflammation (-itis) of blood vessels, so the term is sometimes subject to excessive usage. It should be reserved for those reactive inflammatory conditions that have necrosis, fibrin, or inflammatory cells in the vessel walls. The terms *perivasculitis* or *perivascular dermatitis* (1.109) are used for more common inflammation around vessel walls that does not induce significant vessel damage. Causes of granulomatous vasculitis are listed in 1.51.

1.146 Verrucous lesions

(see also Papillomatosis 1.102)

Acanthosis nigricans (18.5)
Acrokeratosis verruciformis (18.3)
Angiokeratoma circumscriptum (25.2)
Chromomycosis (13.10)
Coccidioidomycosis (13.6)
Condyloma acuminatum (14.1)
Confluent and reticulated papillomatosis (18.5)
Darier's disease (11.3)
Epidermal nevus (18.1)
Epidermodysplasia verruciformis (14.1)
Halogenoderma (3.5)
Ichthyosis (11.1)
Incontinentia pigmenti (second stage, 11.6)
Kyrle's disease (9.12)
Lichen amyloidosus (8.4)
Lichen simplex chronicus and prurigo nodularis (2.3)
Lichen striatus (2.5)
Lipoid proteinosis (8.3)
Lymphangioma circumscriptum
Nevus sebaceus (21.2)
North American blastomycosis (13.8)
Papulosquamous diseases (1.103)
Porokeratosis (18.4)
Scabies, crusted "Norwegian" (15.9)
Sebaceous adenoma (21.3)
Seborrheic keratosis (18.2)
Syringocystadenoma papilliferum (23.3)
Tuberculosis verrucosa cutis (12.10)
Verruca vulgaris (14.1)
Verrucous carcinoma (18.11)
Warty dyskeratoma (18.7)

1.147 Vesicles and bullae

Most vesiculobullous diseases appear in Chapters 5 and 6, but lists are given here because some diseases that primarily appear in other chapters can also produce blisters. Some blistering disorders that are primarily intraepidermal may also produce subepidermal blisters, usually because of papillary dermal edema. Some subepidermal vesicular diseases may also have intraepidermal blisters. Subepidermal blisters may re-epithelialize, giving the false impression of an intraepidermal blister. Clues to this problem include the combination of intraepidermal and subepidermal vesicles, a smooth straight-line base of an "intraepidermal blister", necrosis of the epidermis or neutrophils suggesting an older blister, and evidence of the formation of new migrating epithelium above adnexal structures. *Immunofluorescence* studies looking for autoantibody and complement deposition may be required for definitive diagnosis.[67,70]

A. Subcorneal vesicles (see also Neutrophils pertaining to pustules 1.89)

Bullous impetigo (12.2)
Erythema toxicum neonatorum (5.3)
Friction blister (5.7)
Miliaria crystallina (10.6)
Pemphigus foliaceus and erythematosus (5.4)
Staphylococcal scalded skin syndrome (12.2)

B. Intraepidermal vesicles due to epidermal degeneration

Epidermolytic hyperkeratosis (11.1)
Friction blister (5.7)

C. Intraepidermal spongiotic vesicles (see also Spongiosis 1.132, Eosinophilic spongiosis 1.36)

Arthropod bites (15.7)
Contact dermatitis (2.2)
Eczema (2.1)

D. Intraepidermal vesicles due to ballooning degeneration

Herpes simplex (14.2)
Herpes zoster and varicella (14.2)

E. Intraepidermal acantholytic vesicles (see also Acantholysis 1.2)

Darier's disease (11.3)
Grover's disease (5.6)
Hailey–Hailey disease (5.5)
Herpes virus infection (14.2)
Pemphigus (5.4)

F. Subepidermal cell-poor vesicles

Bullosis diabeticorum (6.9)
Bullous amyloidosis (8.4)
Cell-poor pemphigoid (6.1)
Epidermolysis bullosa (6.6)
Ischemic bullae (6.8)
Porphyria cutanea tarda (8.1)
Pseudoporphyria (8.1)
Scar with blister artifact (27.2)

G. Subepidermal vesicles with neutrophils dominant

Bullous lupus erythematosus (17.6)
Dermatitis herpetiformis (6.5)
Epidermolysis bullosa acquisita, uncommonly
Linear IgA bullous dermatosis (6.4)
Pemphigoid, sometimes (6.1)
Pustular vasculitis (4.1)

Sweet's syndrome (3.7) and *Neutrophilic dermatosis group* (1.89)

H. Subepidermal vesicles with eosinophils dominant

Bullous pemphigoid (6.1)

I. Subepidermal vesicles with lymphocytes mostly

Erythema multiforme (3.2)
Fixed drug eruption (3.5)

J. Vesicles with a hemorrhagic or purpuric appearance

Bullous amyloidosis (8.4)
Disseminated intravascular coagulation (4.14)
Gonococcemia (12.18)
Herpes virus infection (14.2)
Meningococcemia (12.19)
Mucha–Habermann disease (2.14)

K. "Secondarily blistering" diseases (not usually considered to be primary blistering diseases)

Amyloidosis (8.4)
Artifactual blisters over scars
Burns (6.7)
Fixed drug eruption (3.5)
Graft-versus-host disease (17.3)
Lichen planus (2.11)
Lichen sclerosus (9.5)
Mastocytosis (24.17)
Polymorphous light eruption (17.5)
Scabies (15.9)

1.148 Violaceous (purplish) lesions

Chilblains (3.12)
Drug eruptions (3.5)
Hansen's disease (12.12)
Kaposi sarcoma (25.9)
Kaposiform hemangioendothelioma (25.1)
Leukemia cutis, especially myelogenous (24.16)
Lichen planus (2.11)
Lymphoma cutis (24.10)
Lymphomatoid papulosis (24.5)
Morphea (9.3)
Pityriasis lichenoides (2.14)
Purpura (1.120)
Pyoderma gangrenosum (3.7)
Sweet's syndrome (3.7)
Vasculitis (Chapter 4)

1.149 Vulva lesions

Behçet's disease (4.11)
Bowenoid papulosis and Bowen's disease (18.10)
Candidiasis (13.4)

Condyloma acuminatum (14.1)
Contact dermatitis (2.2)
Cysts, Bartholin and others (Chapter 19)
Granuloma inguinale (1.108)
Herpes simplex (14.2)
Hidradenoma papilliferum (23.2)
Lentigo simplex (20.3)
Lichen sclerosus (9.5)
Lichen simplex chronicus (2.3)
Paget's disease (18.13)
Plasma cell vulvitis (2.11)
Pruritic vulvar squamous papillomatosis (14.1)
Psoriasis (2.8)
Syphilis (primary chancre, condyloma lata, 12.13)
Vulvar intraepithelial neoplasia (VIN, 18.10)
Vulvodynia

1.150 White lesions (hypopigmentation, hypomelanosis)

Albinism (11.9)
Chediak–Higashi syndrome
Chemicals (hydroquinone, phenol, etc.)
Cysts (Chapter 19)
Halo nevus (20.5)
Hypomelanosis of Ito (11.7)
Idiopathic guttate hypomelanosis (17.10)
Incontinentia pigmenti (11.6)
Keratosis alba (stucco keratosis, 18.2)
Leprosy (12.12)
Lichen sclerosus (9.5)
Lupus erythematosus, discoid (17.6)
Maceration (hydrated keratin and degenerated soft tissue)
Molluscum contagiosum (14.4)
Morphea and scleroderma (9.3)
Nevus anemicus (17.10)
Nevus depigmentosus (17.10)
Piebaldism (11.9)
Pinta (12.13)

Pityriasis alba (2.6)
Post-inflammatory hypopigmentation (17.10)
Scars, sclerosis, fibrosis (1.125)
Tinea versicolor (13.2)
Tuberous sclerosis (ash leaf macules, 27.3)
Vitiligo (17.2)

1.151 Yellow lesions

(see also White lesions 1.150)

Amyloidosis (8.4)
Calcinosis cutis (usually more white, 8.15)
Carotenemia
Colloid milium (8.2)
Cysts (Chapter 19)
Drugs (quinacrine, canthaxanthin suntan pill, etc., 3.5)
Erythema elevatum diutinum (4.3)
Foam cells in lesions (1.46)
Goltz syndrome (11.8)
Gouty tophus (8.5)
Jaundice from liver disease (1.75)
Juvenile xanthogranuloma (7.10)
Langerhans cell histiocytosis (24.18)
Lichen myxedematosus (8.8)
Lipoid proteinosis (8.3)
Lycopenemia (dietary tomatoes, etc.)
Necrobiosis lipoidica (7.2)
Necrobiotic xanthogranuloma (7.11)
Pseudoxanthoma elasticum (9.8)
Radiodermatitis (9.2)
Sebaceous gland neoplasms (Chapter 21)
Seborrheic keratosis (18.2)
Solar elastosis (9.1)
Tattoo (especially cadmium, 7.6)
Topical substances (tobacco, dihydroxyacetone sunless tanning lotion, chemicals)
Xanthomas (7.9)

CHAPTER 2

Eczematous and Papulosquamous Diseases

Chapter Contents

The diseases in this chapter have dominant epidermal changes (clinical scaling, pathologic changes of spongiosis and parakeratosis), as opposed to rashes in Chapters 3 and 4, which primarily have dermal changes. It has been said by Levine that the diseases in this chapter are "outside jobs", heavily influenced by external factors or contactants. Those in Chapters 3 and 4 are "inside jobs" more heavily influenced by internal antigens. This is an interesting way to think of it, though obviously is oversimplified.

2.1 Eczema (eczematous dermatitis)

(see Fig. 2.1A–G)

The term "eczema" has been criticized as being confusing,[52] and difficult to define, but it is generally used by dermatologists to refer to a group of diseases characterized by diffuse, *ill-defined scaling* in their chronic stages, with spongiosis as an important feature histologically. Papulosquamous diseases (1.103) also have prominent scaling, but lesions are more sharply demarcated and more elevated. There is some overlap between the two groups. Clinicians often use the term "dermatitis" as a synonym for eczema, while others use it as a non-specific term for any inflammatory skin condition (-itis means inflammation of). Patients with eczema often have pruritus (1.114).

The histologic hallmark of eczema is spongiosis (1.9). Eczema in Greek means "to boil over", referring to the small *intraepidermal vesicles* that may occur in eczematous conditions if there is enough spongiosis (intercellular edema). As eczema becomes more chronic, there is a tendency for it to become more acanthotic and less spongiotic. The antiquated terms *"acute dermatitis"* (intraepidermal spongiotic vesicle), *"chronic dermatitis"* (more acanthosis and less spongiosis), and *"subacute dermatitis"* (pathology in between acute and chronic) are best forgotten. In general, eczematous diseases are distinguished clinically rather than histologically, although a few minor helpful features are listed below.

Variations

1. Atopic eczema: *onset in children* after 3 months of age (more likely to be seborrheic dermatitis prior to that age), *extremities*, especially antecubital and popliteal, less involvement of the trunk, prominent on the *face in infants* (1.44), tends to resolve by adulthood in most cases, associated with *asthma* or *allergic rhinitis, inhalant* and *food allergies*, often positive scratch tests or RAST tests, elevated serum IgE, no consistent distinguishing histologic features. Atopic means "out of place", because the rash on the skin is out of place from the allergens that are primarily inhaled or consumed, rather than true allergy to substances in contact with the skin. Compare with contact dermatitis (2.2).

2. Xerotic eczema (dry skin, xerosis, asteatotic eczema, eczema craquele): no consistent distinguishing features.

3. Seborrheic dermatitis: *dandruff, greasy scale of the scalp* (1.124), *eyebrows* (1.42), *eyelids* (1.43), *paranasal folds*, axilla (1.10), or chest (and diaper area in infants), sometimes related to normal flora *Malassezia globosa* yeast overgrowth, sometimes associated with neurologic disorders or HIV virus infection (14.12), no distinguishing histologic features except that it is often more psoriasiform (1.118), but with more spongiosis than is usual for psoriasis (2.8). Lesions with overlapping features of psoriasis are sometimes called *sebopsoriasis*.

- *Focal parakeratosis*, sometimes with crusting (1.104)
- Neutrophils in the stratum corneum if secondarily impetiginized (1.89)
- Acanthosis or hyperkeratosis sometimes (1.61, more if clinically chronic)
- *Spongiosis*, sometimes spongiotic vesicles (more if clinically acute)
- Superficial perivascular lymphocytes (1.109), occasional eosinophils

P

©2012 Elsevier Ltd, Inc, BV
DOI: 10.1016/B978-0-323-06658-7.00002-6

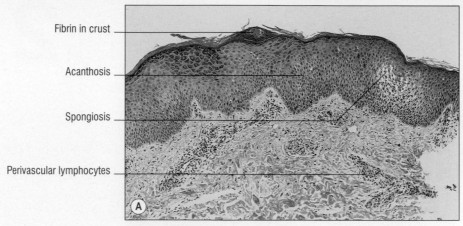

Fibrin in crust

Acanthosis

Spongiosis

Perivascular lymphocytes

Fig. 2.1 A Eczema (low power).

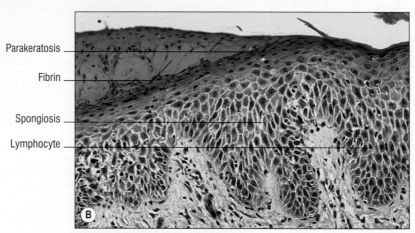

Parakeratosis

Fibrin

Spongiosis

Lymphocyte

Fig. 2.1 B Eczema (medium power).

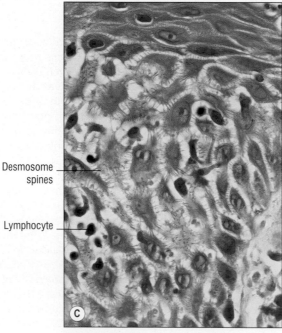

Desmosome spines

Lymphocyte

Fig. 2.1 C Eczema (high-power view of spongiosis).

4. Stasis dermatitis: located on the *lower legs* (1.67), related to vascular stasis and venous valvular dysfunction, often more pigmented clinically (1.18), prone to develop stasis ulcers (1.142), more dilated *papillary dermal small blood vessels* and more *hemosiderin* (1.58); more fibrosis or sclerosing panniculitis in older lesions (16.9).

5. Acroangiodermatitis (pseudo-Kaposi sarcoma): variant of stasis dermatitis in which vascular proliferation is exuberant enough to be impressive clinically, sometimes resembling Kaposi sarcoma histologically (25.9).

6. Contact dermatitis: often included in the eczema group, and is discussed in more detail under 2.2.

7. Dyshidrotic eczema: scaling and microvesicles appear on the *hands, fingers* (1.56), toes, and acral skin (so named because "abnormal sweating" was previously thought to be related), often with "*tapioca-pudding*" *grouped vesicles*, more likely to show spongiosis and vesicles.

8. Id reaction: papules or spongiotic vesicles (often like dyshidrosis) erupt in a remote site such as the palms as a resulting reaction to a predominant rash elsewhere, such as tinea pedis (poorly understood, poorly documented, immunologic phenomenon).

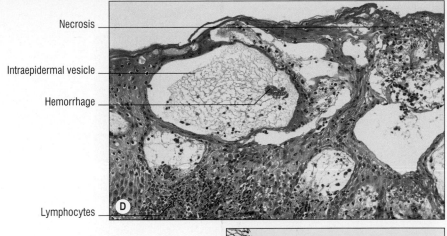

Necrosis

Intraepidermal vesicle

Hemorrhage

Lymphocytes

Fig. 2.1 D Vesicular eczema. Intraepidermal vesiculation or so-called reticular degeneration from severe spongiosis.

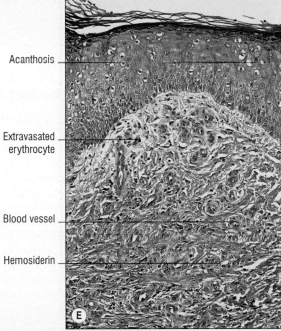

Acanthosis

Extravasated erythrocyte

Blood vessel

Hemosiderin

Fig. 2.1 E Stasis dermatitis.

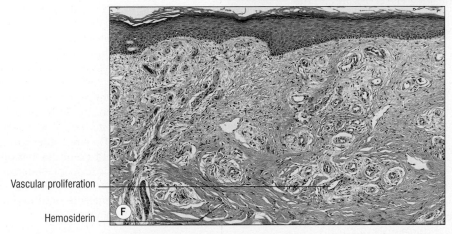

Vascular proliferation

Hemosiderin

Fig. 2.1 F Acroangiodermatitis.

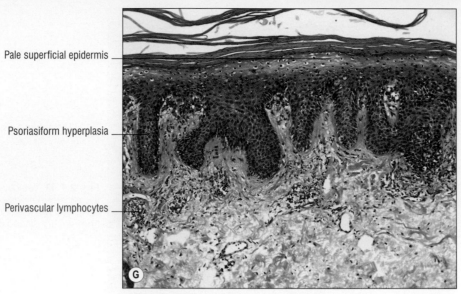

Pale superficial epidermis

Psoriasiform hyperplasia

Perivascular lymphocytes

Fig. 2.1 G Pellagra.

9. Papular eczema, follicular eczema: clinical terms for eczema that presents as tiny papules, resembling folliculitis (1.47), more common in pigmented races.
10. Neurodermatitis: this is a poor clinical term used when "neurosis" is thought to play a prominent role, excoriations often prominent, primary unmanipulated lesions usually not found, no distinguishing histologic features.
11. Nummular eczema: clinical term for rounded or annular (1.5) *coin-shaped* plaques (from same stem word as for numismatists, coin collectors), mostly on extremities, often with more crusting and spongiosis.
12. Wiscott–Aldrich syndrome, Omenn syndrome, and some other immunodeficiencies: often have clinical eczematous lesions and similar histology.
13. Vitamin deficiencies and metabolic disorders such as phenylketonuria, zinc deficiency (17.1), essential fatty acid deficiency, pellagra, Hartnup's disease, biotin deficiency: may present with scaly, red skin like eczema, and have similar histology, but some may have more psoriasiform hyperplasia (1.119) or pale epidermis (1.99).
14. Keratolysis exfoliativa: a variant of palm and sole eczema (1.99) which has a peculiar advancing edge of peeling stratum corneum with central clearing, which patients cannot resist pulling off, and with relatively little or no erythema or inflammation.

Differential diagnosis

1. Tinea (13.1): KOH prep, PAS stain, or culture positive.
2. Other eczematous diseases (1.29), papulosquamous diseases (1.103), and contact dermatitis (2.2).
3. Other spongiotic diseases (1.132), intraepidermal vesicular diseases (1.147), and perivascular dermatitis (1.109).
4. Langerhans microabscesses (pseudo-Pautrier microabscesses, monocyte microabscesses) occur commonly in the epidermis in eczema and contact dermatitis, positive for CD1a or CD68, and can be confused with mycosis fungoides (24.1) and Langerhans cell histiocytosis (24.18).[115]

2.2 Contact dermatitis

Contact dermatitis is defined as a reaction to topical substances, and can be subdivided into *irritant* or *true allergic* (primarily type IV delayed hypersensitivity). It should not be confused with atopic dermatitis (2.1), which is a more systemic allergic problem. Common contactant allergens include neomycin, fragrance, preservatives in creams, rubber, nickel, formaldehyde, plants such as poison ivy, and many others. A careful history and allergy patch tests may be clinically useful to determine the cause. *Juvenile plantar dermatosis* is irritant contact dermatitis of the feet, often thought to be due to irritant contact dermatitis from moisture or occlusion by sweaty tennis shoes. *Diaper dermatitis* is usually an irritant contact dermatitis from feces and urine, but sometimes is due to *Candida*. *Intertrigo* is a term used for dermatitis in intertriginous areas such as the axilla (1.10) or groin (1.55) that is mostly an irritant contact dermatitis to excessive moisture and friction, but some cases can be due to candidiasis (13.4) or erythrasma (12.5). *Angular cheilitis* (*perleche*) is sort of an intertrigo of the angles of the mouth, which is often associated with redundant folds that retain moisture, or poorly fitting dentures. *Chronic actinic dermatitis* (*persistent light reactor*) represents a persistent photocontact dermatitis. After chronic antigenic stimulation, the inflammation can become atypical, developing into *actinic reticuloid*, resembling cutaneous T-cell lymphoma (24.1), since the suffix -oid means resembling reticulosis (an old name for lymphoma). Histology and differential diagnosis for contact dermatitis is similar to eczema (2.1). Severe contact dermatitis and *phytophotodermatitis* (plant allergy in the presence of ultraviolet light, 1.110) may cause necrotic keratinocytes (1.86).

2.3 Lichen simplex chronicus and prurigo nodularis

(see Fig. 2.3A–D)
Lichen simplex chronicus (LSC) is a scaly, erythematous plaque that represents lichenified (thickened) skin due to simple chronic rubbing or irritation. It is lichenoid clinically, not histologically (1.72). Prurigo nodularis (picker's nodule) is the same basic process, except that it is a localized nodule

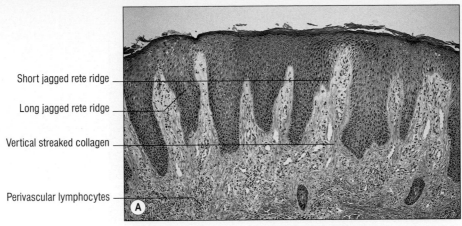

Short jagged rete ridge

Long jagged rete ridge

Vertical streaked collagen

Perivascular lymphocytes

Fig. 2.3 A Lichen simplex chronicus (low mag.).

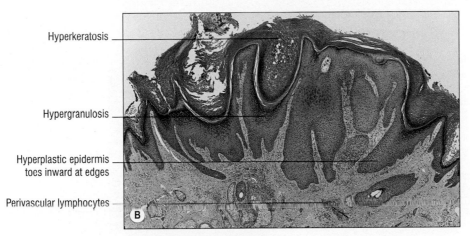

Hyperkeratosis

Hypergranulosis

Hyperplastic epidermis toes inward at edges

Perivascular lymphocytes

Fig. 2.3 B Prurigo nodularis.

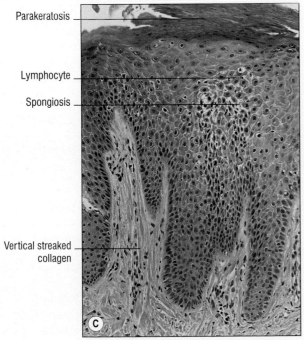

Parakeratosis

Lymphocyte

Spongiosis

Vertical streaked collagen

Fig. 2.3 C Lichen simplex chronicus (high mag.).

instead of a plaque. When many smaller papules are present, the less frequently used designation is prurigo simplex. In all of these patients, excoriations may be prominent also. Both conditions are end-stage lesions that usually start out as some kind of eczema, neurodermatitis, arthropod bite, folliculitis, or some other nuisance that causes the patient to pick or scratch an area of pruritus (1.113).

- Hyperkeratosis with focal parakeratosis (1.104)
- Hypergranulosis (1.60)
- Impressive *irregular acanthosis*
- *Vertical orientation of collagen in dermal papillae*
- Perivascular lymphocytic infiltrate (1.109)
- Prominent fibroblasts sometimes, occasionally multinucleated fibroblasts are seen (Montgomery giant cells) but they may also be seen in any chronic disorder
- Enlarged nerves, occasionally, according to some authorities

P

Variations

1. Corn or callus: compact hyperkeratosis and acanthosis.
2. Frictional lichenoid dermatitis: papules or plaques of the *elbows or knees* from chronic friction. Lymphocytes

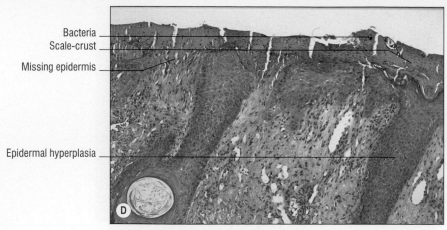

Fig. 2.3 D Trigeminal trophic syndrome. The surface of the epidermis is excoriated and there is epidermal hyperplasia from constant prurigo.

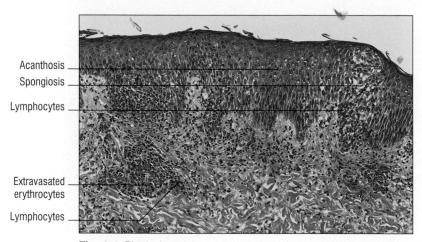

Fig. 2.4 Pityriasis rosea.

more perivascular than lichenoid (it is lichenoid clinically, 1.72).
3. Acanthoma fissuratum ("granuloma" fissuratum): epidermal hyperplasia from chronic rubbing of spectacles on nose or post-auricular areas.

Differential diagnosis

1. Other papulosquamous diseases (1.103) with hyperplasia of epidermis (1.61) or pseudoepitheliomatous hyperplasia (1.116).
2. Psoriasis (2.8): genetic inheritance, characteristic distribution of lesions, sharper clinical lesion demarcation, confluent (not focal) parakeratosis with neutrophils in mounds in stratum corneum, regular clubbed rete ridges that are not as pointed, no vertical orientation of collagen in dermal papillae unless chronically rubbed.
3. Look for the primary lesions or conditions mentioned above, especially itchy ones (1.114).

2.4 Pityriasis rosea (PR)

(see Fig. 2.4)

Common, *papulosquamous*, sometimes papulovesicular, sometimes pruritic (1.114), viral infection (possibly due to herpes virus type 7) of *older children and young adults*, beginning with initial larger lesion (the *herald patch*), often *annular* (1.5) and *resembles tinea*, often *oval-shaped* plaques in a "Christmas tree" distribution on the *trunk* (1.141), skin lesions resolve in 6 weeks.

- Focal parakeratosis (1.104)
- Mild acanthosis sometimes (1.61)
- *Spongiosis* (1.132); rarely spongiotic vesicles (1.147)
- *Perivascular lymphocytes*; rarely eosinophils (1.36)
- Dyskeratosis sometimes (1.27)
- Focal extravasated red blood cells sometimes (1.40)

Differential diagnosis

Mostly is a clinical diagnosis. Not biopsied except in unusual cases.

1. Eczematous diseases (1.29), papulosquamous diseases (1.103).
2. Other diseases with spongiosis (1.132) or perivascular dermatitis (1.109).
3. Secondary syphilis (12.13): positive serology.
4. Parapsoriasis (2.9): persists, does not resolve in 6 weeks.
5. Tinea (13.1): KOH prep, PAS stain, or culture positive.
6. PR-like rashes occur with some drugs (3.5) and with some forms of epidermodysplasia verruciformis (14.1).

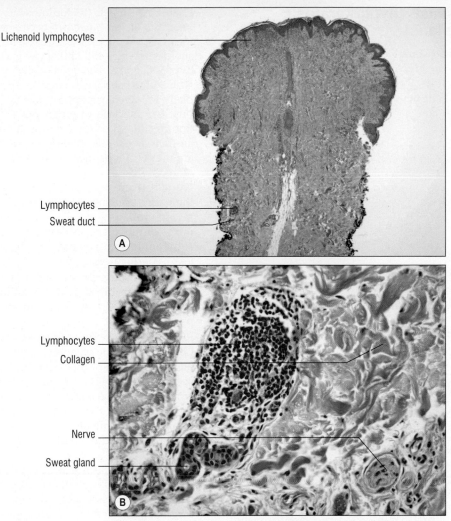

Fig. 2.5 A Lichen striatus (low mag.). **B** Lichen striatus (high mag.).

2.5 Lichen striatus

(see Fig. 2.5)

Uncommon, *linear scaly plaque* (1.73), sometimes hypopigmented (1.150), usually on one *extremity of children*, resolves in months to years.

P
- Focal parakeratosis (1.104)
- Mild acanthosis, sometimes psoriasiform (1.119)
- *Spongiosis*
- *Dyskeratotic keratinocytes* sometimes
- Focal basal layer liquefaction sometimes (1.64)
- *Perivascular* (1.109) or *lichenoid lymphocytes*, often with inflammation around follicles and especially around sweat ducts (*syringocentricity*)

Differential diagnosis

1. "Eczema" (2.1) and other spongiotic diseases (1.132): rarely linear.
2. Other diseases with dyskeratotic keratinocytes (1.27): rarely linear.
3. Of other lichenoid diseases (1.72), linear lichen planus might be most difficult to distinguish (2.11) unless there are multiple other lesions.
4. Epidermal nevus (18.1): also linear, more likely to be congenital, persists indefinitely, more papillomatosis and acanthosis, less spongiosis or dyskeratosis unless irritated.

2.6 Pityriasis alba

Common, *ill defined, scaly patches with hypopigmentation* (1.150), mostly on the face and upper extremities of *children*, often atopic diathesis (2.1).

- Focal parakeratosis (1.104)
- Focal spongiosis
- Perivascular lymphocytes (1.109)

Differential diagnosis

Mostly a clinical diagnosis. Seldom biopsied.
1. Other spongiotic diseases (1.132).
2. Hypopigmented diseases (1.150), especially vitiligo (17.2), tinea versicolor (13.2), and post-inflammatory hypopigmentation (17.10).

2.7 Flegel's disease (hyperkeratosis lenticularis perstans)

Very rare, possibly autosomal dominant, *small disc-like red hyperkeratotic papules* mostly on the *palms, soles, hands, feet, legs,* and *forearms* in adults. Its exact status as a specific entity has been questioned. Well-developed lesions have the following characteristic findings.

- Localized hyperkeratotic mound with parakeratosis (1.104)
- Hypogranulosis (1.63)
- Atrophy of the spinous layer (1.9)
- Lichenoid lymphocytes

Differential diagnosis

1. Perforating disorders, such as Kyrle's disease (9.12), also have localized hyperkeratotic papules, but there is transepidermal elimination, does not involve the palm and sole.
2. Disseminated actinic porokeratosis (18.4): common on the legs, more annular, cornoid lamella.
3. Stucco keratosis (18.2): common on the legs, but has church spire papillomatosis, not red, never on the palm or sole, no inflammation unless irritated.
4. Other lichenoid disorders (1.72).

2.8 Psoriasis

(see Fig. 2.8)

Familial disease in 1–3% of the population. *Papulosquamous* plaques (1.103) that are *sharply demarcated* with *thick silvery scale*, most common on scalp (1.124), trunk (1.141), buttock, elbows (1.32), knees. Least common on the face, probably because ultraviolet light improves the disease. May be annular (1.5). *Nail dystrophy* (1.85): pits, onycholysis, onychauxis. Psoriatic *arthritis* (1.7) in one-third of patients. Pruritus in one-third of patients (1.114).

- *Confluent parakeratosis* (not focal) (1.104), hyperkeratosis (1.61)
- *Neutrophils* in stratum corneum (Munro microabscesses) and in spinous layer (spongiform pustules of Kogoj)
- Hypogranulosis (1.63)
- Suprapapillary thinning of epidermis (epidermis is very thin over dermal papillae)
- *Regular acanthosis* (rete ridges about *same length*), often with *clubbed* rete ridges
- Dilated capillaries in dermal papillae (causes Auspitz sign of pinpoint bleeding if scale picked off)
- Perivascular lymphocytes (1.109)

Variations

1. Psoriasis vulgaris: the classic, common, more *well-developed plaque* form as above.
2. Guttate psoriasis: small *drop-like papules* (1.122), often occurs acutely after an event such as drug exposure, or illness such as streptococcal pharyngitis. Parakeratosis is more focal, less acanthosis.

3. Pustular psoriasis (including several variants). Pustular psoriasis of *von Zumbusch* occurs as a severe generalized form, especially on the trunk, with systemic symptoms such as fever (1.45), leukocytosis (1.69), and hypercalcemia. *Acute generalized exanthematous pustulosis* is pustular psoriasis related to drugs (3.5), and is more likely to have eosinophils. *Impetigo herpetiformis* is pustular psoriasis of pregnancy (1.113), with systemic findings like the von Zumbusch form. *Subcorneal pustular dermatosis of Sneddon–Wilkinson* occurs as annular (1.5) pustules on the trunk more in middle-aged women. *Pustulosis palmaris et plantaris (palmoplantar pustulosis)* and *dermatitis repens* are pustular psoriasis of the palms and soles (1.100). *Acrodermatitis continua* is severe mutilating psoriasis on the fingers (1.56). All forms of pustular psoriasis have neutrophils in stratum corneum forming pustules (1.89), with less acanthosis, less hyperkeratosis.
4. Inverse psoriasis: psoriasis that mainly involves intertriginous areas (1.10, 1.55). Biopsy more likely to be spongiotic (1.132) psoriasiform and less classic for psoriasis.
5. Reiter's disease: tetrad of *psoriasiform* skin lesions (annular circinate balanitis, keratoderma blenorrhagicum of the palms and soles, nail dystrophy), *conjunctivitis* (1.41), *urethritis* or *gastroenteritis* (1.49), and *arthritis* (1.7). Some authorities prefer to call it "reactive arthritis" rather than Reiter's disease, because of Reiter's Nazi affiliation, but it seems unreasonable to advocate a trend of changing an embedded name of a condition based upon politics, and the term reactive arthritis hardly seems like the name of a specific condition. This is a venereal infection associated with chlamydia, or associated with intestinal *Salmonella* or *Shigella*, more in males. Pathology is identical with psoriasis, but more often pustules, more massive hyperkeratosis in keratoderma blenorrhagicum.
6. Geographic tongue: annular (1.5) or serpiginous (1.127) eroded patches on the tongue (1.139), biopsy like psoriasis.

Differential diagnosis

1. Other diseases with neutrophils in the stratum corneum (1.89).
2. Other papulosquamous diseases (1.103) with psoriasiform (regular) acanthosis (1.119).
3. Lichen simplex (2.3): irregular acanthosis (rete ridges not same length), more pointed rete ridges at base (not clubbed), papillary dermal collagen in vertical streaks, fewer neutrophils in stratum corneum.

2.9 Parapsoriasis

Idiopathic *chronic persistent scaly plaques*, usually adults, especially on the trunk, which often *fail to respond* to the usual eczema (2.1) treatments, such as topical corticosteroids. Parapsoriasis is very *controversial*. Dermatologists use different terminology for various forms (many terms have historical significance only). Some consider all examples of parapsoriasis to be mycosis fungoides, while others consider the small plaque type as benign and the large plaque (parapsoriasis en plaque) and variegate (retiform) types as representing early mycosis fungoides. Guttate parapsoriasis is now called pityriasis lichenoides (2.14).

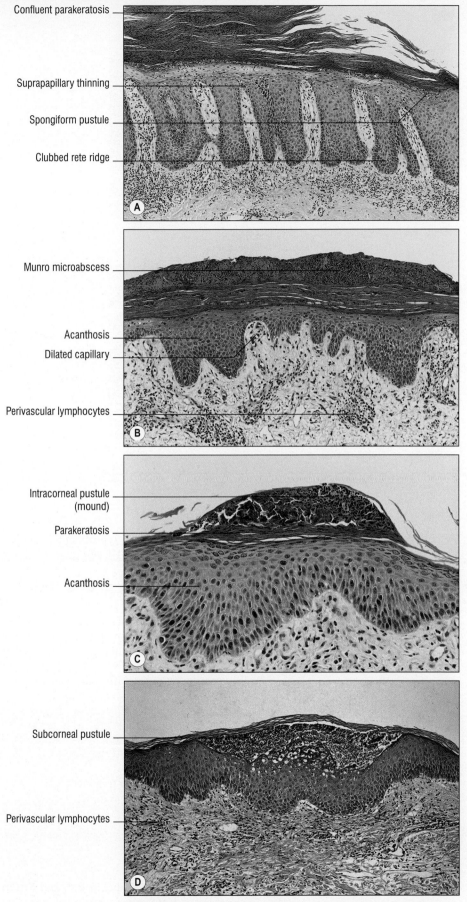

Confluent parakeratosis

Suprapapillary thinning

Spongiform pustule

Clubbed rete ridge

Munro microabscess

Acanthosis

Dilated capillary

Perivascular lymphocytes

Intracorneal pustule (mound)

Parakeratosis

Acanthosis

Subcorneal pustule

Perivascular lymphocytes

Fig. 2.8 A Psoriasis vulgaris. **B** Psoriasis. **C** Pustular psoriasis. **D** Pustular psoriasis.

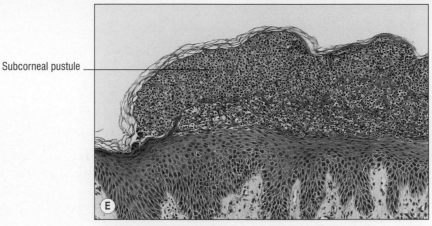

Subcorneal pustule

Fig. 2.8 *Continued* **E** Subcorneal pustular dermatosis.

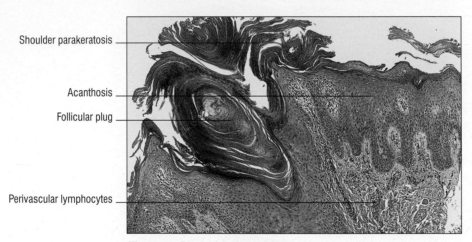

Shoulder parakeratosis

Acanthosis

Follicular plug

Perivascular lymphocytes

Fig. 2.10 Pityriasis rubra pilaris.

P
- Focal parakeratosis (1.104)
- Acanthosis sometimes, atrophy of epidermis (1.9) sometimes
- Spongiosis sometimes
- Focal liquefaction of the basal layer sometimes (1.64)
- Perivascular (sometimes lichenoid) lymphocytes
- Erythrocyte extravasation (1.40) sometimes

Variations

1. Digitate dermatosis: thumb print small plaques.
2. Xanthoerythrodermia perstans: yellowish small plaques.

Differential diagnosis

The diagnosis is primarily clinical, and the histology is nonspecific, unless changes of mycosis fungoides are present.
1. Other eczematous diseases (1.29), papulosquamous diseases (1.103).
2. Other diseases with spongiosis (1.132), perivascular lymphocytes (1.109) or lichenoid lymphocytes (1.72).
3. Pityriasis rosea (2.4): lasts only 6 weeks.
4. Pityriasis lichenoides (2.14): lesions rarely larger than 5 mm, lasts only months to several years, more in children and young adults.
5. Mycosis fungoides (24.1): larger plaques, more epidermotropism, Pautrier microabscesses, more

atypical hyperchromatic lymphocytes, depletion of pan T-cell markers, abnormal T-cell gene rearrangements.

2.10 Pityriasis rubra pilaris (PRP)

(see Fig. 2.10)
Papulosquamous eruption of children or adults, with *psoriasiform plaques with islands of sparing*, often *salmon red* in color, often on the trunk (1.141), often generalized, often with *thick waxy hyperkeratotic palms and soles* (1.100), often with *numerous red follicular papules*, often with nail dystrophy (1.85).

- Follicular plugging often
- "Shoulder parakeratosis" adjacent to follicular plugs, or "sputtering" or "scoreboard parakeratosis" alternated with orthokeratosis (1.104)
- Irregular acanthosis, often psoriasiform
- Acantholysis, focal, sometimes (1.2)
- Perivascular lymphocytes (1.109), occasionally lichenoid (1.72)

Differential diagnosis

1. The diagnosis is primarily clinical, and PRP must be differentiated from other papulosquamous diseases (1.103), especially psoriasis (2.8).
2. Other diseases with follicular plugging (1.47).

3. Other diseases with psoriasiform hyperplasia of epidermis (1.119).

2.11 Lichen planus (LP)

(see Fig. 2.11A–G)

Common idiopathic eruption of *polygonal, planar* (flat-topped), *pruritic* (1.114), *purplish* (1.148) *papules* (five "p"s) and plaques, especially on *wrists*, hands, trunk, legs, often with fine reticulated scale (1.123) over the surface known as *Wickham's striae*, often with *reticulated white plaques in the mouth* (1.82), duration months to years. Less than 10% of cases are associated with hepatitis C (14.7), more commonly if oral lesions.

P
- *Compact hyperkeratosis* (1.61, usually *no parakeratosis* except when rubbed or oral)
- *Hypergranulosis* (1.60), often wedge-shaped
- Irregular acanthosis (1.61) with *"saw-toothed" rete ridges* (rarely epidermal atrophy, 1.9)
- Colloid bodies often (1.27)
- *Liquefaction degeneration* of the basal layer (1.64)
- *Lichenoid* lymphocytes in the papillary dermis
- *Melanin incontinence* often (1.79)
- Direct immunofluorescence reveals immunoglobulin (mainly IgM), complement, and fibrin staining of colloid bodies in the deeper epidermis and superficial dermis. Although the findings are characteristic of LP, direct immunofluorescence of classic LP is not necessary

Variations

1. Hypertrophic LP: more common on the legs (1.67), more epithelial hyperplasia, sometimes to the point of pseudoepitheliomatous hyperplasia (1.116), often squamatized (1.134), more likely to have parakeratosis. May overlap with multiple keratoacanthomas (18.2) or squamous cell carcinomas.
2. Atrophic LP: epidermal atrophy instead of the usual acanthosis.
3. Bullous LP: subepidermal blistering (1.147, Max–Josef cleft).
4. Oral LP: limited to mouth or combined with cutaneous disease, more likely to be erosive or ulcerative (1.142), less of a band of lymphocytes, less hypergranulosis, more parakeratosis (1.104).
5. Plasmacytosis mucosae, Zoon's balanitis (1.107, balanitis plasmacellularis circumscriptum), plasma cell cheilitis (1.74), plasma cell vulvitis (1.149): red plaques on the mucous membranes (uncircumcised penis more common), of uncertain etiology, lichenoid lymphocytes with far more plasma cells (1.111) than LP.
6. Lichen planopilaris (LPP): *scarring alopecia* (1.4) of *scalp* (1.124), lichenoid lymphocytes mostly around *plugged follicles* (1.47), usually sparing the epidermis, otherwise closely resembles discoid lupus erythematosus (17.6). Post-menopausal frontal fibrosing alopecia is probably a frontal scalp variant of LPP.

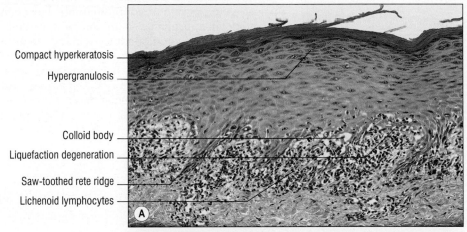

Compact hyperkeratosis
Hypergranulosis
Colloid body
Liquefaction degeneration
Saw-toothed rete ridge
Lichenoid lymphocytes

Fig. 2.11 A Lichen planus.

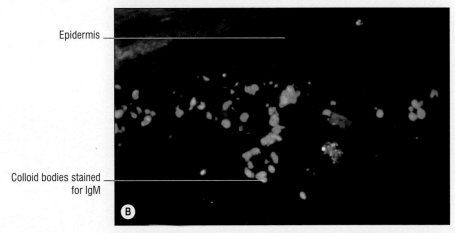

Epidermis
Colloid bodies stained for IgM

Fig. 2.11 B Lichen planus (IgM staining of cytoid bodies).

7. Graham–Little syndrome: LPP and alopecia (1.4) of *axilla and groin* (1.10, 1.55) in addition to *scalp, keratosis pilaris* (10.5) of trunk and limbs.

Differential diagnosis

1. Lupus erythematosus (17.6): more likely to have epidermal atrophy, follicular plugging, dermal mucin, and less likely to have hypergranulosis and colloid bodies. The dermal infiltrate is more perivascular and periadnexal than lichenoid (in LP it tends not to go down the adnexa except in LPP). Clinical, direct immunofluorescence, and serologic findings are different.
2. Lichenoid drug eruption (3.5): more likely to have eosinophils and parakeratosis.
3. Lichenoid keratosis (18.8): may be identical histologically but is solitary and more likely to have parakeratosis.
4. Other forms of lichenoid dermatitis (1.72) and interface dermatitis (1.64).

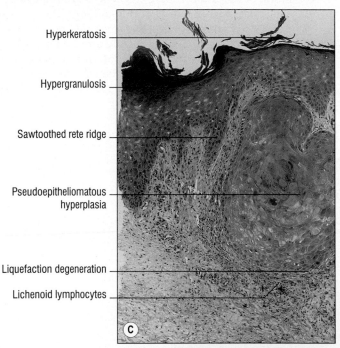

Hyperkeratosis

Hypergranulosis

Sawtoothed rete ridge

Pseudoepitheliomatous hyperplasia

Liquefaction degeneration

Lichenoid lymphocytes

Fig. 2.11 C Hypertrophic lichen planus.

2.12 Lichen nitidus
(see Fig. 2.12)
Uncommon asymptomatic eruption of numerous *tiny 1-mm skin-colored papules* (1.129), more in *children*, especially on the trunk (1.141) or penis (1.107) which lasts months to years.

> ■ Epidermal atrophy (1.9) and often parakeratosis (1.104) overlying a focal ball of papillary dermal lymphocytes. Epidermal rete ridges often form a *collarette* (1.61) that extends around the lymphocytes like a "*ball in clutch*".
> ■ Multinucleated giant cells sometimes (1.84)
> ■ Focal liquefaction degeneration of the basal layer (1.64)
>
> **P**

Differential diagnosis

1. Other lichenoid diseases (1.72): most have larger papules or plaques.
2. Follicular eruptions (1.47): have tiny papules, but are centered upon follicles.
3. "Papular" or "follicular" eczema (2.1): more spongiosis, no "ball in clutch" appearance.
4. Molluscum contagiosum (14.4): more white, may cause clinical difficulty only.

2.13 Keratosis lichenoides chronica (Nekam's disease, lichen ruber moniliformis)

Very rare chronic disorder that has a questionable status as a distinct entity, as published photographs have considerable variability in appearance. It might be a variant of lichen planus (2.11). Red papulonodules with adherent hyperkeratosis, often in a striking linear (1.73) Koebnerized pattern, or reticulated (1.123) pattern (tic tac toe pattern), appear mostly on the extremities and buttocks, sometimes with palmoplantar keratoderma (2.15), sometimes associated with seborrheic dermatitis-like lesions of the face (2.1), nail dystrophy (1.85), and mouth ulcers.

> ■ Focal parakeratosis (1.104)
> ■ Epidermis is acanthotic or atrophic (1.9)
> ■ Liquefaction degeneration of the basal layer (1.64)
> ■ *Lichenoid lymphocytes*
>
> **P**

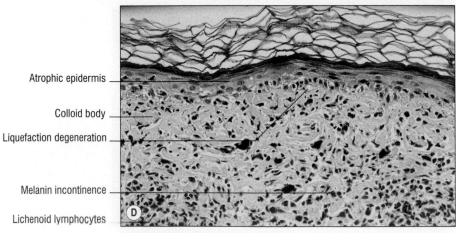

Atrophic epidermis

Colloid body

Liquefaction degeneration

Melanin incontinence

Lichenoid lymphocytes

Fig. 2.11 D Atrophic lichen planus.

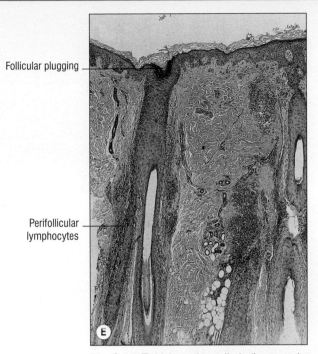

Follicular plugging

Perifollicular
lymphocytes

Fig. 2.11 E Lichen planopilaris (low mag.)

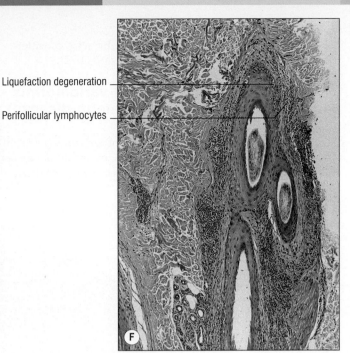

Liquefaction degeneration

Perifollicular lymphocytes

Fig. 2.11 F Lichen planopilaris (high mag.).

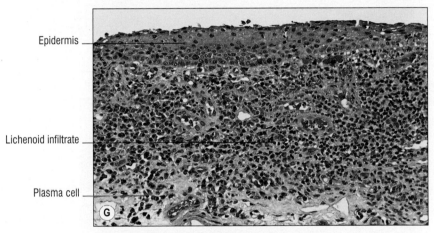

Epidermis

Lichenoid infiltrate

Plasma cell

Fig. 2.11 G Zoon's balanitis.

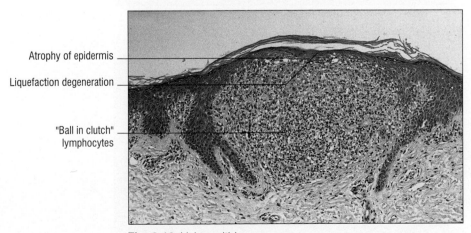

Atrophy of epidermis

Liquefaction degeneration

"Ball in clutch"
lymphocytes

Fig. 2.12 Lichen nitidus.

Differential diagnosis

1. The diagnosis is primarily clinical; otherwise consider other diseases with a lichenoid infiltrate (1.72).

2.14 Pityriasis lichenoides et varioliformis acuta (PLEVA, Mucha-Habermann disease)

(see Fig. 2.14A–C)

Uncommon idiopathic eruption mostly of the *trunk* (1.141) of *older children and young adults*, usually many *small lesions* (1.122) less than 5 mm in diameter which are variable in morphology from scaly papules to *crusted papulovesicles* (1.147), self-limited in months to years.

- Focal parakeratosis (1.104), often with *scale crust*
- Dense wedge-shaped infiltrate centered upon basal layer zone of the papule, with *prominent lymphocytic exocytosis into the epidermis*
- *Necrotic keratinocytes* often
- *Spongiosis* (1.132) with intraepidermal vesicles (1.147) sometimes
- Liquefaction degeneration of the basal layer (1.64)
- *Extravasation of erythrocytes*, often *in the epidermis*

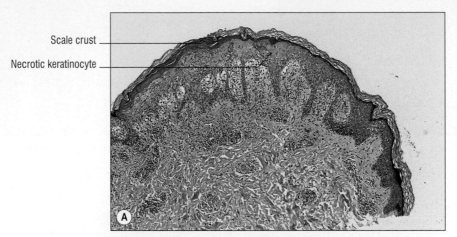

Fig. 2.14 A Pityriasis lichenoides (low mag.).

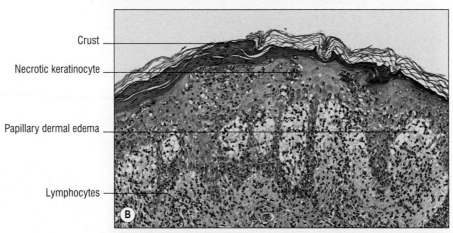

Fig. 2.14 B Pityriasis lichenoides (medium mag.).

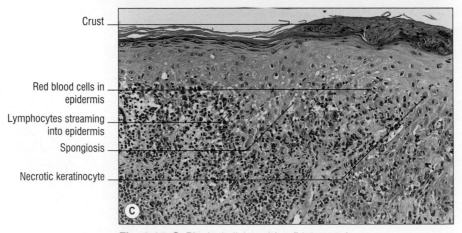

Fig. 2.14 C Pityriasis lichenoides (high mag.).

Variation

1. Pityriasis lichenoides chronica (PLC): a less acute, chronic form which is histologically similar, except that there is less scale crust, fewer neutrophils, less spongiosis, fewer vesicles, and fewer necrotic keratinocytes.

Differential diagnosis

1. Lymphomatoid papulosis ("evil PLEVA", 24.5): atypical lymphocytes.
2. Arthropod bites (15.7): more face and extremities, more eosinophils.
3. Other lichenoid diseases (1.72).
4. Other diseases with necrotic keratinocytes (1.86).
5. Other diseases with extravasated erythrocytes (1.40).

2.15 Palmoplantar keratoderma (hyperkeratosis palmaris et plantaris)

(see Fig. 2.15)

A group of usually genetically inherited conditions with thick hyperkeratotic palms and soles (1.100). The most severe forms are generally autosomal recessive. When the hyperkeratosis extends onto the hands or feet beyond the palms or soles, the term "transgrediens" has been used (Olmsted, Greither, Vohwinkel, and mal de Maleda variants).

- Prominent *hyperkeratosis*, hypergranulosis, acanthosis
- Sparse perivascular lymphocytes (1.109)

Variations

1. Unna–Thost syndrome: autosomal dominant, keratin 1 mutation, *common diffuse form*.
2. Voerner's syndrome (epidermolytic palmoplantar keratoderma): autosomal dominant, keratin 9 defect, common diffuse form, histologic changes identical to the variant of ichthyosis known as *epidermolytic hyperkeratosis* (11.1).
3. Howel–Evans syndrome (tylosis): autosomal dominant, pressure point keratoderma, *esophageal carcinoma* (1.106).
4. Sieman's syndrome: autosomal dominant, *pressure point* keratoderma.
5. Mal de Meleda syndrome: autosomal recessive, SLURP-1 mutation, diffuse transgredient keratoderma, mental retardation.
6. Greither's syndrome: autosomal dominant, keratin 1 mutation, diffuse, transgredient to the *Achilles tendon*, involves *elbows and knees*.
7. Papillon–Lefevre syndrome: autosomal recessive, cathepsin C mutation, diffuse transgredient keratoderma, *periodontitis*, pyodermas, and dural calcification.
8. Vohwinkle syndrome: autosomal dominant, mutation in loricrin gene, diffuse transgredient keratoderma, *mutilating autoamputation* of digits, *starfish-shaped keratoses* on dorsal digits.
9. Olmsted syndrome: diffuse transgredient mutilating keratoderma, *perioral* plaques.
10. Richner–Hanhart syndrome (tyrosinemia II, oculocutaneous tyrosinosis): autosomal recessive, painful hyperkeratotic papules on palms and soles, corneal ulcerations, *refractile eosinophilic deposits in superficial epidermis*.
11. Acrokeratoelastoidosis: autosomal dominant, hyperkeratotic papules mostly on the sides of the hands and feet with *fragmented elastic fibers* (1.31), resembles collagenous and elastotic plaques of the hands (9.1).
12. Pachyonychia congenita: autosomal dominant, defect in keratin 6 and 16, or keratin 17, diffuse keratoderma, extremely *thick subungual hyperkeratosis* (1.85), *leukoplakia* in the mouth (1.82) similar to white sponge nevus (17.11).
13. Punctate keratoderma: autosomal dominant, *small discrete foci* of hyperkeratotic papules, not to be confused with keratosis punctata (a common punctate hyperkeratosis with central depression seen in the palmar creases of black patients). Also resembles porokeratosis punctata palmaris et plantaris (18.4).
14. Hidrotic ectodermal dysplasia (11.2).
15. Bazex syndrome (acrokeratosis paraneoplastica): violaceous keratoderma of the hands and feet with psoriasiform plaques of fingers, toes, ears, nose, arms, or legs, usually preceding an underlying supradiaphragmatic internal malignancy (1.105). Do not confuse with the other Bazex syndrome (follicular atrophoderma, 18.14).

Differential diagnosis

1. Other diseases with hyperplasia of epidermis (1.61) of palms or soles (1.100), especially psoriasis (2.8), pityriasis rubra pilaris (2.10), eczema (2.1), contact dermatitis (2.2), tinea (13.1), crusted scabies (15.9), tripe palm (18.5), and arsenical keratoses (18.9).
2. Syringofibroadenomatosis (23.10) has only a clinical resemblance.

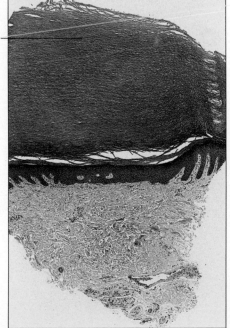

Hyperkeratosis

Fig. 2.15 Acrokeratoelastoidosis.

CHAPTER 3

Reactive Erythemas

The erythemas in this chapter are generally viewed as *reactions to infections, drugs, malignancies,* or other miscellaneous things. They are generally more *dermal,* having *less scale or epidermal changes* than the diseases in Chapter 2. The *erythema blanches,* and there is no purpura or vasculitis as in Chapter 4. When erythemas make rings, they are annular (1.5), and are sometimes called *gyrate erythemas.* When they have an acute onset, are bright red and edematous, and often accompanied by palm and sole involvement or fever, then sometimes clinicians invoke the poorly defined term *toxic erythema.* Toxic erythema can include conditions outside of this chapter, such as scarlet fever (12.2), toxic shock syndrome (12.2), Kawasaki's syndrome (14.10), and acute graft-versus-host disease (17.3).

3.1 Urticaria

(see Fig. 3.1)
Common, occurs in 20% of the population sometime in their lifetime, *evanescent wheals* (hives) that move around hour by hour or at least within 24 hours, very pruritic (1.114), IgE mediated type I hypersensitivity to foods, drugs, infection, or idiopathic factors. May have dermatographism. Airway obstruction due to laryngeal edema may occur in severe cases.

P
- Epidermis normal
- Dermal *edema*
- *Sparse perivascular and interstitial eosinophils, lymphocytes, neutrophils* (1.89), and/or *mast cells* (1.78)

Variations

1. Acute urticaria: usually lasts less than a month, higher chance of specific etiology being found.
2. Chronic urticaria: lasts more than a month, and may last for years, idiopathic in 90% of cases, less likely related to IgE.
3. Cold urticaria: more in children and young adults, related to cold exposure (lesions reproduced with ice cube test).
4. Solar urticaria: appears within hours of sun exposure (photodermatitis, 1.110).
5. Cholinergic urticaria: small papules appear after exercise.
6. Pressure urticaria: pressure on skin of hands, feet, or buttocks induces lesions.
7. Hereditary angioedema: autosomal dominant, prominent facial or lip edema, usually without urticaria, decreased levels or dysfunction of Cl esterase inhibitor.
8. Angioedema with acute urticaria: may have fever, leukocytosis, no family history, less inflammatory cells in skin and more edema, with tendency to extend deeper into subcutaneous fat.
9. Erythema marginatum: variant of urticaria that is faint, very evanescent, occurring with rheumatic fever (12.2).
10. Papular urticaria (15.7): related to arthropod bites.

Differential diagnosis

1. Other diseases with dermal eosinophils (1.36).
2. Other diseases with dermal edema (1.30).
3. Other diseases with normal-appearing histology (1.94), perivascular (1.109), or interstitial dermatitis (1.65).
4. Urticarial vasculitis (4.1): mainly considered clinically when lesions are not evanescent.

3.2 Erythema multiforme (EM)

(see Fig. 3.2A–D)
Common, *acute onset, multiform lesions* (papules, urticarial plaques, *targets* (1.5), blisters), *often recurrent,* especially on acral skin more than the trunk, common on the palms (1.100). Mostly in *children and young adults.* If classic targets are present, it is almost always a reaction to *herpes simplex* infection (14.2). A wide variety of *drugs* (3.5) and infections are the cause in other cases. Although some authors refer to "epidermal" and "dermal" types of erythema multiforme, this is just a function of what type of lesion is biopsied.

©2012 Elsevier Ltd, Inc, BV
DOI: 10.1016/B978-0-323-06658-7.00003-8

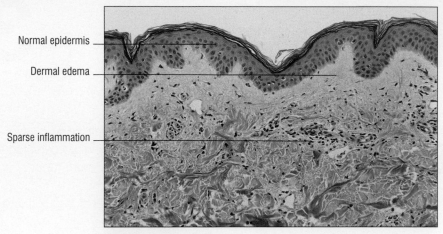

Fig. 3.1 Urticaria.

Normal epidermis

Dermal edema

Sparse inflammation

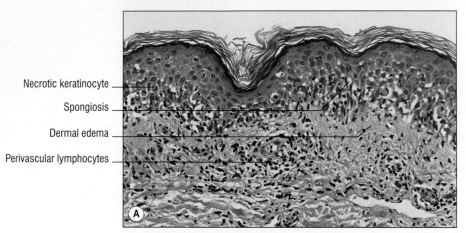

Fig. 3.2 A Erythema multiforme (low mag.).

Necrotic keratinocyte

Spongiosis

Dermal edema

Perivascular lymphocytes

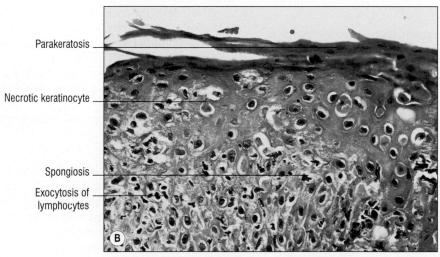

Fig. 3.2 B Erythema multiforme (high mag.).

Parakeratosis

Necrotic keratinocyte

Spongiosis

Exocytosis of lymphocytes

P
- Necrotic keratinocytes
- Sometimes spongiosis (1.132), rarely intraepidermal vesicles
- Basal layer liquefaction (1.64), sometimes subepidermal blister (1.147)
- Edema of the papillary dermis (1.30)
- Perivascular or interface lymphocytes (1.64), rarely with eosinophils (1.36)
- Extravasated erythrocytes sometimes (1.40)

Variations

1. Stevens–Johnson syndrome: more mucous membrane involvement and more epidermal necrosis. Some authorities attempt to define it differently based upon the amount of body surface area involved, making the inane statement that Stevens–Johnson syndrome involves less than 10% body surface area, whereas toxic epidermal necrolysis involves more than 30%, with 10–30% involvement constituting an overlap zone. This is ridiculous

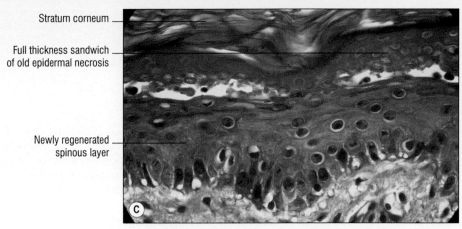

Stratum corneum

Full thickness sandwich
of old epidermal necrosis

Newly regenerated
spinous layer

Fig. 3.2 C Erythema multiforme (re-epithelialization).

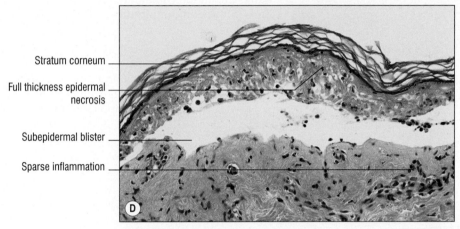

Stratum corneum

Full thickness epidermal
necrosis

Subepidermal blister

Sparse inflammation

Fig. 3.2 D Toxic epidermal necrolysis.

because it makes no sense to change the diagnosis if the disease worsens.

2. Toxic epidermal necrolysis (TEN): extensive sloughing of full-thickness necrotic skin, higher body surface area involved than Stevens–Johnson syndrome, may be life threatening (prognosis calculated by SCORTEN scoring system), usually due to sulfonamides, phenytoin, and other drugs.
3. Necrolytic migratory erythema (glucagonoma syndrome): crusted plaques, especially mouth, perioral, and acral skin, elevated serum glucagon level, psoriasiform (1.119), tendency for only the superficial epidermis to be necrotic and pale (1.99), underlying glucagonoma may not be found in all cases.
4. Fixed drug reaction (3.5): similar to erythema multiforme, but localized to a fixed site, associated with drugs.
5. Erythrodysesthesia syndrome (3.5).

Differential diagnosis

1. Paraneoplastic pemphigus (5.4): necrotic keratinocytes more prominent than acantholysis, so it is easily mistaken for erythema multiforme clinically and histologically.
2. Rowell syndrome (17.6): lupus erythematosus with necrotic keratinocytes resembling erythema multiforme.
3. Other diseases with necrotic keratinocytes (1.86) or perivascular lymphocytes (1.109).

3.3 Erythema annulare centrifugum (EAC)

(see Fig. 3.3A,B)

Uncommon, *annular plaques* (if rings are not present, then it is not EAC!), often with half-rings with a collarette of *trailing scale*, usually of the *trunk* (1.141) of adults. Usually idiopathic, sometimes a cause such as tinea pedis is found.

- Occasional focal spongiosis (1.132) or parakeratosis (1.104)
- Sharply demarcated *"coat-sleeve" lymphocytes* densely arranged around dilated superficial and deep blood vessels

P

Differential diagnosis

1. Other annular diseases (1.5), especially gyrate erythemas.
2. Erythema multiforme (3.2): more necrotic keratinocytes.
3. Secondary syphilis (12.13): plasma cells, positive serology.
4. Other diseases with superficial and deep perivascular dermatitis (1.109).

3.4 Erythema gyratum repens (EGR)

Very rare, *impressive wood-grain appearance* of pruritic, red, scaly rash most common on trunk (1.141), changing daily, usually associated with *underlying systemic malignancy* (1.105), especially carcinomas, most commonly of the lung.

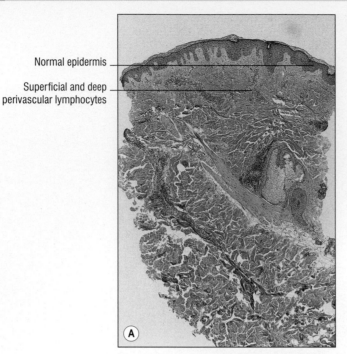

Normal epidermis

Superficial and deep perivascular lymphocytes

Fig. 3.3 A Erythema annulare centrifugum (low mag.).

- Mild focal spongiosis (1.132) and parakeratosis (1.104)
- Perivascular lymphocytes (1.109), sometimes with eosinophils (1.36)

P

Differential diagnosis

1. Diagnosis is made from characteristic clinical "wood-grain" appearance. Other annular rashes (1.5) rarely have such a striking clinical appearance. Histology is non-specific, resembling other diseases with perivascular dermatitis (1.109).

3.5 Drug eruptions

(see Fig. 3.5A–I)
Drugs are all too commonly used nowadays, and drug reactions in the skin can produce *almost any clinical and histologic pattern.*

Variations

1. Maculopapular (1.81, morbilliform, exanthematous) rashes: the most common drug reaction pattern, generalized small red papules and macules without

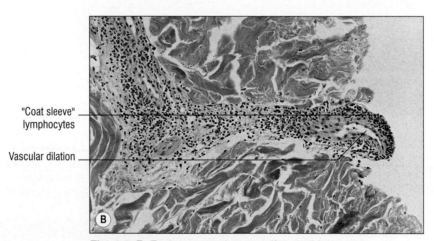

"Coat sleeve" lymphocytes

Vascular dilation

Fig. 3.3 B Erythema annulare centrifugum (high mag.).

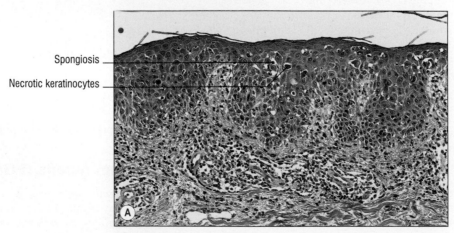

Spongiosis

Necrotic keratinocytes

Fig. 3.5 A Fixed drug eruption.

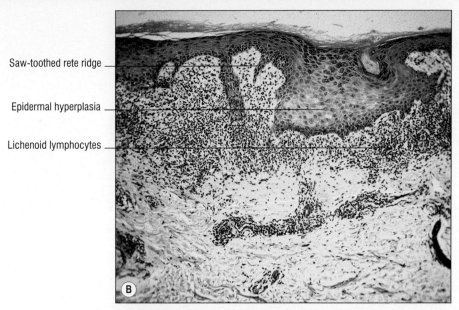

Fig. 3.5 **B** Lichenoid drug eruption.

Saw-toothed rete ridge

Epidermal hyperplasia

Lichenoid lymphocytes

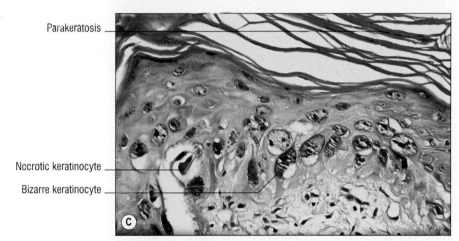

Fig. 3.5 **C** Chemotherapy often induces bizarre changes in keratinocytes (such as so-called "busulfan" cells), especially in photodistributed actinic keratoses.

Parakeratosis

Necrotic keratinocyte

Bizarre keratinocyte

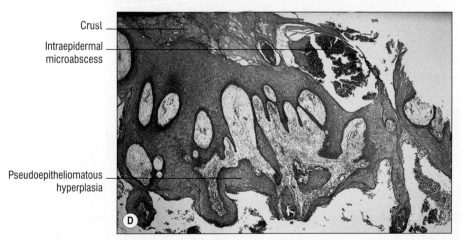

Fig. 3.5 **D** Bromoderma (low mag.).

Crust

Intraepidermal microabscess

Pseudoepitheliomatous hyperplasia

scale initially, perivascular lymphocytes (1.109), often with eosinophils (1.36), sometimes interface dermatitis (1.64), usually minimal epidermal changes.
2. Urticaria (3.1).
3. Drug-induced vasculitis (4.1).

4. Erythema multiforme, Stevens–Johnson syndrome, toxic epidermal necrolysis (3.2).
5. Fixed drug eruption: often due to acetaminophen, sulfonamides, tetracyclines, and many others. Clinically a bright red plaque, with or without blistering, fixed in

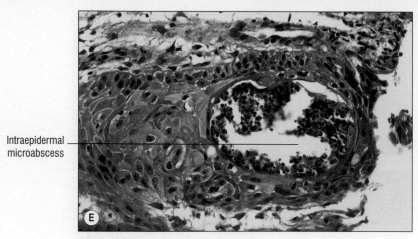

Intraepidermal microabscess

Fig. 3.5 E Bromoderma (high mag.).

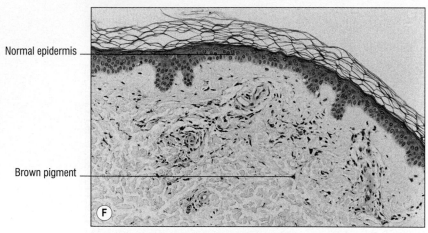

Normal epidermis

Brown pigment

Fig. 3.5 F Minocycline pigmentation.

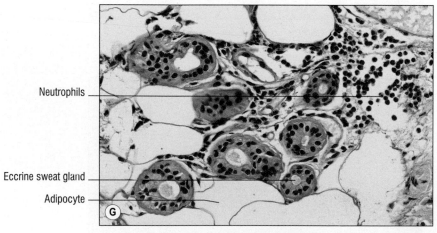

Neutrophils

Eccrine sweat gland

Adipocyte

Fig. 3.5 G Neutrophilic eccrine hidradenitis.

one place consistently when challenged with the drug, heals with hyperpigmentation, histology similar to erythema multiforme (3.2), but more likely to have eosinophils.

6. Lichenoid drug eruption: often due to gold salts, beta blockers, antimalarials, thiazides, furosemide, tumor necrosis factor inhibitors, interferon, and many others. Histology similar to lichen planus (1.72, 2.11), but more likely to have parakeratosis (1.104) and eosinophils.

7. Eczematous (spongiotic) drug reaction: uncommon, as most drug reactions primarily cause dermal changes (1.132, 2.1).

8. Psoriasiform drug reactions: uncommon, more with beta blockers (1.119).

9. Drug-induced photodermatitis: varying degrees of spongiosis, necrotic keratinocytes (1.86) and perivascular dermatitis, resembling other causes of photodermatitis (1.110).

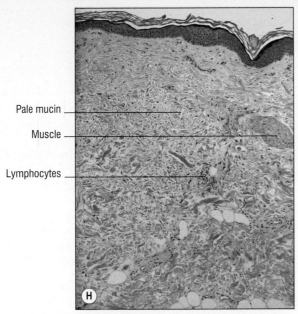

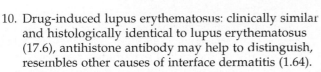

Fig. 3.5 H Eosinophilia myalgia syndrome.

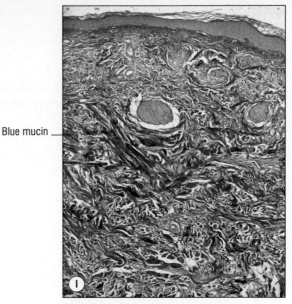

Fig. 3.5 I Eosinophilia myalgia syndrome (colloidal iron stain for mucin).

10. Drug-induced lupus erythematosus: clinically similar and histologically identical to lupus erythematosus (17.6), antihistone antibody may help to distinguish, resembles other causes of interface dermatitis (1.64).

11. Drug-induced dermatomyositis: clinically similar and histologically identical to dermatomyositis (17.7). Hydroxyurea is the most common cause.

12. Drug-induced pseudoporphyria: identical to porphyria cutanea tarda (8.1).

13. Drug-induced pemphigus (due to penicillamine, etc.): identical to pemphigus (5.4).

14. Linear IgA bullous drug reaction (due to vancomycin, captopril, etc.): identical to IgA bullous dermatosis (6.4).

15. Bullous drug reactions: overlap clinically and histologically with erythema multiforme (3.2), immunofluorescence negative.

16. Halogenodermas (bromoderma, iododerma): due to excessive consumption of bromides (such as in medications) or iodides (such as in SSKI or kelp), extensive acneiform lesions with histology like acne (10.1), often pseudoepitheliomatous hyperplasia with intraepidermal microabscesses (1.117) and granulomatous inflammation.

17. Acute generalized exanthematous pustulosis (AGEP): similar to pustular psoriasis (2.8), but is almost always due to drugs, and is more likely to have papillary dermal edema, necrotic keratinocytes, and eosinophils.

18. Drug-induced acne (10.1).

19. Interstitial granulomatous drug reaction:[143] rare, similar to granuloma annulare, but may also have interface dermatitis changes (7.1).

20. Erythrodysesthesia syndrome:[140] an acute erythema multiforme-like eruption with painful acral red plaques ("hand–foot syndrome") usually due to chemotherapy (3.2). Don't confuse it with the "one hand–two feet syndrome" related to tinea (13.1), which is more chronic rather than acute, and is more scaly and less bright red.

21. Eosinophilia–myalgia syndrome: disease of the past, due to tryptophan ingestion (when it was contaminated during manufacture), eosinophilia (1.34), myalgias, sclerodermoid changes (1.125), perivascular lymphocytes with eosinophils, sometimes dermal mucinosis (1.83).

22. Drug-induced hyperpigmentation (1.18): argyria (8.18), minocycline (brown dermal pigment positive with iron and/or melanin stains), gold (chrysiasis pigment appears as black particles), bleomycin (increased melanin in basal layer), clofazimine (brown lipofuscin stains with PAS), amiodarone (brown pigment stains with PAS).

23. Drug-induced pseudolymphoma (phenytoin, antihistamines, etc.): may be nearly identical to lymphocytoma cutis (24.14).

24. Drug-induced Sweet's syndrome: (3.7).

25. Neutrophilic eccrine hidradenitis (10.15): usually associated with chemotherapy, neutrophils around eccrine sweat glands.

26. Syringosquamous metaplasia: associated with chemotherapy, papules coalesce into plaques, spongiosis or interface dermatitis with sweat duct squamous metaplasia (1.61).

27. DRESS syndrome (drug reaction with eosinophilia and systemic symptoms): a more severe drug reaction in which the rash (usually morbilliform) is associated with fever, malaise, pharyngitis, lymphadenopathy, hepatitis, nephritis, pneumonitis, and/or eosinophilia. May overlap with drug-induced pseudolymphoma mentioned above.

Differential diagnosis

Since drugs can induce almost any inflammatory pattern, the list of alternative possibilities is endless, and few patterns are specific. The presence of eosinophils (1.36) is often overemphasized, when actually not all drug reactions have eosinophils, and rashes other than drug reactions can also have eosinophils. A skin biopsy usually cannot prove that a rash *is* a drug reaction, and often cannot prove that it is *not*. Ideal proof of drug reaction requires that the rash resolves after discontinuation of the drug, and then recurs after rechallenge (if rechallenge is dared attempted!). A common reason to biopsy suspected drug reactions is to also look for other possible diagnoses.

3.6 Pruritic urticarial papules and plaques of pregnancy (PUPPP, polymorphous eruption of pregnancy, PEP)

(see Fig. 3.6)
Most common pregnancy rash, papular and urticarial (rarely vesicular, 1.147) rash of *third trimester primigravidas*, *very pruritic* (1.114), usually *begins in abdominal striae*, resolves after delivery, increased rate of twins or rapid abdominal distention, no increased fetal problems.

Differential diagnosis

1. This is primarily a clinical diagnosis, and it is mainly biopsied to rule out pemphigoid gestationis (6.3), which

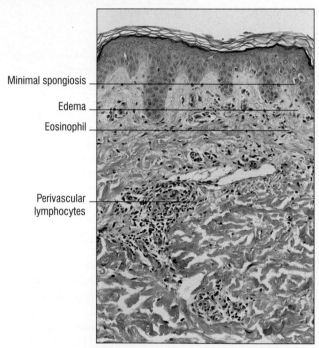

Fig. 3.6 Pruritic urticarial papules and plaques of pregnancy (PUPPP).

Minimal spongiosis

Edema

Eosinophil

Perivascular lymphocytes

- Mild focal parakeratosis (1.104) and spongiosis (1.132)
- Edema of dermis (1.30)
- *Perivascular lymphocytes with eosinophils*
- Negative direct immunofluorescence for immunoglobulins and complement

usually blisters and has C3 deposition at the basement membrane zone.

2. Other diseases with dermal eosinophils (1.36) or perivascular dermatitis (1.109).
3. Prurigo gestationis of Besnier: second trimester, excoriated papules mostly on extremities, may be related to atopy (2.1), biopsy like PUPPP.
4. Papular dermatitis of Spangler: rare questionable entity with increased fetal problems, widespread papules, elevated human chorionic gonadotropin and decreased estriol, biopsy like PUPPP.
5. Other pregnancy rashes (1.113).

3.7 Sweet's syndrome (acute febrile neutrophilic dermatosis)

(see Fig. 3.7A–C)
Uncommon neutrophilic dermatosis of acute onset, *painful* (1.97) *dark red or hemorrhagic* (1.120) *crusted plaques or bullae* (1.147), especially on the face or extremities, resembles vasculitis or infection clinically, but is a *diagnosis made after excluding infection* in the skin lesions with special stains and cultures, responds to systemic corticosteroids. Sometimes fever (1.45) and leukocytosis (1.69). Associated with *myelogenous leukemia* (24.16), *arthritis* (1.7), *inflammatory bowel disease* (1.49), previous upper respiratory infection, or drugs (3.5).

- Epidermal changes variable, sometimes epidermal necrosis I (1.86)
- *Superficial dermal edema often* (1.30), sometimes subepidermal blister (1.147)
- *Diffuse dermal neutrophils*, but also lymphocytes, histiocytes, and a few eosinophils (1.36)
- Traditionally *no true vasculitis* (no vessel wall necrosis, but occasionally has been reported as present), but nuclear dust is common
- Sometimes extravasated erythrocytes (1.40)

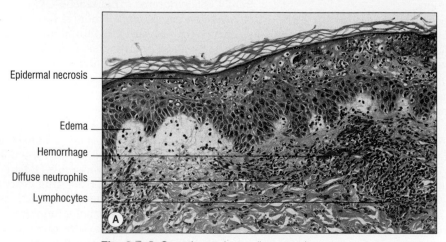

Epidermal necrosis

Edema

Hemorrhage

Diffuse neutrophils

Lymphocytes

A

Fig. 3.7 A Sweet's syndrome (low mag.).

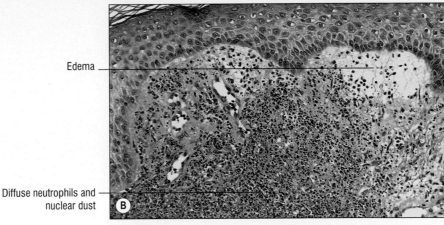

Edema

Diffuse neutrophils and
nuclear dust

B

Fig. 3.7 B Sweet's syndrome (medium mag.).

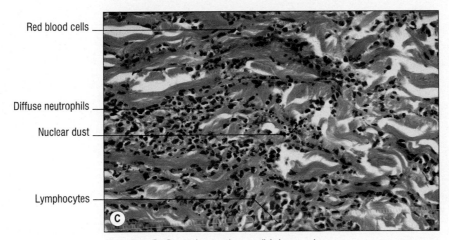

Red blood cells

Diffuse neutrophils

Nuclear dust

Lymphocytes

C

Fig. 3.7 C Sweet's syndrome (high mag.).

Variations

1. Rheumatoid neutrophilic dermatitis: a "neutrophilic dermatosis" similar to Sweet's syndrome, with papules, plaques, and rarely vesicles on extensor surfaces, associated with *rheumatoid arthritis*. Do not confuse with rheumatoid papules, which are a true leukocytoclastic vasculitis.
2. Neutrophilic dermatosis of the hands: a localized variant of Sweet's syndrome localized to the hands (mostly dorsal, but may also involve lateral digital or palmar aspects).

Differential diagnosis

1. Other diseases with neutrophils in the dermis (1.89). The other non-infectious "neutrophilic dermatoses" include pyoderma gangrenosum (4.12, more ulcerative), and rheumatoid neutrophilic dermatitis, Behçet's disease (4.11, different clinically), and bowel bypass syndrome (4.1, follows ileojejunal bypass surgery which is rarely performed today).
2. Vasculitis (Chapter 4): necrosis of vessel walls, or fibrin and inflammatory cells (usually neutrophils) in vessel walls, and the neutrophils are mostly vasocentric and less diffuse in the dermis.

3.8 Well's syndrome (eosinophilic cellulitis)

(see Fig. 3.8A–B)

Rare *bright red*, idiopathic, painful or pruritic, non-infectious *indurated plaques resembling infectious cellulitis* (12.3), sometimes with blisters, usually resolving in several days or weeks, often with peripheral eosinophilia. Responds to systemic corticosteroids.

- Intraepidermal or subepidermal blisters (1.147), sometimes
- *Diffuse dermal eosinophils*, lymphocytes, and histiocytes
- *Flame figures* in the dermis (bright eosinophilic areas of collagen encrusted with eosinophil granules)

P

Differential diagnosis

1. Flame figures rarely may be confused with necrosis of the dermis (1.87), or with other eosinophilic materials (1.35). Flame figures are most characteristic of Well's syndrome, but are sometimes seen in other diseases with eosinophils (1.36), and are sometimes absent in Well's syndrome.

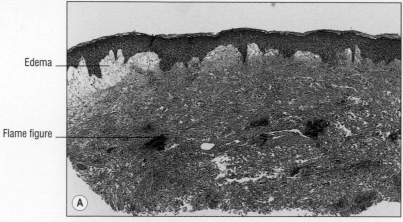

Edema

Flame figure

Fig. 3.8 A Well's syndrome (low mag.).

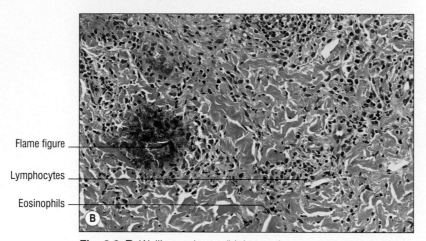

Flame figure

Lymphocytes

Eosinophils

Fig. 3.8 B Well's syndrome (high mag.).

2. Arthropod bites (15.7): usually are more clinically localized into papules and nodules, and rarely are large plaques.

3.9 Erythema ab igne

Uncommon, *reticulated*, *red–brown* (1.18) patches related to chronic heat exposure, especially from excessive *use of heating pads* for back pain, or on the legs from sitting next to a fire ("ab igne" means "from fire"), commonly seen in females with hypothyroidism (1.138). Telangiectasias or, rarely, squamous cell carcinomas may occur.

P
- Epidermal atrophy (1.9), sometimes
- Keratinocyte atypia, sometimes
- Liquefaction degeneration of the basal layer (1.64), focal, sometimes
- *Dilated dermal blood vessels*
- Elastosis in the dermis (1.31)
- *Melanin incontinence* (1.79) and *hemosiderin* (1.58) in the dermis

Differential diagnosis

1. This is primarily a clinical diagnosis. Consider other reticulated diseases (1.123), or other diseases with telangiectasia (1.136).

3.10 Livedo reticularis and cutis marmarata

(see Fig. 3.10)
Uncommon fixed *reticulated* red patches, often idiopathic, sometimes associated with autoimmune rheumatologic diseases, calciphylaxis (8.15), dysproteinemia (1.80) or emboli (4.16).

P
- Vascular dilation or normal appearance on biopsy
- Sparse or no inflammation; not a true vasculitis

Variation

1. Sneddon's syndrome: livedo reticularis associated with systemic arterial thrombi in the brain, heart, kidney, or peripheral vascular system.

Differential diagnosis

1. Cutis marmarata: more in infants, evanescent and not fixed, physiologic change related to temperature changes, harmless, without significant systemic associations, often resolves spontaneously.
2. Cutis marmarata telangiectactica (phlebectasia): congenital purplish localized or generalized patch, persistent and not evanescent, sometimes associated with nevus flammeus, skeletal malformations, and glaucoma.

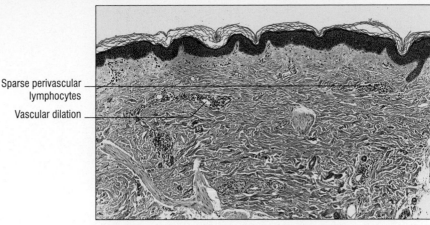

Fig. 3.10 Livedo reticularis.

Sparse perivascular lymphocytes

Vascular dilation

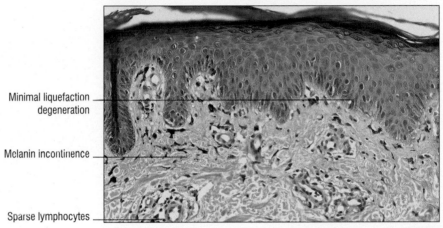

Minimal liquefaction degeneration

Melanin incontinence

Sparse lymphocytes

Fig. 3.11 Erythema dyschromicum perstans (EDP).

3. Other reticulated disorders (1.123), such as livedo vasculitis (4.13).

3.11 Erythema dyschromicum perstans (ashy dermatosis, dermatitis cenicienta)

(see Fig. 3.11)

Uncommon, considered by some to be a variant of lichen planus (2.11), idiopathic, asymptomatic, *blue–gray macules* (1.14) persist especially on the face and trunk (1.141), sometimes generalized, especially in Latin Americans.

- Liquefaction degeneration of the basal layer (1.64), colloid bodies (1.27), mild or absent
- *Melanin incontinence* (the more commonly biopsied older lesions often have only this)
- Perivascular (1.109) or interface lymphocytes (usually sparse, only in early lesions)

Differential diagnosis

1. Other diseases with melanin incontinence (1.79).
2. Other diseases with interface dermatitis (1.64).

3.12 Chilblains (perniosis)

Somewhat common *purplish* (1.148) macules or plaques of acral skin, especially *feet* (1.48), associated with *cold injury* (less severe than frostbite). The diagnosis is primarily clinical.

- Epidermis usually normal, rarely necrotic (1.86) or ulcerated l (1.142)
- Dermal edema (1.30) often
- Perivascular lymphocytes (1.76), sometimes around sweat ducts
- Thrombi sometimes (1.137)

3.13 Erythromelalgia (erythermalgia)

Recurrent, *painful erythema* of *hands* (1.56) and *feet* (1.48), or distal extremities, *worsens with exercise or heat* (opposite of Raynaud's phenomenon), associated with peripheral vascular disease, rheumatologic disorders, thrombocythemia or *myeloproliferative disease*. It is primarily a clinical diagnosis.

- Mild vascular dilation with thickened basement membrane and endothelial swelling
- Arteriolar thrombi sometimes (1.137)
- Perivascular dermal edema (1.30)
- Sparse perivascular lymphocytes (1.109)

Vasculitis and Other Purpuric Diseases

These diseases are all characterized by vascular damage of some type. Extravasated erythrocytes (1.40) often produce the appearance of *purpura* (1.120). Some of these diseases are considered to be true vasculitis. Vasculitis (literally, inflammation of the blood vessels) cannot be diagnosed with certainty unless there is visible vessel wall damage (*necrosis, hyalinization,* or *fibrin in the wall*) and inflammatory cells in vessel walls. *Red blood cell extravasation, thrombi,* and *nuclear dust* from leukocytoclasia of neutrophils are secondary, less specific findings frequently seen in vasculitis, but are not as important as finding vessel damage. Nuclear dust can be seen in any lesion that has many neutrophils (1.89). Vessel wall changes without the inflammation is often called vasculopathy instead of vasculitis. Extravasation of erythrocytes (1.40) can be seen in many diseases without vasculitis. Thrombi (1.137) are also frequently seen in diseases other than vasculitis. Vasculitis is often imperfectly classified based upon the clinical presentation, type of *predominant inflammatory cell* (neutrophils, lymphocytes, or macrophages) and the *type and caliber of vessels* involved (small vessels, arteries, or veins). Most cases of cutaneous vasculitis involve small blood vessels and are neutrophilic (4.1). Causes of *granulomatous vasculitis* are listed in 1.51. Consider that overlap exists between these disorders.

In addition to the diseases listed in this chapter, vasculitis may be seen in several other diseases, as well (1.145).

1. Erythema induratum (nodular vasculitis, 16.6)
2. Erythema nodosum leprosum (12.12)
3. Herpes virus infections (14.2)
4. Lymphomatoid granulomatosis (24.6)

4.1 Leukocytoclastic vasculitis (LCV, neutrophilic vasculitis, necrotizing vasculitis)

(see Fig. 4.1A–D)
This is the most common type of vasculitis found in skin. Classically, *palpable purpura* appears on the *legs* (1.67), and may be painful (1.97). Vasculitis is often idiopathic, but may be caused by *infections, drugs,* or *rheumatologic* disorders. Systemic vasculitis may involve the kidneys (1.66), brain, or other organs.

©2012 Elsevier Ltd, Inc, BV
DOI: 10.1016/B978-0-323-06658-7.00004-X

■ Epidermis varies from normal to necrotic, sometimes with vesicles or pustules
■ *Vasculitis* of mostly small venules, with a predominant number of *neutrophils*; sometimes eosinophils, lymphocytes, or histiocytes
■ *Nuclear dust* often
■ *Red blood cell extravasation* often
■ *Thrombi* sometimes
■ Direct immunofluorescence: usually not needed for diagnosis, reveals IgG, IgM, or complement in a granular pattern in the superficial blood vessels of early lesions of LCV. Fibrin deposits ("splash pattern") may be seen in young or old lesions.

Variations

1. Henoch–Schönlein purpura: distinct syndrome in *children*, rarely in adults, often idiopathic or due to streptococcal pharyngitis. *Abdominal pain* (1.49), bloody diarrhea, arthralgia or arthritis, hematuria, and palpable purpura more likely to become confluent, immunofluorescence more likely to show granular *IgA in the superficial dermal blood vessels*, usual self-limited *benign course*, resolves in a few weeks.

2. Urticarial vasculitis: clinical lesions more urticarial (3.1) than purpuric, *persist in one place longer than urticaria,*

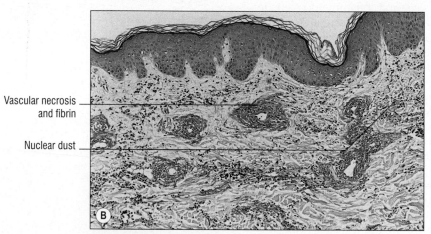

Vascular necrosis
and fibrin

Nuclear dust

Neutrophils

Extravasated
red blood cells

Fig. 4.1 A Leukocytoclastic vasculitis (low mag.).

may be related to rheumatologic disorder or hypocomplementemia, biopsy more likely to show eosinophils than other types of vasculitis. Often has very little vessel changes, so that overlap with urticaria is a difficult diagnostic problem. In many cases there are only the usual pathologic changes of urticaria combined with red blood cell extravasation.

3. Septic vasculitis, acute and subacute bacterial endocarditis (SBE): vasculitic changes due to actual bacteria, fungi, or immune complexes in the skin lesions from a disseminated infection. Histology identical to ordinary LCV, must find infectious agent. *Janeway's lesions* are acute, small, edematous red macules on acral skin from septic emboli, and *Osler's nodes* are more chronic and painful nodules of acral skin. Gonococcemia (12.18) and meningococcemia (12.19) are also examples of septic vasculitis.

4. Bowel bypass syndrome: follows ileojejunal bypass (procedure generally no longer performed), more likely to have epidermal changes or pustules; true vasculitis not always present.

5. Pustular vasculitis:[146] intraepidermal or subepidermal pustules in addition to usual changes of leukocytoclastic vasculitis.

Vascular necrosis
and fibrin

Nuclear dust

Fig. 4.1 B Leukocytoclastic vasculitis (high mag.).

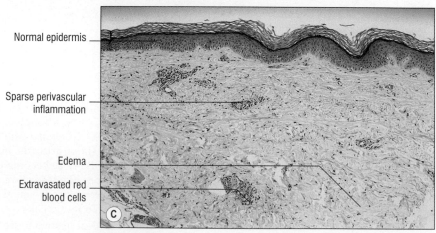

Normal epidermis

Sparse perivascular
inflammation

Edema

Extravasated red
blood cells

Fig. 4.1 C Urticarial vasculitis (low mag.).

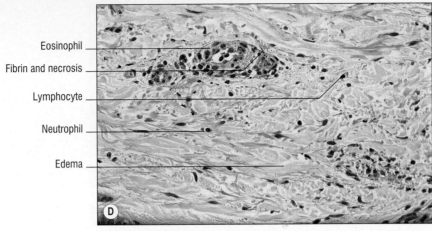

Eosinophil

Fibrin and necrosis

Lymphocyte

Neutrophil

Edema

Fig. 4.1 D Urticarial vasculitis (high mag.).

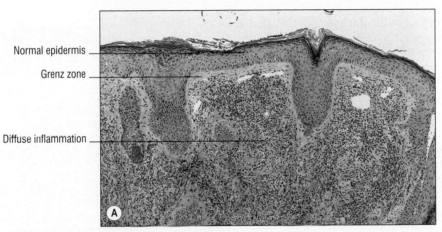

Normal epidermis

Grenz zone

Diffuse inflammation

Fig. 4.2 A Granuloma faciale (low mag.).

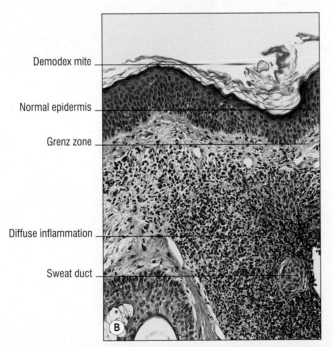

Demodex mite

Normal epidermis

Grenz zone

Diffuse inflammation

Sweat duct

Fig. 4.2 B Granuloma faciale (medium mag.).

6. Eosinophilic vasculitis:[120] eosinophils prominent.
7. Acute hemorrhagic edema of infancy: *children* up to 3 years old, fever, edema of *face* and extremities, *bright red purpuric ears*, resolves spontaneously within 3 weeks like Henoch–Schönlein purpura, but no IgA is present.

Differential diagnosis

1. Other diseases with purpura (1.120).
2. Other disease with neutrophils in the dermis (1.89).
3. Other diseases with thrombi (1.137) or extravasation of erythrocytes (1.40).
4. Other diseases with vasculitis in this chapter.

4.2 Granuloma faciale (GF)

(see Fig. 4.2A–C)
Uncommon, idiopathic brown–red plaques (1.18) on the face (1.44) of adults. GF is a misnomer, as there is no granuloma formation as defined in Section 1.35.

- Epidermis is usually unremarkable
- Grenz zone (1.49) above a *diffuse* mixed dermal *neutrophils*, *eosinophils*, *lymphocytes*, and *histiocytes*, sometimes with plasma cells or mast cells
- Often leukocytoclastic *vasculitis* (4.1)
- Often hemosiderin in dermis (1.58)

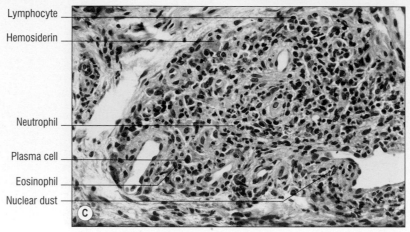

Lymphocyte
Hemosiderin
Neutrophil
Plasma cell
Eosinophil
Nuclear dust

Fig. 4.2 C Granuloma faciale (high mag.).

Differential diagnosis

1. Other diseases with neutrophils in the dermis (1.30).
2. Other diseases with eosinophils in the dermis (1.31).
3. Other diseases with nodular or diffuse dermatitis (1.91).

4.3 Erythema elevatum diutinum (EED)

(see Fig. 4.3A–C)
Rare, *firm red to yellow–brown plaques* (1.151), usually on *extensor extremities*, especially on the elbows (1.32), knees, and dorsal hands and feet (1.56). It is usually not associated with systemic vasculitis, but sometimes can occur with rheumatologic disorders or HIV infection (14.12). Some patients have monoclonal gammopathy (1.80).

- Epidermis usually unremarkable
- *Leukocytoclastic vasculitis* (less apparent in older lesions)
- *Fibrosis* or lipid deposits (cholesterol clefts or "extracellular cholesterolosis") in older lesions

Differential diagnosis

1. Other diseases with neutrophils in the dermis (1.30) or fibrosing disorders (1.125).

4.4 Polyarteritis nodosa (periarteritis nodosa, PAN)

(see Fig. 4.4A–C)
Uncommon systemic illness, with constitutional symptoms, or limited to skin (*cutaneous PAN*). The systemic form of the disease may involve severe *kidney*, *heart*, *brain*, or *abdominal arteritis* or *aneurysms* (detected by arteriography), potentially resulting in death. Skin lesions include urticarial lesions, purpura (1.120), painful red nodules (1.96), livedo reticularis (3.10), or digital infarctions. Patients with systemic disease often have hepatitis B or C (14.7), cryoglobulinemia (4.9), or autoantibodies such as ANCA.

- Epidermis normal, necrotic, or ulcerated
- Leukocytoclastic *vasculitis of small to medium arteries* of deep dermis or subcutaneous fat
- Intimal proliferation and thrombi sometimes (1.137)
- Fibrosis in older lesions

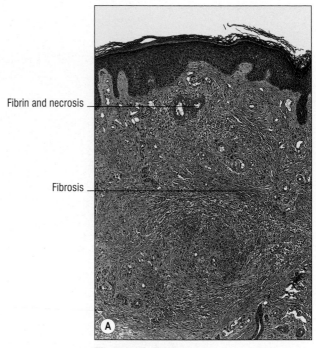

Fibrin and necrosis
Fibrosis

Fig. 4.3 A Erythema elevatum diutinum (low mag.).

Differential diagnosis

1. Churg–Strauss syndrome (4.5): asthma, p-ANCA antibodies (perinuclear antineutrophil cytoplasmic antibodies), more eosinophils in blood and skin, smaller vessels involved, and more granulomatous.
2. Wegener's granulomatosis and microscopic polyarteritis (4.6).
3. Kawasaki's disease (14.10): has PAN-like arteritis in the coronary arteries, but not in the skin.
4. Other causes of vasculitis (1.145).
5. Panniculitis (1.101) can be similar if the involved artery is not found. Erythema induratum (16.6) is more granulomatous and involves veins instead of arteries. Superficial thrombophlebitis (16.7) also involves veins.

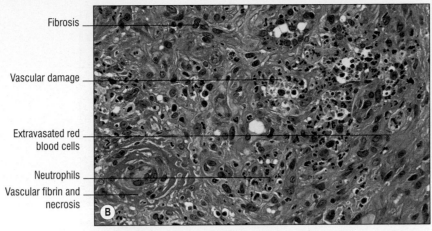

Fibrosis

Vascular damage

Extravasated red
blood cells

Neutrophils

Vascular fibrin and
necrosis

Fig. 4.3 B Erythema elevatum diutinum (high mag.).

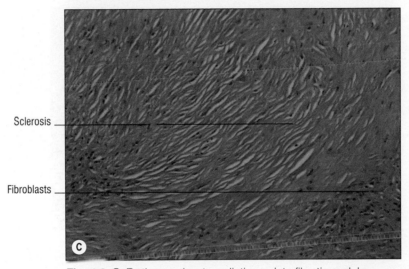

Sclerosis

Fibroblasts

Fig. 4.3 C Erythema elevatum diutinum, late fibrotic nodule.

4.5 Churg–Strauss syndrome (CSS, allergic granulomatosis)

Uncommon vasculitis of young adults, with *asthma*, *peripheral eosinophilia* (1.34), *p-ANCA*. Skin lesions vary: petechiae, *purpura* (1.120), red nodules, or ulcers (1.142).

P
- Epidermis normal, necrotic, or ulcerated
- *Neutrophilic vasculitis* (4.1) of small vessels
- *Many eosinophils* in the dermis
- *Granulomatous* inflammation and necrosis within blood vessels and in surrounding dermis and subcutaneous tissue, often *palisading*
- Thrombi (1.137) or extravasated erythrocytes sometimes (1.40)

Differential diagnosis

1. Polyarteritis nodosa (4.4).
2. Wegener's granulomatosis (4.6).
3. Systemic granuloma annulare (7.1): considerable overlap with CSS.
4. Other granulomatous diseases (1.51), especially those that palisade (1.51) and granulomatous vasculitis (1.51).
5. Well's syndrome (3.8).

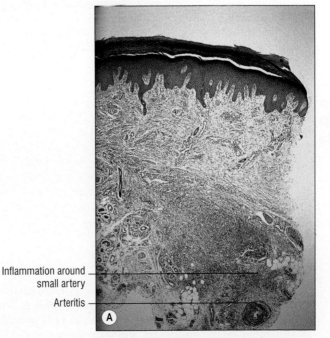

Inflammation around
small artery

Arteritis

Fig. 4.4 A Polyarteritis nodosa (low mag.).

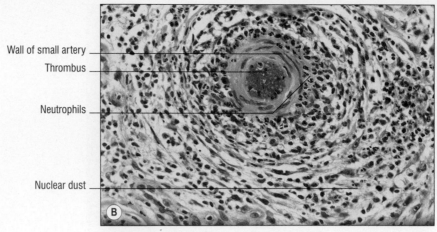

Wall of small artery

Thrombus

Neutrophils

Nuclear dust

B

Fig. 4.4 B Polyarteritis nodosa (high mag.).

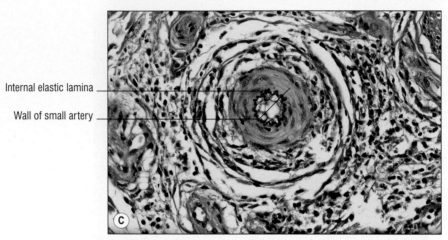

Internal elastic lamina

Wall of small artery

C

Fig. 4.4 C Polyarteritis nodosa (VVG stain demonstrating internal elastic lamina of artery).

4.6 Wegener's granulomatosis (WG)

(see Fig. 4.6A,B)

Uncommon systemic granulomatous vasculitis mainly with *sinusitis*, *pulmonary* disease, *nephritis*, and *c-ANCA* antibodies (cytoplasmic antineutrophil cytoplasmic antibodies). Cutaneous palpable purpura (1.120), necrotic nodules, or ulcers (1.141) occur in one-third of patients.

P
- Epidermis often necrotic or ulcerated
- Non-specific perivascular inflammation in some cases
- *Vasculitis* of small arteries and veins involving neutrophils, lymphocytes, plasma cells, and (rarely) eosinophils
- *Granulomatous* inflammation in blood vessels and in surrounding dermis often, sometimes palisading
- Thrombi often (1.137), resulting in extensive necrosis
- Extravasation of erythrocytes (1.40)

Variation

1. Microscopic polyarteritis (microscopic polyangiitis): acute viral-like syndrome of adults, neutrophilic vasculitis of arterioles as well as venules (4.1) mainly separated as an "entity" by regular presence of p-ANCA (c-ANCA antibodies are also common), and kidney disease. Pulmonary disease and palpable purpura of

skin occur in one-third of patients. Perhaps is an artificial category.

Differential diagnosis

Skin lesions of WG may be pathologically indistinguishable from other types of vasculitis (often just like any ordinary non-granulomatous leukocytoclastic vasculitis), and prominent sinopulmonary involvement with c-ANCA may be needed to make a distinction.

1. Allergic granulomatosis of Churg–Strauss (4.5): asthma, no sinus involvement, more likely to have p-ANCA than c-ANCA, more palisading granulomas, more eosinophils both in blood and skin usually.
2. Palisading granulomas, granulomatous vasculitis, and other granulomas (1.51).
3. Polyarteritis nodosa (4.4): no sinopulmonary disease, less likely to have ANCA, involves small and medium arteries, less granulomatous.
4. Lymphomatoid granulomatosis (24.6): clinical features different, CD56 positive atypical lymphocytes, less granulomatous.

4.7 Lymphocytic vasculitis

(see Fig. 4.7)

This nebulous term has been used for diseases in which there is a predominant lymphocytic infiltrate within or tightly

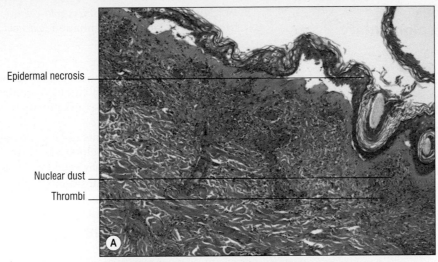

Epidermal necrosis

Nuclear dust

Thrombi

Fig. 4.6 A Wegener's granulomatosis (low mag.).

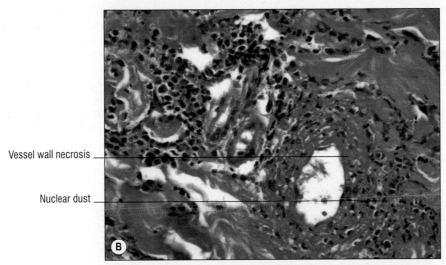

Vessel wall necrosis

Nuclear dust

Fig. 4.6 B Wegener's granulomatosis (high mag.).

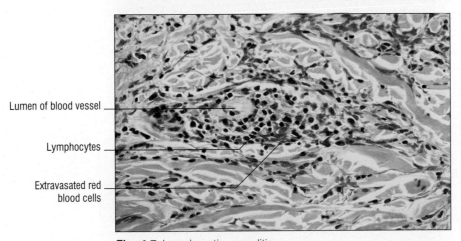

Lumen of blood vessel

Lymphocytes

Extravasated red blood cells

Fig. 4.7 Lymphocytic vasculitis.

arranged around vessel walls in combination with red blood cell extravasation (as opposed to the more usual neutrophilic vasculitis (4.1). Examples include purpura pigmentosa chronica, erythema multiforme, pityriasis lichenoides, some drug eruptions, Sjögren's syndrome, some viral exanthems, some Rickettsial infections, and lymphomatoid papulosis.

There is only a vague difference between lymphocytic vasculitis and any other perivascular dermatitis (1.109) with extravasated erythrocytes (1.40). Because vessel wall damage as defined at the beginning of this chapter rarely occurs in lymphocytic vasculitis, we prefer to use the term rarely or not at all.

4.8 Purpura pigmentosa chronica (progressive pigmentary purpura, capillaritis)

(see Fig. 4.8A,B)
Common, idiopathic, usually *macular purpuric eruption* of the *legs* (1.67), harmless, and not associated with systemic disease.

- Epidermis usually normal, sometimes spongiosis or focal parakeratosis
- *Extravasated erythrocytes*, endothelial swelling, and *perivascular lymphocytes* (so-called lymphocytic vasculitis, 4.7)
- Hemosiderin in older lesions (1.58)

Variations

1. Schamberg's disease: *cayenne pepper* appearance of petechiae and brown speckles.
2. Purpura annularis telangiectodes (Majocchi's disease, not to be confused with Majocchi's granuloma, 13.1): *annular* (1.5) purpuric macules.
3. Pigmented purpuric lichenoid dermatitis of Gougerot and Blum: *lichenoid* inflammatory reaction (1.72) instead of perivascular.
4. Eczematid-like purpura of Doucas and Kapetanakis: more *scale and spongiosis* (1.132).

5. Lichen aureus: more solitary, *gold-colored*, often *solitary* macule or plaque, inflammation *lichenoid*.

Differential diagnosis

1. Stasis dermatitis (2.1): more edema, venous insufficiency spongiosis or acanthosis, vascular proliferation mainly in superficial dermis, less inflammation, more fibrosis in late lesions.
2. Leukocytoclastic vasculitis (4.1): more palpable, more neutrophils, necrosis of blood vessel walls.
3. Other diseases with extravasated erythrocytes (1.40).
4. Other diseases with hemosiderin deposits (1.58).
5. Other diseases with perivascular lymphocytes (1.109).

4.9 Cryoglobulinemia

(see Fig. 4.9)
Uncommon, palpable purpura (1.120), urticarial papules, livedo reticularis (3.10), acral cyanosis, *painful ulcers* (1.142), or digital gangrene, especially on legs (1.67) and *acral skin*, associated with polyarthralgia, kidney disease, and involvement of other organs. Due to cryoglobulins, which are immunoglobulins that precipitate when serum is cooled, redissolving when warmed. Cryoglobulins and closely related cryofibrinogens can both be measured by generally available lab testing. Histology depends upon the type of cryoglobulins. Type I (monoclonal) cryoglobulinemia has the histologic findings below, and is usually associated with underlying lymphoma

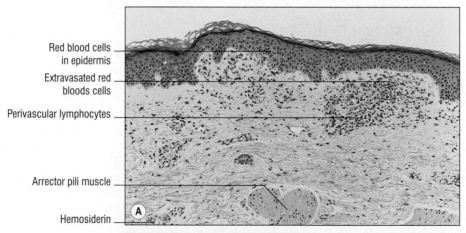

Red blood cells in epidermis
Extravasated red bloods cells
Perivascular lymphocytes
Arrector pili muscle
Hemosiderin

Fig. 4.8 A Schamberg's disease.

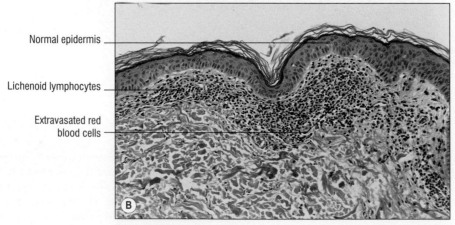

Normal epidermis
Lichenoid lymphocytes
Extravasated red blood cells

Fig. 4.8 B Lichen aureus.

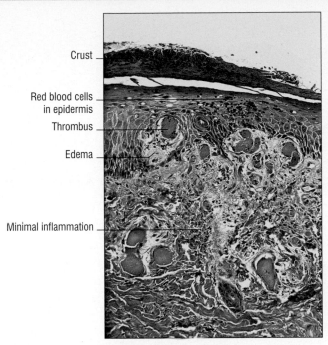

Crust

Red blood cells
in epidermis

Thrombus

Edema

Minimal inflammation

Fig. 4.9 Cryoglobulinemia.

(Chapter 24), myeloma (24.12), Waldenstrom's macroglobulinemia (24.12), or chronic lymphocytic leukemia (24.16). Type II (mixed monoclonal and polyclonal) and type III (polyclonal) cryoglobulinemia have histologic features identical to leukocytoclastic vasculitis (4.1), and are usually associated with rheumatologic disorders, hepatitis, and Epstein–Barr virus.

- Epidermis normal, necrotic (1.86), or ulcerated (1.142)
- *Thrombi* and precipitated cryoglobulin in dermal blood vessels
- Extravasated erythrocytes (1.40)
- Sparse perivascular lymphocytes sometimes (usually not a true vasculitis in the monoclonal type of cryoglobulinemia)

Differential diagnosis
1. Other diseases with thrombi (1.137) or vasculitis (1.145).

4.10 Degos disease (malignant atrophic papulosis)

(see Fig. 4.10A–C)
Rare idiopathic thrombotic disorder with small (average less than 5 mm), red macules eventually healing as *white, atrophic papules*, mostly on the *trunk* (1.141). Associated with *bowel or brain infarcts*, with a 50% mortality rate.

- *Atrophic epidermis* in old lesions (1.9), sometimes with hyperkeratosis
- *Wedge-shaped dermal infarct* with broad base toward epidermis
- Necrotic or absent adnexal structures
- *Mucin* in dermis in *early red macules*, or around edges of early white papules, sclerosis in older lesions (1.125)
- *Thrombosed arteriole* (usually in subcutaneous fat) with minimal inflammation, endothelial swelling, or intimal fibrosis. Difficult to find without serial sections

Differential diagnosis
1. Other white papules (1.150), especially scars (27.2), idiopathic guttate hypomelanosis (17.10), and early vitiligo (17.2).
2. Other diseases with mucin in the dermis (1.83).
3. Other diseases with dermal necrosis (1.88).

4.11 Behçet's syndrome (Adamantiades–Behçet's disease)

Rare idiopathic syndrome of *oral and genital ulcers* (1.82), *uveitis* (1.41) or other ocular findings, meningoencephalitis, superficial thrombophlebitis (16.7), gastrointestinal ulcers, and *cutaneous pustules* (may be induced by minor trauma, known as *pathergy*), most common in the Middle East and Asia. Genetic susceptibility appears to be increased with HLA B51.

- Epidermis with ulceration or pustule formation
- *Diffuse dermal neutrophils*, lymphocytes, and/or histiocytes, sometimes with vasculitis

Differential diagnosis
1. Behçet's syndrome is primarily diagnosed clinically rather than histologically.
2. Other diseases with neutrophils in the dermis or pustules (1.89), particularly Sweet's syndrome (3.7).

4.12 Pyoderma gangrenosum (PG)

(see Fig. 4.12A,B)
Uncommon "neutrophilic dermatosis" with violaceous nodules (1.148) resulting in *ulcers* with *undermined rolled edges*. Associated with inflammatory bowel disease (1.49), arthritis (1.7), and myelogenous leukemia (24.16). Pyogenic granuloma, a completely different entity (25.3), is also commonly abbreviated PG.

- Epidermis necrotic (1.86) or *ulcerated*, occasionally with pustules
- Pseudoepitheliomatous hyperplasia at edge of ulcer, sometimes (1.117)
- *Diffuse infiltrate of neutrophils*, lymphocytes, and histiocytes in the dermis, sometimes with vasculitis

Variations
1. Pyoderma vegetans (blastomycosis-like pyoderma): vegetating plaques with pustules, especially on intertriginous areas, face, legs, related to *Staphylococcus aureus*, or as a variant of pyoderma gangrenosum (4.12) with potential secondary infection, pseudoepitheliomatous hyperplasia with intraepithelial microabscesses with neutrophils and eosinophils (1.117), resembles pemphigus vegetans (5.4), except that direct immunofluorescence is negative.
2. Pyostomatitis vegetans: rare vegetating mucosal pustules associated with inflammatory bowel disease (1.49), considered to be a mucosal form of pyoderma vegetans.

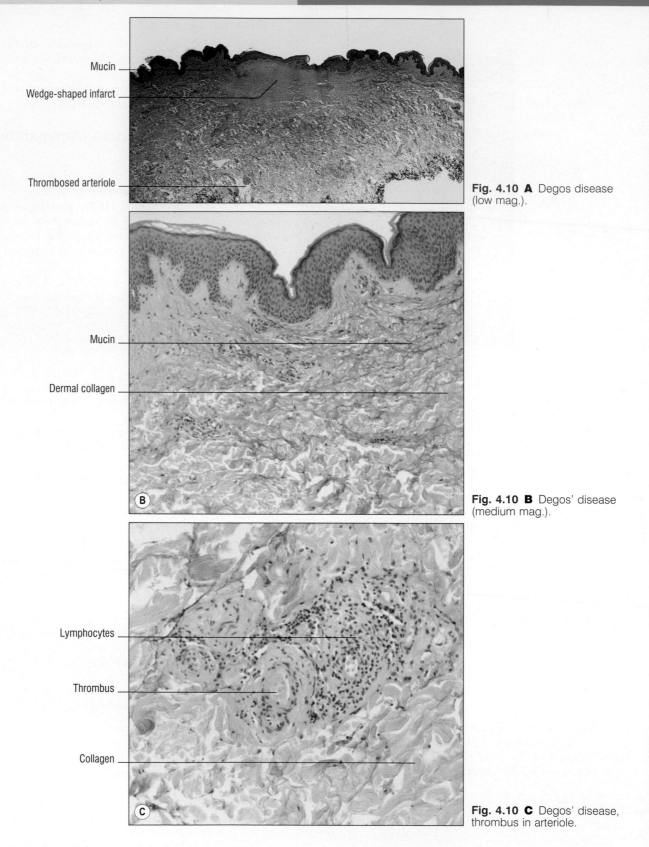

Mucin

Wedge-shaped infarct

Thrombosed arteriole

Fig. 4.10 A Degos disease (low mag.).

Mucin

Dermal collagen

Fig. 4.10 B Degos' disease (medium mag.).

Lymphocytes

Thrombus

Collagen

Fig. 4.10 C Degos' disease, thrombus in arteriole.

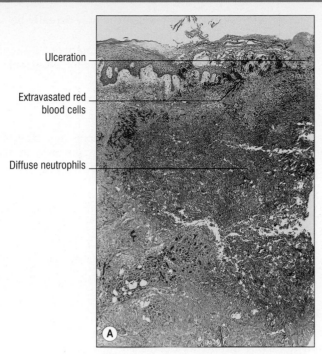

Fig. 4.12 A Pyoderma gangrenosum (low mag.).

Differential diagnosis

1. Pyoderma gangrenosum is primarily a clinical diagnosis, after excluding other causes of ulcers (1.142), especially infectious causes such as ecthyma gangrenosum (12.17).
2. Other diseases with neutrophils in the dermis (1.30), especially the closely related, but less ulcerative, Sweet's syndrome (3.7).

4.13 Atrophie blanche (segmental hyalinizing vasculopathy, livedoid vasculopathy)

(see Fig. 4.13A–C)
Uncommon disorder of the lower *legs* (1.67) in middle-aged to older females. Purpuric macules, often purplish (1.148) and reticulated (1.123), results in punched-out ulcers, healing with atrophic white (1.150) scars (1.125).

Differential diagnosis

1. Livedo reticularis (3.10): also has reticulated purplish macules, but classically has no vascular necrosis or ulceration.

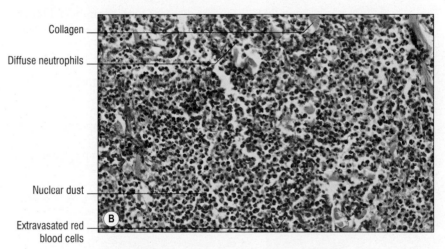

Fig. 4.12 B Pyoderma gangrenosum (high mag.).

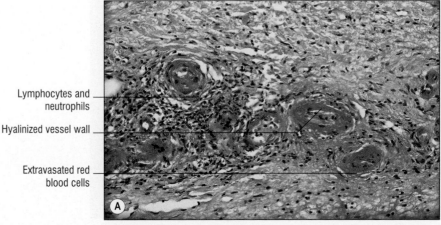

Fig. 4.13 A Atrophie blanche.

- *Atrophic* (1.9), necrotic (1.86), or *ulcerated* (1.142) epidermis
- *Hyalinized dermal blood vessel walls* prominent
- *Thrombi* often
- Extravasation of erythrocytes (1.40)
- Dermal fibrosis in older lesions
- Sparse perivascular lymphocytes or neutrophils (since inflammation is minimal, this condition is often considered to be a vasculopathy rather than a vasculitis)
- Direct immunofluorescence of perilesional skin reveals heavy homogeneous deposits of immunoglobulins, complement, and fibrin in dermal blood vessels

2. Stasis dermatitis and ulcer (2.1): larger ulcers instead of the small punched-out ones, associated with vascular insufficiency and edema, fibrin cuffing around vessel walls mainly in ulcer bed may resemble the hyalinized vessels of atrophie blanche, and may also heal with

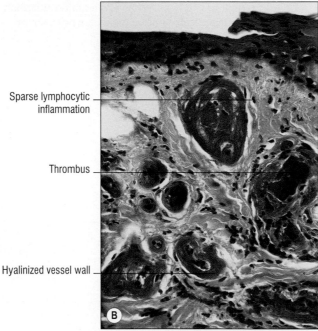

Sparse lymphocytic inflammation

Thrombus

Hyalinized vessel wall

Fig. 4.13 B Atrophie blanche.

similar white scars. Atrophie blanche may actually be related to stasis in some cases.
3. Other causes of vasculitis (1.145) or thrombi (1.137) usually do not have such prominent hyalinized vessel walls, healing with white scars on legs.

4.14 Coagulopathies

(see Fig. 4.14)
Several different types of coagulation problems may result in bleeding diatheses and non-inflammatory purpura in the skin (1.120).

P
- Epidermis is normal or necrotic (1.86)
- Subepidermal blister sometimes (1.147)
- *Thrombi* in dermal blood vessels, dermal necrosis in late-stage lesions (1.88)
- *Extravasated erythrocytes* in the dermis (1.40)
- Little or *no inflammation*

Variations

1. Idiopathic thrombocytopenic purpura (ITP).
2. Thrombotic thrombocytopenic purpura (TTP).
3. Disseminated intravascular coagulation (DIC, purpura fulminans).

Differential diagnosis

1. Other diseases with thrombi (1.137) or extravasated erythrocytes (1.40), such as thrombotic and embolic diseases (4.16).
2. Deep fungal infections (Chapter 13) and ecthyma gangrenosum (12.17).

4.15 Solar purpura

Common purpura (1.120), especially on the forearms (1.6), in sun-damaged skin, worse with corticosteroid or non-steroidal anti-inflammatory drug therapy, other drugs with anticoagulant effects.

P
- Atrophic epidermis, sometimes (1.9)
- *Solar elastosis* (9.1)
- *Extravasated erythrocytes* in the dermis (1.40)
- *No inflammation*

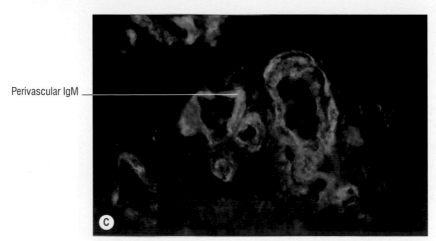

Perivascular IgM

Fig. 4.13 C Atrophie blanche (IgM immunofluorescence).

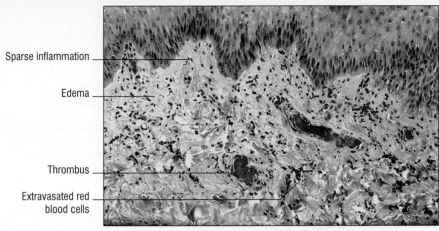

Fig. 4.14 Disseminated intravascular coagulation (DIC).

Labels: Sparse inflammation, Edema, Thrombus, Extravasated red blood cells

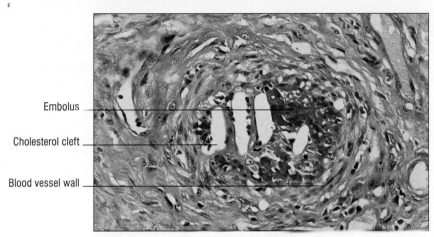

Fig. 4.16 Cholesterol emboli.

Labels: Embolus, Cholesterol cleft, Blood vessel wall

4.16 Thrombotic and embolic diseases

(see Fig. 4.16)
There are a variety of disorders with thrombi (1.137) or emboli in cutaneous or subcutaneous vessels. Skin lesions vary: livedo reticularis (3.10), purpura (1.120), foci of necrosis (1.86, 1.88), ulcers (1.142).

Variations

1. Lupus anticoagulant syndrome (17.6).
2. Cholesterol emboli: often occur after arteriography in older patients with atherosclerosis, often with livedo reticularis, cholesterol clefts (1.23) are found in vessels.
3. Sclerosing lymphangitis of the penis: cord-like (1.21) thrombosed vein near coronal sulcus, likely related to trauma from sexual activity.
4. Mondor's disease: superficial thrombophlebitis in a cord-like lesion (1.21) of the chest, either idiopathic or associated with trauma or rheumatologic disease.
5. Superficial thrombophlebitis of the legs (16.7).
6. Migratory thrombophlebitis (Trousseau's syndrome): this differs from the usual superficial thrombophlebitis of the legs (16.7) in that it is more migratory, is more common on the upper extremities and trunk, and is associated with internal malignancy (1.105).

4.17 Scurvy

(see Fig. 4.17)
Vitamin C (ascorbic acid) deficiency, often presenting as *perifollicular purpura* (1.120) with *corkscrew hairs*. Other vitamin deficiencies may coexist (2.1).

- Follicular plugging (1.47)
- Perifollicular erythrocyte extravasation (1.40)
- Mild to absent perifollicular lymphocytic infiltrate
- Hemosiderin (1.58) in older lesions

4.18 Coumarin-induced necrosis

Rare, acute onset of localized purpura, often with black necrotic eschars or blistering, especially in fatty areas of the trunk and lower limbs, as an idiosyncratic reaction to loading-dose treatment with coumarin or heparin, associated with protein C deficiency. May be severe and fatal, but may spontaneously resolve, and does not progress with continued coumarin treatment.

- Epidermal necrosis (1.86)
- Subepidermal blister (1.147) sometimes
- *Thrombi* in dermal blood vessels, dermal necrosis (1.88)
- *Sparse or no inflammation*
- Extravasation of erythrocytes in the dermis (1.40)

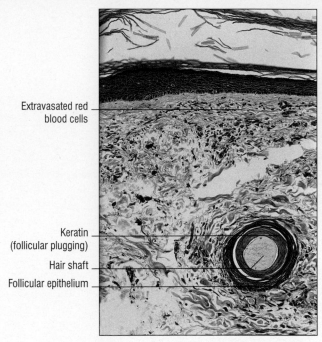

Extravasated red
blood cells

Keratin
(follicular plugging)

Hair shaft

Follicular epithelium

Fig. 4.17 Scurvy.

Differential diagnosis

1.Other diseases with purpura (1.120) or thrombi (1.137), especially DIC (4.14).

4.19 Buerger's disease (thromboangiitis obliterans)

Rare ischemic disease of upper and lower extremities in young male tobacco smokers, resulting in ulcers (1.142), gangrene, and frequent need for amputation.

- Thrombi (1.137) of medium sized arteries with occlusion of lumina
- Ischemia, necrosis, ulcers
- Mixed inflammatory cells in vessel walls

P

Differential diagnosis

1. Peripheral vascular disease from arteriosclerosis.

CHAPTER 5

Intraepidermal Vesicular and Pustular Diseases

The classification of vesicles and bullae are discussed in general in Section 1.147. Many of them are not discussed in this chapter. Some subepidermal diseases can appear to be intraepidermal when they have re-epithelialized. Intraepidermal diseases can also appear subepidermal if the blister blows out into the subepidermal zone or if there is prominent papillary dermal edema. The *most common causes* of intraepidermal vesicles are *eczema* (2.1) and *contact dermatitis* (2.2), but these diseases are in the chapter on eczematous diseases because they also commonly have that morphology. To diagnose an intraepidermal vesicular disorder, the pathologist pays particular attention to three things: (1) the site of the blister (*subcorneal, midepidermis,* or *suprabasal*); (2) the type of inflammatory cells involved (*neutrophils, lymphocytes,* or *eosinophils*); and (3) the mechanism of blister formation (*spongiosis* 1.132, *acantholysis* 1.2, *ballooning degeneration,* or *epidermolysis*). See 1.89 for other diseases with pustules in the epidermis (many are subcorneal).

5.1 Acropustulosis of infancy

(see Fig. 5.1)
Uncommon idiopathic *pustules on acral skin* of infants is a diagnosis made only after other causes of pustules have been excluded. It usually resolves within 2 years.

> **P**
> - Subcorneal pustule of neutrophils
> - Perivascular (1.109) neutrophils and lymphocytes

Differential diagnosis

1. Other subcorneal pustules (1.89), especially scabies (15.9), impetigo (12.1), candidiasis (13.4), and tinea (13.1).

5.2 Transient neonatal pustular melanosis

Uncommon idiopathic *pustular* eruption of newborns, mainly on the *chest*, often heals with *hyperpigmentation* (1.18) in patients with heavily pigmented skin.

Differential diagnosis

1. Erythema toxicum neonatorum (5.3): may be a related disorder, usually has more eosinophils.
2. Other subcorneal pustules (1.89).

> **P**
> - *Subcorneal pustule*, sometimes with eosinophils as well as neutrophils
> - Perivascular (1.109) neutrophils, lymphocytes, and eosinophils

5.3 Erythema toxicum neonatorum

Common idiopathic *vesiculopustular* eruption, especially on the *face and trunk* of *neonates*, often with bright red erythematous macular base, resolves in a few weeks. Rarely biopsied because pediatricians know what it is clinically.

> **P**
> - Subcorneal vesicle often centered upon a hair follicle, containing mostly eosinophils
> - Perivascular (1.109) infiltrate of mostly eosinophils

Differential diagnosis

1. Incontinentia pigmenti (11.6): rare, almost always female infants, vesicles more linear on the extremities, more warty in second stage, more spongiosis and the vesicles are deeper in the epidermis, more dyskeratosis in older lesions, not centered on follicles.
2. Transient neonatal pustular melanosis (5.2): more on the trunk, usually more neutrophils.
3. Eosinophilic pustular folliculitis (10.2): may be a related disorder, deeper involvement of the follicle, more chronic.
4. Other diseases with eosinophils (1.36) or pustules (1.89).

5.4 Pemphigus

(see Fig. 5.4A–E)
Group of *autoimmune* blistering diseases with acantholysis, most common in middle-aged adults.

Variations

1. Pemphigus vulgaris: almost always with *mouth* (1.82) erosions or ulcers, *flaccid fragile vesicles* on the skin, antibodies mainly to desmoglein 3 (finding not usually

©2012 Elsevier Ltd, Inc, BV
DOI: 10.1016/B978-0-323-06658-7.00005-1

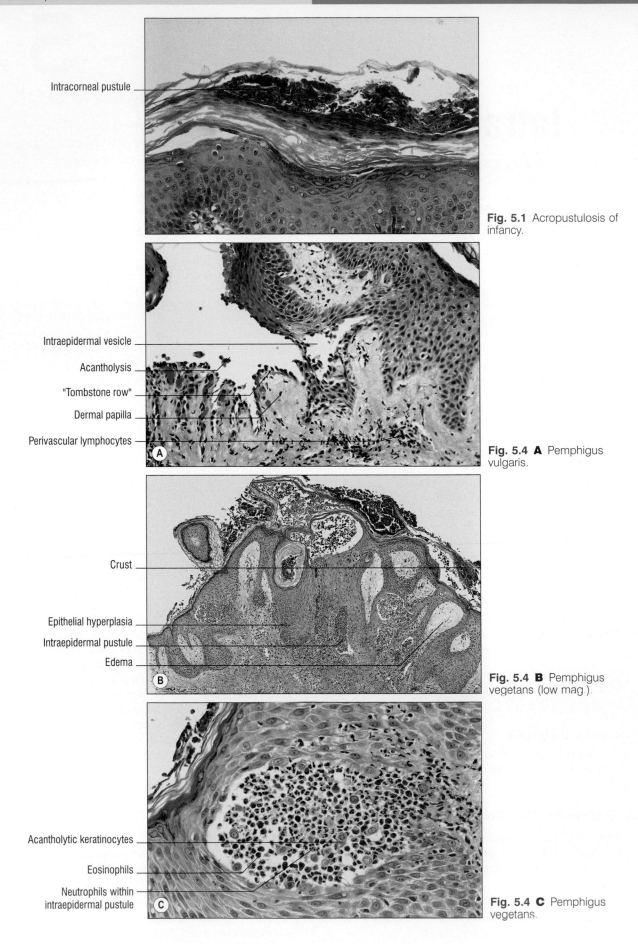

Intracorneal pustule

Fig. 5.1 Acropustulosis of infancy.

Intraepidermal vesicle
Acantholysis
"Tombstone row"
Dermal papilla
Perivascular lymphocytes

A

Fig. 5.4 A Pemphigus vulgaris.

Crust

Epithelial hyperplasia
Intraepidermal pustule
Edema

B

Fig. 5.4 B Pemphigus vegetans (low mag.).

Acantholytic keratinocytes

Eosinophils

Neutrophils within intraepidermal pustule

C

Fig. 5.4 C Pemphigus vegetans.

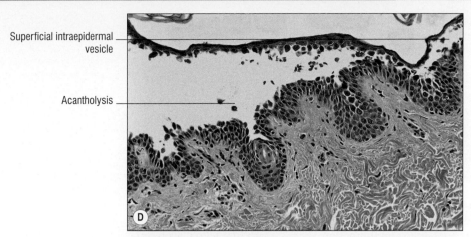

Superficial intraepidermal vesicle

Acantholysis

Fig. 5.4 D Pemphigus foliaceus.

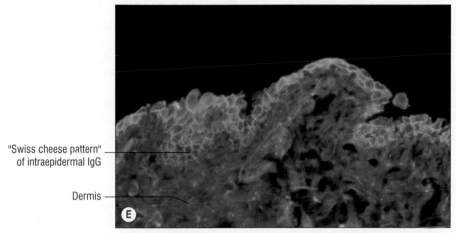

"Swiss cheese pattern" of intraepidermal IgG

Dermis

Fig. 5.4 E Pemphigus foliaceus (IgG immunofluorescence).

P

- *Acantholysis* in the epidermis, the exact location of which depends upon the variant
- Usually no dyskeratotic or very few necrotic keratinocytes
- Perivascular lymphocytes (1.109), *eosinophils* (1.36), sometimes neutrophils or plasma cells
- *Direct immunofluorescence* with IgG and complement within the intercellular spaces (*Swiss cheese pattern*), with staining most intense in areas of acantholysis. Deposits in pemphigus vulgaris and vegetans tend to be more prominent in the deeper layers of the epidermis, just above the basal cells, while those in pemphigus foliaceus and erythematosus are sometimes more intense in the superficial epidermis, near the granular layer

evaluated as a routine lab test), acantholytic vesicle in *suprabasal location*, leaving a *"tombstone row"* of basal cells attached to the dermal papillae (resembling gastrointestinal "villi"). The name tombstone may also refer to the frequent death of these patients prior to the corticosteroid era.

2. Pemphigus vegetans: rare, variant of pemphigus vulgaris, *vegetating purulent plaques*, usually in *axilla* (1.10), *groin* (1.55), or *inframammary* areas, with *pseudoepitheliomatous hyperplasia* (1.117), intraepidermal pustules filled mostly with neutrophils and eosinophils and a few hidden acantholytic keratinocytes.

3. Pemphigus foliaceus: uncommon less severe form of more *superficial pemphigus*, antibodies mainly to desmoglein 1, and sometimes also desmoglein 3, *"crushed cornflake"* plaques mostly on the *trunk*. (1.141) that may look papulosquamous (1.103) with occasional subtle flaccid vesicles, mostly on the trunk, usually without mouth involvement, with subcorneal vesicle or pustule with acantholytic cells (can be very subtle, fusiform or sparse at times).

4. Pemphigus erythematosus: rare variant of pemphigus foliaceus that involves the *face*, with bright red erythema and crusting, photosensitivity, *overlapping clinical features with lupus erythematosus* (LE), such as positive antinuclear antibody, direct immunofluorescence may also exhibit positive staining at the dermal–epidermal junction similar to LE, in addition to the usual intercellular epidermal staining.

5. Paraneoplastic pemphigus (paraneoplastic autoimmune multiorgan syndrome): antibodies to desmoplakin, or other plakins, or desmoglein 1 or 3, associated with *systemic malignancy* (1.105), prominent *mouth* involvement, often *resembles erythema multiforme* (3.2) clinically and histologically necrotic keratinocytes and less impressive acantholysis, immunofluorescence also *positive on rat bladder epithelium*, unlike other forms of pemphigus.

6. IgA pemphigus: very rare, antibodies to desmocollin, minimal mouth involvement, subcorneal or intraepidermal vesicles or pustules with minimal

acantholysis, immunofluorescence with intercellular epidermal IgA. Antibodies to desmoglein 1 and 3, and desmocollin 1 have been found.

7. Fogo selvagem (wild fire, endemic pemphigus foliaceus): endemic in rural Brazil, acute onset, sometimes familial, antibodies to desmocollin 1 or desmoglein 1.

Differential diagnosis

1. Other diseases with acantholysis (1.2).
2. Other intraepidermal vesicular diseases (1.147).
3. Pustular diseases (1.89).
4. Bullous pemphigoid (6.1) is more common, has larger tense subepidermal bullae, appears mostly in the elderly, and has a linear dermal–epidermal junction staining pattern.

5.5 Hailey–Hailey disease (benign familial pemphigus)

(see Fig. 5.5A,B)

Uncommon, *autosomal dominant*, deficiency of desmoplakin and plakoglobin, crusted *eroded plaques* on the *axilla* (1.10) or neck (1.86), occasionally more widespread. Vesicles are rarely seen. Related to calcium pump protein mutation ATP2C1 on chromosome 3 (compare with Darier disease ATP2A2).

■ Extensive acantholysis throughout the epidermis ("dilapidated brick wall")
■ Dyskeratotic keratinocytes sometimes (1.27)
■ Perivascular lymphocytes (1.109); eosinophils absent or rare
■ Direct immunofluorescence for immunoglobulins and complement is negative

Differential diagnosis

1. Other acantholytic diseases (1.2) are usually not accentuated in the axilla and neck, most are not genetically inherited, do not present as large crusted plaques, and usually do not have extensive acantholysis to the degree seen in Hailey–Hailey disease.

5.6 Grover's disease (transient acantholytic dermatosis, TAD)

(see Fig. 5.6)

Common *acneiform* (1.3) papulovesicular (1.147) to pustular eruption (1.89) of the *trunk* (1.141) resembling a *"heat rash"*, often idiopathic or occurring after sun or heat exposure, or fever, or in bedridden patients with occluded backs. Usually *self-limited* in a few weeks or months, but sometimes persistent and refractory to treatment.

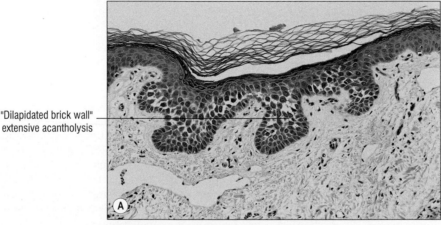

"Dilapidated brick wall" extensive acantholysis

Fig. 5.5 A Hailey–Hailey disease (low mag.).

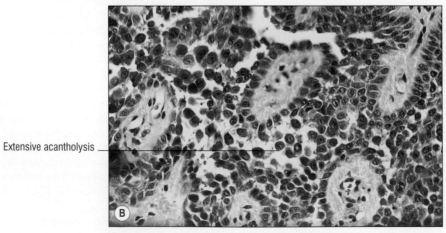

Extensive acantholysis

Fig. 5.5 B Hailey–Hailey disease (high mag.).

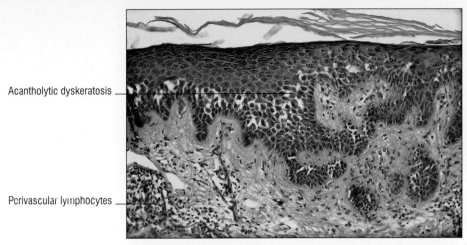

Acantholytic dyskeratosis

Perivascular lymphocytes

Fig. 5.6 Grover's disease.

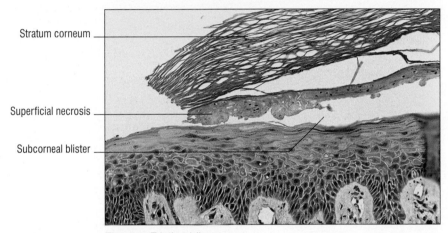

Stratum corneum

Superficial necrosis

Subcorneal blister

Fig. 5.7 Friction blister.

- *Small foci* of acantholysis (rarely extensive acantholysis), usually suprabasal, rarely subcorneal
- Dyskeratotic cells (1.27) often ("*acantholytic dyskeratosis*")
- Spongiosis (1.132) sometimes
- Perivascular lymphocytes (1.109), sometimes eosinophils (1.36)
- Direct immunofluorescence for immunoglobulin and complement is negative

Differential diagnosis

1. Clinical information may be needed to distinguish TAD from other acantholytic disorders (1.2), especially pemphigus (5.4), Darier's disease (11.3), and Hailey–Hailey disease (5.5) since the histology can be identical to any of these.

5.7 Friction blister

(see Fig. 5.7)
Common, but rarely biopsied, blister after friction, especially acral skin.

- Blister in superficial epidermis near granular layer (1.147)
- Degenerated keratinocytes adjacent to blister (1.86)
- Inflammation mild or absent

CHAPTER 6

Subepidermal Vesicular Diseases

A list of vesiculobullous diseases appears in section 1.147. Some subepidermal diseases can appear to be intraepidermal when they have re-epithelialized. Usually, the blister will have a smooth base in that case. The following diseases may sometimes produce subepidermal blisters, but are not discussed in this chapter.

1. Erythema multiforme (3.2).
2. Porphyria (8.1).
3. Lichen planus (2.11).
4. Amyloidosis (8.4).
5. Mastocytosis (24.17).
6. Lupus erythematosus (17.6).
7. Lichen sclerosus (9.5).
8. Graft-versus-host disease (17.3).

6.1 Bullous pemphigoid (BP)

(see Fig. 6.1A–D)
Somewhat common, autoimmune disorder mostly of the *elderly*, with pruritic (1.114) *urticarial plaques* leading to *tense bullae*. Antibodies are directed toward BP1 antigen (230 kD) or BP2 antigen (180 kD, type XVII collagen). Mouth and mucous membranes uncommonly involved.

- *Eosinophilic spongiosis* (1.36) sometimes, especially in early non-blistered red plaques
- *Subepidermal blister*
- Viable roof over blister, necrotic only in old blisters
- Perivascular lymphocytes (1.109) and *eosinophils* (eosinophils sometimes numerous); sometimes very sparse infiltrate (cell-poor pemphigoid). If numerous eosinophils are found in the dermis in an elderly patient, even without blistering, the diagnosis of pemphigoid is highly likely
- Superficial dermal edema (1.30)
- Microabscesses of neutrophils and eosinophils in the dermal papillae sometimes, as in dermatitis herpetiformis (6.5)
- *Direct immunofluorescence* of perilesional skin reveals linear IgG (usually IgG4) and complement deposits at the basement membrane zone in the lamina lucida (usually on the roof of blister, including salt-split skin preparations, but there are exceptions). Sometimes complement is seen in the absence of IgG

Variations

1. Localized Brunsting–Perry cicatricial pemphigoid (6.2): lesions are localized to a specific site on the skin, such as the scalp, with scarring and fewer eosinophils.
2. Pemphigoid gestationis (6.3): very similar disease, occurs in pregnancy by definition.

Differential diagnosis

1. Early lesions without blisters may resemble urticaria or other diseases with eosinophils in the dermis (1.36). Elderly patients with numerous eosinophils in their dermis, even without blistering, usually have pemphigoid rather than a drug reaction or other dermatosis with eosinophils.
2. Other diseases with subepidermal blisters should be considered (1.147), especially those with eosinophils, those with neutrophils, and those that sometimes are cell poor. Only epidermolysis bullosa acquisita (EBA) (6.6), cicatricial pemphigoid (6.2), and pemphigoid gestationis (6.3) have an immunofluorescence pattern similar to pemphigoid. Pemphigoid and pemphigoid gestationis deposits occur within the lamina lucida, while EBA deposits occur in the superficial dermis. With salt-split skin preparations, which produce separation through the lamina lucida, and with biopsies from the edge of blisters, bullous pemphigoid fluorescence is usually found on the roof of the blister, while in EBA, fluorescence is found on the floor of the blister.

6.2 Mucous membrane pemphigoid (cicatricial pemphigoid)

Rare autoimmune scarring erosions, *ulcers*, and *blisters* of *mucosal surfaces* (mucosal pemphigoid), especially the *eyes* (1.41) and *mouth* (1.82). The term mucous membrane pemphigoid is preferred by some over "cicatricial pemphigoid" because of the confusion with the Brunsting–Perry type. This probably is a heterogeneous group of disorders, and autoantigens vary, usually localizing to the lamina densa, with the blister in the lamina lucida.

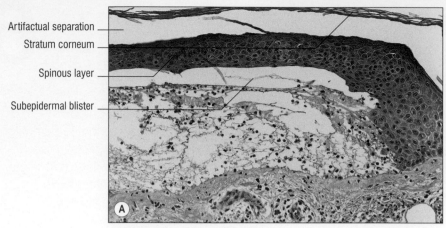

Artifactual separation
Stratum corneum
Spinous layer
Subepidermal blister

Fig. 6.1 A Bullous pemphigoid.

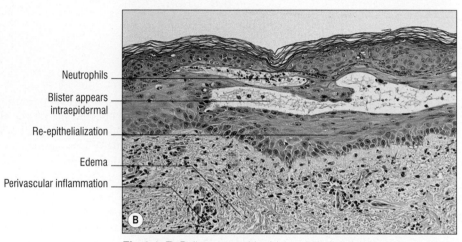

Neutrophils
Blister appears intraepidermal
Re-epithelialization
Edema
Perivascular inflammation

Fig 6.1 B Bullous pemphigoid (re-epithelialization).

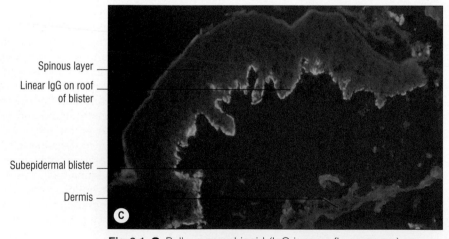

Spinous layer
Linear IgG on roof of blister
Subepidermal blister
Dermis

Fig 6.1 C Bullous pemphigoid (IgG immunofluorescence), staining on roof of blister, in contrast to EBA.

P
- Subepidermal blister
- Viable or eroded roof over the blister
- Perivascular lymphocytes (1.109) with variable eosinophils (1.36), neutrophils (1.89), or plasma cells (1.111, if on mucous membrane)
- Direct immunofluorescence is identical to bullous pemphigoid (6.1)

Variations

1. Localized Brunsting–Perry cicatricial pemphigoid: blistering, eroded, and scarring plaques limited to localized areas of the skin instead of mucous membranes.
2. Anti-epiligrin mucous membrane pemphigoid: antibodies are directed against alpha subunit of epiligrin (laminin-5), with probable increased association with internal malignancy. Immunofluorescence positive on floor of blister instead of the roof.

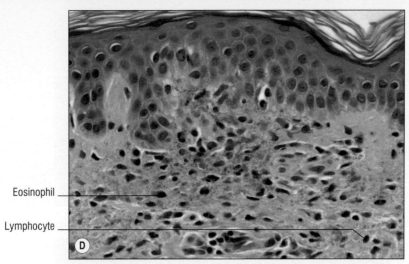

Eosinophil ___

Lymphocyte ___

Fig 6.1 D Pemphigoid prior to blistering. Many eosinophils are in the dermis.

Differential diagnosis

1. Other subepidermal blistering diseases should be considered (1.147), but bullous pemphigoid (6.1) resembles it most closely.

6.3 Pemphigoid gestationis (herpes gestationis, HG)

(see Fig. 6.3A,B)

The misnomer "herpes" is unfortunate, as it has nothing to do with herpes virus. Rare autoimmune disease associated with HLA DR3 and DR4, antibodies directed to BP2 antigen (180 kD, in lamina lucida and hemidesmosome) *vesicles, bullae, or urticarial plaques in the second or third trimester of pregnancy* on trunk and extremities, often *periumbilical* (1.143), controversial increased fetal morbidity or mortality is thought to occur, usually resolves within a few weeks of delivery. About 5% of infants born to affected mothers have self-limited blisters.

- Spongiosis (1.132), sometimes eosinophilic spongiosis (1.36) or intraepidermal vesicle
- Necrotic keratinocytes sometimes (1.86), especially at basal layer
- Marked papillary dermal edema (1.30), often *subepidermal blister*
- Perivascular lymphocytes (1.109) with *eosinophils* (1.36)
- *Direct immunofluorescence* is identical to bullous pemphigoid (see Section 6.1) except that IgG is present less often than *complement alone*

Differential diagnosis

1. Other diseases with subepidermal blisters (1.147).
2. Other pregnancy rashes (1.113).

6.4 Linear IgA bullous dermatosis

(see Fig. 6.4A,B)

Rare autoimmune bullous disorder with tense *blisters* often present along *annular red rings* (1.5), like a *string of pearls*, especially in the groin. Antibodies are usually found in the

lamina lucida (rarely sublamina densa), directed against portions of BP1 or BP2 antigens or type VII collagen as in EBA.

- Subepidermal blister (1.147)
- Sometimes microabscesses of neutrophils in the dermal papillae, as in dermatitis herpetiformis (6.5)
- Perivascular lymphocytes (1.109) and eosinophils (1.36) sometimes
- Direct immunofluorescence of perilesional skin shows linear staining of IgA (seldom with IgG also) with or without complement at the dermal–epidermal junction.
- Staining is in the roof of the blister with salt-split skin preparations.

Variations

1. Chronic bullous dermatosis of childhood: *childhood* form of the disease.
2. Drug-induced linear IgA bullous dermatosis (3.5). Vancomycin is one of the most common culprits.

Differential diagnosis

1. Other blistering diseases with neutrophils in the dermal papillae (1.147) include dermatitis herpetiformis (6.5), bullous lupus erythematosus (LE) (17.6), pemphigoid (sometimes, 6.1), and the neutrophilic dermatosis group (1.89).

6.5 Dermatitis herpetiformis (DH)

(see Fig. 6.5A–C)

Uncommon autoimmune vesicular disease, associated with HLA haplotypes B8 and DR3, presenting most commonly in *middle-aged men* with *very pruritic* (1.114) *papulovesicles* (often not apparent because they are quickly excoriated) on extensor surfaces such as *elbows* (1.32), *knees*, and *buttock*. Patients have *gluten-sensitive enteropathy* (1.49), often asymptomatic, and small bowel villous atrophy. Treatment is dapsone and/or gluten-free diet. Serum antibodies to epidermal transglutaminase are found in 95%, and to tissue transglutaminase in 80%,

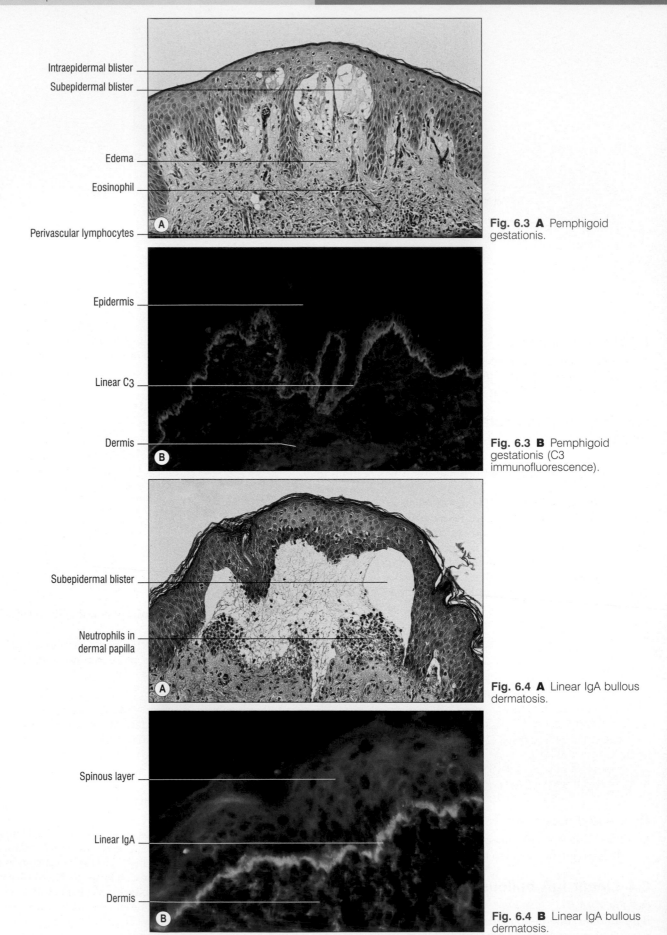

Intraepidermal blister

Subepidermal blister

Edema

Eosinophil

Perivascular lymphocytes

Fig. 6.3 A Pemphigoid gestationis.

Epidermis

Linear C3

Dermis

Fig. 6.3 B Pemphigoid gestationis (C3 immunofluorescence).

Subepidermal blister

Neutrophils in dermal papilla

Fig. 6.4 A Linear IgA bullous dermatosis.

Spinous layer

Linear IgA

Dermis

Fig. 6.4 B Linear IgA bullous dermatosis.

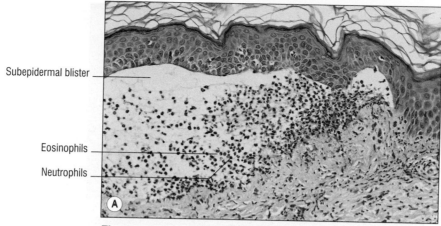

Subepidermal blister

Eosinophils

Neutrophils

Fig. 6.5 A Dermatitis herpetiformis (low mag.).

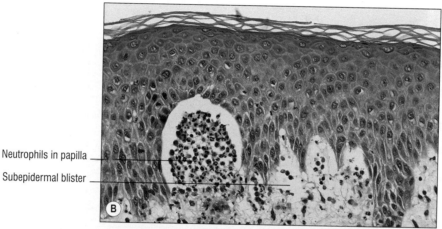

Neutrophils in papilla

Subepidermal blister

Fig. 6.5 B Dermatitis herpetiformis (high mag.).

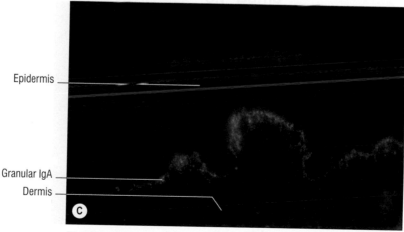

Epidermis

Granular IgA

Dermis

Fig. 6.5 C Dermatitis herpetiformis (IgA immunofluorescence).

of patients with active disease not on gluten-free diet. Patients with refractory pruritus of unknown origin sometimes are biopsied for direct immunofluorescence to search for DH.

- Neutrophilic microabscesses in the dermal papillae, with few eosinophils
- Small subepidermal vesicles
- Direct immunofluorescence taken from normal-appearing skin or perilesional skin has granular deposits of IgA in the tips of dermal papillae

Differential diagnosis

1. Other blistering diseases with neutrophils in the dermal papillae (1.147) include bullous LE (17.6), linear IgA bullous dermatosis (6.4), and pemphigoid (sometimes, 6.1) and the neutrophilic dermatosis group (1.89). LE almost never has eosinophils.

6.6 Epidermolysis bullosa (EB)

(see Fig. 6.6A–C)

Uncommon to rare group of blistering disorders that starts at birth or in *early childhood*, except for the EBA type.

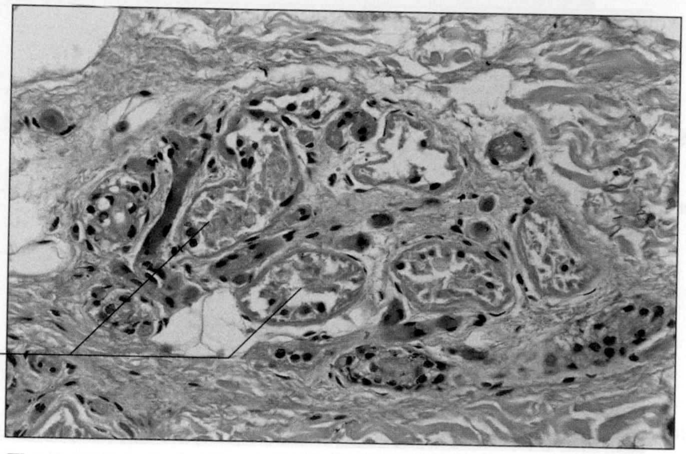

Necrotic sweatglands

Fig. 6.8 Sweat gland necrosis in ischemic bulla.

Variations

1. Coma bullae.
2. Phenobarbital bullae (other drugs also).
3. Pressure bullae.
4. Carbon monoxide bullae.

6.9 Bullosis diabeticorum

Uncommon, poorly defined disorder with tense bullae on legs, feet, or hands of patients with diabetes mellitus (1.26).

- Blister varies from subcorneal, intraepidermal, to subepidermal (intraepidermal location may be due to re-epithelialization)
- Inflammation usually sparse
- Negative direct immunofluorescence

Differential diagnosis

1. Other cell-poor subepidermal blisters (1.147).

CHAPTER 7

Non-infectious Granulomas

A discussion of granulomas and their differential diagnoses appears in section 1.51. Granulomas can occasionally resemble other non-granulomatous diseases with epithelioid cells (1.38).

7.1 Granuloma annulare (GA)

(see Fig. 7.1A–E)
Common idiopathic *non-scaly annular plaques* (1.5) and erythematous papules, most common on *hands* (1.56), *feet* (1.48), *elbows* (1.32), mostly children and young adults, spontaneously resolve in several years.

- Epidermis normal
- *Palisading granulomas* (histiocytes, giant cells) around small foci of mild connective tissue degeneration (*necrobiosis*) and *mucin* accumulation
- Often single-filing (1.128) or *subtle interstitial pattern* of histiocytes (macrophages) or giant cells between collagen bundles
- Perivascular lymphocytes often. Sometimes neutrophils or eosinophils are present

Variations

1. Perforating GA: keratotic papules or plaques, transepidermal elimination (1.140) of degenerated collagen and mucin through a canal in the epidermis.
2. Deep GA (pseudorheumatoid nodule): palisading granuloma deep in dermis or subcutaneous fat identical to rheumatoid nodule, but often in children, sometimes adults, with no evidence of rheumatoid arthritis.
3. Disseminated GA: numerous lesions disseminated, possible association with diabetes mellitus (1.26).
4. Systemic GA[157] (interstitial granulomatous dermatitis, palisaded neutrophilic and granulomatous dermatitis, extravascular necrotizing granuloma, Winkelmann granuloma): uncommon, macules, patches or plaques, sometimes annular or linear, associated with systemic diseases such as rheumatologic diseases, drug reactions,[143] HIV infection, and myeloproliferative disorders (1.105), may have interface dermatitis or neutrophilic vasculitis combined with the interstitial macrophages and giant cells, sometimes thick collagen bundles with basophilic hue, may overlap with Churg–Strauss granulomatosis (4.5).
5. Patch GA:[150] macules or patches may resemble morphea or patch stage mycosis fungoides.
6. Papular GA: unusual clinical appearance of papules instead of the usual annular plaque.
7. Actinic granuloma (7.4): often considered to be a GA variant rather than a separate entity.
8. Interstitial GA: the interstitial macrophages are present without much palisading or necrobiosis, so is more difficult to diagnose for the inexperienced.

Differential diagnosis

1. Necrobiosis lipoidica (7.2): mostly on the shins, less annular, more yellowish–brown, mostly with diabetes, more likely to have larger, more prominent areas of necrobiosis parallel to epidermis, more multinucleated giant cells, more sclerosis, plasma cells, epidermal atrophy, and no mucin.
2. Rheumatoid nodule (7.3): location over joints, often with rheumatoid arthritis, more likely to contain fibrin rather than mucin and is larger and deeper.
3. Other palisading granulomas and caseating granulomas (1.51).
4. Other forms of interstitial dermatitis (1.65).

©2012 Elsevier Ltd, Inc, BV
DOI: 10.1016/B978-0-323-06658-7.00007-5

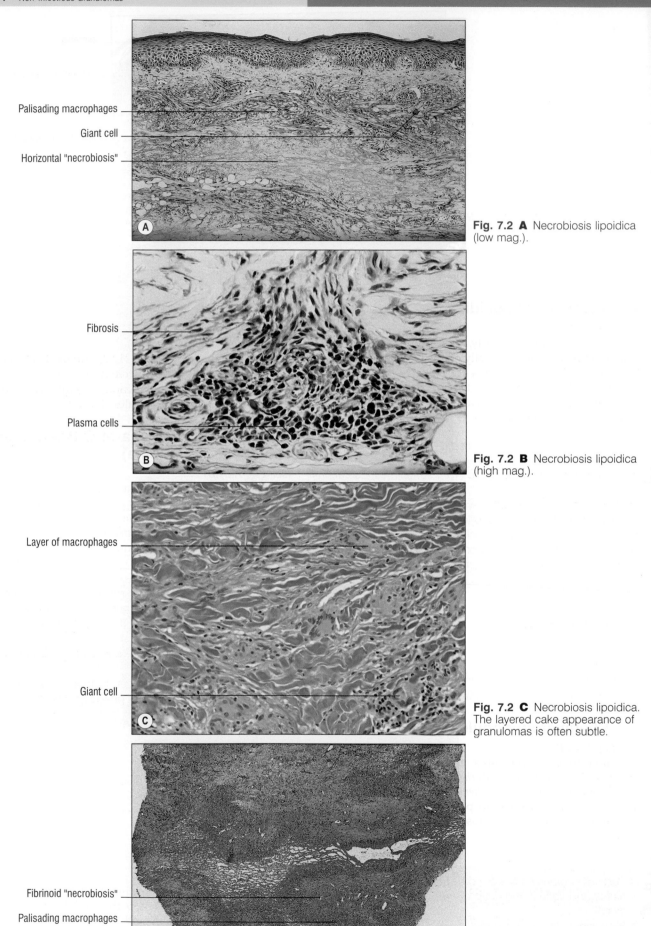

Palisading macrophages

Giant cell

Horizontal "necrobiosis"

Fig. 7.2 A Necrobiosis lipoidica (low mag.).

Fibrosis

Plasma cells

Fig. 7.2 B Necrobiosis lipoidica (high mag.).

Layer of macrophages

Giant cell

Fig. 7.2 C Necrobiosis lipoidica. The layered cake appearance of granulomas is often subtle.

Fibrinoid "necrobiosis"

Palisading macrophages

Fig. 7.3 A Rheumatoid nodule (low mag.).

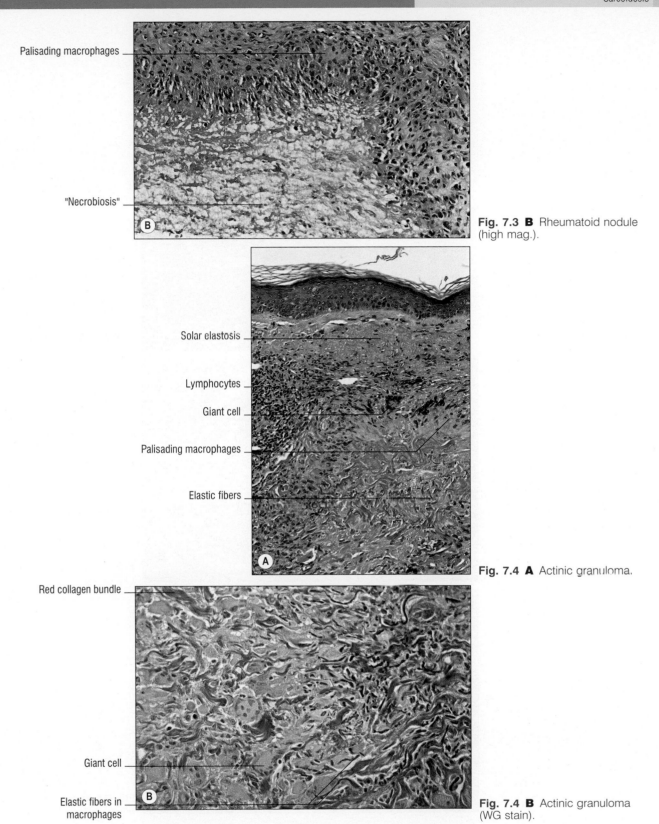

Palisading macrophages

"Necrobiosis"

Fig. 7.3 B Rheumatoid nodule (high mag.).

Solar elastosis

Lymphocytes

Giant cell

Palisading macrophages

Elastic fibers

Fig. 7.4 A Actinic granuloma.

Red collagen bundle

Giant cell

Elastic fibers in macrophages

Fig. 7.4 B Actinic granuloma (WG stain).

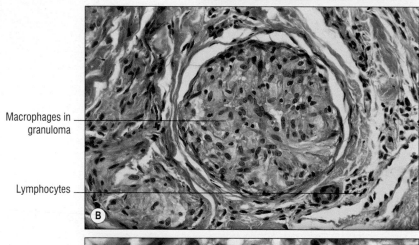

"Naked" granuloma

Sparse lymphocytes

Fig. 7.5 A Sarcoidosis (low mag.).

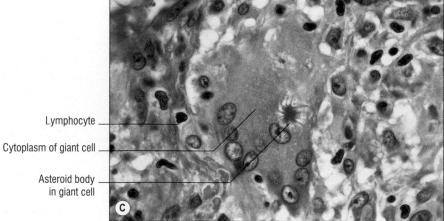

Macrophages in granuloma

Lymphocytes

Fig. 7.5 B Sarcoidosis (high mag.).

Lymphocyte

Cytoplasm of giant cell

Asteroid body in giant cell

Fig. 7.5 C Sarcoidosis (asteroid body).

material in some of the granulomas.[141] The *skin lesions are highly variable* (*a great mimic*), including papules, nodules, subcutaneous nodules (Darier–Roussy variant), annular plaques (1.5), ulcers, ichthyosis (11.1) with granulomas in the dermis beneath the epidermal changes. *Lupus pernio* refers to nose, cheek and ear plaques resembling perniosis (3.12). Other findings include polyclonal gammopathy on serum protein electrophoresis, elevated serum angiotensin converting enzyme (ACE) levels, hypercalcemia, and hypercalciuria. The Kveim skin test is generally no longer used.

- Epidermis usually normal, sometimes parakeratosis, hyperkeratosis, or acanthosis, such as in the ichthyotic variant
- *Non-caseating* (rarely caseating) well-demarcated, *granulomas* in the dermis or subcutaneous tissue, often (but not always) "*naked*" (relatively few lymphoid cells around the epithelioid cells)
- *Schauman bodies* (round, blue, calcified, laminated inclusions) or *asteroid bodies* (stellate, intracytoplasmic eosinophilic inclusions) sometimes present within multinucleated giant cells, but these are not specific for sarcoidosis. Don't confuse with asteroid bodies of sporotrichosis (13.11)

Variation

1. Loefgren's syndrome: a more acute, yet transient form of sarcoidosis with erythema nodosum (16.1), hilar adenopathy, fever (1.45), polyarthritis (1.7), and iritis (1.41).

Differential diagnosis

1. Of the granulomas listed in Section 1.51, lupus vulgaris (12.10), foreign body reactions (7.6) to zirconium, beryllium, or silica, granulomatous rosacea (10.1), late secondary syphilis (12.13) and tuberculoid leprosy (12.12) most closely resemble sarcoidosis. Since sarcoidosis granulomas tend to occur in old scars, the presence of foreign material may cause a misdiagnosis as foreign body granuloma.[141] There is no specific test for sarcoidosis, so it is a diagnosis of exclusion, especially after ruling out infectious granulomas.

7.6 Foreign body granuloma

(see Fig. 7.6A–N)

The most common "foreign body" granulomas in skin are those related to ruptured cysts or follicles (*keratin or hair* often identified). Most *tattoo pigments* appear black with H&E, 1.12), with granulomatous reaction only if there is an allergic reaction to them. Some foreign materials, such as *silica* from dirt or glass, *talc* from some deodorants or powdered gloves, and most *suture materials* are doubly refractile and become more apparent with polariscopic examination, while other materials such as *zirconium* (from some deodorants of the past) and *beryllium* (from fluorescent light bulbs of the past) cannot be identified without more sophisticated techniques, such as spectrographic analysis. *Starch* from most current examination gloves and deodorants is PAS and GMS stain

positive and produces a Maltese cross configuration with polarized light. Some foreign bodies result in more fibrosis with very little inflammation or granuloma formation. Exogenous lipid deposits from injected material produce "Swiss cheese" holes in the dermis because the lipid material is largely removed during processing of the tissue. Such lesions are called *paraffinomas* or *sclerosing lipogranulomas*, and lipid stains using frozen tissue, such as oil-red-O are positive.

- Caseating or non-caseating *granulomas* with *foreign material*
- *Fibrosis* or sclerosis (1.125) replaces granulomas in older lesions

Variations

1. Collagen-injection granulomas: *palisading granuloma* around collagen injected for cosmetic purposes.
2. Amalgam tattoo: pigmented lesion in the mouth from dental use of alloy containing mercury, silver, tin, copper, and/or zinc (8.18). *Black–brown (1.12) granules stain the collagen*, usually with very little inflammation.
3. Monsel's solution tattoo: *brown–black deposits (1.17)* of iron-containing pigment in the dermis from the use of ferric subsulfate (also known as ferric sulfate or ferrous subsulfate) for hemostasis, resembles melanocytic neoplasms (Chapter 20), but stains positive with stains used for hemosiderin (1.58). Ferric chloride is said to have a lesser propensity for staining the skin brown.
4. Aluminum chloride: applied for hemostasis, *macrophages contain cytoplasmic basophilic aluminum particles*, negative staining for PAS, GMS, Giemsa, or Gram stains, resembles parasitized histiocytes (15.1).
5. Paraffinoma: injection of oils, vitamin E, paraffin, or grease gun lubricant results in a *Swiss cheese appearance of holes* containing lipids that may stain with lipid stains on frozen section. There is variable fibrosis and granulomatous inflammation.
6. Sclerosing lipogranuloma: similar to paraffinoma, but this usually occurs on male genitalia (1.107, 1.126) after injection of paraffin or other oils, with more *sclerosis and granulomatous* inflammation along with the Swiss cheese holes.
7. Mercury: most often from a broken thermometer, spherical black globules (1.12).
8. Silicone: from ruptured breast implants or injected for cosmetic purposes, most of the dimethicone dissolves out during processing, leaving Swiss cheese holes with variable granulomatous or fibrotic reaction.
9. Black dermatographism: black or green discoloration (1.13) of the surface of the skin from the metal of jewelry.
10. Wood splinters: these appear brownish (1.17), with prominent cell walls, and variable suppurative granulomatous reaction. Sometimes fungi, especially dematiaceous fungi are found within the splinter.

Differential diagnosis

1. Other granulomatous diseases (1.51).

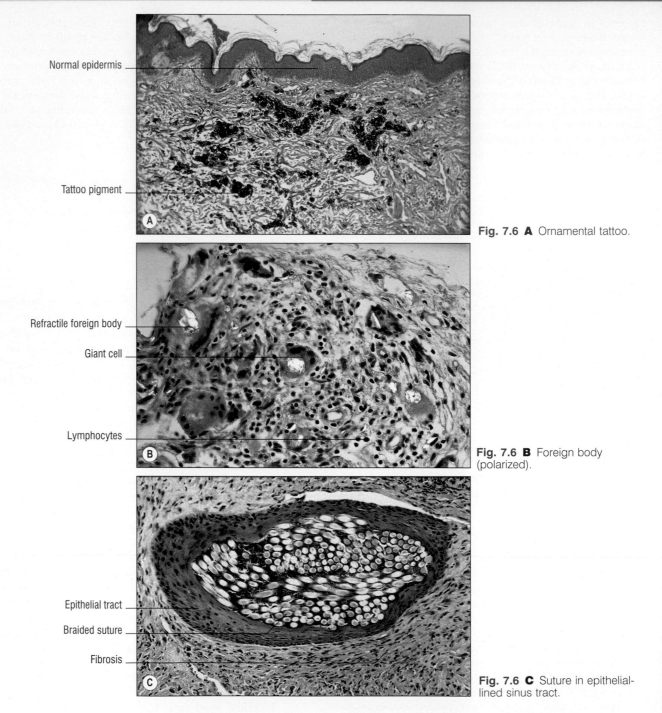

Normal epidermis

Tattoo pigment

Fig. 7.6 A Ornamental tattoo.

Refractile foreign body

Giant cell

Lymphocytes

Fig. 7.6 B Foreign body (polarized).

Epithelial tract

Braided suture

Fibrosis

Fig. 7.6 C Suture in epithelial-lined sinus tract.

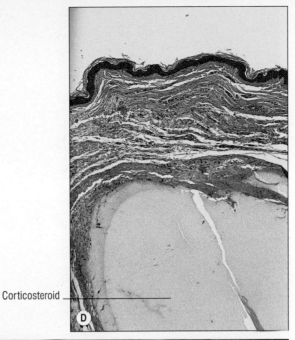

Corticosteroid

Fig. 7.6 D Injected triamcinolone.

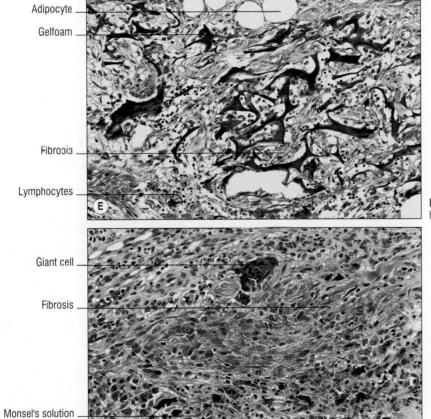

Adipocyte

Gelfoam

Fibrosis

Lymphocytes

Fig. 7.6 E Gelfoam used for hemostasis.

Giant cell

Fibrosis

Monsel's solution

Fig. 7.6 F Monsel's solution tattoo.

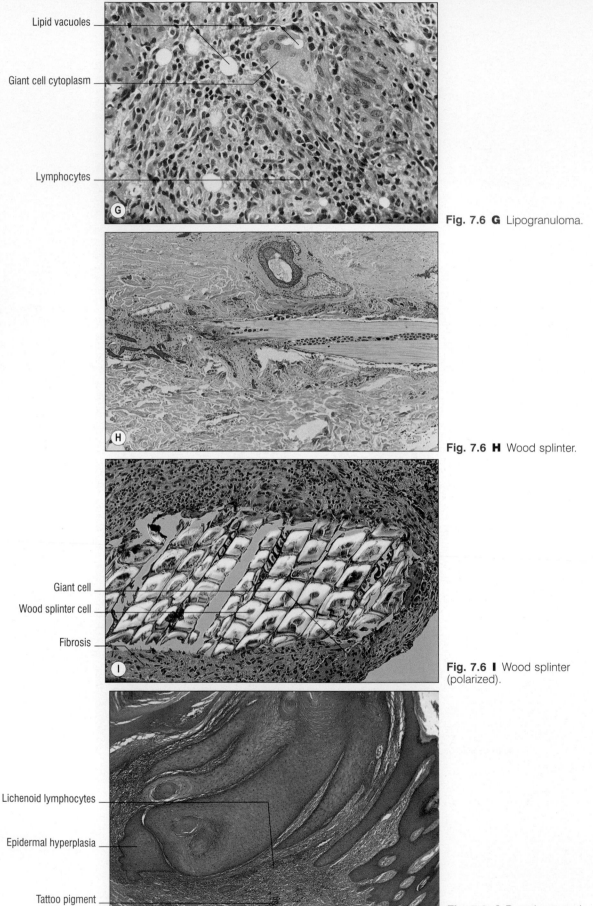

Lipid vacuoles

Giant cell cytoplasm

Lymphocytes

G

Fig. 7.6 G Lipogranuloma.

H

Fig. 7.6 H Wood splinter.

Giant cell

Wood splinter cell

Fibrosis

I

Fig. 7.6 I Wood splinter (polarized).

Lichenoid lymphocytes

Epidermal hyperplasia

Tattoo pigment

J

Fig. 7.6 J Reaction to red tattoo with epithelial hyperplasia and lichenoid inflammation.

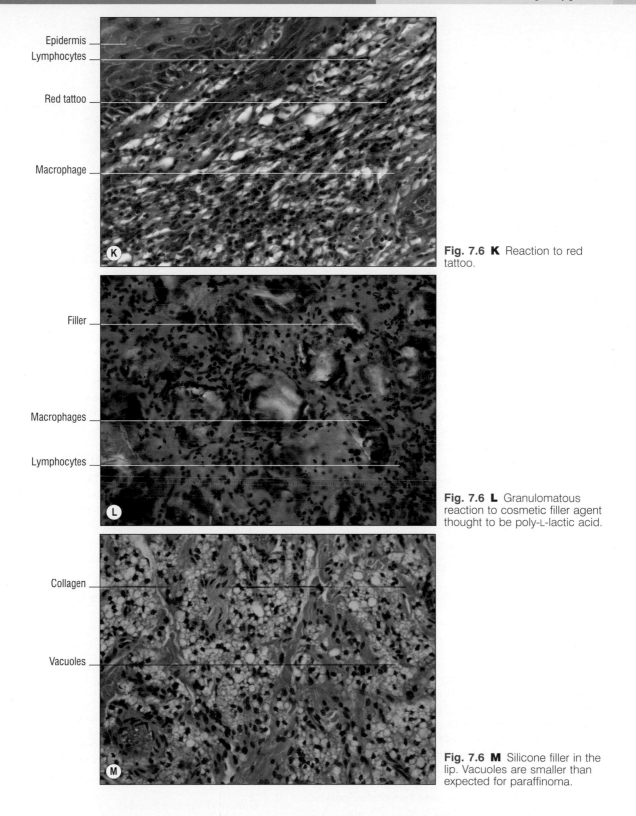

Epidermis
Lymphocytes

Red tattoo

Macrophage

Fig. 7.6 K Reaction to red tattoo.

Filler

Macrophages

Lymphocytes

Fig. 7.6 L Granulomatous reaction to cosmetic filler agent thought to be poly-L-lactic acid.

Collagen

Vacuoles

Fig. 7.6 M Silicone filler in the lip. Vacuoles are smaller than expected for paraffinoma.

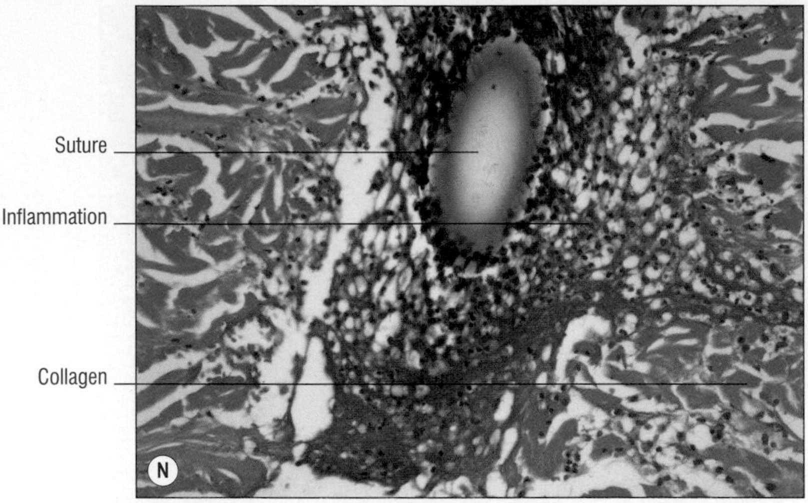

Fig. 7.6 **N** Reaction to monofilament nylon or polypropylene suture.

7.7 Cheilitis granulomatosa

(see Fig. 7.7A,B)

The *Melkersson–Rosenthal syndrome* is the rare triad of large puffy lips (1.74, cheilitis granulomatosa), lingua plicata (fissured scrotal tongue, 1.139), and facial nerve palsy. Many patients do not have the complete triad. The term *orofacial granulomatosis* is used as an encompassing term for the spectrum of localized lip swelling through orofacial swelling and mucosal ulceration.

P
- Epidermis or mucosa usually normal
- Interstitial or nodular infiltrate of lymphocytes and plasma cells (1.111) in an *edematous stroma* (1.30)
- *Tuberculoid granulomas sometimes subtle*, not always present, may impinge upon adjacent dilated blood vessels and lymphatics

Differential diagnosis

1. Cheilitis glandularis: this is a completely different disease, despite the similar name, lip swelling produces beads of mucus on the surface, sometimes with pain and a purulent discharge. Lymphocytes or neutrophils are found within or around dilated or metaplastic salivary ducts. Spongiosis may be present.
2. Cutaneous Crohn's disease: this can cause nearly identical lip swelling, with similar histologic findings, in addition to perianal lesions (1.108), and rare distant "metastatic" cutaneous lesions, but Crohn's disease involves the gastrointestinal tract (1.49), and patients with cheilitis granulomatosa deserve an evaluation of the GI tract, realizing that the skin lesions can precede intestinal involvement.
3. Sarcoidosis (7.5) can also have nearly identical lip swelling and histology, so other clinical findings may be needed to make the distinction.
4. Actinic cheilitis (18.8) and plasma cell cheilitis (2.11).
5. Ascher's syndrome: onset in childhood, acute swelling of lip (due to redundant salivary gland tissue), and swelling of upper eyelids (1.43, blepharochalasis and lacrimal gland inflammation), sometimes with thyroid enlargement (1.138).
6. Mucosal neuroma syndrome (26.3).
7. Other granulomatous diseases (1.51), including granulomatous rosacea (10.1), and collagen injection granulomas (7.6).

7.8 Multicentric reticulohistiocytosis (MRH)

(see Fig. 7.8A–C)

Rare systemic rheumatologic disease with *papular or nodular* skin lesions, and severe, sometimes *mutilating arthritis* (1.7). It is paraneoplastic in 30% of cases (1.105), with a wide variety of associated malignancies.

P
- *Nodular infiltrate of large true histiocytes* with abundant eosinophilic non-foamy *"ground glass" cytoplasm*, and positive histiocyte stains
- *Bizarre multinucleated giant cells*, often polygonal, with irregularly distributed nuclei in older lesions
- Mixed diffuse infiltrate of lymphocytes, and sometimes neutrophils or eosinophils

Variation

1. Reticulohistiocytic granuloma (reticulohistiocytoma): rare solitary dermatofibroma-like nodule, without systemic disease, histology identical to MRH.

Differential diagnosis

1. Other diseases with epithelioid cells (1.38).
2. Juvenile xanthogranuloma (7.10): children, foamier.
3. Dermatofibroma (histiocytoma variant, 27.1): histiocytes not so large.
4. Self-healing reticulohistiocytosis is a completely different misnamed disease, and is a variant of Langerhans cell histiocytosis (24.18).
5. Other histiocytoses (7.13).
6. Other juxta-articular nodules (1.91).

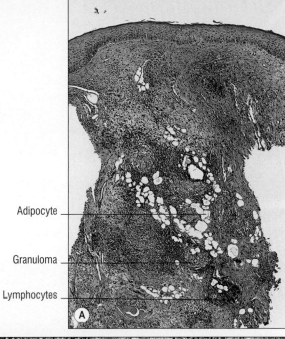

Adipocyte

Granuloma

Lymphocytes

Fig. 7.7 A Cheilitis granuloma-tosa (low mag.).

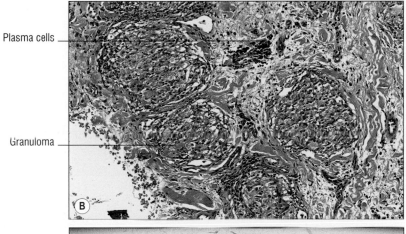

Plasma cells

Granuloma

Fig. 7.7 B Cheilitis granuloma-tosa (high mag.).

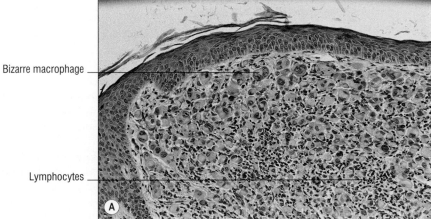

Bizarre macrophage

Lymphocytes

Fig. 7.8 A Multicentric reticulo-histiocytosis (low mag.).

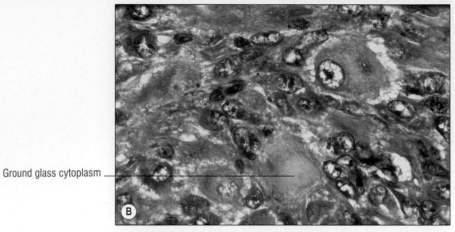

Ground glass cytoplasm ⎯⎯⎯

Fig. 7.8 B Multicentric reticulohistiocytosis (high mag.).

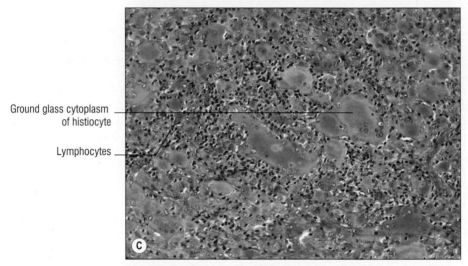

Ground glass cytoplasm
of histiocyte ⎯⎯⎯

Lymphocytes ⎯⎯⎯

Fig. 7.8 C Solitary reticulohistiocytoma.

7.9 Xanthoma

(see Fig. 7.9A–C)
Common *yellowish* (1.151) macule, papule, or plaque, often
multiple, often associated with *hyperlipidemia*.

■ *Foam cells in dermis* (positive for lipid with special stains
  such as oil-red-O)
■ Touton giant cells (1.46) sometimes
■ Small numbers of lymphocytes or neutrophils in younger
  lesions, especially in eruptive xanthomas
■ Fibrosis or cholesterol clefts in older lesions

Variations

1. Tuberous xanthoma: *nodules* of elbows, knees, buttocks,
   or fingers, which mostly contain cholesterol esters
   (positive with Schultz stain and refractile when frozen
   sections are polarized), resembles other juxta-articular
   nodules (1.91).
2. Tendon xanthoma: similar to tuberous xanthoma, fixed
   to *tendon* (Achilles or fingers), associated with
   hypercholesterolemia.

3. Xanthelasma: *eyelids* (1.43), associated with
   hypercholesterolemia in 50% of cases.
4. Plane xanthoma: macules or plaques in the axilla, groin,
   or palms, associated with hypercholesterolemia.
5. Normolipemic plane xanthoma: more widespread
   macules and patches around face or periocular, usually
   without hyperlipidemia, sometimes *paraproteinemia*
   (1.80) or myeloma (24.12).
6. Eruptive xanthoma: multiple *reddish–yellow* papules,
   especially of trunk or thighs, more rapid onset, more
   capable of spontaneous regression than the other types,
   contain mostly *triglycerides* which is sometimes
   extracellular, and more lymphocytes and neutrophils.

Differential diagnosis

1. Granular cell tumor (26.4): more granular (PAS positive)
   than foamy, cell boundaries less distinct, pustulo-ovoid
   bodies.
2. Lepromatous leprosy (12.12): different clinical
   presentation, holes at sites of globi, AFB stain positive,
   plasma cells usually found.
3. Other diseases with foam cells (1.46).

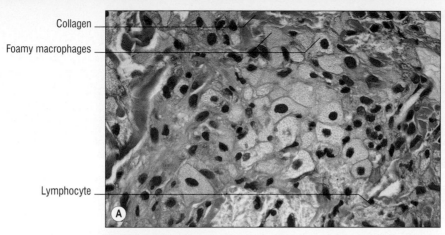

Collagen

Foamy macrophages

Lymphocyte

Fig. 7.9 A Xanthoma.

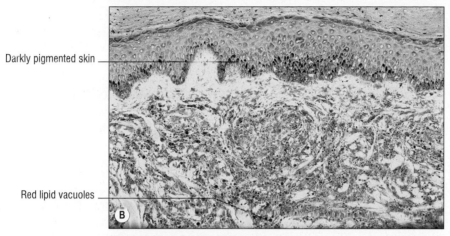

Darkly pigmented skin

Red lipid vacuoles

Fig. 7.9 B Xanthoma (oil-red-O stain).

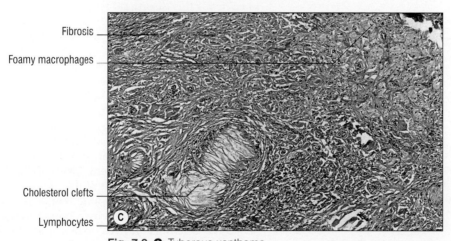

Fibrosis

Foamy macrophages

Cholesterol clefts

Lymphocytes

Fig. 7.9 C Tuberous xanthoma.

7.10 Juvenile xanthogranuloma (JXG)

(see Fig. 7.10)

Uncommon, idiopathic, solitary or multiple red to *yellow–brown nodules* (1.151), *mostly in children*, sometimes adults, *without hyperlipidemia*. Usually no systemic disease, rarely eye (1.41) or other organ involvement. Skin lesions usually spontaneously regress. Multiple JXGs plus café-au-lait macules can indicate neurofibromatosis type I (26.1), the combination of which creates a 20-fold increased incidence of childhood chronic myelogenous leukemia (24.16).

- Nodular or diffuse mixed infiltrate of histiocytes, lymphocytes, and *eosinophils* (1.36, eosinophils more common in younger lesions)
- *Foamy histiocytes and Touton giant cells* (1.46) in older lesions
- Fibrosis prominent in some older lesions
- Positive staining with CD68 and HAM56 (macrophages), and factor XIIIa (dermal dendrocytes)

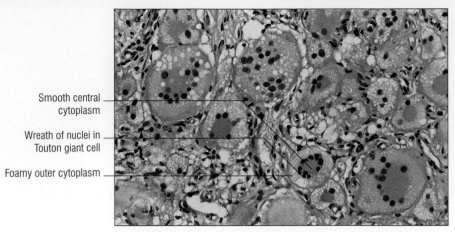

Smooth central cytoplasm

Wreath of nuclei in Touton giant cell

Foamy outer cytoplasm

Fig. 7.10 Juvenile xanthogranuloma (JXG).

Differential diagnosis

1. Other nodules in childhood (1.93).
2. Touton giant cells (1.84), if numerous, are characteristic for JXG, but are occasionally seen in other diseases with foam cells (1.46).
3. Langerhans cell histiocytosis (24.18): epidermotropism, reniform nuclei, positive for S-100 and CDla, unlike JXG.
4. Some of the other rare histiocytoses (7.13) are thought to be JXG variants.

7.11 **Necrobiotic xanthogranuloma (NXG)**

(see Fig. 7.11)
Rare, idiopathic, usually large, *yellow–brown to red–brown plaques*, may ulcerate, especially on *eyelids* (1.43) and trunk, associated with *paraproteinemia* (1.80).

- *Palisading granulomas* with areas of *necrosis* (more severe degeneration than the "necrobiosis" seen with GA or NLD)
- Cholesterol clefts common (1.23)
- *Foamy histiocytes*, *Teouton giant cells* (1.84) and foreign body giant cells, lymphocytes, plasma cells (1.111), neutrophils

Differential diagnosis

1. Necrobiosis lipoidica (7.2): usually on the shins, often with diabetes mellitus, more sclerosis than necrosis, usually no foamy cells, no Touton giant cells, no paraproteinemia.
2. Juvenile xanthogranuloma (7.10): usually children, more nodules than plaques, no necrosis or palisading.
3. Other diseases with foam cells (1.46), dermal necrosis (1.87), or palisading granulomas (1.51).

7.12 **Verruciform xanthoma**

(see Fig. 7.12A,B)
Rare, idiopathic, solitary plaque in the *mouth* (1.82), rarely on the scrotum or genitals, *no hyperlipidemia*.

- Hyperkeratosis, acanthosis, *papillomatosis* (verrucous)
- *Foamy histiocytes limited to submucosal or dermal papillae*

Differential diagnosis

1. Other diseases with papillomatosis (1.102), or foam cells (1.46). The few foam cells beneath the epidermis may be subtle and easy to miss.

7.13 **Other rare histiocytoses**

(see Fig. 7.13A,B)
There are several rare overlapping disorders of proliferating histiocytes.

Variations

1. Benign cephalic histiocytosis: children, red–yellow nodules mainly on the *head* (1.44), resolve in a few years. Diffuse dermal *non-foamy histiocytes* with sparse lymphocytes and eosinophils. The *worm-like or comma-shaped bodies* described by electron microscopy are not specific for this disorder. Probably a less lipidized JXG variant (7.10).
2. Progressive nodular histiocytosis: children or adults, widespread papulonodules, may involve the conjunctiva, mouth, or larynx, *without spontaneous resolution*. Foamy histiocytes, Touton giant cells, fibrosis, hemosiderin (1.58), *resembles disseminated dermatofibromas* (27.1), may be a JXG variant (7.10).
3. Generalized eruptive histiocytosis: *mostly adults*, disseminated brownish papulonodules, may involve mucous membranes, spontaneously resolves, but may recur, no internal involvement, histology like *non-foamy* JXG, probably a JXG variant (7.10).
4. Xanthoma disseminatum: young adults or children, disseminated yellow–red–brown papules, especially in *flexural areas* such as neck, axilla, antecubital fossa, groin, perianal area, may become confluent, may involve conjunctiva, mouth, or larynx, persists for years and then remits, *diabetes insipidus* common, rarely osteolytic bone lesions, histiocytes quite foamy, hemosiderin may be present (1.58), histology like JXG, probably a JXG variant (7.10).
5. Rosai–Dorfman disease (sinus histiocytosis with massive lymphadenopathy): rare, possibly due to herpes type 6 (14.7). Fever, anemia, leukocytosis, *cervical adenopathy*, polyclonal gammopathy, mostly in *male children*, with skin papules or nodules in 10% of patients. *Very large histiocytes* with abundant cytoplasm in masses (*S-100*+, CD4+, CD68+, CD25+, lysozyme+,

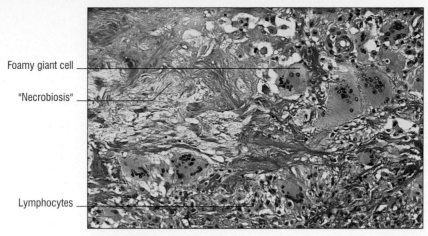

Foamy giant cell

"Necrobiosis"

Lymphocytes

Fig. 7.11 Necrobiotic xanthogranuloma.

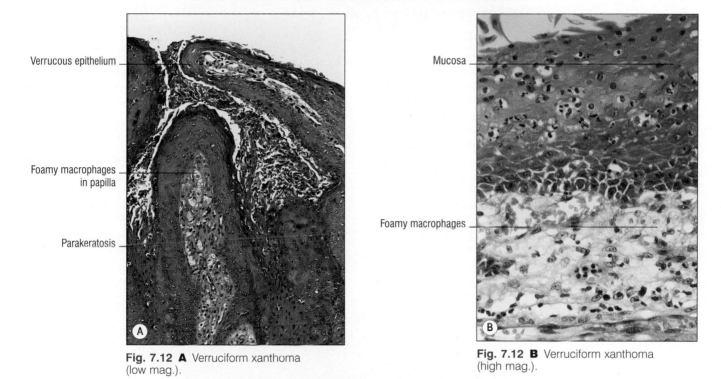

Verrucous epithelium

Foamy macrophages in papilla

Parakeratosis

Fig. 7.12 A Verruciform xanthoma (low mag.).

Mucosa

Foamy macrophages

Fig. 7.12 B Verruciform xanthoma (high mag.).

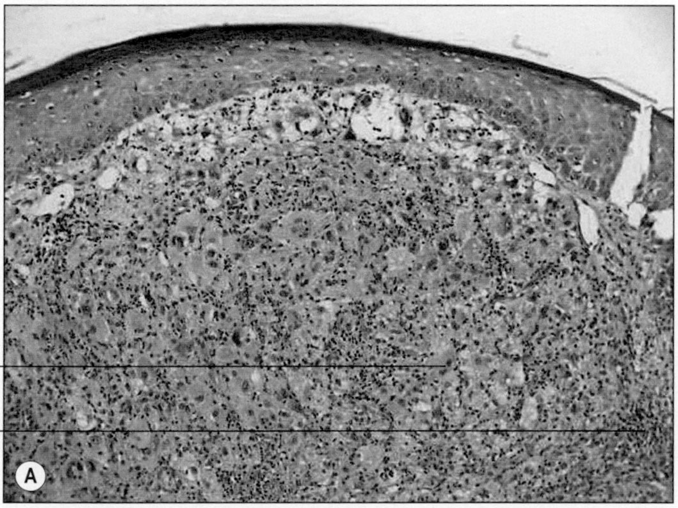

Histiocyte

Lymphocytes

Fig. 7.13 A Rosai–Dorfman disease.

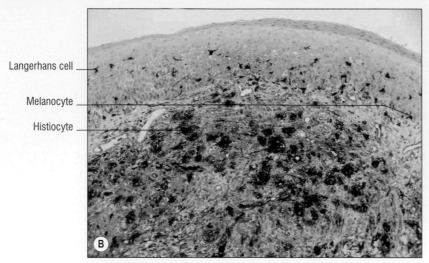

Langerhans cell

Melanocyte

Histiocyte

Fig. 7.13 B Rosai–Dorfman disease (S-100 stain).

CD1a-neg), multinucleated giant cells (1.84), *plasma cells* (1.110), *nodular aggregates of lymphocytes*, vascular dilation with polymorphous infiltrate in the lumina, *emperipolesis* (phagocytosis of nuclear debris, which is also seen in cytophagic histiocytic panniculitis 24.1, and rarely in melanoma and squamous cell carcinoma).

6. Multinucleate cell angiohistiocytoma: very rare, papules on the *extremities* and *dorsum of the hands* (1.56), more in *middle-aged females*, prominent *dilated blood vessels*, *floret-type giant cells* (1.84), perivascular lymphocytes, plasma cells, or neutrophils. The multinucleated cells are positive for vimentin, but negative for MAC387,

alpha-1 antitrypsin, factor XIIIa, S-100, and CD1a), but the stromal histiocytes are positive for vimentin, factor XIIIa, and CD68. The blood vessels are positive for the usual vascular markers.

Differential diagnosis

1. The above disorders are all considered to be non-Langerhans cell (non-X) histiocytoses, because the proliferating cells are true histiocytes (1.76), Langerhans cell histiocytosis and its variants (24.18) are S-100+ and CD1a+. Rosai–Dorfman disease is S-100+, CD1a-neg.
2. Other disorders with epithelioid cells (1.38).

Deposition and Metabolic Diseases

8.1 Porphyria

(see Fig. 8.1A–F)
Uncommon to rare group of porphyrin metabolism disorders. Most of them present as *photodermatitis* (1.110) with papules or vesicles mostly on sun-exposed skin.

Variations

1. Porphyria cutanea tarda (PCT): most common type of porphyria, uroporphyrin decarboxylase deficiency, uroporphyrins highly elevated in the urine, "tarda" refers to "late" (adult) onset of *vesicles*, papules, crusts, and *milia* in areas of scarring, most common on the *dorsum of the hands* (1.56), *malar hypertrichosis* (1.62), associated with *hepatitis* C (14.7), *alcohol* abuse, and *liver disease* (1.75):
    a. Subepidermal blister with viable roof, *festooning* of dermal papillae (very well-preserved papillae projecting into blister), and very little inflammation (*cell poor*).
    b. Caterpillar bodies (eosinophilic, linear, segmented basement membrane material resembling dyskeratotic cells, 1.27) sometimes found in the roof of the blister, not specific for porphyria.
    c. Sparse *hyalinized material around blood vessels* (PAS positive, diastase resistant), especially in papillary dermis, sometimes throughout dermis.
    d. Dermal sclerosis in late stages sometimes (1.125).
    e. Direct immunofluorescence: IgG and C3 around papillary dermal vessels with lesser staining at dermal–epidermal junction in the lamina lucida.
2. Acute intermittent porphyria (AIP): rare, porphobilinogen deaminase (hydroxymethylbilane synthase) deficiency, increased porphobilinogen (PBG) in the blood, acute abdominal pain, psychosis, neurologic disease, *no skin lesions*.
3. Variegate porphyria (VP): protoporphyrinogen oxidase deficiency, combined features of *AIP plus PCT*.
4. Hereditary coproporphyria (HCP): rare, mutation in CPOX gene, coproporphyrinogen oxidase deficiency, combined features of *AIP plus PCT*.
5. Erythropoietic protoporphyria (EPP): rare, ferrochelatase deficiency, photodermatitis with very few blisters begins in *childhood*, occasional fatal liver disease, free erythrocyte protoporphyrin elevated in the blood, *impressive deposits of hyalinized material* in the dermis, less blistering.
6. Congenital erythropoietic porphyria (CEP, EP, Günther's disease): very rare, uroporphyrinogen III synthase deficiency, severe *congenital mutilating "werewolf"* form with onset in infancy, red fluorescent teeth, extensive hypertrichosis, hemolytic anemia, splenomegaly, more hyalinized material in dermis than other forms of porphyria (1.35).
7. Pseudoporphyria: related to *hemodialysis* or certain *drugs* (3.5), especially non-steroidal anti-inflammatory drugs, tetracycline, and furosemide, nearly identical to PCT histologically.

Differential diagnosis

1. Other diseases with abundant dermal eosinophilic amorphous pink material (1.35) may resemble EPP, especially lipoid proteinosis (8.3) and amyloidosis (8.4).
2. Other subepidermal blistering diseases (1.147, Chapter 6), especially the more cell-poor ones such as epidermolysis bullosa (6.6), bullous amyloidosis (8.4), and some examples of bullous pemphigoid (6.1).

8.2 Colloid milium

(see Fig. 8.2)
Uncommon *grouped whitish papules* on *sun-exposed* skin (1.110) on the *dorsum of the hands* (1.56), face, neck, or ears in adults, or on the face in the very rare childhood form.

©2012 Elsevier Ltd, Inc, BV
DOI: 10.1016/B978-0-323-06658-7.00008-7

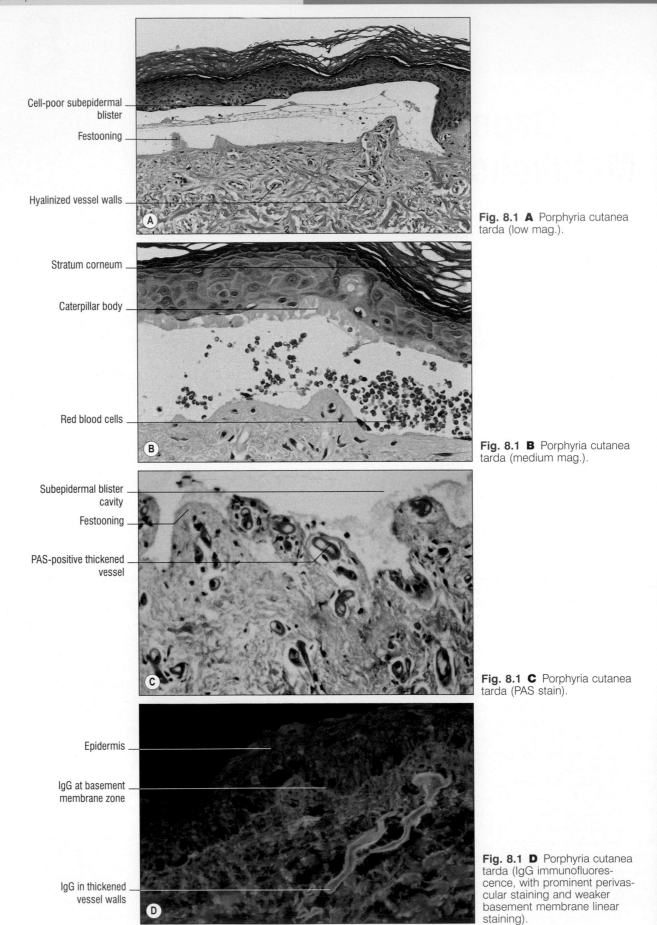

Cell-poor subepidermal blister

Festooning

Hyalinized vessel walls

Fig. 8.1 A Porphyria cutanea tarda (low mag.).

Stratum corneum

Caterpillar body

Red blood cells

Fig. 8.1 B Porphyria cutanea tarda (medium mag.).

Subepidermal blister cavity

Festooning

PAS-positive thickened vessel

Fig. 8.1 C Porphyria cutanea tarda (PAS stain).

Epidermis

IgG at basement membrane zone

IgG in thickened vessel walls

Fig. 8.1 D Porphyria cutanea tarda (IgG immunofluorescence, with prominent perivascular staining and weaker basement membrane linear staining).

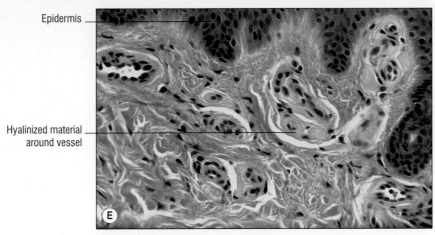

Epidermis

Hyalinized material around vessel

Fig. 8.1 E Erythropoietic protoporphyria.

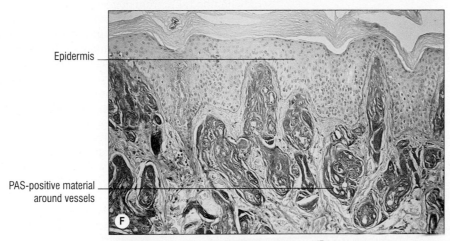

Epidermis

PAS-positive material around vessels

Fig. 8.1 F Erythropoietic protoporphyria (PAS stain).

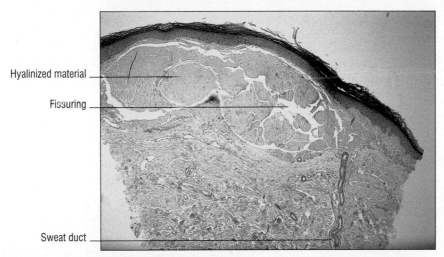

Hyalinized material

Fissuring

Sweat duct

Fig. 8.2 Colloid milium.

P
- Often epidermal atrophy (1.9) with hyperkeratosis
- *Nodular fissured masses* (1.23) of *amorphous eosinophilic material* in the superficial dermis
- Separation between the masses by a thin rim of collagen, elastic tissue, or collarette of epidermal rete ridges
- Special stains of the eosinophilic material (Congo red and crystal violet) often stain positive, as in amyloidosis
- Solar elastosis common

Differential diagnosis

1. Other diseases with amorphous pink material (1.35), especially amyloidosis (8.4) and nodular colloid degeneration (9.1).

8.3 Lipoid proteinosis (hyalinosis cutis et mucosae, Urbach–Wiethe disease)

(see Fig. 8.3A,B)

Very rare autosomal recessive deposition disorder, related to mutation in the extracellular matrix protein 1 gene (ECM1), beginning in childhood with laryngeal papules resulting in *hoarseness*, and *beaded papules of the eyelids* (1.43) and nose, and *verrucous plaques* (1.146) of other areas of skin, especially over joints (1.92).

> **P**
> - Hyperkeratosis, papillomatosis (1.102) sometimes
> - *Amorphous eosinophilic deposits* beginning around the vessels, later diffuse throughout the dermis, with a tendency to be perpendicular to the epidermis and to arrange around adnexal structures and blood vessels
> - Positive staining with colloidal iron, Alcian blue, Sudan black, *PAS with or without diastase*. Sudan black oil-red-O variably positive. Amyloid stains usually weakly positive or negative

Differential diagnosis

1. Juvenile hyaline fibromatosis: very rare, autosomal recessive, due to CMG2 (capillary morphogenesis gene-2) or ANTXR2 (anthrax toxin receptor) mutation, deposition disorder affecting young children, mental retardation, no hoarseness, *flexural contractures*, *gingival hypertrophy*, papules or nodules on the *lips* (1.74), nose (1.95), ears (1.28), and perianal areas (1.108). PAS and Alcian blue positive hyalinized dermal deposits with a *chondroid* appearance.

2. Infantile systemic hyalinosis: somewhat like juvenile hyaline fibromatosis, with same genetic defect reported, but there is more systemic involvement.

3. Other diseases with amorphous pink material (1.35), especially amyloidosis (8.4) and erythropoietic protoporphyria (8.1).

8.4 Amyloidosis

(see Fig. 8.4A–I)

Uncommon deposits of eosinophilic amyloid protein, due to systemic disease involving kidney, heart, or liver, or in rubbed or lichenified skin from degeneration of keratinocytes without systemic disease (macular and lichen amyloid). Amyloid is a beta-pleated sheet by X-ray diffraction and infrared spectroscopy, and non-branching filaments with a diameter of 6–10 nm are seen by electron microscopy. The amyloid fibrils themselves can consist of a variety of proteins, and the deposits in the skin also contain small amounts of other substances such as glycosaminoglycans, apolipoprotein E (apoE), and serum amyloid P (SAP). In macular and lichen amyloidosis, there is evidence of keratin (immunostains EKH4 or EAB-903) or tonofilaments (by electron microscopy) in the papillary dermal amyloid deposits, which are thought to originate from the damaged keratinocytes in the epidermis.

> **P**
> - Deposits of amorphous, eosinophilic, fissured material (1.23)
> - Special stains positive: crystal violet, Congo red, thioflavin T, pagoda red 9 (Dylon), scarlet red (RIT). PAS is moderately positive but is not used for this purpose. Immunostains for amyloid are available
> - Keratin stains such as EAB-903 may be positive in lichen and macular amyloidosis

Variations

1. Primary systemic amyloidosis: AL types of amyloid with immunoglobulin light chains (usually lambda) deposited, associated with *myeloma* (24.12), *yellowish* (1.151) or *purpuric* (1.120) macules or plaques, mostly in

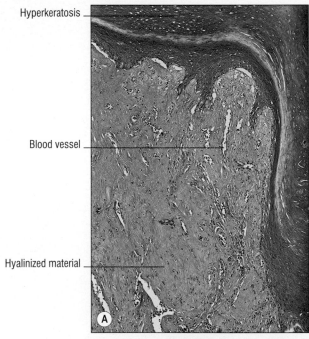

Hyperkeratosis

Blood vessel

Hyalinized material

Fig. 8.3 A Lipoid proteinosis.

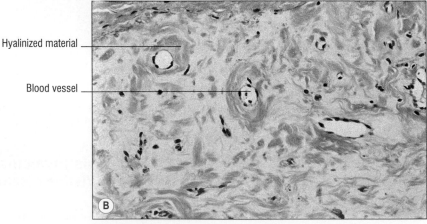

Hyalinized material

Blood vessel

Fig. 8.3 B Juvenile hyaline fibromatosis.

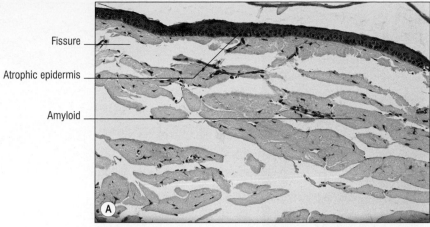

Fissure

Atrophic epidermis

Amyloid

Fig. 8.4 A Primary systemic amyloidosis, eyelid, in patient with myeloma.

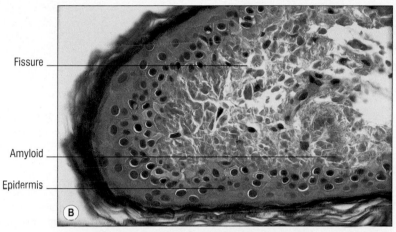

Fissure

Amyloid

Epidermis

Fig. 8.4 B Primary amyloidosis (Congo red stain).

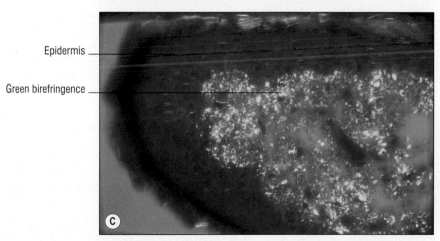

Epidermis

Green birefringence

Fig. 8.4 C Primary amyloidosis (Congo red stain, polarized).

the *elderly*, especially on the *eyelids* (1.43), deposits diffuse in dermis and/or especially *around blood vessels*, sweat glands, and adipocytes, often with scattered lymphocytes, plasma cells (1.111), and extravasated erythrocytes (1.40). Special immunostains for light chains usually positive, but can also be positive by non-specific absorption in macular and lichen amyloidosis.

2. Secondary systemic amyloidosis: AA type of amyloid (serum derived) associated with chronic systemic diseases such as rheumatoid arthritis or leprosy, *no skin*

lesions usually present clinically, but patients have deposits of amyloid in other organs. Dermatologists are sometimes asked to biopsy "normal" lower abdomen skin to find subtle amyloid around blood vessels, sweat glands, or fat cells, obviating the need for rectal biopsy or internal organ biopsy.

3. Nodular amyloidosis: *large waxy nodule* of diffuse light chain AL amyloid in the dermis, plasma cells usually present (1.111), with systemic amyloidosis or myeloma in a minority of cases.

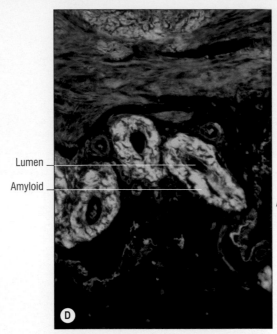

Fig. 8.4 D Primary amyloidosis (thioflavin-T staining of blood vessels).

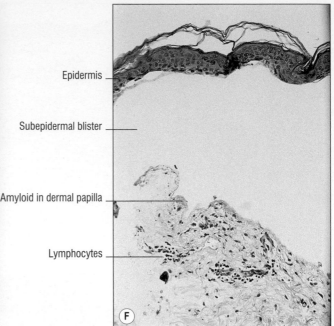

Fig. 8.4 F Bullous amyloidosis (low mag.).

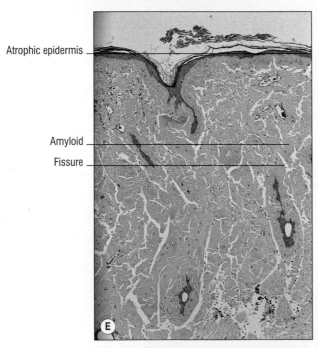

Fig. 8.4 E Nodular amyloidosis.

4. Bullous amyloidosis: rare form of systemic amyloidosis with *hemorrhagic* (1.120) *cell-poor blisters* (1.147), amyloid deposits may be subtle or prominent. Amyloid can act as a sponge for IgM or C3, which may cause confusion with autoimmune blistering disorders such as pemphigoid when direct immunofluorescence is performed.

5. Lichen amyloidosus (technically the only form of amyloid spelled with the ending –us due to Latin derivation): pebbled lichenified plaques, mostly on the *shins*, or scattered *grouped papules* in areas that are chronically rubbed, without systemic disease, small deposits of *amyloid limited to dermal papillae*, often melanin incontinence (1.79), may resemble or may be a variant of lichen simplex chronicus (2.3).

6. Macular amyloidosis: *brown macules* (1.17) with a *rippled* appearance ("hammered brass" or "corduroy pants"), most common on the *upper back* (1.141), without systemic disease, nearly normal epidermis, *very subtle amyloid blobs in the papillary dermis* in areas of *melanin incontinence* (1.79), biopsy may appear nearly normal (1.94).

7. Muckle–Wells syndrome: rare, autosomal dominant, mutation in *CIAS* gene encoding cryopyrin, urticaria, deafness, and AA amyloid in kidney.

8. Familial Mediterranean fever: rare, autosomal recessive, fever, peritonitis, pleurisy, arthritis, cellulitis-like plaques of the legs, AA amyloid in kidney.

Differential diagnosis

1. Other diseases with amorphous pink material (1.35), especially porphyria (8.1), colloid milium (8.2), lipoid proteinosis (8.3), and Waldenström's macroglobulinemia (24.12). Because special stains can be variable, electron microscopy may be desirable if proof of amyloid deposits is desired.

8.5 Gout

(see Fig. 8.5A–E)

Common *whitish–red nodules* (1.150), especially on the *digits and over joints*, associated with uric acid accumulation and a metabolic defect. Patients often have *arthritis* (1.7).

Differential diagnosis

1. Most of the other amorphous pink materials in Section 1.35 are not surrounded by a giant cell infiltrate, and do not show the subtle needle-shaped crystals.

2. Other juxta-articular nodules (1.92), especially calcinosis cutis (8.15) rheumatoid nodules (7.3).

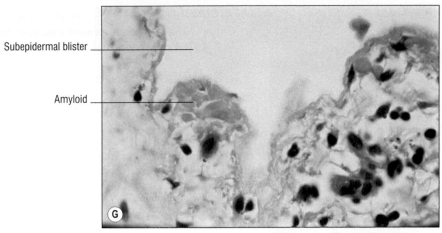

Fig. 8.4 G Bullous amyloidosis (high mag.).

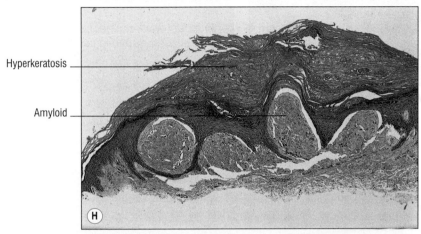

Fig. 8.4 H Lichen amyloidosis.

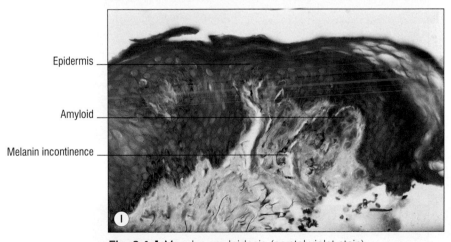

Fig. 8.4 I Macular amyloidosis (crystal violet stain).

P
- Amorphous deposits of *eosinophilic material in dermis* and subcutaneous tissue with formalin-fixed tissue
- *Brownish* (1.17), doubly-refractive needle-shaped crystals in *clefts* (1.23) if alcohol fixed, or in the deeper aspects of incompletely fixed or processed tissue
- Lymphocytes, histiocytes, and multinucleated giant cells around the deposits
- Positive staining with von Kossa, but *de Galantha* is more specific for urates

8.6 Generalized myxedema

Uncommon changes in the skin from *hypothyroidism* (1.138). Patients have skin that may look normal, but often is *edematous* (especially *periorbital*), *xerotic*, or eczematous (1.29). Skin *looks nearly normal* with H&E; rarely, the collagen bundles appear slightly separated by clear spaces or bluish deposits of mucin. Slightly increased acid mucopolysaccharide can sometimes be demonstrated between collagen bundles by special stains such as Alcian blue, colloidal iron, or toluidine blue.

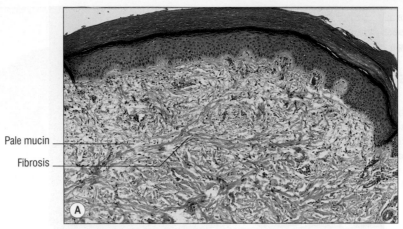

Pale mucin
Fibrosis

Fig. 8.8 A Scleromyxedema.

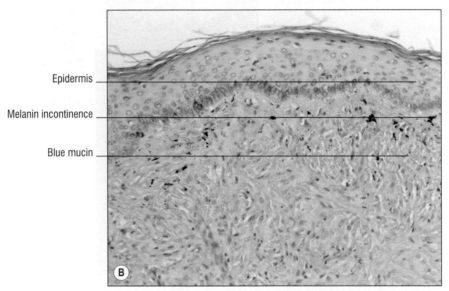

Epidermis

Melanin incontinence

Blue mucin

Fig. 8.8 B Scleromyxedema (Alcian blue stain).

Differential diagnosis

1. Other diseases with mucin in the dermis (1.83) should be considered, but most do not have such an impressive amount of mucin on the legs.
2. Diseases causing dermal edema can produce spaces between collagen bundles (1.30), but mucin stains are negative.

8.8 Papular mucinosis (lichen myxedematosus)

(see Fig. 8.8A,B)
Rare, *grouped papules*, especially on the face or arms, may be associated with *monoclonal gammopathy* (1.80).

P
- Circumscribed *deposits of abundant acid mucopolysaccharide* between collagen bundles in the *superficial dermis*, positive with Alcian blue, colloidal iron, or toluidine blue stains
- Fibrosis sometimes
- Increased mast cells (1.78)

Variation

1. Scleromyxedema: severe condition with *extensive induration* of skin (1.125), internal organ involvement like scleroderma, may cause death, more fibrosis than ordinary papular mucinosis (positive for CD34 and procollagen-1).

Differential diagnosis

1. Other diseases with mucin deposits in the dermis (1.83).
2. Other diseases with fibrosis or alteration of connective tissue, such as scleroderma (9.3), and nephrogenic systemic fibrosis (8.19).
3. Pretibial myxedema (8.7) has less fibroblast proliferation and more mucin, not just in the upper dermis.
4. Scleredema (8.12).

8.9 Digital mucous cyst (digital myxoid pseudocyst, digital synovial cyst)

(see Fig. 8.9A,B)
Somewhat common translucent papule or nodule of the *dorsal proximal nail fold* of a digit (1.56), containing gelatinous material. Some of these lesions represent herniation of the joint space, but many do not, and the latter are thought to be due to local synthesis of mucin by fibroblasts.

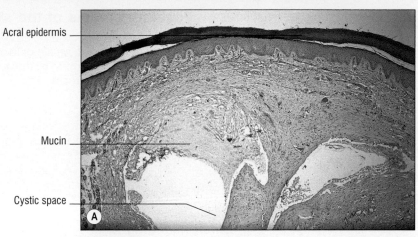

Acral epidermis

Mucin

Cystic space

Fig. 8.9 A Digital mucous cyst.

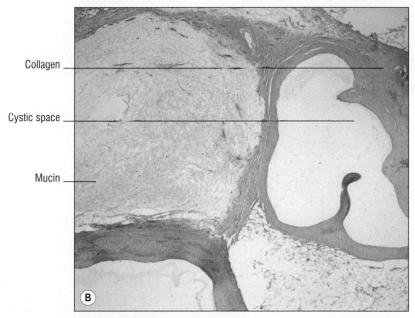

Collagen

Cystic space

Mucin

Fig. 8.9 B Ganglion cyst.

 P
- Hyperplasia of epidermis sometimes
- Localized increased *mucin* in clefts *between collagen bundles* or in a cystic space, coalescing into one large cystic space in older lesions. Sometimes mucin extrudes into the epidermis, giving the appearance of a cyst there. Often considered not a true cyst because there is no epithelial lining, although a collarette of epidermal rete ridges may clutch the cyst
- Sometimes there is a synovial lining, but most of the time the cells lining the mucin cavity are flattened fibroblasts
- Positive staining with acid mucopolysaccharide stains

Variation

1. Ganglion cyst (synovial cyst): usually larger and deeper, not usually excised by dermatologists, connects to joint space, especially around the wrist.

Differential diagnosis

1. Other diseases with increased mucin in the dermis (1.83).
2. Other cysts (1.25).

3. Focal mucinosis (8.11): identical except for location and less tendency to form a large cystic space.

8.10 Mucocele (mucous cyst of the mouth)

(see Fig. 8.10A,B)

Somewhat common *translucent papule* or nodule, especially of the mucosal surface of the *lip* (1.74), due to minor salivary gland trauma.

- Ruptured minor salivary duct or gland **P**
- One or several spaces (1.25) filled with sialomucin, lined by granulation tissue or a mixed infiltrate of fibroblasts, lymphocytes, and histiocytes
- Sialomucin is positive with staining for both neutral mucopolysaccharide (PAS positive, diastase resistant) and acid mucopolysaccharide

Differential diagnosis

1. Other diseases with increased mucin in the dermis (1.83) are unlikely in this location. The mucin may be subtle, and non-specific granulation tissue and a mixed inflammatory infiltrate may be predominant.

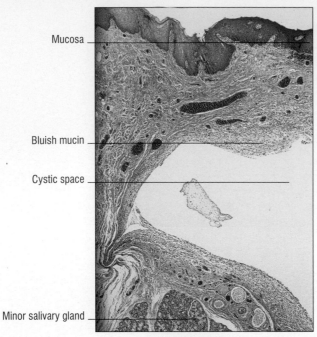

Mucosa

Bluish mucin

Cystic space

Minor salivary gland

Fig. 8.10 A Mucocele.

8.11 Focal mucinosis of the skin

(see Fig. 8.11)

Uncommon *solitary localized papule* or nodule, unassociated with systemic disease, thought to be due to a localized fibroblast synthesis of excessive mucin.

- Localized increased dermal mucin
- Normal or slightly increased numbers of S100 negative fibroblasts
- Positive staining with acid mucopolysaccharide stains (Alcian blue, toluidine blue, or colloidal iron)

Differential diagnosis

1. Other diseases with increased mucin in the dermis (1.83).
2. Digital mucous cyst (8.9).
3. Lichen myxedematosus (8.8) is not a solitary lesion, and has more fibrosis, more fibroblasts, and less mucin.
4. Myxoma (27.17).

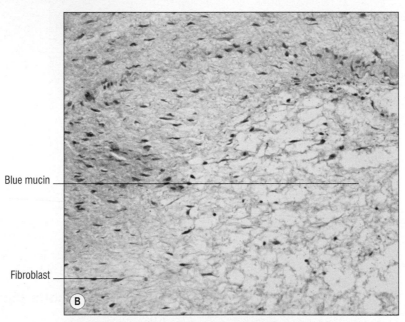

Blue mucin

Fibroblast

Fig. 8.10 B Mucocele. It is common not to see a discrete cyst.

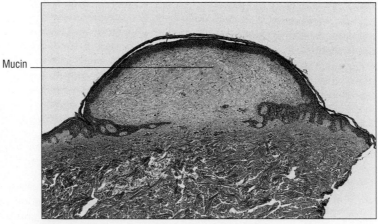

Mucin

Fig. 8.11 Focal mucinosis of the skin.

Pigmented epidermis

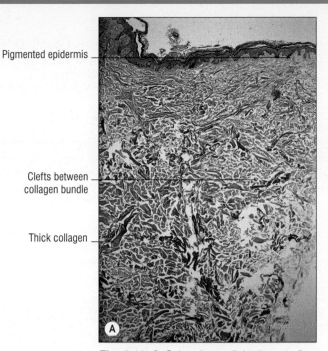

Clefts between
collagen bundle

Thick collagen

Fig. 8.12 A Scleredema diabeticorum (low
mag.).

8.12 **Scleredema of Buschke**

(see Fig. 8.12A–C)

Tremendous thickening and *induration of the upper trunk* (1.141), without systemic sclerosis, may be associated with *paraproteinemia* (1.80).

- *Dermis markedly thicker* than normal, extending below sweat gland coils, with very *thick collagen bundles separated by clefts* (1.23)
- *Normal or decreased number of fibroblasts*
- Increase in *acid mucopolysaccharide between collagen bundles* (stains with Alcian blue, colloidal iron, or toluidine blue)

P

Variations

1. Respiratory infection type (true Buschke type): very rare, follows an *upper respiratory infection*, may spontaneously resolve.
2. Scleredema diabeticorum: most common type, associated with *diabetes mellitus* (1.26), persistent.

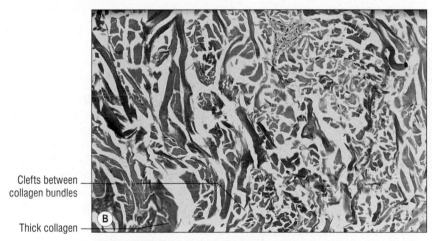

Clefts between
collagen bundles

Thick collagen

Fig. 8.12 B Scleredema diabeticorum (high mag.).

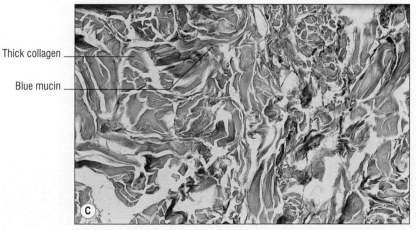

Thick collagen

Blue mucin

Fig. 8.12 C Scleredema diabeticorum (colloidal iron stain for mucin).

Differential diagnosis

1. Other diseases with mucin in the dermis (1.83).
2. May resemble normal back skin (1.94), which is already quite thick, on cursory examination.
3. Scleroderma (9.3) or other sclerosing disorders (1.125).

8.13 Reticular erythematous mucinosis syndrome (REM syndrome)

(see Fig. 8.13A,B)
Rare *reticulated macules* (1.123), usually of the *chest* of women.

P
- Perivascular and perifollicular lymphocytes
- Very subtle to moderate amount of mucin between collagen bundles
- Mucin is positive with acid mucopolysaccharide stains (Alcian blue, toluidine blue, and sometimes mucicarmine)

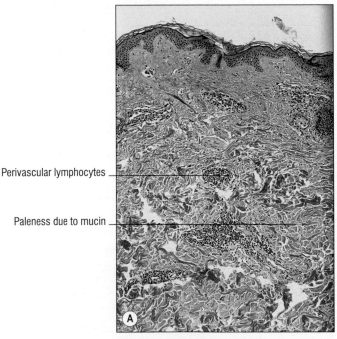

Perivascular lymphocytes

Paleness due to mucin

Fig. 8.13 A Reticular erythematous mucinosis syndrome (low mag.).

Differential diagnosis

1. Most of the other diseases with increased mucin (1.83) do not have the inflammatory infiltrate.
2. This diagnosis is only made after excluding dermatomyositis (17.7) and lupus erythematosus (17.6).

8.14 Mucopolysaccharidoses

Very rare group of at least ten lysosomal storage disorders in which dermatan sulfate, heparan sulfate, or keratan sulfate accumulate in the tissues. They are usually diagnosed by testing for mucopolysaccharides in the *blood* or *urine*, or by *fibroblast cultures*. There are skeletal abnormalities, short stature, mental retardation, corneal clouding, deafness, gargoyle facies, arteriosclerosis, or hepatosplenomegaly, depending upon the syndrome. Skin lesions include *eczema* (1.29) and *hypertrichosis* (1.62). Skin-colored *waxy papulonodules* are most common on the *upper back*.

P
- *Granules within cytoplasm of fibroblasts or histiocytes* ("gargoyle cells") and occasionally within keratinocytes that can be stained with Giemsa, toluidine blue, Alcian blue, or colloidal iron. The cells may appear vacuolated prior to special stains. Special fixation in alcohol may be needed. Peripheral blood lymphocytes also contain these granules
- *Mucin* (1.83) in middle or deep dermis in the papulonodules

Variations

1. Hurler's syndrome (MPS I): autosomal recessive, alpha-L-iduronidase deficiency (assayed in cultured leukocytes or fibroblasts), sclerodermoid plaques (1.125) and furrows, worst prognosis. Urinary dermatan sulfate and heparan (not heparin) sulfate are elevated.
2. Hunter's syndrome (MPS II): X-linked recessive, iduronate sulfatase deficiency.

8.15 Calcinosis cutis

(see Fig. 8.15A–E)
Somewhat common, often *whitish* (1.150) *papules or nodules*, often with erythema.

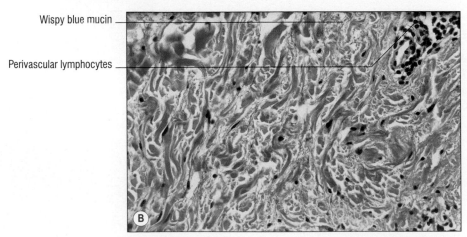

Wispy blue mucin

Perivascular lymphocytes

Fig. 8.13 B Reticular erythematous mucinosis syndrome (high mag.).

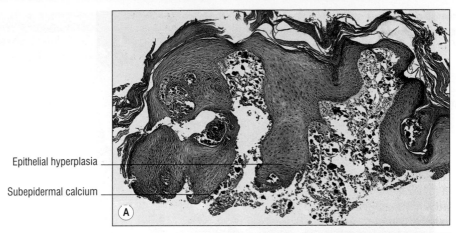

Epithelial hyperplasia

Subepidermal calcium

Fig. 8.15 A Subepidermal calcified nodule.

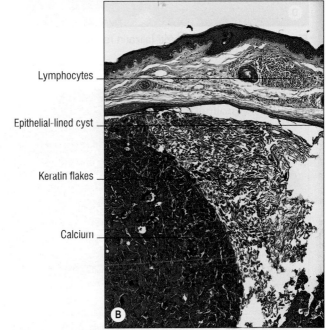

Lymphocytes

Epithelial-lined cyst

Keratin flakes

Calcium

Fig. 8.15 B Calcinosis scroti.

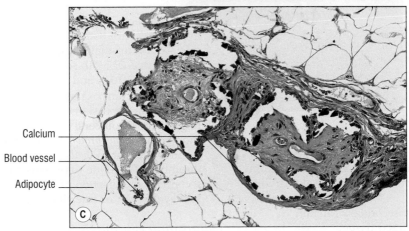

Calcium

Blood vessel

Adipocyte

Fig. 8.15 C Calciphylaxis.

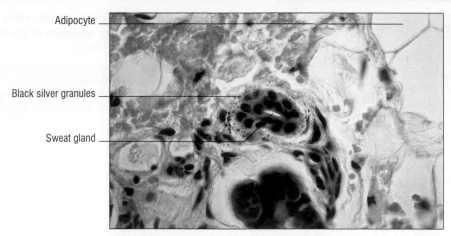

Fig. 8.18 Argyria.

Variation

1. Amalgam tattoo (7.6).

Differential diagnosis

1. Other heavy metal deposits or black deposits (1.12) usually do not show particles of such uniform size. Do not confuse with brown histologic deposits (1.17).

8.19 Nephrogenic systemic fibrosis (nephrogenic fibrosing dermopathy, scleromyxedema-like fibromucinosis of renal disease)

(see Fig. 8.19A–C)
New but rare condition found exclusively in renal failure (1.66), wherein gadolinium used for MRI scans accumulates in skin causing fibrosing dermatitis (1.125), sometimes with severe associated contractures and weakness. Red plaques may progress to woody induration with peau d'orange change and calcification (1.19). Calciphylaxis may coexist (8.15). Extremities are most commonly involved, with less truncal involvement. Internal organs may become involved. The disease is a common focus of litigation.

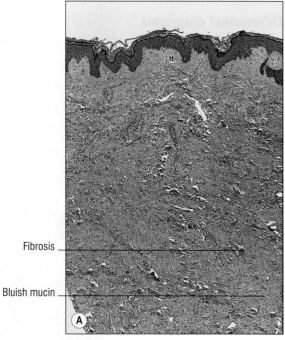

Fig. 8.19 A Nephrogenic systemic fibrosis (low mag.).

 ■ Fibrosing changes in dermis, sometime more subtle than the impressive clinical findings, often extending into deep subcutaneous tissue
■ Positive staining for CD34 and procollagen-1. Sometimes factor XIIIa is positive
■ Sometimes mucin increased between collagen bundles in dermis (positive for Alcian blue or colloidal iron)
■ Usually no inflammation, but in some cases can be present
■ Gadolinium demonstrated in skin lesions with quantitative scanning electron microscopy and energy dispersive X-ray spectroscopy.

Differential diagnosis

1. Other diseases with fibrosing changes (1.125), especially scleromyxedema (8.8), scleroderma (9.3), and pretibial myxedema (8.7). Scleromyxedema is more likely to have

paraproteinemia, facial involvement, a papular surface change, and no association with renal failure. Scleroderma has more collagen and decreased fibroblasts, no mucin or CD34 staining, sparse lymphocytes and plasma cells, no renal disease until late stages, and is more likely to have positive ANA and Scl-70 antibodies. Fibrosing wounds and scleromyxedema also commonly stain for CD34 and procollagen-1.
2. Other diseases with mucinosis (1.83). Mucin is usually less than with scleromyxedema and pretibial myxedema.

8.20 Miscellaneous deposition diseases

(see Fig. 8.20)
Other rare conditions are beyond the scope of this book, but dermatopathologists are sometimes asked to evaluate skin biopsies for Lafora disease.

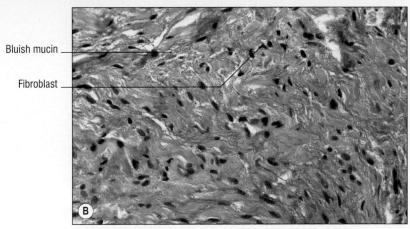

Bluish mucin

Fibroblast

Fig. 8.19 B Nephrogenic systemic fibrosis (high mag.).

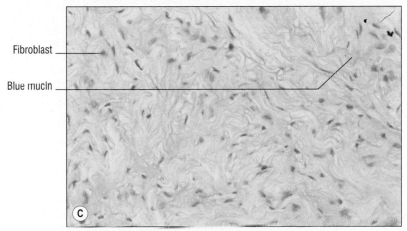

Fibroblast

Blue mucin

Fig. 8.19 C Nephrogenic systemic fibrosis (Alcian blue).

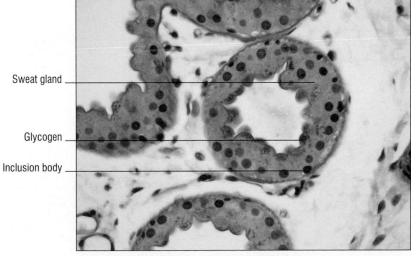

Sweat gland

Glycogen

Inclusion body

Fig. 8.20 Lafora disease, with PAS-positive inclusion bodies. (courtesy Shane Meehan MD).

Variation

1. Lafora disease (Lafora progressive myoclonic epilepsy): autosomal recessive disorder with inclusion bodies (Lafora bodies) in the neurons, heart, liver, skeletal muscle, and skin. Mutations of two known genes, EPM2A and EPM2B, code for the protein laforin. Seizures develop around age 10–17 years old, with death by age 25. PAS-positive, diastase resistant inclusion bodies of polyglycan are found in the cytoplasm of axillary apocrine sweat gland myoepithelial cells, or forearm eccrine ducts, from clinically normal skin. Misreading of the inclusion bodies has caused misdiagnosis.[111] DNA sequencing is recommended for definitive diagnosis.

CHAPTER 9

Alterations of Connective Tissue

9.1 Solar elastosis

(see Fig. 9.1A,B)
Very common parched or wrinkled skin due to sun damage (dermatoheliosis) with degeneration of connective tissue (increased abnormal elastic tissue and less collagen).

P
- Amorphous, fibrous, or globular basophilic material in the dermis
- Elastic fibers (1.31) become bluish–gray, and stain positively with elastic tissue stains (Chapter 30)

Variations

1. Nodular colloid degeneration: papule or nodule of histologically clumped areas of solar elastosis, often resembling amyloid (8.4). Rarely found in non-sun-damaged areas.
2. Elastotic globes: small (less than 40 microns), round basophilic to eosinophilic blobs of elastotic material in the dermis.
3. Weathering nodules of the ears, elastotic nodules of the ears: firm papules on the ears, degenerated cartilage or elastic tissue, fibrosis, not painful like chondrodermatitis (17.9).
4. Favre–Racouchot syndrome: solar elastosis, cysts (19.1) and comedones (1.24), especially on the malar area.
5. Collagenous and elastotic plaques of the hands: linear plaques (1.73) along the sides of the hands, with degenerated elastic tissue, resembling acrokeratoelastoidosis (2.15, which is familial, has an earlier age of onset, and involves both hands and feet).

Differential diagnosis

1. Other diseases with blue deposits (1.15), especially mucin (1.83): mucin is more stringy, smudged, or granular, while even in smudged areas of solar elastosis, individual bluish elastic fibers can be identified.

9.2 Radiodermatitis

(see Fig. 9.2A,B)
Acute radiodermatitis presents as red patches (1.121), sometimes with desquamation or blistering. Chronic radiodermatitis presents as atrophic (1.9) indurated plaques, often whitish (1.150) or yellowish (1.151), with telangiectasia (1.136), sometimes with hyperkeratosis (1.61), sometimes squamous cell carcinoma or sarcoma can develop years after exposure.

A. Acute radiodermatitis

P
- Pale (1.99), vacuolated (1.144), or *necrotic keratinocytes* (1.86)
- Subepidermal blister (1.147) or ulceration (1.142) sometimes
- Superficial *dermal edema* (1.30)
- Endothelial proliferation, vascular dilation, thrombi (1.137)
- Degeneration of dermal connective tissue

B. Chronic radiodermatitis

P
- Epidermal hyperplasia (1.61) or atrophy (1.9), sometimes ulceration (1.142)
- Keratinocytes pale (1.99), atypical, or necrotic (1.86)
- Telangiectatic blood vessels, sometimes surrounded by hyperplastic rete ridges
- Thrombi sometimes (1.137)
- Decreased adnexal structures
- *Degenerated dermis* (mainly *hyalinized*, sometimes basophilic)
- Sometime atypical, bizarre fibroblasts

Variation

1. Eosinophilic polymorphic pruritic eruption associated with radiotherapy (EPPER): papular, sometime vesicular, eruption that extends beyond area of radiotherapy, with spongiosis, superficial and deep lymphocytes and eosinophils.[165]

©2012 Elsevier Ltd, Inc, BV
DOI: 10.1016/B978-0-323-06658-7.00009-9

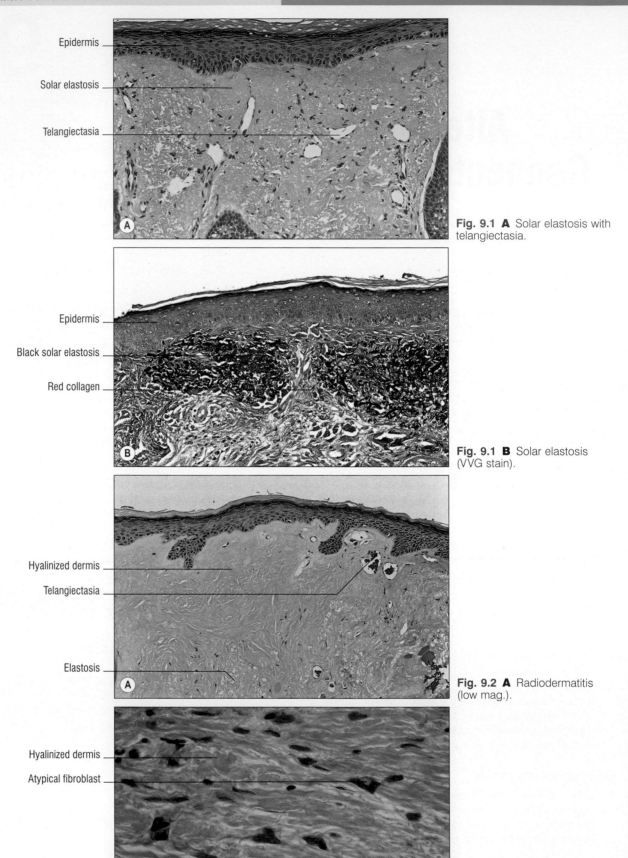

Epidermis

Solar elastosis

Telangiectasia

Fig. 9.1 A Solar elastosis with telangiectasia.

Epidermis

Black solar elastosis

Red collagen

Fig. 9.1 B Solar elastosis (VVG stain).

Hyalinized dermis

Telangiectasia

Elastosis

Fig. 9.2 A Radiodermatitis (low mag.).

Hyalinized dermis

Atypical fibroblast

Fig. 9.2 B Radiodermatitis (high mag.).

Differential diagnosis

1. Other diseases with hyalinization (1.35) or dermal sclerosis (1.125), especially lichen sclerosus (9.5) and scleroderma (9.3).
2. Solar elastosis (9.1) and actinic keratosis (18.8): dermis more basophilic and degeneration not as deep.

9.3 Scleroderma

(see Fig. 9.3A–D)

Somewhat common chronic systemic disease with *indurated skin*, especially of trunk, extremities, perioral face, and fingers (sclerodactyly, 1.56), often with hypopigmentation (1.150) or hyperpigmentation (1.18), often with "salt and pepper" appearance, associated with Raynaud's phenomenon, hypertension, gastrointestinal disease (especially esophageal dysmotility, 1.49), pulmonary fibrosis, and kidney disease (1.66), sometimes with overlapping features with other rheumatologic diseases. A minority of patients have *Scl-70 antibody*. ANA with a speckled or characteristic *antinucleolar* pattern may be present.

- Epidermis normal or atrophic (1.9)
- *Hyalinized dermis* and subcutaneous fat, more prominent in late lesions
- Sparse perivascular lymphocytes, sometimes plasma cells (1.111), in dermis or subcutaneous fat, more prominent in early lesions and in morphea than in systemic scleroderma
- *Decreased adnexal structures*; eccrine glands are entrapped by collagen and higher up in the dermis than usual because of increased collagen in subcutaneous fat

Variations

1. Morphea: localized sclerotic plaques of the skin, especially on the *trunk* (1.141), controversial relationship to tick bites and Borrelia (12.14), often with a violaceous halo (1.148) in active new lesions, sometimes whitish, with overlapping histologic features of lichen sclerosus (9.5), *no systemic disease*.
2. Systemic scleroderma (progressive systemic sclerosis, PSS): described above.
3. Eosinophilic fasciitis (Shulman's syndrome): *acute onset after vigorous exercise*, hyalinized, thickened *fascia* more than dermal sclerosis, more on the *extremities*, associated with peripheral *eosinophilia* (1.34) more than eosinophils in the fascia (therefore some prefer to call it fasciitis with eosinophilia), polyclonal gammopathy, occasional aplastic anemia, response to prednisone.
4. Linear scleroderma: linear form of morphea, without systemic disease, *linear plaques* (1.73) on the *extremities*, or on the forehead (1.44) or scalp appearing like a slash of a saber (en coup de sabre), sometimes with underlying bony disease (1.16).
5. CREST syndrome: calcinosis (1.19), Raynaud's phenomenon, esophageal abnormalities, sclerodactyly and telangiectasias (1.136), with *anticentromere* antibody, better prognosis with regard to kidney disease than other forms of systemic scleroderma.

Differential diagnosis

1. Other sclerosing or fibrosing conditions (1.125), hyalinized conditions (1.35), especially scleredema (8.12), chronic graft-versus-host disease (17.3), chronic

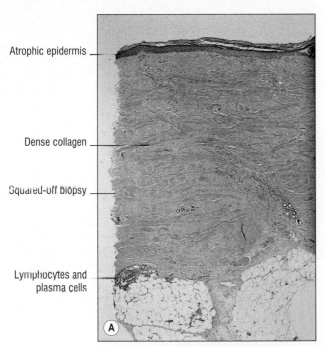

Atrophic epidermis

Dense collagen

Squared-off biopsy

Lymphocytes and plasma cells

Fig. 9.3 A Morphea (low mag.).

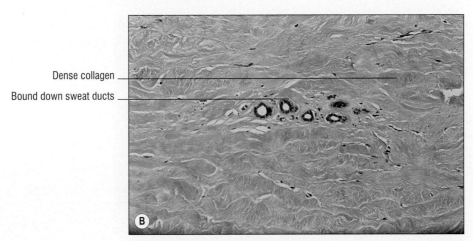

Dense collagen

Bound down sweat ducts

Fig. 9.3 B Morphea (high mag.).

jack-hammer use, polyvinyl chloride exposure, sclerodermoid porphyria cutanea tarda (8.1), scleromyxedema (8.8), nephrogenic fibrosing dermopathy (8.20), normal thick skin in areas such as the back, and lichen sclerosus (9.5).

9.4 Atrophoderma of Pasini and Pierini

Rare prominently depressed large atrophic *"cliff-drop" plaque*, usually on the *lower back*, often with prominent blood vessels seen within it.

P
- Hyalinized dermis (1.35), often subtle, requiring fusiform excision of adjacent normal skin for comparison to appreciate the *dermal atrophy* in the involved skin (1.8)
- Perivascular lymphocytes (1.109) in early lesions

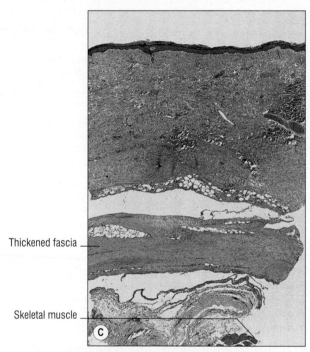

Thickened fascia

Skeletal muscle

Fig. 9.3 C Eosinophilic fasciitis (low mag.).

Differential diagnosis

1. Atrophoderma may be an atrophic end-stage lesion of morphea (9.3).
2. Anetoderma has a similar name, but is completely different (9.11).
3. Acrodermatitis chronica atrophicans: has a similar atrophic depressed appearance, but is located on the legs, associated with borreliosis (12.14).

9.5 Lichen sclerosus (lichen sclerosus et atrophicus, LS&A)

(see Fig. 9.5)

Somewhat common *indurated white plaques* (1.150) of the *vulva* (1.149) and perianal area (1.108), mostly in females, sometimes involving other cutaneous sites, without systemic disease. Pruritus (1.114) can be prominent, erythema, erosions or ulcers may occur, and rarely carcinoma can develop.

P
- Hyperkeratosis (1.61) often, but usually with atrophy of the spinous layer of the epidermis (1.9)
- Follicular plugging (1.47)
- Liquefaction degeneration of the basal layer (1.64), rare subepidermal blister (1.147)
- Edematous *homogenized superficial dermis* (1.35) with vascular dilation
- *Lichenoid lymphocytes* (1.72) in early lesions (near basal layer in very early lesions, mid-dermis beneath homogenized zone later)
- Vascular dilation

Differential diagnosis

1. Other diseases with amorphous pink material (1.35) or dermal sclerosis (1.125).
2. Scleroderma (9.3): less epidermal atrophy, less liquefaction degeneration of the basal layer, less dermal edema, less follicular plugging, less subepidermal bulla formation, and a deeper extension of hyalinized collagen.
3. Morphea (9.3): may have identical histology, but there is no vulvar or perianal disease, and the plaques are typically larger on the trunk, sometimes with a violaceous border when active.

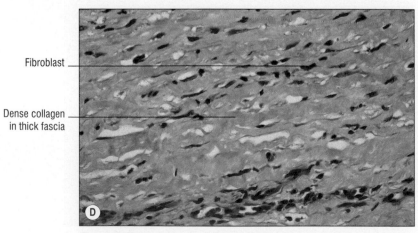

Fibroblast

Dense collagen in thick fascia

Fig. 9.3 D Eosinophilic fasciitis (high mag.).

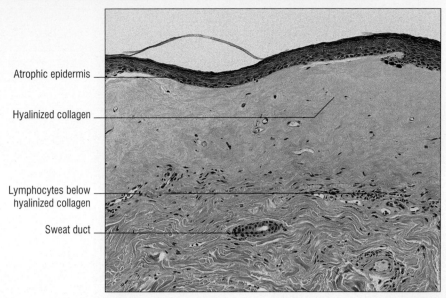

Fig. 9.5 Lichen sclerosus.

9.6 Progeria

Very rare group of autosomal recessive premature aging syndromes which can be related to de novo heterozygous mutations in the lamin A gene (LMNA). The childhood form is known as *Hutchinson–Gilford syndrome*, and begins in the first year of life as growth retardation. The adult form begins in the teens and is known as *Werner's syndrome* (pangeria), related to mutations in the RECQL2 gene. Patients with both forms develop bird-like facies, hypogonadism or absent sexual maturation, alopecia, and sclerodermoid skin. Diabetes mellitus (1.26) is common in Werner's syndrome. Premature death occurs from atherosclerosis by age 20 years in the childhood form, and by age 50 in Werner's syndrome. A third autosomal recessive premature aging syndrome, *acrogeria*, may be a variant of Ehlers–Danlos syndrome type IV (9.9). Those patients have sclerodermoid changes mainly on acral extremities (hence, acrogeria), and do not develop premature atherosclerosis, diabetes mellitus, or a decreased life expectancy.

- Epidermal atrophy (1.9)
- *Dermal fibrosis or sclerosis* (1.125)
- *Decreased adnexal structures*
- *Decreased subcutaneous fat*

Differential diagnosis

1. Ataxia–telangiectasia (11.12), Cockayne syndrome (11.10), scleroderma (9.3) and other sclerodermoid conditions (1.125).
2. Lipodystrophy (16.11).

9.7 Pachydermoperiostosis

Very rare autosomal recessive or dominant heterogeneous group of diseases, some due to mutation in the HPGD gene, with *clubbing of the digits* (1.85), *soft tissue hyperplasia* and *periosteal proliferation* (1.16) of forearms and legs, and furrowing of the skin of face and scalp (*cutis verticis gyrata*, CVG). CVG has been found in 4% of institutionalized psychiatric patients, mostly males.

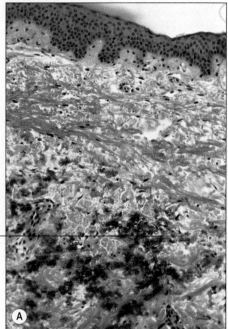

Fig. 9.8 A Pseudoxanthoma elasticum (low mag.).

- Increased *dense collagen* and increased fibroblasts in the dermis (1.125)
- Increased *acid mucopolysaccharide* between collagen bundles (1.125)
- CVG may have normal histology, or dermal fibrosis with pilosebaceous hyperplasia

9.8 Pseudoxanthoma elasticum (PXE, Gronblad–Strandberg syndrome)

(see Fig. 9.8A–C)

Rare autosomal recessive elastic tissue disorder due to mutation in the ABCC6 gene, with grouped, "*plucked-chicken*", pseudoxanthomatous *yellowish papules* (1.151) in flexural

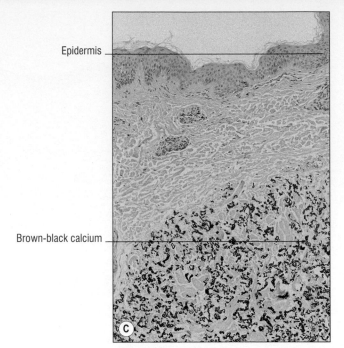

Fig. 9.8 B Pseudoxanthoma elasticum (VVG stain for elastic tissue).

Fig. 9.8 C Pseudoxanthoma elasticum (von Kossa stain for calcium).

areas such as the *neck* (1.86), *axilla* (1.10), groin (1.55), antecubital, and popliteal areas. Systemic elastic tissue problems, especially eye problems (1.41) such as *angioid streaks*, *retinal hemorrhages*, and blindness. Calcified peripheral arteries may result in gastrointestinal hemorrhage and peripheral vascular occlusion.

- *Clumped*, *calcified elastic fibers* in the dermis (positive staining for calcium with alizarin red or von Kossa stains, or for elastic tissue with Verhoeff stain)

Variations

1. Perforating PXE: transepidermal elimination in PXE (1.140).
2. Periumbilical perforating calcific elastosis: not related to PXE, a different disorder usually in multiparous obese black females, with a plaque of keratotic papules in the periumbilical area, no systemic disease, histology like perforating PXE.

Differential diagnosis

1. PXE is not often confused with anything else once biopsied. Consider other calcified conditions (1.19), elastic tissue disorders (1.31), and connective tissue alterations (Chapter 9).

9.9 Ehlers–Danlos syndrome (EDS)

A group of at least ten uncommon to rare diseases with connective tissue alteration mainly involving collagen, fragile, *hyperextensible*, *soft*, *velvety skin* with impaired wound healing and *fish mouth scars*, fragile blood vessels which may result in *hematomas or pseudotumors*, and *joint hypermobility*. Some patients have a normal life expectancy, but premature death

may occur in others from arterial or intestinal rupture. Biochemical and genetic defects have been discovered in some of the variants, and a detailed description is beyond the scope of this book.

- *Normal-appearing skin* by light microscopy (1.93) in most cases
- Collagen fibers may have subtle thinning, with slight increase in elastic fibers
- Dermal atrophy may be present (1.8)
- Pseudotumors at sites of trauma show hemorrhage early, and fibrosis, multinucleated histiocytes, and vascular proliferation late

Differential diagnosis

1. Osteogenesis imperfecta: autosomal dominant group of disorders in type I collagen, defects of COL1A1 or COL1A2 genes, *bone fragility* (this disease is mainly an orthopedic problem), short stature, loose joints, blue sclera (1.14), deafness, soft, thin skin, sometimes dermal atrophy (1.8) or *normal-appearing skin* (1.93) on H&E biopsy.
2. Marfan syndrome: autosomal dominant defect in elastic tissue fibrillin (fibrillin-1 gene mutation), *tall stature*, *arachnodactyly*, *lens dislocation* (ectopia lentis), *aortic aneurysms*, *mitral valve prolapse*, striae, sometimes dermal atrophy (1.8), thin collagen or elastic fibers, or *normal-appearing skin* on H&E biopsy (1.93).

9.10 Cutis laxa

Very rare heterogeneous group of autosomal dominant or recessive congenital elastic tissue disorders, related to mutations in the elastin gene ELN, or ATP6V0A2, PYCR1, FBLN5 or FBLN4 genes. *Loose, pendulous skin*, especially of face and neck, bloodhound facies, emphysema, GI or bladder diverticula, rectal prolapse, and inguinal, umbilical, and hiatal hernias. *Acquired cutis laoca* in children or adults is not inherited, and begins following a hodgepodge of inflammatory erythematous or vesicular diseases, or drug therapy.

- Skin looks normal with H&E stain (1.93)
- Elastic stain shows *decreased*, *thinned*, *degenerated*, or *nearly normal elastic fibers* in the dermis (1.31)
- Lymphocytes, multinucleated giant cells rarely in dermis

Differential diagnosis

1. Granulomatous slack skin (24.1): lax skin like cutis laxa, but has a lymphomatous infiltrate and giant multinucleated cells.
2. Sagging skin can also be found in some forms of Ehlers–Danlos syndrome (type IX is also known as X-linked cutis laxa), neurofibromatosis (26.1), weight loss, blepharochalasis (idiopathic eyelid laxity), Ascher's syndrome (7.7), acrodermatitis chronica atrophicans (12.14), and anetoderma (9.11).

9.11 Anetoderma (macular atrophy)

(see Fig 9.11)
Rare atrophic patches of skin with a *bleb-like herniated appearance*, usually on the *upper trunk* (1.141) in young adults. Most patients have no systemic disease, but some have had ocular or skeletal problems.

- Normal epidermis
- Perivascular lymphocytes, histiocytes, neutrophils, or eosinophils (early lesions only)
- Decreased or completely *absent elastic tissue in the dermis* (1.31) with Verhoeff–van Gieson stain, but skin looks nearly normal with H&E (1.93)

Variations

1. Primary Jadassohn–Pellizzari type: inflammatory red macules or papules precede the atrophic stage.
2. Primary Schweninger–Buzzi type: non-inflammatory from the beginning.
3. Secondary type: syphilis, lupus erythematosus, leprosy, HIV infection, or other preceding disease gives rise to the atrophic lesions.

Differential diagnosis

1. Despite the similar name, do not confuse anetoderma with atrophoderma (9.4), which is completely different.
2. Elastic fibers can be decreased in ordinary scars (27.2) and in some other sclerosing conditions (1.125).

9.12 Kyrle's disease (hyperkeratosis follicularis et parafollicularis in cutem penetrans)

(see Fig. 9.12)
Uncommon condition usually associated with *pruritus* (1.114) related to systemic diseases (see below), resulting in

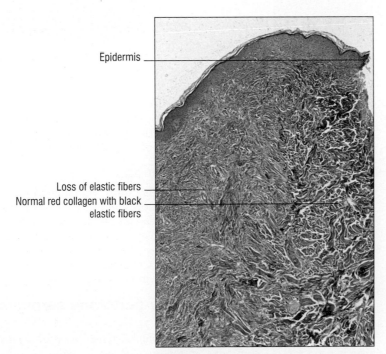

Fig. 9.11 Anetoderma. Note loss of black elastic fibers on one side compared to the other (Verhoeff–van Gieson stain).

Epidermis

Loss of elastic fibers
Normal red collagen with black elastic fibers

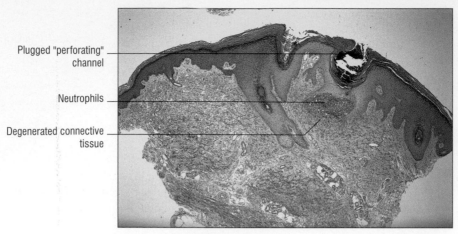

Plugged "perforating" channel

Neutrophils

Degenerated connective tissue

Fig. 9.12 Kyrle's disease.

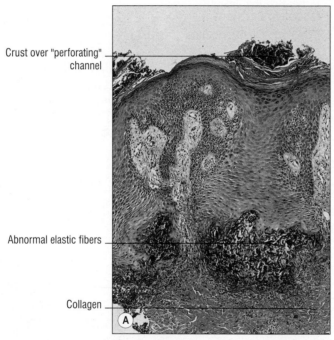

Crust over "perforating" channel

Abnormal elastic fibers

Collagen

Fig. 9.13 A Elastosis perforans serpiginosa (low mag.).

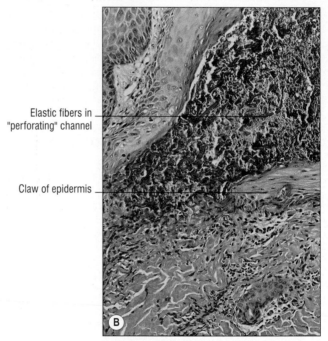

Elastic fibers in "perforating" channel

Claw of epidermis

Fig. 9.13 B Elastosis perforans serpiginosa (high mag.).

hyperkeratotic papules with central keratotic craters (1.47), most common on the *legs* (1.67), or generalized.

P
- *Hyperkeratotic plug* containing degenerated material, sometimes associated with follicular orifices, sometimes completely perforating the epidermis or follicle, sometimes with neutrophils or crust
- Parakeratosis and dyskeratotic keratinocytes (1.27)
- Epidermal hyperplasia (1.61) around the plug
- No increase in elastic fibers in the dermis and *no elastic fibers or collagen fibers within the plug*
- Foreign body giant cells (1.84) in the dermis at perforation site sometimes

Variation

1. Acquired perforating dermatosis: this term is used for those adults with perforating skin lesions as above, related to diabetes mellitus (1.26), kidney failure (1.66),

or rarely liver disease. The histology may be that of Kyrle's disease, acquired reactive perforating collagenosis (9.14), perforating folliculitis (10.3) or very rarely elastosis perforans serpiginosa (9.13).

Differential diagnosis

1. Kyrle's disease is poorly defined and many reported cases actually represent other transepidermal elimination diseases (1.140). Some authors consider it to be an end-stage epithelial hyperplasia of perforating folliculitis. Many of the patients also have prurigo nodularis (2.3). Consider other diseases with pseudoepitheliomatous hyperplasia (1.116).

9.13 Elastosis perforans serpiginosa (EPS)
(see Fig. 9.13A–D)

Rare *annular* (1.5) *hyperkeratotic plugged papules* (1.47), most common on the *neck* (1.86) in children or young adults, often *associated with a variety of genetic conditions*, including Down syndrome, Ehlers–Danlos syndrome, osteogenesis

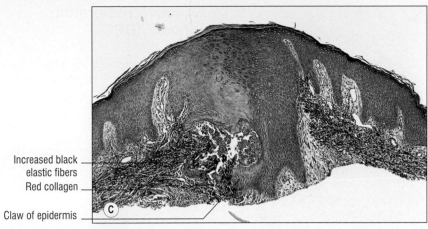

Increased black
elastic fibers

Red collagen

Claw of epidermis

Fig. 9.13 C Elastosis perforans serpiginosa (VVG stain, low mag.).

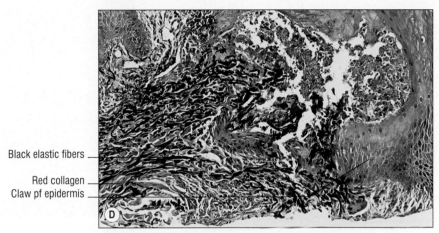

Black elastic fibers

Red collagen
Claw pf epidermis

Fig. 9.13 D Elastosis perforans serpiginosa (VVG stain, high mag.).

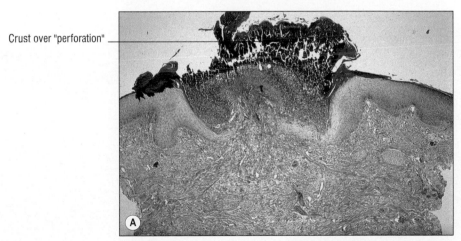

Crust over "perforation"

Fig. 9.14 A Reactive perforating collagenosis (RPC, low mag.).

imperfecta, Marfan syndrome, pseudoxanthoma elasticum, Rothmund–Thomson syndrome, and acrogeria.

Differential diagnosis

1. Other transepidermal elimination diseases (1.140).
2. Elastic fibers may be found within the epidermis at the base of keratoacanthoma (8.12), or any condition with

pseudocarcinomatous hyperplasia (1.116), especially healing wounds.

- Hyperkeratotic plug with transepidermal elimination of elastic fibers
- Hyperplastic epidermis that often appears to clutch the dermis at the site of perforation like a crab claw, elephant snout, or vacuum cleaner

P
- Increased brightly eosinophilic elastic fibers in dermis (1.31) near perforation (black with Verhoeff–van Gieson stain)
- Bramble bush lumpy-bumpy elastic fibers with lateral buds in penicillamine-induced EPS
- Macrophages, multinucleated giant cells, lymphocytes, or neutrophils in the plug or dermis at site of perforation

9.14 Reactive perforating collagenosis (RPC)

(see Fig. 9.14A–D)

Rare, genetically inherited, recurrent *hyperkeratotic papules* that *appear after superficial trauma*, spontaneously resolving in

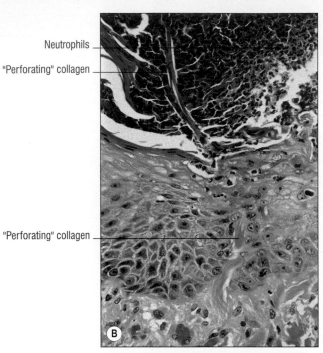

Fig. 9.14 **B** Reactive perforating collagenosis (RPC, high mag.).

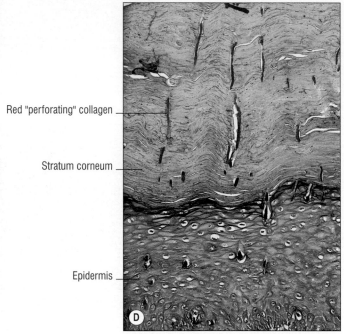

Fig. 9.14 **D** Reactive perforating collagenosis (RPC, VVG stain).

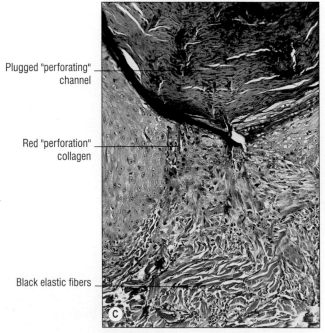

Fig. 9.14 **C** Reactive perforating collagenosis (RPC, VVG stain).

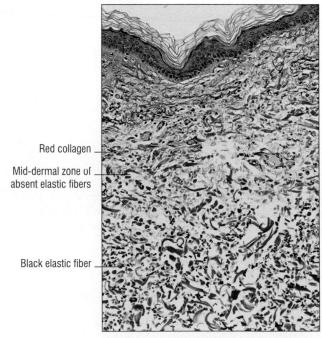

Fig. 9.15 Mid-dermal elastolysis (VVG stain).

several weeks, especially on the arms and hands. RPC more commonly occurs anywhere on the body in the acquired form (9.12).

- *Hyperkeratotic plug* in the epidermis, often "perforating" through the epidermis
- *Transepidermal elimination of collagen fibers* (red with Verhoeff–van Gieson stain) in the plug
- Macrophages, multinucleated giant cells, lymphocytes, or *neutrophils* (1.89) in the plug or dermis at site of perforation

Differential diagnosis

1. Other transepidermal elimination diseases (1.140).

9.15 Mid-dermal elastolysis

(see Fig. 9.15)

Very rare disease, persistent *fine wrinkling* of the upper extremities, trunk, or neck of adult women. Sometimes there is a preceding erythema of the area.

- Normal-appearing skin with H&E stain (1.93)
- *Mid-dermal loss of elastic fibers* (1.31) seen with Verhoeff–van Gieson stain
- Macrophages with elastic fiber phagocytosis sometimes (7.4)

Differential diagnosis

1. Pseudoxanthoma elasticum (9.8): yellowish papules, clumped elastic fibers.
2. Solar elastosis (9.1).

CHAPTER 10

Adnexal Inflammatory Diseases

These are inflammatory diseases involving sweat glands or pilosebaceous units.

10.1 Acne

(see Fig. 10.1A–E)

Very common disorder, *open comedones* (blackheads), *closed comedones* (whiteheads), *red papules, pustules, cysts* (ruptured inflamed sebaceous glands without an epithelial lining as in most "true cysts", 1.25), and nodules. More in teenagers and young adults, more on face and trunk, related to increased keratinization of the infundibulum of the follicle, increased sebum production related to hormones, secondary normal flora bacterial overgrowth, and inflammation related to bacterial products and lipids. Acne vulgaris is the prototype. The term vulgaris in the ancient dermatology literature was often applied in this way, so that psoriasis vulgaris is standard plaque psoriasis, verruca vulgaris is the standard wart of the fingers, and lupus vulgaris was a standard type of tuberculosis seen on the face more commonly years ago.

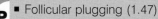

- Follicular plugging (1.47)
- Sometimes intraepidermal pustules (1.89) overlying follicles, or within follicles
- Frequently ruptured pilosebaceous apparatus with perifollicular mixed infiltrate of neutrophils, lymphocytes, plasma cells (1.111), histiocytes, and/or multinucleated giant cells (1.84)
- Sometimes abscesses, sinus tracts, and fibrosis

Variations

1. Follicular occlusion triad: term used for the closely related diseases acne conglobata (nodulocystic acne of the face and trunk), *folliculitis decalvans* of the scalp (*perifolliculitis capitis abscedens et suffodiens, dissecting cellulitis of the scalp*) (10.2), and *hidradenitis suppurativa* (acne inversa) of the axilla, inframammary, or groin areas (distribution like inverse psoriasis). Hidradenitis is really a follicular occlusion problem rather than an apocrine gland disease (despite synonym apocrinitis), as the apocrine glands drain into the follicles.
   The histology of all of these conditions is similar, with frequent abscesses, suppurative granulomas, and sinus tracts.
2. Rosacea: mainly in adults, with a *telangiectatic type* that is mostly macular erythema, with frequent flushing with exposure to heat, certain foods and other flare factors, and a true acne rosacea in which there are typical acneiform papules and pustules (but fewer comedones than acne vulgaris), more on the central face, sometimes producing blepharitis (ocular rosacea), sometimes producing sarcoidal or tuberculoid granulomas (granulomatous rosacea), rarely with caseation. Persisting papules of granulomatous rosacea (for 1 or 2 years or more) has also been called lupus miliaris disseminatus faciei or acne agminata because it resembles military tuberculosis. Rosacea and other forms of acne have a relationship with *Demodex* mites (15.8).
3. Erythema and edema of the face (solid facial edema, Morbihan's disease):[122] clinical form of severe acne in which there is impressive redness and swelling of the central face.
4. Chloracne: mostly comedones, less inflammation, mostly due to oils or chemical exposures.
5. Other clinical variants: drug-induced or aggravated acne may be due to steroids, lithium, phenytoin, iodides, and bromides. Acne fulminans is a severe form of nodulocystic acne most common in males, with fever, leukocytosis, proteinuria, arthritis, or osteolysis. Acne mechanica is related to friction from hats, helmuts, chin straps, etc. Neonatal acne is present in many normal newborns, often blamed on *Pityrosporum* yeast, resolving by 3 months of age.
6. Acne excoriee (including acne excoriee des jeunes filles, meaning more common in "young women"): prominent excoriations from picking acne lesions are dominant.

©2012 Elsevier Ltd, Inc, BV
DOI: 10.1016/B978-0-323-06658-7.00010-5

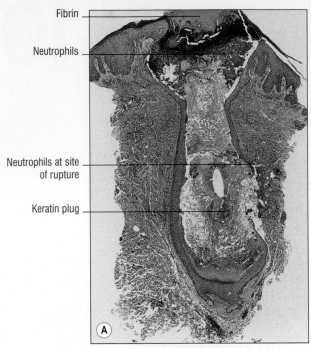

Fig. 10.1 A Ruptured comedo.

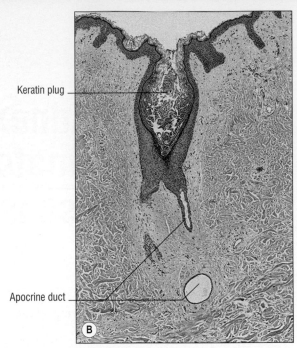

Fig. 10.1 B Hidradenitis suppurativa (low mag.).

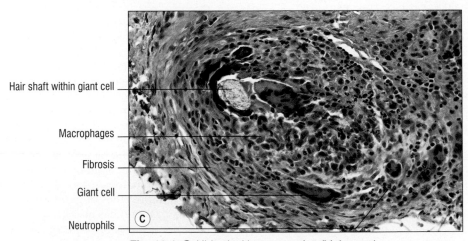

Fig. 10.1 C Hidradenitis suppurativa (high mag.).

7. Perioral dermatitis and periocular dermatitis: acneiform lesions with coexisting eczema-like (dermatitis) changes, often due to or aggravated by topical steroid abuse, usually around the mouth or eyes.
8. Pyoderma faciale: severe form of nodulocystic acne of the face, more in females.
9. Familial dyskeratotic comedones:[130] rare inherited condition with comedones (1.24) on the trunk, at the base of which is acantholytic dyskeratosis (1.2, 1.27).
10. Chalazion: red papule or nodule of the inner eyelid, with granulomatous inflammation around a Meibomian sebaceous gland. Sty and hordeolum are similar, but these terms are more commonly used for lesions of the cutaneous surface of the eyelid.
11. Pilonidal sinus or cyst: suppurative granulomatous reaction to follicular unit, with many hair shafts embedded in fibrosis, may become quite large, usually in hairy or obese adult males on the sacral area, resembles a ruptured cyst but has no epithelial lining, although sinus tracts may be present.

Differential diagnosis

1. Other acneiform (1.3), follicular (1.47) or comedonal (1.24) diseases.
2. Other diseases with neutrophils (1.89).
3. Other granulomas (1.51).

10.2 Folliculitis

(see Fig. 10.2A,B)

Common *papulopustular eruption*, especially on the scalp (1.124), trunk (1.141), and legs (1.67) of women from shaving irritation.

- *Perifollicular or intrafollicular mixed infiltrate* of lymphocytes, histiocytes, or plasma cells, sometimes resulting in a ruptured follicle surrounded by neutrophils and multinucleated giant cells
- Look for *causative organisms:* most folliculitis is due to follicular occlusion with normal flora, but some cases are due to *Staphylococcus*, Gram negatives (Gram-negative folliculitis, especially in patients on chronic antibiotics), *Tinea* (13.10), *Candida* (13.4), *Malassezia*, *Pityrosporum*, or *Demodex* (15.8)
- Perifollicular fibrosis in older lesions

Variations

1. Pseudofolliculitis barbae (PFB): razor bumps from shaving the beard and neck (1.86), more in black skin, with *inward-coiling hairs* producing folliculitis (not really a "pseudo").

2. Perifolliculitis capitis abscedens et suffodiens (dissecting cellulitis of the scalp): *severe clinical disease*, more in black skin, more abscess and sinus tract formation on *scalp*.

3. Folliculitis decalvans: *deeper folliculitis on scalp*, more common in black skin, which may progress to dissecting cellulitis.

4. Disseminate infundibulofolliculitis of Hitch and Lund: characteristic clinical appearance of multiple *smooth papules* resembling gooseflesh, mostly on the *upper trunk in black skin*, spongiosis and lymphocytes in superficial part (infundibulum) of follicle and sweat ducts.

5. Eosinophilic pustular folliculitis (Ofuji's disease): form of folliculitis in which papulopustules may become confluent into plaques, more common in HIV disease (14.12) or as a childhood scalp disorder, *many eosinophils* (1.36) in or around follicles along with lymphocytes.

6. Folliculitis keloidalis nuchae: *posterior scalp and neck* ("nuchae"), more in black skin, more scarring (*keloid* formation, 27.2).

7. Hot tub folliculitis: due to *Pseudomonas* from exposure to hot tubs with inadequate bromine, self-limited.

8. Erosive pustulosis of the scalp: idiopathic condition with pustules, erosions of scalp.

9. Epidermal growth factor inhibitor (EGFRI) drug reaction. The drugs lapatinib, cetuximab, erlotinib, and panitumumab are used for solid tumors, often resulting in folliculitis.

Differential diagnosis

1. Acne (10.1). The difference between acne and folliculitis is sometimes moot because the follicle and sebaceous gland are all part of a pilosebaceous unit.

2. Special stains and cultures can help to rule out bacterial or fungal folliculitis.

3. Other diseases with follicular plugging (1.47), neutrophils in the dermis (1.89), or granulomas (1.51).

10.3 Perforating folliculitis

Uncommon papular eruption with hyperkeratotic plugs or pustules in the center of lesions, distinguished from ordinary folliculitis by some authorities because of the rupture of the follicular walls, but this may not really be different than any other form of folliculitis (10.2).

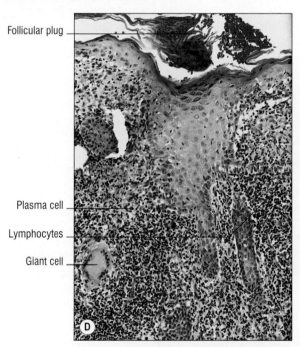

Follicular plug

Plasma cell

Lymphocytes

Giant cell

Fig. 10.1 D Granulomatous rosacea.

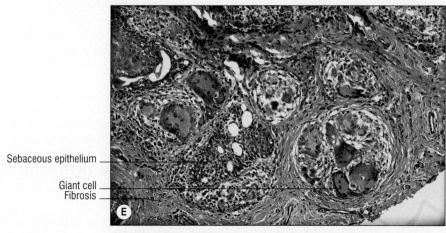

Sebaceous epithelium

Giant cell
Fibrosis

Fig. 10.1 E Chalazion.

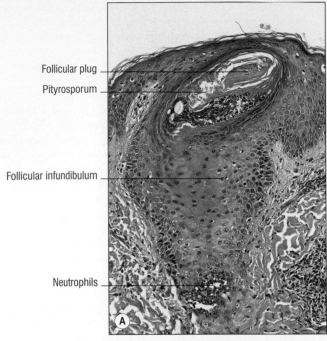

Fig. 10.2 A Folliculitis.

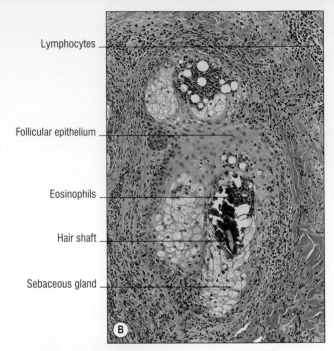

Fig. 10.2 B Eosinophilic folliculitis.

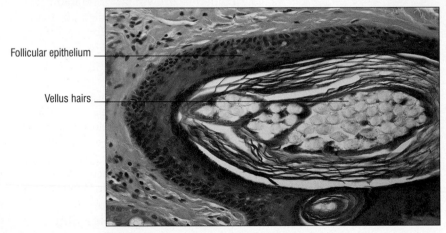

Fig. 10.4 Trichostasis spinulosa.

P
- Follicular plugging
- *Perforation of the follicle* by degenerating elastic and collagen fibers
- Perifollicular neutrophils (1.89), lymphocytes, or plasma cells (1.111) often

Differential diagnosis

1. Other perforating diseases (1.140) or follicular diseases (1.47).

10.4 Trichostasis spinulosa

(see Fig. 10.4)
Common as an incidental histologic finding in some other lesion such as a melanocytic nevus, or presenting as multiple black open comedones (1.24), especially on the nose (1.95) or face (1.44), sometimes associated with acne (10.1).

P
- Numerous vellus hairs within a follicle

Differential diagnosis

1. Pili multigemini: terminal hairs are clumped within a follicle instead of vellus hairs, arising from multiple divisions within the hair matrix, or several hair papillae may converge into one follicle, most common on the beard of males. Hairs may adhere to one another, then become separate, then adhere again (pili bifurcati). Compound hairs, where two or three hairs come forth from a follicle, is similar, considered to be normal on the occipital scalp.
2. Tufted hair or tufted folliculitis (polytrichia, doll's hair deformity) occurs in cicatricial alopecia, where inflammation damages a follicle or multiple adjacent follicles so that multiple hairs come out of one orifice.

10.5 Keratosis pilaris (KP) and lichen spinulosus

(see Fig. 10.5)
Keratosis pilaris is a common eruption of *spiny follicular papules*, especially on the *lateral arms and anterior thighs* of

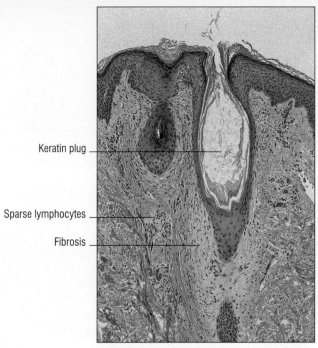

Fig. 10.5 Keratosis pilaris.

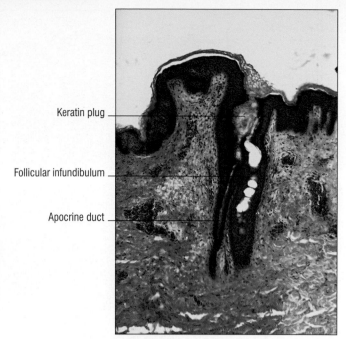

Fig. 10.7 Fox Fordyce disease.

children and young adults. Lichen spinulosus appears as a localized plaque of grouped spiny papules, mostly on the trunk, found in the same age group. Both conditions are associated with atopic dermatitis (2.1).

- Follicular plugging
- Sparse perifollicular lymphocytes or neutrophils sometimes

Variations

1. Ulerythema ophryogenes (KP atrophicans): KP of *cheeks and eyebrows*, beginning in childhood, with *epidermal atrophy and madarosis* (1.77), more perifollicular fibrosis.
2. Atrophoderma vermiculata: *perifollicular atrophy* following KP of the *cheeks* produces a honeycombed *worm-eaten* appearance, resembling severe acne scarring. Associated with Rombo syndrome (atrophoderma vermiculata with basal cell carcinomas, 18.14).

Differential diagnosis

1. Follicular atrophoderma: rare, onset in early childhood, widened follicular ostia with perifollicular fibrosis, without as much keratin plugging as KP. Associated with Conradi syndrome (11.1), palmoplantar keratoderma (2.15), and Bazex syndrome (follicular atrophoderma with basal cell carcinomas of face, 18.14). Don't confuse with atrophoderma of Pasini and Pierini (9.4).
2. Other diseases with follicular plugging (1.47).

10.6 Miliaria

Common, but rarely biopsied "*heat rash*" or "prickly heat", with tiny papules, vesicles, or pustules after heat exposure, sweating, fever, or occlusion. Don't confuse with milia (19.1).

Variations

1. Miliaria crystallina: hundreds of mostly clear, minute, subcorneal vesicles (1.147), which contain no inflammatory cells over sweat duct.
2. Miliaria rubra: red papules, spongiosis of intraepidermal sweat duct, sometimes producing intraepidermal vesicles, perivascular lymphocytes or neutrophils (1.89).
3. Miliaria profunda (miliaria pustulosa): red nodules or pustules, deeper and denser inflammation.

Differential diagnosis

1. Red papular diseases (1.122), especially follicular diseases (1.47), acne (1.3, 10.1), folliculitis (10.2).
2. Neutrophilic eccrine hidradenitis (3.5).

10.7 Fox–Fordyce disease (apocrine miliaria)

(see Fig. 10.7)

Rare, extremely *pruritic* (1.114) eruption of *papules in the axilla* (1.10) and anogenital area of *women*, responds to estrogen therapy. Don't confuse with Fordyce spots (21.1) or angiokeratomas of Fordyce (25.2).

- Spongiosis or vesicle in plugged follicle near connection with apocrine duct
- Perivascular or peri-sweat duct lymphocytes or neutrophils
- Perifollicular foamy histiocytes

Differential diagnosis

1. Hidradenitis suppurativa: more impressive tender nodules or sinus tracts rather than many small pruritic papules.

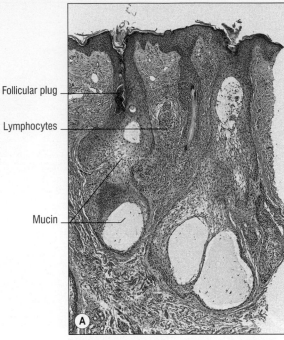

Fig. 10.8 A Follicular mucinosis (low mag.).

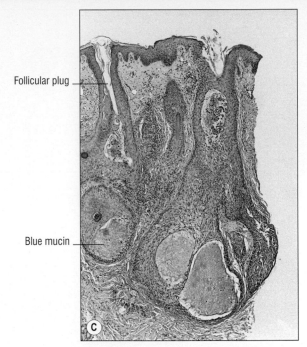

Fig. 10.8 C Follicular mucinosis (Alcian blue stain).

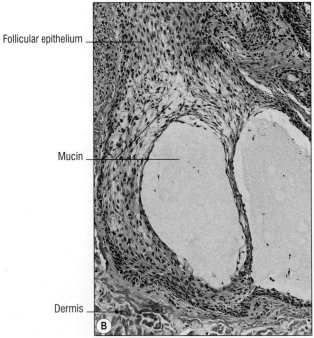

Fig. 10.8 B Follicular mucinosis (high mag.).

- Acid *mucopolysaccharide deposition* (1.83, positive with Alcian blue or colloidal iron stains) *in hair follicle* between keratinocytes, resembling spongiosis
- Perivascular or lichenoid lymphocytes, histiocytes, or eosinophils, with exocytosis into the follicles
- Coexisting *mycosis fungoides* sometimes (24.1). Most studies show that there is no consistent immunoprofile or gene rearrangement finding that accurately predicts which patients will develop MF. Patients under 40 years of age usually have a benign course.

Differential diagnosis

1. Spongiotic diseases (1.132) of the hair follicle lack the mucin deposition.
2. Other alopecias (1.4) or eczematous eruptions (1.29).

10.9 Alopecia areata (AA)

(see Fig. 10.9)

Common autoimmune *non-scarring* alopecia mostly found in children and young adults, resulting in *smooth round patches* of alopecia most commonly on the scalp, but sometimes in the beard. It uncommonly results in complete scalp alopecia (*alopecia totalis*), or alopecia of the entire body, including eyebrows, eyelashes, axilla, and pubic area (*alopecia universalis*). Spontaneous regrowth can occur, especially in localized forms. Involvement of a continuous band from the temple to the occiput is called *ophiasis*, and this has a poor prognosis for regrowth. *Diffuse alopecia areata* is a term used for general thinning of the scalp, instead of the more common localized round patches of alopecia, which may resemble telogen effluvium or androgenetic alopecia. *Exclamation point hairs* that are tapered at the base may persist in localized patches. Nail pits (1.85) resembling hammered brass may occur.

2. Folliculitis (10.2), candidiasis (13.4), contact dermatitis (2.2), miliaria (10.6), other conditions with foamy cells (1.46) and other follicular plugging eruptions (1.47).

10.8 Follicular mucinosis (MF, alopecia mucinosa)

(see Fig. 10.8A–C)

Rare, *red edematous plaques* or *dry scaly patches* with *follicular plugging* (1.47), especially on the head or scalp (1.124), sometimes more extensive.

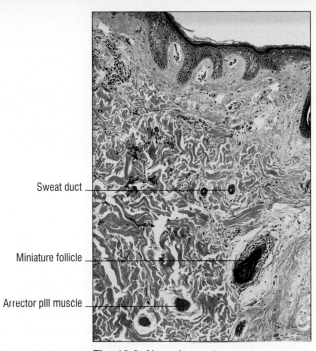

Sweat duct

Miniature follicle

Arrector pill muscle

Fig. 10.9 Alopecia areata.

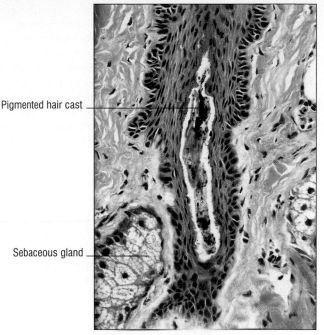

Pigmented hair cast

Sebaceous gland

Fig. 10.11 Traction alopecia.

P • CD4+ lymphocytes, sometimes eosinophils, around hair bulb lower portion of follicle (not the infundibulum or isthmus) in early lesions, said to resemble a "*swarm of bees*"
• Increased numbers of *miniature* ("*nanogen*") *telogen and catagen follicles* or sometimes early anagen hair follicles in the superficial dermis
• Fibrous tract remnants (follicular streamers, follicular stelae) of destroyed follicles may be present, but this can overlap with scarring alopecia[133]

Differential diagnosis

1. Non-scarring alopecia such as trichotillosis (10.11), telogen effluvium (10.14), and androgenetic alopecia (10.12) most closely resemble alopecia areata, and are primarily distinguished clinically but some overrated histologic findings may help somewhat. Trichomalacia and pigmented hair casts have sometimes been reported in alopecia areata biopsies, but perhaps this is because some of the patients also pull their hair or because the finding is just not very specific, like many of the hair loss histologic findings.
2. Other alopecias (1.4).

10.10 Pseudopelade of Brocq

Rare form of scarring alopecia that probably represents the *end-stage* "burned-out" result of a variety of conditions. Sometimes used as a specific diagnosis because of its characteristic clinical appearance of islands of clumps of terminal hairs that persist in a background of severe sclerosis ("*footprints in the snow*"). Pelade is a French term for alopecia areata (10.9), so pseudopelade is supposed to resemble alopecia areata somewhat, but the latter is non-scarring.

P • Lymphocytes mainly around follicles in early lesions
• *Fibrosis and absent follicles* in older lesions

Differential diagnosis

1. Other scarring alopecias (1.4), such as lupus erythematosus, lichen planopilaris, scleroderma, and folliculitis decalvans. Whether pseudopelade is a specific entity or merely an end result of other scarring alopecias is controversial.

10.11 Follicular trauma
(see Fig. 10.11)
Trauma to the follicular unit, either from the habit of pulling, twisting, or otherwise manipulating the hair (*trichotillosis*, a better term than telling people they have *trichotillomania*), or traction from braiding, straightening, and other grooming habits (*traction alopecia, hot comb alopecia*), eventually can scar and cause considerable alopecia. The histologic findings depend greatly upon the stage of development of the lesions biopsied.[110]

• Deformed hair shafts and follicles (*trichomalacia*)   **P**
• *Pigmented casts* (blobs of melanin) in follicles
• *Empty follicles* (hair shafts pulled out), with increased catagen or telogen follicles
• Perifollicular lymphocytes, plasma cells, or neutrophils usually sparse or absent
• Perifollicular hemorrhage sometimes
• Perifollicular fibrosis; if follicle is destroyed, a vertical fibrous tract often remains

Variation

1. Central centrifugal cicatricial alopecia (CCCA): this is the latest popular term for an idiopathic type of scarring hair loss that is poorly understood, a common form of alopecia most common in black women on the central scalp. It is placed here because traction or other hair trauma was thought to play a role, but it may be more

of a genetic problem. It is more of a clinical diagnosis than a pathologic one, because all of the reported histologic findings can be seen in other forms of alopecia. It overlaps with *folliculitis decalvans* (10.1), which is more likely to have neutrophilic pustules or perifollicular granulomas. It was previously called *follicular degeneration syndrome*, because premature desquamation of the inner root sheath below the isthmus was claimed to be particularly characteristic, but this has been debated because that finding is thought by some to be just a sectioning artifact or a non-specific finding. Concentric fibrosis is often seen around the follicles.

Differential diagnosis

1. Other alopecias (1.4).
2. Folliculitis (10.2) is also common in the scalp, particularly in black patients, and trauma of any kind can produce changes just like folliculitis.
3. Lichen planopilaris: more intense perifollicular inflammation along entire follicle, hypergranulosis, follicular plugging, liquefaction degeneration along the follicle.

10.12 Androgenetic alopecia (AGA)

Common *"pattern baldness"*, most common in *men on the bitemporal areas and crown of the scalp*, and less common in women usually as a diffuse, milder, non-scarring alopecia. Related to homones (andro-) and genetic factors. Castrated males apparently do not develop this alopecia. It is only biopsied when not classic clinically (BOOF – biopsy out of frustration). In the opinion of this author, the biopsy is typically non-specific, but may help to reassure the absence of some other condition.

- Miniaturized vellus follicles in late stages (but most forms of chronic alopecia have this!)
- Increased telogen hairs in late stages (but most forms of chronic alopecia have this!)
- Vertical fibrous stelae of destroyed follicles may be present, but this can overlap with scarring alopecia and alopecia areata[133]

Differential diagnosis

1. Alopecia areata (10.9): more in children, more acute onset, more rounded patches of alopecia with different distribution in the scalp.

2. Trichotillomania (10.11).
3. Other alopecias (1.4).

10.13 Lipedematous alopecia

Rare form of alopecia (1.4) in which there is a *boggy thickened edematous-appearing scalp*, usually in *black women*.

- Decreased follicles, increased telogen
- *Increased thickness of adipose tissue*

Differential diagnosis

1. Lipoma (29.2): more localized into a nodule, usually no alopecia.

10.14 Telogen effluvium (TE)

Common condition in which a patient *acutely "molts"* considerable hair, usually from the scalp, often 3 months after a *stressful event* such as major surgery, childbirth, or febrile illness. Due to cycling of growing anagen hairs into the telogen phase. Usually not biopsied unless it is not classic clinically, and often can be diagnosed with a trichogram (examination of hair shafts microscopically) instead of a biopsy.

- Increased telogen hair count
- No miniaturized follicles

Differential diagnosis

1. Other causes of alopecia (1.4), especially diffuse alopecia areata (10.9), trichotillomania, traction alopecia (10.11), and androgenetic alopecia (10.12).

10.15 Neutrophilic eccrine hidradenitis

There are two main forms of this, usually presenting as red painful macules, plaques, or nodules on the palms or soles. One form is associated with chemotherapy (3.5) or bacterial infection. The other occurs mostly in children, sometimes adults (palmoplantar hidradenitis).

- Neutrophils around eccrine sweat glands. Bacteria cannot be demonstrated.
- Syringosquamous metaplasia may occur in the chemotherapy-induced type.

Differential diagnosis

1. Other conditions with dermal neutrophils (1.89).

Some Genodermatoses

11.1 Ichthyosis

(see Fig. 11.1A–D)

Although ichthyosis (fish skin) has traditionally been divided into four major groups (the first four listed below), this is an oversimplification. Most present as *scaly skin* (1.29) at *birth or early childhood*. There are *many syndromes* associated with ichthyosis. Ichthyosis vulgaris, epidermolytic hyperkeratosis, and Refsum's disease show distinctive pathology; the others are less specific histologically.

- *Compact hyperkeratosis* (instead of normal "basket-weave") in most forms of ichthyosis
- Normal or thickened granular layer in most variants, except decreased granular layer (hypogranulosis) in ichthyosis vulgaris and acquired ichthyosis
- Varying degrees of acanthosis, usually not much parakeratosis

Variations

1. Ichthyosis vulgaris: *most common* type of ichthyosis, autosomal dominant, with defect in filaggrin synthesis (FLG gene). Milder *fine whitish scales* begin in childhood, but not usually present at birth, *spares antecubital* and *popliteal flexural* areas. Associated with atopic dermatitis (2.1, which tends to involve flexural creases and is more spongiotic, without a decreased granular layer), and keratosis pilaris (10.5).

- *Compact orthokeratosis* and acanthosis (1.61)
- Decreased or *absent granular layer* (1.63)
- Follicular plugging sometimes (1.47)

2. Epidermolytic hyperkeratosis (EHK, bullous congenital ichthyosiform erythroderma, BCIE): autosomal dominant, defect in keratin 1 (KRT1) or 10 (KRT10, suprabasal keratins), *brownish, verrucous*, scaly skin with appearance of *furrows* and mud on the skin, prominent flexural involvement, *vesicles and bullae* may occur early in life.

- Compact orthokeratosis and acanthosis
- *Hypergranulosis* (1.60)
- Distinct type of degeneration of keratinocytes (1.144) called "*epidermolytic hyperkeratosis*" (superficial epidermis degenerated, appearing as if "blown out by a shotgun")
- Sometimes intraepidermal blisters (1.147) in the degenerated areas, early in infancy (not later in life)

3. X-linked ichthyosis: *brownish scaly* eruption begins in early childhood in *males*. Associated with steroid sulfatase deficiency (STS gene). More likely to involve the flexural creases than ichthyosis vulgaris, but sometimes flexures are spared.

4. Lamellar ichthyosis: autosomal recessive (possibly there is a rare autosomal dominant form), *severe thick plates* of scale resemble reptile scales, onset usually at birth. Variants have been associated with keratinocyte transglutaminase, ABCA12, or CYP4F22 genes. Involves flexures, palms, and soles. May present as a collodion baby. Associated with mutation in keratinocyte transglutaminase. Lamellar ichthyosis has been separated from *non-bullous recessive congenital ichthyosiform erythroderma* (NCIE), on the basis of the former being less severe, and improving with age, but there may not be overlap between these conditions.

5. Collodion baby: ichthyosis of the *newborn*, representing initial presentation of lamellar ichthyosis, or less commonly one of the other forms.

6. Harlequin fetus: rare, mutation in ABCA12 gene (also causes some forms of lamellar ichthyosis), a more severe form of collodion baby infant born encased in thick horny skin with deep fissures, *marked ectropion* and *eclabium, rudimentary ears*, usually *fatal*, massive compact orthokeratosis, sometimes with parakeratosis, absence of lamellar bodies with electron microscopy.

7. Conradi–Hunermann syndrome: rare, mutation in gene encoding delta(8)-delta(7) sterol isomerase emopamil-binding protein (EBP), X-linked dominant, linear (1.73)

©2012 Elsevier Ltd, Inc, BV
DOI: 10.1016/B978-0-323-06658-7.00011-7

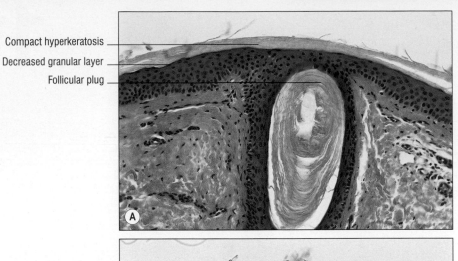

Compact hyperkeratosis
Decreased granular layer
Follicular plug

Fig. 11.1 A Ichthyosis vulgaris.

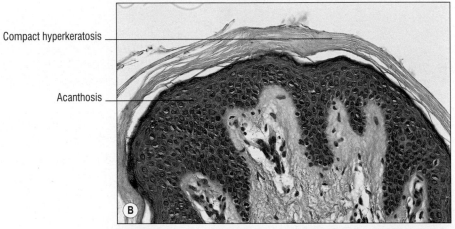

Compact hyperkeratosis

Acanthosis

Fig. 11.1 B X-linked ichthyosis.

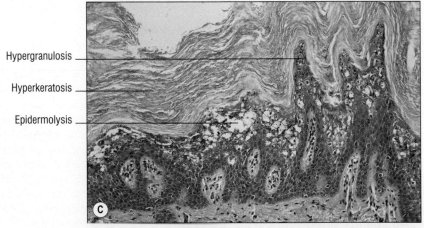

Hypergranulosis

Hyperkeratosis

Epidermolysis

Fig. 11.1 C Epidermolytic hyperkeratosis.

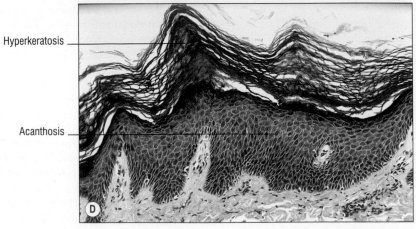

Hyperkeratosis

Acanthosis

Fig. 11.1 D Erythrokeratodermia variabilis.

or whorled ichthyosis with hyperpigmentation, cataracts, and skeletal defects such as *chondrodysplasia punctata* (stippled epiphyses).

8. Netherton's syndrome: rare, but one of the more common ichthyotic syndromes, autosomal recessive, mutation in gene encoding serine protease inhibitor Kazal-type 5 (SPINK5), failure to thrive in infancy, generalized erythroderma, mild alopecia with hair defect (1.4) known as *trichorrhexis invaginata* (*bamboo hair*). About half of the patients develop a peculiar migratory *ichthyosis linearis circumflexa* (*annular* (1.5) to serpiginous (1.127), psoriasiform (1.119) plaques, that have *double-edged borders* described by Comel, so sometimes is called Comel–Netherton syndrome), PAS-positive exudative material in the granular layer has been emphasized, but is not so specific.

9. Erythrokeratodermia variabilis (Mendes da Costa syndrome): rare, autosomal dominant, mutation in genes for gap junction proteins GJB3 (encoding connexin 31) and GJB4 (encoding connexin 30.3), onset within 1 year of age, *polycyclic to annular* (1.5) *migrating* red scaly plaques, often palmoplantar keratoderma (2.15).

10. Refsum's disease: Rare, autosomal recessive, generalized ichthyosis, cerebellar ataxia, peripheral neuropathy, retinitis pigmentosa, and elevated CSF protein without increase in cells. Classic adult form has a mutation in gene encoding phytanoyl-CoA hydroxylase (PHYH, or PAHX), or gene for peroxin-7 (PEX7). Infantile form has mutation in PEX1, PEX2, or PEX 26 genes. *Lipid vacuoles in suprabasal cells, phytanic acid* accumulation.

11. Sjögren–Larsson syndrome: rare, mutation in ALDH3A2 gene for fatty aldehyde dehydrogenase, autosomal recessive, seizures, retinitis pigmentosa, lamellar ichthyosis, mental retardation, *and spastic paresis*.

12. Keratitis–ichthyosis–deafness (KID) syndrome: rare, sporadic or autosomal dominant, mutation in gap junction protein GJB2 (encoding connexin-26), face, elbows, knees, palm and sole ichthyosis, sparing trunk.

13. CHILD syndrome (congenital hemidysplasia with ichthyosiform erythroderma and limb defects): rare, probably X-linked, mutation in gene encoding NSDHL, almost always females, *unilateral* ichthyosis with *underdeveloped limbs* on same side.

14. Ichthyosis hystrix: autosomal dominant, *form of epidermal nevus* with *whorling* (18.1), may have epidermolytic hyperkeratosis.

15. Ichthyosis bullosa of Siemens: rare, autosomal dominant, blistering ichthyosis similar to epidermolytic hyperkeratosis, except that hyperkeratosis is mild, the *epidermolysis involves mostly the granular layer* and is less extensive, and the gene defect is keratin 2e.

16. Acquired ichthyosis: onset in adulthood, often as a *paraneoplastic* syndrome (1.105), especially with lymphoma, histology usually like ichthyosis vulgaris.

17. Pityriasis rotunda: rare, *perfectly round*, sharply demarcated, scaly plaques, more common in pigmented races, sometimes familial or associated with underlying malignancy, sometimes considered a localized form of ichthyosis vulgaris or acquired ichthyosis.

Differential diagnosis

1. Other diseases with hyperplasia of epidermis (1.61), especially eczema (2.1).
2. The histologic finding of epidermolytic hyperkeratosis can be seen in some forms of hyperkeratosis palmaris et plantaris (2.16), some forms of epidermal nevi (18.1), epidermolytic acanthoma and, occasionally, as an incidental finding in a variety of disorders, especially dysplastic nevi.[144] Normally it is not mistaken for spongiosis (1.132), koilocytosis (14.1), or artifactual vacuolization of keratinocytes (1.144).

11.2 Ectodermal dysplasia

Very rare heterogeneous group of more than 150 disorders of skin and its appendages, mainly involving *hair, teeth, nails, and sweating*. It is a misnomer because the ectoderm is hypoplastic, not dysplastic (if dysplasia is defined as cytologic atypia of epithelium). Traditionally, patients were imperfectly placed into hidrotic and anhidrotic groups.

- Decreased number and hypoplasia of sebaceous glands and hair follicles
- Decreased number or absent sweat glands in patients with the anhidrotic form

P

Variations

1. Hidrotic ectodermal dysplasia: autosomal dominant, mutation in GJB6 gene encoding connexin-20, milder disease than anhidrotic, patients retain relatively *normal sweating*, alopecia (1.4), dystrophic nails (1.85), and *palmoplantar keratoderma* (2.15), dental defects sometimes.
2. Anhidrotic (hypohidrotic) ectodermal dysplasia: X-linked recessive, mutation in gene encoding ectodysplasin-A (EDA), mostly *males, characteristic facies*, with frontal bossing and a depressed nasal bridge, decreased or *absent sweating*, alopecia (1.4), dystrophic nails (1.85), and marked dental defects.
3. Schoepf syndrome: alopecia, nail dystrophy, teeth defects, *eyelid hidrocystomas*, basal cell carcinoma, palmoplantar keratoderma associated with *syringofibroadenomatosis* (23.10).

Differential diagnosis

1. Ectodermal dysplasia is primarily a clinical diagnosis, and biopsies of palms or soles are mainly helpful by showing absent sweat glands in the anhidrotic form, or associated findings such as syringofibroadenomatosis.

11.3 Darier's disease (Darier–White disease, keratosis follicularis)

(see Fig. 11.3A–C)

Uncommon *autosomal dominant* disorder, related to calcium pump protein mutation ATP2A2 (compare with Hailey–Hailey disease, ATP2C1), with *ground nutmeg dirty verrucous appearance of skin of the trunk* (1.141), and sometimes the face, flaring with sun or heat exposure (1.110), *palmar pits* (1.100), *nails* with longitudinal ridges and triangular distal defects

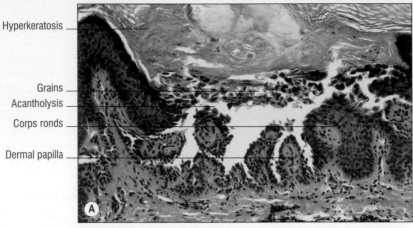

Hyperkeratosis

Grains
Acantholysis
Corps ronds

Dermal papilla

Fig. 11.3 A Darier's disease (low mag.).

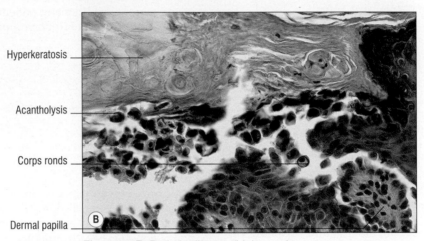

Hyperkeratosis

Acantholysis

Corps ronds

Dermal papilla

Fig. 11.3 B Darier's disease (high mag.).

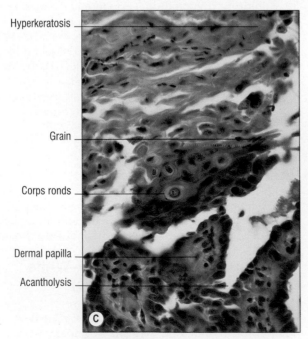

Hyperkeratosis

Grain

Corps ronds

Dermal papilla

Acantholysis

Fig. 11.3 C Darier's disease (high mag.).

(1.85), *white plaques in the mouth* (1.82). *Acrokeratosis verruciformis* may occur (18.3) on the dorsum of hands and feet.

- *Hyperkeratosis*, parakeratosis sometimes, pseudoepitheliomatous hyperplasia sometimes (1.116), basaloid hyperplasia sometimes. "Follicularis" is partially a misnomer because the hyperkeratosis is not preferentially over follicles, but sometimes follicular plugging is indeed present (1.47)
- Papillomatosis and acanthosis
- *Acantholytic dyskeratotic keratinocytes*, often forming "*corps ronds*" and "grains" (1.27)
- Clefts (1.23) or *lacunae* forming in suprabasal location due to acantholysis; dermal papillae lined by basal cells stick up into the lacunae, resembling *villi*. Rarely this can appear clinically vesiculobullous (1.147)

Differential diagnosis

1. Other diseases with acantholysis (1.2), especially those that also show dyskeratosis: transient acantholytic dermatosis (TAD, 5.2), warty dyskeratoma (18.7), and sometimes Hailey–Hailey disease (5.5). TAD can be identical histologically and sometimes must be

distinguished clinically. Pemphigus (5.4) is usually not dyskeratotic, without corps ronds, and tends to have eosinophils. Linear epidermal nevus (18.1) may have acantholytic dyskeratosis, and some forms of this have been called localized, linear, or zosteriform Darier's disease. The rare familial dyskeratotic comedones has a clinically comedonal appearance with acantholysis at the base of the comedones.

11.4 Dyskeratosis congenita (DKC)

Very rare X-linked recessive disorder due to mutation in gene encoding dyskerin (DKC1). There is an autosomal dominant form related to mutation in the gene encoding telomerase RNA component (TERC). There is a recessive form due to mutation in NOLA3 gene (NOP10), or NOLA2 (NHP2). The X-linked form is mostly in *males*, with *reticulated* (1.123), *poikilodermatous* (1.112), grayish (1.54) *hyperpigmentation* (1.18) of the *neck* (1.86), thighs, and trunk, *leukoplakia* in the mouth (1.82), especially on the buccal mucosa, that may become carcinoma, nail dystrophy (1.85), aplastic anemia, and internal malignancies (1.105).

- Epidermis normal or atrophic (1.9)
- *Melanin incontinence*
- Absent or minimal interface lymphocytes (1.64)

Differential diagnosis
1. The pathology is non-specific, and the diagnosis is primarily made clinically. Consider other disorders with melanin incontinence (1.79).

11.5 Rothmund–Thomson syndrome (poikiloderma congenitale)

Very rare, autosomal recessive, mutation in DNA helicase gene RECQL4, *photodermatitis* (1.110), with *poikiloderma* (1.112), *dwarfism, hypogonadism,* saddle nose, congenital bone defects, mental retardation, *cataracts* (1.41), predisposed to actinic keratosis and squamous cell carcinoma.

- Epidermal atrophy (1.9)
- Liquefaction degeneration of the basal layer in early lesions
- *Melanin incontinence*
- Perivascular or lichenoid lymphocytes in early lesions
- Dilated blood vessels

Differential diagnosis
1. Other diseases with liquefaction degeneration of the basal layer (1.64) or melanin incontinence (1.79).
2. Bloom's syndrome (11.10): less melanin incontinence.

11.6 Incontinentia pigmenti (IP, Bloch–Sulzberger syndrome)

(see Fig. 11.6A,B)
Rare X-linked dominant disorder mainly found in *female* infants (thought to be mostly lethal in males), related to IKK-gamma gene (inhibitor of kappa-B kinase) of the NEMO (NF-kappa-B essential modulator) complex. The first stage of skin lesions are *linear vesicles* (1.73) mostly on extremities. The second stage is *verrucous papules* and plaques (1.146) on extremities, lasting several months. The third stage is *whorled hyperpigmentation on the trunk*. Sometimes hypopigmented or atrophic patches are considered to be a fourth stage in adults. It is associated with bone and teeth abnormalities (1.16), eye disease (1.41), and central nervous system disease (seizures, mental retardation).

1. First stage

- Eosinophilic spongiosis and intraepidermal vesicles containing eosinophils
- Dyskeratotic keratinocytes
- Perivascular lymphocytes and eosinophils

2. Second stage

- Papillomatosis, hyperkeratosis, and acanthosis
- Pale glassy keratinocytes, often dyskeratotic and forming squamous eddies
- Minimal perivascular lymphocytes
- Melanin incontinence

3. Third stage

- Melanin incontinence, sometimes with basal cell degeneration or basal cell hyperpigmentation

Differential diagnosis
1. Other diseases with eosinophilic spongiosis (1.36) resemble the first stage, but the presence of dyskeratosis (1.27) combined with eosinophilic spongiosis is nearly pathognomonic.
2. Other diseases with prominent verrucous changes with dyskeratosis and squamous eddies (1.27) may resemble the second stage.
3. Other diseases with melanin incontinence (1.79) may resemble the third stage.

11.7 Hypomelanosis of Ito (incontinentia pigmenti achromians)

(see Fig. 11.7)
Rare, sporadic, and rarely familial *whorled hypopigmentation of the trunk* (1.141) since birth or early childhood, in the same pattern seen in the hyperpigmented patches of incontinentia pigmenti (11.6). Online Mendelian Inheritance in Man (OMIM) states that it is not a distinct entity and is a symptom of many different states of mosaicism. Usually related to X-chromosome. Patients often have mental retardation, seizures, skeletal anomalies, abnormal teeth and eyes.

- *Decreased melanocytes and melanin* at the basal layer (special stains for melanin needed)

Differential diagnosis
1. Vitiligo (17.2) and other hypopigmented disorders (1.150) are usually not whorled, so the diagnosis is primarily clinical.

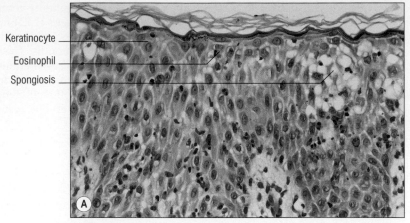

Keratinocyte
Eosinophil
Spongiosis

Fig. 11.6 A Incontinentia pigmenti (vesicular stage).

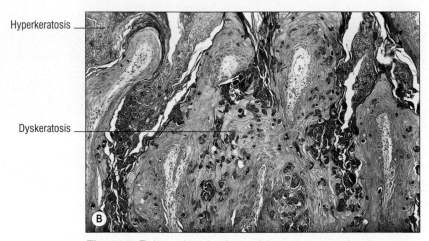

Hyperkeratosis

Dyskeratosis

Fig. 11.6 B Incontinentia pigmenti (verrucous stage).

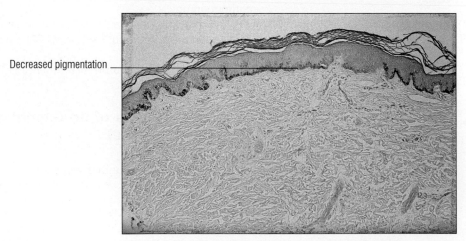

Decreased pigmentation

Fig. 11.7 Hypomelanosis of Ito (Fontana melanin stain).

11.8 Goltz syndrome (focal dermal hypoplasia)

(see Fig. 11.8)

Very rare X-linked dominant disorder found mostly in *females*, related to mutation in the PORCN gene. *Linear* plaques (1.73) of *atrophic skin* resembling striae, hypopigmentation or hyper-pigmentation, telangiectasia (1.136), *yellowish nodules* (1.151), and ulcers, syndactyly or *malformation of digits* ("lobster

claw"), eye defects (1.41), hypoplasia of hair, teeth, and nails. Parallel, vertical striations in the metaphyses of long bones (*osteopathia striata*, 1.16) are characteristic.

- Severe dermal atrophy so that the *subcutaneous fat may reach the epidermis* (or perhaps is a fatty hamartoma in the dermis instead)

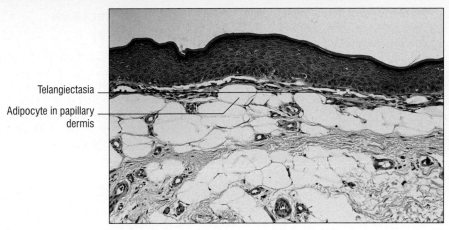

Telangiectasia

Adipocyte in papillary dermis

Fig. 11.8 Goltz syndrome.

Differential diagnosis

1. Other diseases with dermal atrophy (1.8) rarely cause confusion because they are much different clinically and the dermal atrophy is not as severe. See nevus lipomatosus (29.1) for a list of other diseases that have adipose located in the superficial dermis.

11.9 Albinism (oculocutaneous albinism)

Uncommon, group of genetic conditions, almost all autosomal recessive, with *congenital, generalized lack of melanin* pigment in *skin, hair,* and *eyes* (1.41). *Nystagmus* may be present. *Tyrosinase-positive* patients may produce small amounts of pigment in their hair, eyes, or skin (such as *solar lentigines* in sun-exposed areas), whereas the *tyrosinase-negative* patients have more severe albinism without this capacity. *Actinic keratoses, basal cell carcinomas, squamous cell carcinomas,* and *melanomas* can become quite problematic in these patients without pigmentation. Protection from the sun is critical for these patients, especially those living in the tropics.

- *Melanocytes are present* at the basal layer, but do not actively produce melanin
- *Decreased or absent melanin* demonstrated with Fontana melanin stain

Variations (some of these are really separate conditions from albinism)

1. Piebaldism (formerly called partial albinism): autosomal dominant, KIT mutation, congenital localized patches of depigmentation of skin and hair (poliosis is decreased hair pigmentation), especially on the forehead (white forelock) and usually elsewhere also. Melanocytes are absent or reduced, sometimes with few large melanocytes.
2. Waardenburg's syndrome: autosomal dominant, at least four different types, mutation of MITF, PAX3, or other genes, depigmentation of localized skin or hair (poliosis), especially white forelock like piebaldism, iris heterochromia, dystopia canthorum (increased inner canthi distance with normal interpupillary distance) and congenital deafness. Pathology like piebaldism.

3. Nevus depigmentosus (17.10): normal number of melanocytes with short dendrites.

Differential diagnosis

1. Albinism is primarily a clinical diagnosis. Other hypopigmented disorders (1.150) are rarely confused with it, and biopsies are rarely performed except on the skin neoplasms that may occur.

11.10 Bloom syndrome (congenital telangiectatic erythema)

Rare autosomal recessive disorder, mutation in gene encoding DNA helicase RecQ protein-like-3, *chromosome instability,* thin face with prominent nose, butterfly-distributed erythematous *photodermatitis* of the cheeks (1.110) with onset in infancy, *dwarfism,* normal mental development, severe respiratory infections, carcinoma of skin, *leukemia and lymphoma.* Sometimes there can be serum IgA or IgM deficiency.

- Interface dermatitis (1.64) or perivascular lymphocytic dermatitis (1.109)
- Telangiectasia (1.136)

Differential diagnosis

1. Cockayne syndrome: rare, autosomal recessive, DNA repair disorder caused by mutation in ERCC8 or ERCC6 genes, mostly males, photodermatitis, progeria-like (9.6) "Mickey-mouse" facies, with prognathism and sunken eyes, large ears, feet and hands, dwarfism, mental retardation, deafness.
2. Rothmund–Thomson syndrome (11.5): more pigmentary changes, hypogonadism, cataracts, no IgA or IgM deficiency, no chromosome breakage, no increase in leukemia and lymphoma.
3. Other forms of photodermatitis (1.110), especially lupus erythematosus (17.6).

11.11 Xeroderma pigmentosum (XP)

Rare autosomal recessive heterogeneous group of disorders causing *photosensitivity* (1.110), with a variety of genetic defects of DNA repair following ultraviolet radiation, numerous *solar lentigines* (20.4), *poikiloderma* (1.112) in sun-exposed areas, xerosis, scarring, and many *actinic keratoses, basal cell carcinomas, squamous cell carcinomas*, and *melanomas* develop in childhood.

- Epidermis may be atrophic (1.9) or hyperkeratotic (1.61)
- Necrotic keratinocytes (1.86) sometimes
- *Solar elastosis* (9.1), *telangiectasia* (1.136)
- Basal layer decreased or increased melanin, dermal *melanin incontinence* (1.79)
- Perivascular lymphocytes (1.109)
- *Neoplasms* as above

Variation

1. DeSanctis–Cacchione syndrome: microcephaly, dwarfism, choreoathetosis, cerebellar ataxia, and mental retardation.

11.12 Ataxia–telangiectasia (Louis–Bar syndrome)

Rare, autosomal recessive, mutation in ataxia–telangiectasia mutated gene (ATM), *chromosomal breakage, cerebellar ataxia* beginning in infancy, *telangiectasias* (1.136) of *skin and bulbar conjunctiva* (1.41) later in childhood, sclerodermoid progeria-like changes (11.9), nystagmus, mental retardation, frequent *IgA or IgE deficiency, increased serum alpha-fetoprotein, sinopulmonary infections, leukemia or lymphoma.*

- Dilated blood vessels in the dermis
- Café-au-lait macules sometimes (20.2)

CHAPTER 12

Bacterial Diseases

12.1 Impetigo

(see Fig. 12.1A–D)
Common superficial infection with *Staphylococcus aureus* and/or *Streptococcus pyogenes*. Most common in children, especially around mouth, nose (1.95), axilla, or groin (1.55). *Honey-colored crusts* and an acute onset are typical. Glomerulonephritis (1.66) is a rare complication.

P
- *Subcorneal pustule* filled with neutrophils and sometimes occasional acantholytic cells
- Spongiosis often (1.132)
- Dermal perivascular lymphocytes and neutrophils
- *Gram-positive cocci* sometimes found in the pustule (but culture is more helpful)

Variations

1. Bullous impetigo (12.2).
2. Furuncle: deeper infection, usually by *Staphylococcus aureus*, often centered upon a follicular unit, dermal abscess formation, sometimes with subcorneal pustule.
3. Furunculosis: multiple furuncles, often associated with chronic staphylococcal carrier state, may closely resemble hidradenitis (10.1).
4. Ecthyma: punched-out ulcers usually associated with *Streptococcus pyogenes*.
5. Pyoderma vegetans (blastomycosis-like pyoderma, 4.12).

Differential diagnosis

1. Most other diseases with subcorneal pustules (1.89) cannot be distinguished without clinical correlation, special stains, or cultures.
2. Superficial acantholytic conditions (1.2) such as pemphigus (5.4), or herpes virus (14.2).

12.2 Toxin-induced bacterial diseases

(see Fig. 12.2)
Uncommon infections with toxin-producing bacteria that are usually found at sites remote from the skin lesions. The prototype, *staphylococcal scalded skin syndrome* (SSSS, Ritter's disease), occurs mostly in children, and is due to *Staphylococcus aureus* in phage group II. Fever (1.45), mild constitutional symptoms, and conjunctivitis (1.43), appear along with *flaccid bullae* with fragile roofs on *red skin appearing like a burn*, especially of the face and neck, later elsewhere.

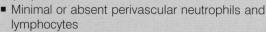

P
- *Subcorneal blister* (1.147) containing only *rare inflammatory cells* and sometimes some acantholytic cells (1.2)
- Minimal or absent perivascular neutrophils and lymphocytes
- Bacteria not present in the blistering toxin-induced lesions (culture may be positive from the nares, groin, or conjunctiva)

Variations

1. Bullous impetigo: toxin-producing staphylococci cause *subcorneal blisters* (1.147), with absent or rare cocci, occasional acantholytic keratinocytes (1.2), and papillary dermal edema with *very little inflammation*.
2. Scarlet fever: fever, acute generalized bright red rough *"sandpaper" rash* in children (1.81), accentuation in skin folds (*Pastia's lines*), post-erythema desquamation later, due to *Streptococcus pyogenes* that is usually in the pharynx, pharyngitis, *strawberry tongue* (1.139). Complications include myocarditis (1.57) and glomerulonephritis (1.66). Diagnosis made clinically rather than by biopsy. Biopsy varies, with spongiosis, necrotic keratinocytes (sometimes inclusion bodies

©2012 Elsevier Ltd, Inc, BV
DOI: 10.1016/B978-0-323-06658-7.00012-9

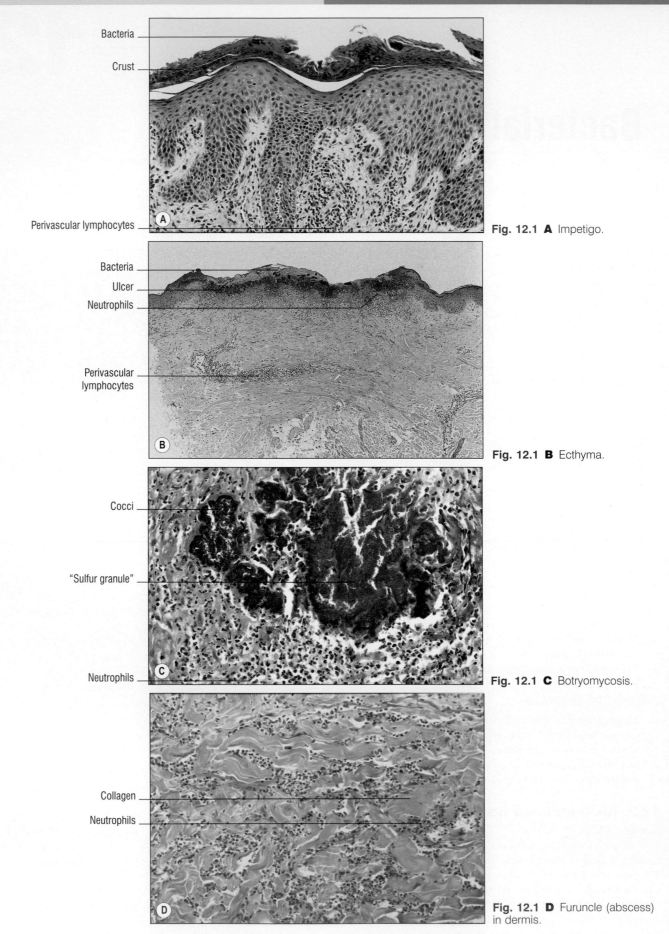

Fig. 12.1 **A** Impetigo.

Fig. 12.1 **B** Ecthyma.

Fig. 12.1 **C** Botryomycosis.

Fig. 12.1 **D** Furuncle (abscess) in dermis.

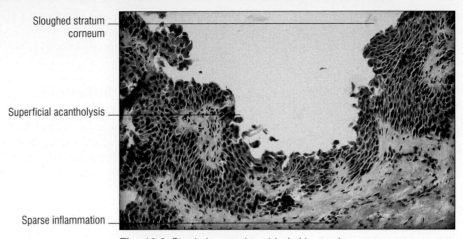

Sloughed stratum corneum

Superficial acantholysis

Sparse inflammation

Fig. 12.2 Staphylococcal scalded skin syndrome.

called Mallory's bodies), exocytosis of lymphocytes or neutrophils into the epidermis, and perivascular lymphocytes and neutrophils.

3. Rheumatic fever: acute febrile illness, mostly in children, due to *Streptococcus pyogenes*, usually present in the pharynx. The five major criteria are erythema marginatum rheumaticum that are evanescent, annular (1.5), red macules with histology like urticaria (3.1), carditis (1.57), polyarthritis (1.7), chorea, and rheumatic fever nodules that are palisading granulomas (1.51).

4. Toxic shock syndrome: rare acute illness, *high fever*, sunburn-like rash, post-erythema desquamation later, *hypotension*, and involvement of at least three organ systems, due to *Staphylococcus aureus* (phage group I) or *Streptococcus pyogenes* toxin. The bacteria proliferate in *tampons*, abscesses or surgical wounds. Biopsy like scarlet fever.

5. Typhoid fever: due to *Salmonella typhi* gastroenteritis (1.49), few red macules or papules called *rose spots* appear on the trunk, especially periumbilical (1.143), dilated blood vessels infiltrated by *macrophages* (1.76) that may contain the Gram-negative bacteria.

Differential diagnosis

1. Other morbilliform eruptions (1.81), and fever with rash (1.45), especially Kawasaki's syndrome (14.10) and drug eruption (3.5).

2. Toxic epidermal necrolysis (3.2) also has sloughing of skin, but there is epidermal necrosis and the sloughing is subepidermal rather than subcorneal. An emergency frozen section is sometimes recommended, but usually the difference is obvious clinically because SSSS mostly occurs in children and the blisters are much more superficial than toxic epidermal necrolysis.

3. Other diseases with perivascular dermatitis (1.109), spongiosis (1.132), or necrotic keratinocytes (1.86).

12.3 Infectious cellulitis

(see Fig. 12.3)

Common infection of the skin usually presenting as *bright red tender erythema*. Cellulitis is defined in the dictionary simply as inflammation of tissue but is commonly used to mean infectious cellulitis, usually due to group A streptococci (*Streptococcus pyogenes*), *Staphylococcus aureus*, or other bacteria.

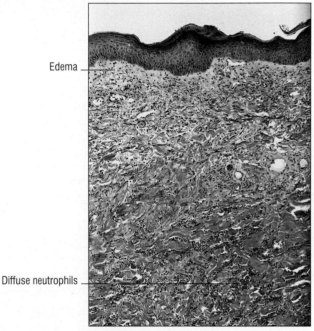

Edema

Diffuse neutrophils

Fig. 12.3 Infectious cellulitis.

- Epidermis usually normal; sometimes with necrosis (1.86)
- Dermal edema
- *Diffuse or interstitial infiltrate of predominantly neutrophils* in the dermis, sometimes sparse
- Bacteria uncommonly can be seen with Gram stain
- Culture of biopsy positive in less than 10% of cases

Variations

1. Erysipelas: cellulitis of the *face* (1.44) due to group A streptococci, usually presenting as a red edematous plaque with a *sharply demarcated elevated border*, histology with *edema* often more prominent than inflammation.

2. Erysipeloid: rare red macules or plaques of the hand (1.56) due to infection with *Erysipelothrix rhusiopathiae*, in those who handle fish or other animal products.

3. Paronychia: infection of periungual region (1.56), with tender erythema, crusting, or pustules, associated with

Staphylococcus aureus in most acute infections, and with *Candida* (13.4) in some chronic infections.

4. Blistering distal dactylitis: infection of the distal finger (1.56) with *Streptococcus pyogenes* or *Staphylococcus aureus* results in tender erythema, edema, crusting, or blistering, mostly in children or adolescents, sometimes with an upper respiratory infection also.

5. Necrotizing fasciitis: acute, rapidly progressive, deep infection of fascia and soft tissue often related to injury, diabetes, alcoholism, peripheral vascular disease, drug abuse, or immunosuppression. A variety of synergistic bacteria may grow in culture. Biopsies have diffuse infiltration of soft tissue with neutrophils and lymphocytes, often with necrosis (1.87), hemorrhage (1.40), and thrombosis (1.137).

6. Perianal streptococcal cellulitis: due to group A beta-hemolytic streptococci, perianal area (1.108), almost always in infants.

Differential diagnosis

1. Other diseases with neutrophils in the dermis (1.89) or edema of the dermis (1.30).

12.4 Anthrax

Infection usually related to contact with infected animals, such as *goats and sheep*, rare except in undeveloped countries, due to *Bacillus anthracis*. About 5% of cases are inhalation anthrax (wool sorter's disease), but 95% occur after primary skin inoculation, usually on the hands (1.56). Lesions are red macules that become pustular ("*malignant pustule*"), later ulcerating with a *black eschar*, healing spontaneously or resulting in systemic infection.

P
- *Epidermal necrosis* or ulceration (1.142)
- Dermal edema (1.30)
- Extravasated erythrocytes (1.40)
- Diffuse dermal neutrophils or minimal inflammation
- *Large Gram-positive rods* (average 1–8 microns) often visible with H&E

Differential diagnosis

1. Sweet's syndrome (3.7), staphylococcal infections (12.1), erysipeloid (12.3), atypical mycobacteria (12.11),

sporotrichosis (13.11), herpetic whitlow (14.2), orf (14.5), and tularemia (12.6).

2. Other diseases with epidermal necrosis (1.86) or diffuse dermal neutrophils (1.89).

12.5 Corynebacterial infections

(see Fig. 12.5)
Some corynebacteria are considered normal flora in the follicles, but some species are pathogenic, and overgrowth of normal flora in moist conditions can also cause disease.

Variations

1. Erythrasma: *red–brown patches* in *intertriginous areas* (1.10, 1.55) with only slight scale, due to *Corynebacterium minutissimum*, *coral-red fluorescence* with Wood's light exam. Gram-positive coccobacilli or filaments in the stratum corneum may be barely visible with H&E, or stained better with PAS or Giemsa stain, with minimal host inflammatory reaction.

2. Trichomycosis: *yellowish nodular concretions on axillary or pubic hairs*, associated with *Corynebacterium tenuis* (1 micron or less), which may be confused with white piedra (*Trichosporon beigelii* or other *Trichosporon sp*) or black piedra (*Piedraia hortae*), both of which are fungi with larger organisms (4–8 microns).

3. Pitted keratolysis: *numerous 1-mm pits* occur in the *macerated stratum corneum of the soles*, associated with *Corynebacterium* species, *Micrococcus sedentarius*, *Dermatophilus congolensis*, or *Actinomyces*. Biopsy like erythrasma.

4. Diphtheria: *Corynebacteria diphtheriae* causes pharyngitis with a pseudomembrane in unimmunized patients in undeveloped countries, with complications due to the toxin that is produced. It rarely can cause a *secondary skin infection complicating eczema or scabies*, usually presenting as necrotic ulcers with considerable fibrin, and neutrophils. Sometimes the Gram-positive bacilli are found. It can be cultured with special media.

12.6 Tularemia

Very rare infection by *Francisella tularensis* occurs after contact with *wild rabbits*, deer flies, tick feces, or other animals. The most common type of infection is *ulcero-glandular*. A red papule on the *finger or hand* (1.56) evolves into an ulcer (1.142)

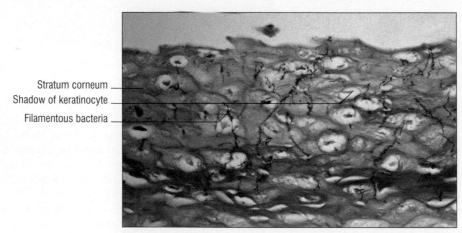

Stratum corneum
Shadow of keratinocyte
Filamentous bacteria

Fig. 12.5 Erythrasma (Giemsa stain).

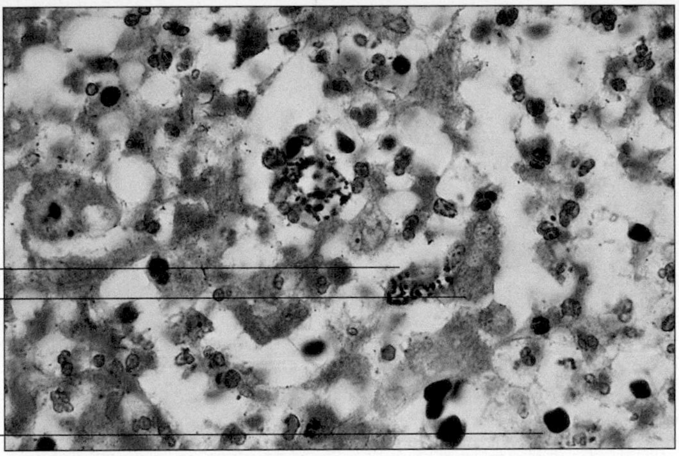

Bacteria

Histiocyte

Lymphocyte

Fig. 12.8 Granuloma inguinale (Warthin–Starry stain).

with a black eschar, with prominent lymphadenopathy. Other less common types of infection include oculoglandular, oropharyngeal, gastrointestinal, pulmonary, and typhoidal presentations. The *diagnosis is usually made serologically.* Cultures are hazardous. Polymerase chain reaction (PCR) has been used.

P
- Epidermal necrosis (1.86) or *ulceration*
- *Mixed diffuse infiltrate of neutrophils*, lymphocytes, histiocytes, and multinucleated giant cells
- *Granulomas* may be tuberculoid or sarcoidal, sometimes with caseation
- Gram-negative coccobacilli usually cannot be identified by special stains (Dieterle silver stain or fluorescent antibody stains may be helpful)

Differential diagnosis

1. Other hand infections (12.4).
2. Other suppurative granulomas (1.51).

12.7 Chancroid

Uncommon *painful genital ulcer* (1.107, 1.149, *non-indurated "soft chancre"*), often multiple, due to venereal infection with *Haemophilus ducreyi*. Prominent regional *lymphadenopathy* is common. Cultures are difficult; PCR is starting to become used.

P
- *Three zones of inflammation* under an *ulceration* (1.142) are not as specific as implied in the literature:
  - Necrotic debris, fibrin, and neutrophils on the surface
  - Granulation tissue in the middle zone
  - Lymphocytes and plasma cells (1.111) deep
- Gram-negative coccobacilli (1.5 × 0.2 microns) can rarely be demonstrated in tissue with Gram or Giemsa stains, and are best seen on *smears*

Differential diagnosis

1. Other genital ulcers (12.13). Syphilis ulcer more likely to be painless and solitary.

12.8 Granuloma inguinale (donovanosis)
(see Fig. 12.8)

Uncommon venereal disease caused by *Klebsiella granulomatis* (formerly *Calymmatobacterium* or *Donovania granulomatis*), name changed repeatedly mainly to ensure microbiologist full employment, even though it is usually not cultured. *Ulcers* on genitals (1.107, 1.149) or perianal area (1.108) often have beefy red *exuberant granulation tissue*, often resulting in considerable destruction (esthiomene). Adenopathy is less prominent than with chancroid or lymphogranuloma venereum. The diagnosis is usually made clinically or by smears. PCR not readily available and serologic testing not very accurate.

P
- Ulceration with granulation tissue
- Pseudoepitheliomatous hyperplasia at the ulcer border sometimes
- Diffuse mixed infiltrate in the dermis made up of histiocytes, plasma cells, and a few lymphocytes; small neutrophilic abscesses
- The 1.2-micron Gram-negative organisms (Donovan bodies) can sometimes be seen within histiocytes with Giemsa or Warthin–Starry stains, but are best seen on smears. Bipolar staining at two ends of the organism may produce a safety pin appearance

Differential diagnosis

1. Other genital ulcers (12.13).
2. Other diseases with pseudoepitheliomatous hyperplasia (1.116) and ulceration (1.142).
3. Other diseases with "parasitized histiocytes" with small organisms of 1–2 microns (15.1) are not generally found in the genital area.
4. Malakoplakia (12.21) occurs in the groin and perianal areas, but the macrophages contain 5–15-micron granules that stain positive with PAS, von Kossa, and Perl's stains, but is most common in the groin and perianal areas.

12.9 Rhinoscleroma

(see Fig. 12.9A,B)

Very rare infection by *Klebsiella rhinoscleromatis* is often called scleroma, because it can affect other portions of the

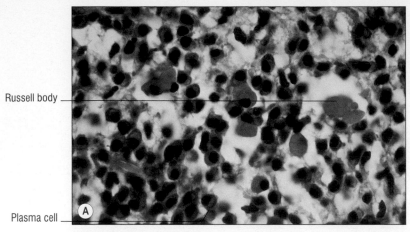

Russell body

Plasma cell

Fig. 12.9 A Rhinoscleroma.

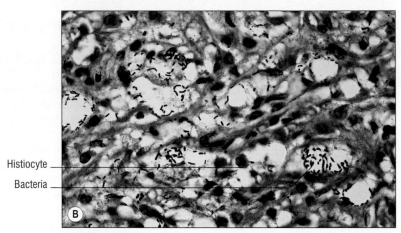

Histiocyte

Bacteria

Fig. 12.9 B Rhinoscleroma (Warthin–Starry stain).

respiratory tract besides the *nose* (1.95). It mainly occurs in Central America, Indonesia, and Egypt. Nasal congestion later evolves into *impressive tissue proliferation* and *indurated scarring*. Cultures positive in only half of cases.

- Pseudoepitheliomatous hyperplasia (1.116) sometimes in older lesions
- *Dense diffuse infiltrate* (1.91) of many *plasma cells*, *Russell bodies* (1.111), histiocytes, neutrophils, and lymphocytes
- Gram-negative rods (2–3 microns) seen within large vacuolated histiocytes (*Mikulicz cells*) with H&E stain, or better with *Giemsa, PAS, Warthin–Starry, or immunostains*
- *Marked fibrosis* in older lesions

Differential diagnosis

1. Other diseases with numerous plasma cells (1.111).
2. Other diseases with small organisms of 2–3 microns within histiocytes, including granuloma inguinale (12.8), leishmaniasis (15.1), and histoplasmosis (13.9). Only the latter two are likely to occur near the nose, the usual location for rhinoscleroma.

12.10 Tuberculosis
(see Fig. 12.10A–C)
Mycobacterium tuberculosis is common in some parts of the world. It primarily infects the lungs, but can involve many

other organs. Skin lesions vary greatly morphologically, and almost always indicate systemic infection, except for the very rare primary inoculation TB. Infection can be detected by a positive *PPD skin test* (tuberculin-purified protein derivative), Ziehl–Neelsen *acid-fast bacilli* (*AFB*) *stain*, culture, or by PCR. *Tuberculids* are hypersensitivy reactions to active TB elsewhere, and improvement of the tuberculids following treatment of TB is helpful confirming evidence.

Variations

1. Miliary TB: rare, *papulopustular* (1.89) eruption from hematogenous dissemination resulting from poor immunity or corticosteroid treatment, diffuse dermal mixed infiltrate with many neutrophils, with variable granulomatous component later, AFB often present.
2. Primary inoculation TB: rare, *crusted ulcer with regional lymphadenopathy*, usually following laboratory accidents, performance of autopsies, or tattooing, histology like miliary TB.
3. Tuberculosis cutis orificialis: *mucosal ulcers* (1.82) in patients with poor immunity, histology like miliary TB.
4. Scrofuloderma: nodular swelling or ulceration resulting from direct extension of underlying *bone* (1.16) *or lymph node TB*, histology like miliary TB.
5. Tuberculosis verrucosa cutis: solitary purulent verrucous plaque (1.146) seen in patients with high immunity, *epithelial hyperplasia, intraepithelial neutrophilic microabscesses* (1.117), diffuse dermal infiltrate with

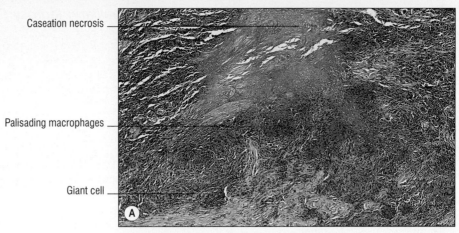

Caseation necrosis

Palisading macrophages

Giant cell

Fig. 12.10 A Tuberculosis.

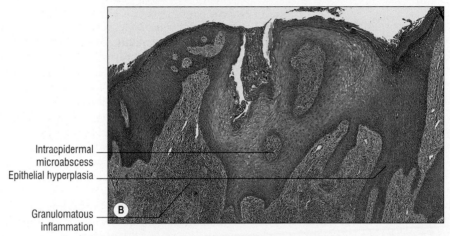

Intracpidermal microabscess
Epithelial hyperplasia

Granulomatous inflammation

Fig. 12.10 B Tuberculosis verrucosa cutis.

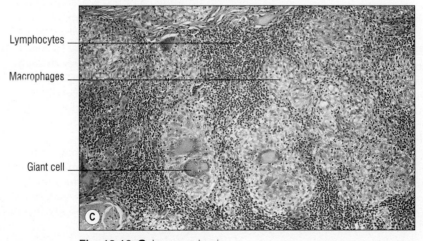

Lymphocytes

Macrophages

Giant cell

Fig. 12.10 C Lupus vulgaris.

neutrophils prominent, tuberculoid granulomas, sometimes with caseation, AFB sometimes demonstrated.

6. Lupus vulgaris: red–brown "*apple jelly*" patches or plaques, usually on the *face* (1.44), resulting from reactivation in a patient with good immunity, epidermis may be atrophic, hyperplastic, or ulcerated, dermal tuberculoid *granulomas with little or no caseation*, predominant Langhans giant cells (1.84), AFB usually cannot be demonstrated.

7. Papulonecrotic tuberculid: multiple crusted papules, lymphocytic or neutrophilic vasculitis (Chapter 4), frequent *microthrombi* (1.137), wedge *of dermal necrosis* (1.87).

8. Lichen scrofulosorum: a tuberculid with *follicular* (1.47) or *annular* (1.5) papules, mostly on the trunk, granulomatous inflammation with or without caseation.

9. Erythema induratum (Bazin's disease): *a panniculitis tuberculid of the legs* (16.6).

Differential diagnosis

1. Other diseases with granulomas (1.51), predominant neutrophils (1.89).

12.11 Atypical mycobacterial infections

(see Fig. 12.11A–D)

Uncommon infections with various "atypical" *Mycobacterium* species other than *M. tuberculosis* (12.10) and *M. leprae* (12.12) usually results in solitary or multiple *red nodules* (1.92), *abscesses*, *ulcers* (1.142), verrucous plaques (1.146), or sinus tracts, sometimes with a sporotrichoid distribution (1.133), usually from direct cutaneous inoculation. Some distinctive organisms include *M. marinum* ("swimming pool granuloma"), *M. ulcerans* (Buruli ulcer in South America and Central Africa, organisms usually numerous), *M. avium-intracellulare* (MAI, especially with AIDS), and *M. fortuitum* and *M. chelonae* ("rapid growers").

- *Epidermis hyperplastic* or ulcerated, sometimes with neutrophilic *microabscesses*
- *Diffuse dermal mixed infiltrate* of neutrophils, histiocytes, and plasma cells (1.110)
- *Tuberculoid granulomas* often present, usually without caseation
- *Acid-fast bacilli* found by AFB stain, culture, or PCR
- Prominent fibrosis sometimes

Differential diagnosis

1. Other diseases with granulomas (1.51), predominant neutrophils (1.89), pseudoepitheliomatous hyperplasia with intraepithelial microabscesses (1.117), especially deep fungal infections (Chapter 13).

12.12 Hansen's disease (leprosy)

(see Fig. 12.12A–H)

Rare, except in certain parts of the world, due to *Mycobacterium leprae*, and recently attributed also to *M. lepromatosis*, subdivided into two polar forms depending upon the immune status: lepromatous (multibacillary) and tuberculoid (paucibacillary). It does not grow in routine cultures. It grows in the footpads of mice or in armadillos. Lepromatous patients have many non-scaly *red plaques* with many organisms because of poor immunity. *Leonine facies* (1.68) or madarosis (1.42) may occur. Tuberculoid patients have fewer lesions with rare organisms because of good immunity. Hypoesthetic, hypopigmented (1.150), scaly, or annular patches (1.5) or plaques are found. Leprosy infects multiple organs, especially eyes (1.41) and peripheral nerves. Thickened nerves may be palpable (greater auricular, ulnar, radial, peroneal, posterior tibial). Neuropathies may result in deformities of the distal extremities.

A. Lepromatous (multibacillary) leprosy (LL)

- Many non-scaly red plaques with many organisms because of poor immunity
- Diffuse infiltrate (1.91) of predominantly foamy histiocytes, separated from the epidermis by a Grenz zone (1.53)
- Acid-fast bacilli seen with Fite stain, sometimes in clumps called globi

B. Tuberculoid (paucibacillary) leprosy (TT)

- *Tuberculoid granulomas* that may reach the epidermis (*no Grenz zone*), with a tendency to be *linear along cutaneous nerves*, and usually without caseation
- *Acid-fast bacilli rare or not present* with Fite stain

Variations

1. Borderline leprosy (BB, BT or BL): clinical and histologic findings in between tuberculoid and lepromatous leprosy.
2. Indeterminant leprosy: leprosy that cannot decide what kind it wants to be. *Hypopigmented* (1.150) or erythematous macules, mostly recognized in endemic countries as a manifestation of leprosy, histology indeterminant and usually non-diagnostic, with mostly perivascular lymphocytes (1.109), sometimes with perineural inflammation or scattered histiocytes, but usually without organisms.
3. Histoid leprosy: nodule that is fibrous, less foamy, many organisms with Fite stain as in lepromatous leprosy, may resemble a dermatofibroma (27.1).
4. Lepra reaction (type I reaction): this is called a reversal reaction when the patient is under treatment and has shifted toward the tuberculoid spectrum with greater immunity. It is called a downgrading reaction when untreated patients shift toward the lepromatous pole. *Existing lesions become swollen*, with constitutional symptoms, histology like borderline leprosy.
5. Erythema nodosum leprosum (ENL, type II reaction): *tender new nodules* (1.96) and plaques occur in lepromatous or borderline lepromatous patients, related to immune complexes, accompanied by constitutional symptoms (1.45). Histology of lepromatous leprosy combined with *leukocytoclastic vasculitis* (4.1).
6. Lucio's phenomenon (type III reaction): patients with diffuse lepromatous leprosy develop *hemorrhagic plaques* (1.120) on the face, extremities, or buttocks that eventually can ulcerate, usually without constitutional symptoms. Histology is like a severe type II reaction, with more severe *vasculitis*, *thrombosis* (1.137), *necrosis* (1.86), and *ulceration* (1.142).
7. Diffuse leprosy: patients have diffuse, shiny, waxy infiltration of the face, sometimes with a red to cyanotic hue. The loss of hair and eyebrows, and loss of wrinkles in older patients, can give their face a smooth appearance called lepra bonita (beautiful leprosy).

Differential diagnosis

1. Other diseases with granulomas (1.51). For paucibacillary cases with negative stains, PCR may be needed for diagnosis (available from National Hansen's Disease Center in Baton Rouge, LA).
2. Other diseases with foam cells (1.46).

12.13 Syphilis

(see Fig. 12.13A–I)

Venereal infection with *Treponema pallidum*, evolving in three stages. *Primary syphilis* occurs as a painless indurated genital (1.107, 1.149) or lip *ulcer* (1.142). *Secondary syphilis* is a *great*

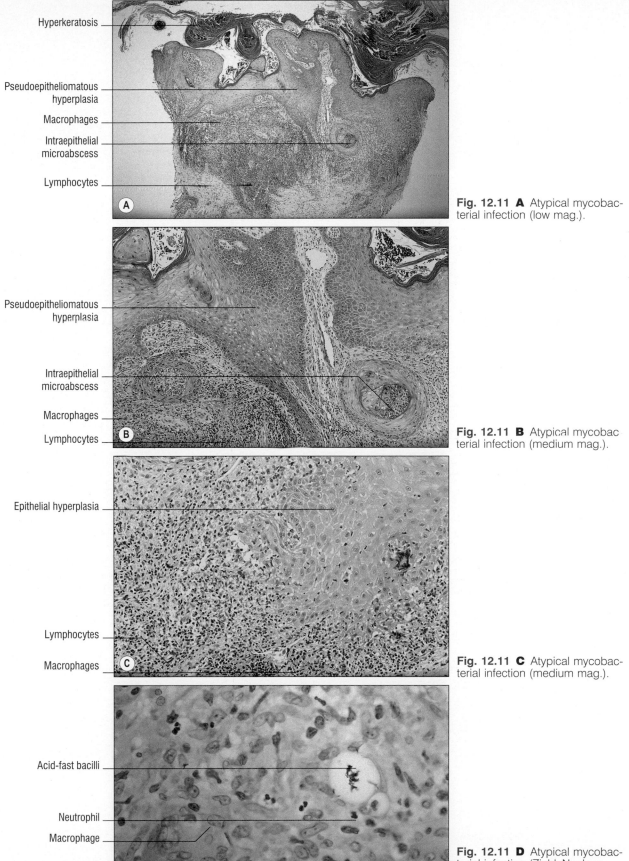

Hyperkeratosis

Pseudoepitheliomatous hyperplasia

Macrophages

Intraepithelial microabscess

Lymphocytes

Fig. 12.11 A Atypical mycobacterial infection (low mag.).

Pseudoepitheliomatous hyperplasia

Intraepithelial microabscess

Macrophages

Lymphocytes

Fig. 12.11 B Atypical mycobacterial infection (medium mag.).

Epithelial hyperplasia

Lymphocytes

Macrophages

Fig. 12.11 C Atypical mycobacterial infection (medium mag.).

Acid-fast bacilli

Neutrophil

Macrophage

Fig. 12.11 D Atypical mycobacterial infection (Ziehl–Neelsen stain). It is common for organisms to be sparsely hidden within holes in the sections like this.

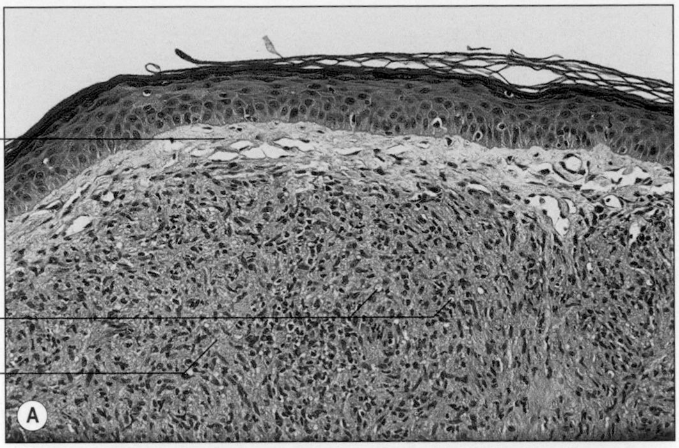

Grenz zone

Globi

Foamy macrophages

Fig. 12.12 A Lepromatous Hansen's disease (low mag.).

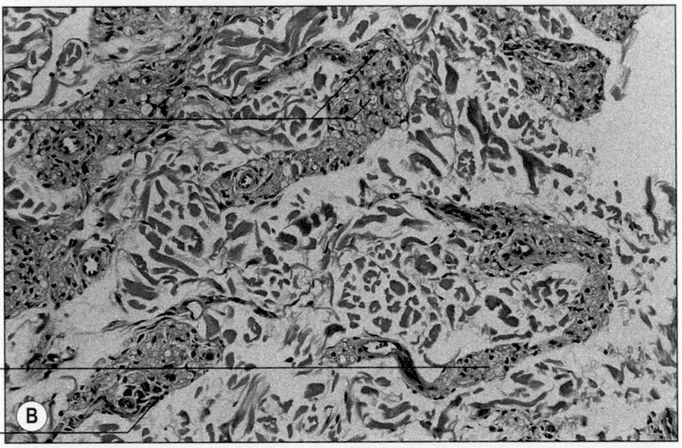

Globi

Linear foamy granulomas

Plasma cell

Fig. 12.12 B Lepromatous Hansen's disease (high mag.).

Globi

Foamy macrophage

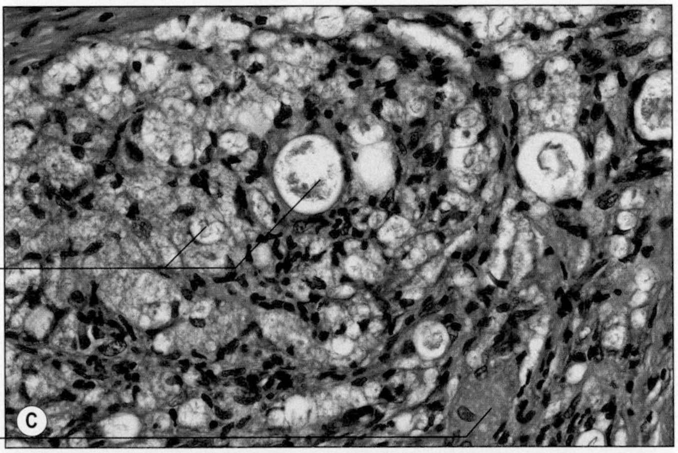

Fig. 12.12 C Lepromatous Hansen's disease (high mag.).

Acid-fast bacilli

Globi

Macrophage

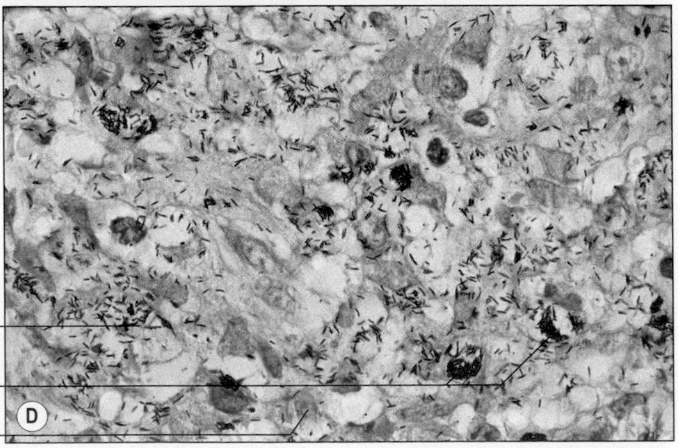

Fig. 12.12 D Lepromatous Hansen's disease (Fite stain).

Granuloma

Sweat duct

Granuloma

Fig. 12.12 E Tuberculoid Hansen's disease (low mag.).

mimic, with various lesions: the most common non-pruritic *morbilliform* eruption (1.81) with constitutional symptoms (1.45), lymphadenopathy, common *palm and soles lesions* (1.100), *alopecia* (1.4), papulosquamous plaques (1.103), annular plaques (1.5, especially of the face in pigmented races), folliculitis (1.47), pustules (1.89), genital plaques (1.55, condyloma lata), hypertrophic crusted "rupioid" or "ostra-ceous" oyster shell plaques, mucous patches in the mouth (1.82). The rare *tertiary syphilis* presents as solitary or multiple plaques, sometimes annular, or as ulcers. *Congenital syphilis* can present with any of the above lesions, and is generally the only form that can be vesiculobullous with any significant frequency. The diagnosis of syphilis is more often made sero-logically with the *RPR, VDRL, MHA–TP,* or *FTA–ABS* tests than by biopsy.

A. Primary syphilis

- *Ulceration* of epidermis (1.142)
- Diffuse infiltrate of many *plasma cells*, lymphocytes, and histiocytes
- Endothelial swelling and proliferation
- *Spirochetes* often present with *Warthin–Starry stain*, but the stain is difficult to use. An immunostain is commercially available.

P

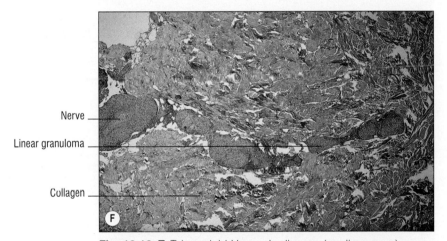

Nerve

Linear granuloma

Collagen

Fig. 12.12 F Tuberculoid Hansen's disease (medium mag.).

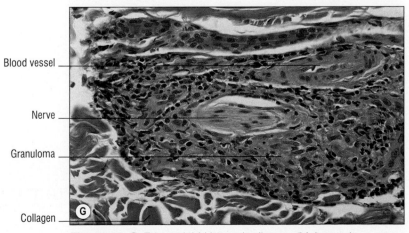

Blood vessel

Nerve

Granuloma

Collagen

Fig. 12.12 G Tuberculoid Hansen's disease (high mag.).

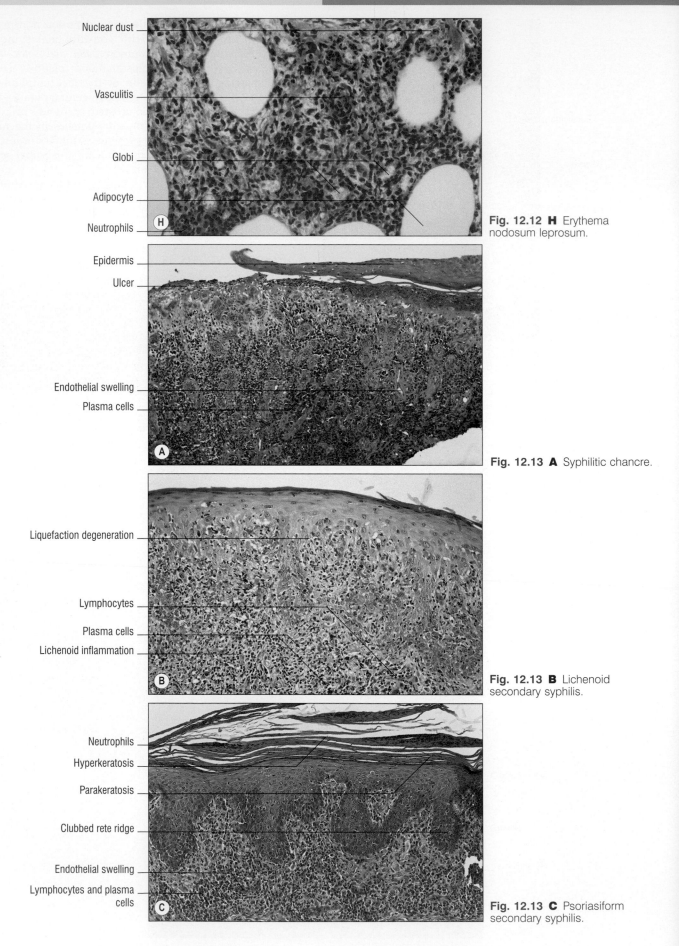

Nuclear dust

Vasculitis

Globi

Adipocyte

Neutrophils

H

Fig. 12.12 H Erythema nodosum leprosum.

Epidermis

Ulcer

Endothelial swelling

Plasma cells

A

Fig. 12.13 A Syphilitic chancre.

Liquefaction degeneration

Lymphocytes

Plasma cells

Lichenoid inflammation

B

Fig. 12.13 B Lichenoid secondary syphilis.

Neutrophils

Hyperkeratosis

Parakeratosis

Clubbed rete ridge

Endothelial swelling

Lymphocytes and plasma cells

C

Fig. 12.13 C Psoriasiform secondary syphilis.

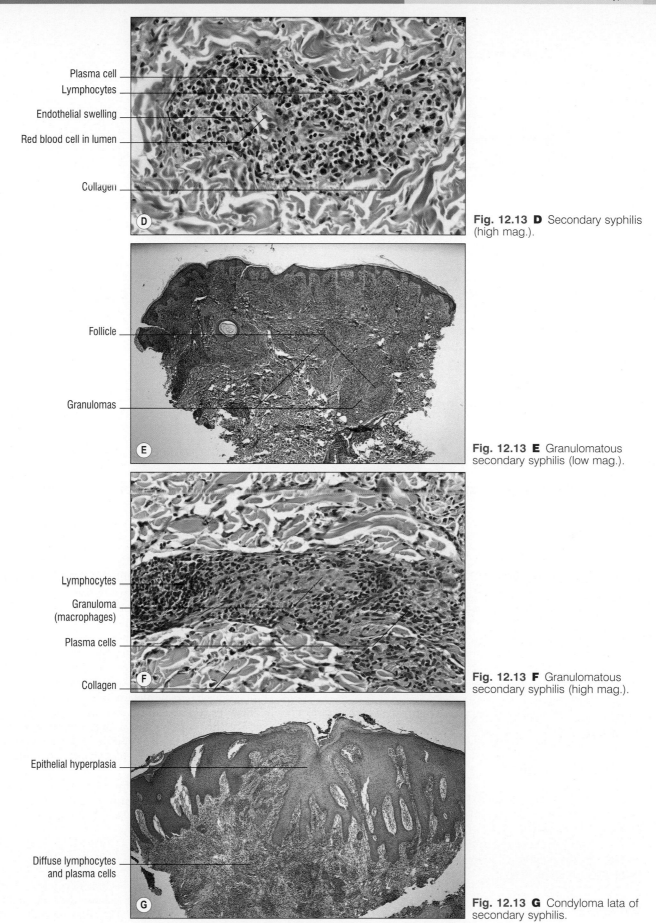

Plasma cell
Lymphocytes
Endothelial swelling
Red blood cell in lumen

Collagen

Fig. 12.13 D Secondary syphilis (high mag.).

Follicle

Granulomas

Fig. 12.13 E Granulomatous secondary syphilis (low mag.).

Lymphocytes
Granuloma (macrophages)
Plasma cells

Collagen

Fig. 12.13 F Granulomatous secondary syphilis (high mag.).

Epithelial hyperplasia

Diffuse lymphocytes and plasma cells

Fig. 12.13 G Condyloma lata of secondary syphilis.

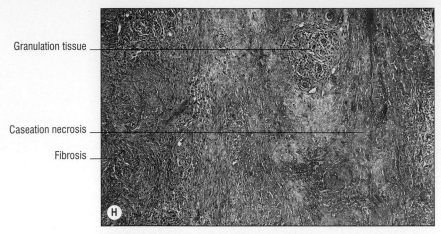

Fig. 12.13 **H** Gumma of tertiary syphilis.

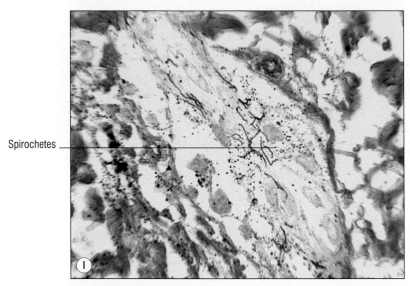

Fig. 12.13 **I** Syphilis (spirochetes with Warthin–Starry stain).

B. Secondary syphilis

- Epidermis may be normal, hyperkeratotic, psoriasiform, necrotic, or ulcerated
- Neutrophils or pustules may be in the epidermis
- *Perivascular or lichenoid infiltrate* of many *plasma cells*, lymphocytes, and histiocytes
- *Granulomatous* infiltrate may be present in older lesions
- Endothelial swelling and proliferation
- Spirochetes present in epidermis or dermis in one-third of cases

C. Tertiary syphilis

- Epidermis normal, atrophic, hyperplastic, or ulcerated
- *Tuberculoid granulomas* with or without caseation, often with plasma cells
- Endothelial swelling and proliferation
- Spirochetes usually not identified with Warthin–Starry stain
- Fibrosis in some lesions

Variations

1. Lues maligna: severe form of secondary syphilis with ulceration and vasculitis.

2. Yaws: non-venereal infection with *Treponema pertenue* in tropical climates. Primary *mother yaw* (crusted nodule with satellite pustules due to primary inoculation) progresses to secondary smaller *daughter yaws* (especially periorificial papules and morbilliform eruption), and later *tertiary abscesses and ulcers*. Yaws can be diagnosed serologically. Histology like syphilis.

3. Pinta: non-venereal infection with *Treponema carateum* in Central America. *Primary inoculation papule* with halo or satellites, may become a large plaque, progresses to *secondary* pintids (small papules and plaques), and *tertiary hypopigmented macules* (1.150). Histology like syphilis.

4. Endemic syphilis (bejel): found in Arabia and the Sahara, non-venereal infection due to *Treponema pallidum endemicum*, histology like syphilis.

Differential diagnosis

1. Other diseases with perivascular dermatitis (1.109), interface dermatitis (1.64), lichenoid dermatitis (1.72), or psoriasiform dermatitis (1.119). Plasma cells (1.111) are a valuable clue.

2. Other diseases with granulomas (1.51).

3. Other genital ulcers: chancroid (12.7), granuloma inguinale (12.8), herpes simplex (14.2), lymphogranuloma venereum (14.14).

12.14 Borreliosis

Infection with *Borrelia burgdorferi* and other species produce a variety of skin lesions.

Variations

1. Lyme disease. due to tick bites (usually *Ixodes*) containing *Borrelia burgdorferi* spirochetes. There may be co-infection with *Ehrlichia* species and *Babesia microti*. Most common in north-eastern US (such as Lyme, Connecticut) and Wisconsin. Local annular red macule with central clearing advances after the bite (*erythema chronicum migrans*), or may disseminate with multiple lesions. *Arthritis* (1.7) and other systemic involvement are common. Diagnosis often made clinically or with serology (sometimes unreliable). Vaccine now available:
   a. Sometimes spongiosis (1.132).
   b. Perivascular lymphocytes and *plasma cells* or eosinophils (1.36).
   c. *Spirochetes* with silver stains (rarely found) or with molecular biologic techniques.
2. Acrodermatitis chronica atrophicans: mainly found in Europe. Erythema of an upper or lower extremity (1.67) results in end-stage lesions with prominent atrophy or sclerodermoid changes, through which blood vessels are easily seen. Serology or PCR helps in diagnosis:
   a. Epidermal atrophy.
   b. Perivascular or lichenoid lymphocytes, plasma cells, or eosinophils in early lesions.
   c. Dermal edema (1.30) in early lesions, severe dermal atrophy or sclerosis later.
   d. Decreased or absent adnexa in older lesions.
3. Lymphocytoma cutis (24.14).
4. Primary cutaneous immunocytoma (24.12).
5. Relapsing fever: epidemics due to *Borrelia recurrentis*, or endemic disease in Africa due to *B. duttoni* or *B. hermsi*, intermittent attacks of high fever, headache, vomiting, respiratory symptoms, hepatosplenomegaly, and a petechial or purpuric rash mostly on the trunk, spirochetes are best found in the blood.

Differential diagnosis

1. Other diseases with annular lesions (1.5), perivascular dermatitis (1.109), plasma cells (1.111), epidermal atrophy (1.9), dermal atrophy (1.8), sclerosis (1.125).
2. Lupus erythematosus (17.6), scleroderma (9.3), eosinophiliamyalgia syndrome (3.5), erythema annulare centrifugum (3.3).

12.15 Bartonella infections

(see Fig. 12.15A–C)
1. Oroya fever (Carrion's disease): rare infection due to Gram-negative *Bartonella bacilliformis*, limited to the region around Peru, resulting in an acute *febrile illness*, secondarily developing nodules known as *verruga peruana*, with histology identical to bacillary angiomatosis (see below). Rocha–Lima inclusions in the endothelial cells contain the organisms.
2. Cat scratch disease: uncommon infection with *Bartonella* (formerly *Rochalimaea*) *henselae*, usually begins from a cat scratch or bite, mostly in children. The primary skin lesion is not impressive, and often heals uneventfully. *Painful lymphadenopathy* develops several weeks later as the usual chief complaint. Conjunctivitis and preauricular lymphadenopathy is *Parinaud's oculoglandular syndrome*, which is also seen in Chagas disease (15.14). Skin lesions may have perivascular or lichenoid infiltrates of lymphocytes, plasma cells, neutrophils, or eosinophils, sometimes forming *palisading granulomas* (1.51). In rare cases, Warthin–Starry stain will demonstrate bacilli. An immunostain is commercially available. Lymph nodes are more commonly biopsied, and these have stellate microabscesses with subcapsular foci of necrosis, later becoming more granulomatous.
3. Bacillary angiomatosis: rare infection with *B. henselae* or *B. quintana*, primarily found in patients with AIDS (14.12) or other immunosuppression, probably spread by the cat flea, *Ctenocephalides felis*. Red friable cutaneous *nodules resembling pyogenic granuloma* (25.3) or *Kaposi sarcoma* (25.9). Sometimes associated with systemic disease of many other organs, such as in the gastrointestinal tract or bacillary peliosis of the liver or spleen. Serologic testing or PCR may help identify the organism. Papules or nodules sometimes have pseudocarcinomatous hyperplasia (1.116), usually with *granulation tissue with neutrophils*, and *smudgy amphophilic areas* that contain numerous bacilli easily demonstrated with the *Warthin–Starry or Giemsa stain*. Fibrosis occurs later, factor XIIIa positive, negative for HHV-8 and CD31.
4. Trench fever: rare *recurrent fevers and a truncal morbilliform eruption* (1.81) due to infection with *B. quintana*, spread by the body louse.

12.16 Actinomycosis

(see Fig. 12.16A,B)
Uncommon infection with *Actinomyces israelii* bacteria, considered normal flora in the mouth and GI tract, but causes nodules or abscesses in the mouth (1.82) following trauma, or dental infections.

Variations

1. Cervicofacial actinomycosis ("lumpy jaw"): nodule, indurated woody plaque, draining sinus tract or abscess of the submandibular region (1.86), with primary infection in the mouth.
2. Actinomycetoma (13.14).
3. Thoracic actinomycosis: infection of the lung, often from aspiration.
4. Gastrointestinal actinomycosis: infection of the GI tract:
   a. *Diffuse infiltrate* (1.91) in dermis or subcutaneous tissue consisting of granulation tissue and sinus tracts, mixed inflammatory infiltrate, *neutrophilic microabscesses*, and fibrosis later.
   b. *Sulfur granules* (clumps of organisms up to 10 mm in diameter, usually 2–3 mm, which may be seen grossly) are basophilic, often an eosinophilic border known as the *Splendore–Hoeppli phenomenon*.

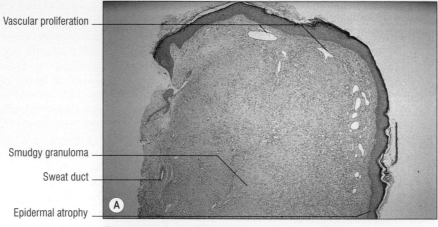

Vascular proliferation

Smudgy granuloma

Sweat duct

Epidermal atrophy

Fig. 12.15 A Bacillary angiomatosis (low mag.).

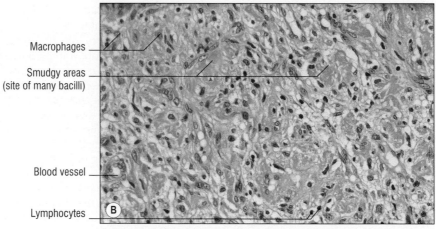

Macrophages

Smudgy areas
(site of many bacilli)

Blood vessel

Lymphocytes

Fig. 12.15 B Bacillary angiomatosis (high mag.).

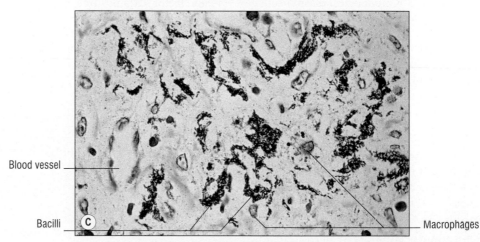

Blood vessel

Bacilli

Macrophages

Fig. 12.15 C Bacillary angiomatosis (Warthin–Starry stain).

c. *Filamentous bacteria only 1 micron in diameter*.
d. Organisms are *positive with Gram, Giemsa, GMS, or PAS stains*.

Differential diagnosis

1. Botryomycosis: sulfur granules due to bacteria such as *Staphylococcus*, *Pseudomonas*, or *Proteus* have cocci or small bacilli usually visible in the granules rather than filaments, will grow in culture.
2. Nocardiosis (12.17).
3. Eumycetoma (13.15): due to true fungi, usually has sulfur granules that are brown to black instead of white to yellow, hyphae are fatter.
4. Other diseases with dermal and subcutaneous abscesses (1.89).

12.17 Nocardiosis

(see Fig. 12.17A–C)

Uncommon infection with *Nocardia brasiliensis*, *N. asteroides*, or *N. otitidiscaviarum*. Skin lesions are usually nodules, *abscesses*, or draining sinuses. The organisms grow in routine

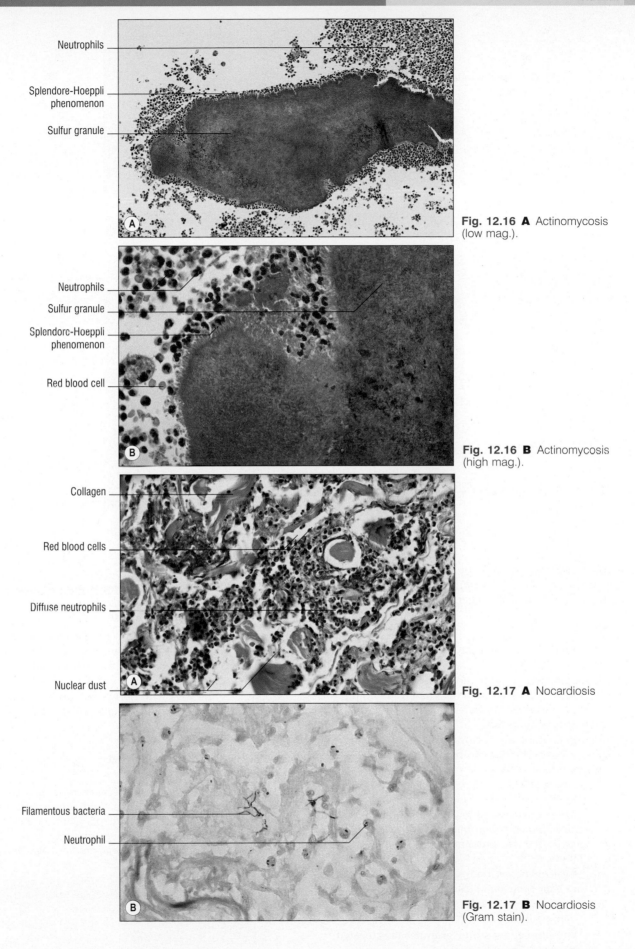

Neutrophils

Splendore-Hoeppli phenomenon

Sulfur granule

Fig. 12.16 A Actinomycosis (low mag.).

Neutrophils

Sulfur granule

Splendore-Hoeppli phenomenon

Red blood cell

Fig. 12.16 B Actinomycosis (high mag.).

Collagen

Red blood cells

Diffuse neutrophils

Nuclear dust

Fig. 12.17 A Nocardiosis

Filamentous bacteria

Neutrophil

Fig. 12.17 B Nocardiosis (Gram stain).

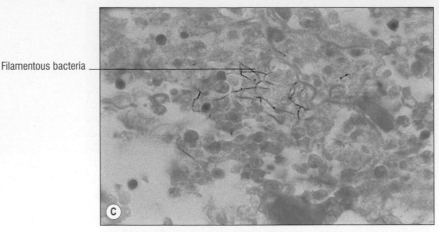

Filamentous bacteria

Fig. 12.17 C Nocardiosis (GMS stain).

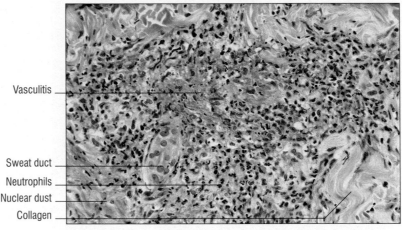

Vasculitis

Sweat duct
Neutrophils
Nuclear dust
Collagen

Fig. 12.18 Gonococcemia.

aerobic bacterial cultures, but the lab should be alerted of the suspicion, because *Nocardia* grows more slowly, and the culture should be held longer.

Variations

1. Pulmonary or CNS nocardiosis: disease may be limited to these organs.
2. Disseminated systemic nocardiosis: often in immunosuppressed patients, disseminated disease occurs in multiple organs (especially lung and brain), disseminating to skin.
3. Lymphocutaneous nocardiosis: traumatic inoculation of the skin results in sporotrichoid nodules (1.132) with lymphadenopathy.
4. Mycetoma (13.14):
   a. *Diffuse infiltrate* (1.91) in dermis or subcutaneous tissue consisting of granulation tissue and sinus tracts, mixed inflammatory infiltrate, *neutrophilic microabscesses*, sometimes granulomas, and fibrosis later.
   b. *Filamentous bacteria* resemble thin fungal hyphae, but are *only 1 micron in diameter*.
   c. Organisms stain with *AFB, GMS, PAS stains*, and are *Gram-positive*.
   d. White to yellow sulfur granules (aggregated organisms) may be present.

Differential diagnosis

1. Tuberculosis (12.10), and atypical mycobacterial infection (12.11) are acid-fast, but are less filamentous.
2. Actinomycosis (12.16): organisms are anaerobic, respond to penicillin instead of sulfonamides, are not acid-fast, more likely to form less fragmented sulfur granule aggregates.
3. Other diseases with dermal or subcutaneous abscesses (1.89), sporotrichoid lesions (1.133), and less often granulomas (1.51).

12.18 Gonococcemia

(see Fig. 12.18)
Gonorrhea, due to *Neisseria gonorrhoeae*, is a common cause of acute purulent urethritis, and less commonly proctitis, oropharyngitis, or endocervicitis. Gonococcemia (*dermatitis–arthritis syndrome*) usually presents with fever (1.45), *oligoarthritis* (1.7), and *few acral necrotic hemorrhagic pustules*.

- Pustules and epidermal necrosis (1.86) often
- *Septic neutrophilic vasculitis*
- Extravasated erythrocytes (1.40) and thrombi (1.137)
- Gram-negative diplococci seldom demonstrated

Differential diagnosis

1. Other causes of vasculitis (Chapter 4), pustules (1.89), fever, and rash (1.45).

12.19 Meningococcemia

Neisseria meningitidis causes epidemics of bacteremia and meningitis. Acute disseminated meningococcemia causes acute systemic illness, with fever (1.45), *petechiae, and ecchymoses* (1.120). Adrenocortical insufficiency (Waterhouse–Friderichsen syndrome) may result in shock. In the rare chronic meningococcemia, patients have fever, arthritis (1.7), and recurrent morbilliform (1.81) or petechial eruptions.

- Pustules and epidermal necrosis sometimes
- *Septic neutrophilic vasculitis*, with more lymphocytes in the chronic form
- Extravasated erythrocytes (1.40) and thrombi (1.137)
- Gram-negative diplococci seldom demonstrated

Differential diagnosis

1. Other causes of vasculitis (Chapter 4), morbilliform eruptions (1.81), fever and rash (1.45), rickettsial infections (14.13).

12.20 Ecthyma gangrenosum

(see Fig. 12.20)

This is defined as *sepsis* with *Pseudomonas aeruginosa*, not to be confused with the generic ecthyma described previously (12.1). Red macules, pustules, or bullae eventually become *ulcers with black eschars*.

- Epidermal necrosis (1.86) or ulceration
- *Dermal necrosis* or infarction
- *Sparse inflammation* with lymphocytes or neutrophils
- *Numerous Gram-negative bacilli* in dermis stain poorly with H&E
- *Vasculitis and thrombi* common

Differential diagnosis

1. Other diseases with ulceration (1.142), extensive dermal necrosis (1.87), vasculitis (Chapter 4), or thrombi (1.137).

12.21 Malakoplakia

Ulcerating *furuncles, abscesses,* or *sinus tracts,* especially *groin* (1.55) *or perianal* (1.108) areas in *immunosuppressed patients,* an unusual reaction to infection, especially to *Escherichia coli,* with poor ability of macrophages to digest the organisms, may affect internal organs such as the urinary tract.

- Diffuse infiltrate of *granular von Hansemann histiocytes* containing *Michaelis–Gutmann bodies* (5–15-micron granules that stain positive with PAS, von Kossa, and Perl's stains)
- Diffuse neutrophils (1.89), plasma cells (1.111), or lymphocytes may be present

Differential diagnosis

1. Foreign body granuloma (7.6) or other granulomas (1.51).
2. Parasitized macrophage disorders (15.1), especially granuloma inguinale (12.8).

12.22 Brucellosis

Human infection by *Brucella* species occurs after ingesting infected milk or food, or inhalation of *animal products*. Most patients have an acute *multisystem febrile illness*. Skin lesions occur in 10% of patients: morbilliform rashes (1.31), petechiae, erythema multiforme, bullae, or ulcers. Primary inoculation brucellosis presents as erythema, papules, or pustules on the hands or arms (12.4) of veterinarians and other animal workers, especially after handling infected placentas. Some of these patients have a contact hypersensitivity (2.2) to *Brucella* antigens rather than actual infection. The *diagnosis of brucellosis is usually made serologically*, because laboratory cultures are hazardous. Serum antibodies may cross-react with those found in cholera, plague, and yersiniosis.

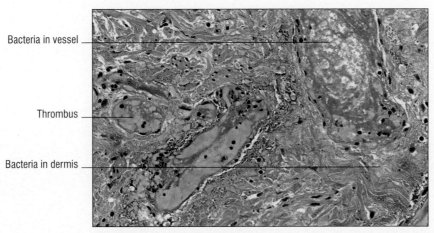

Bacteria in vessel

Thrombus

Bacteria in dermis

Fig. 12.20 Ecthyma gangrenosum.

- Histology like anthrax (12.4) or tularemia (12.6).
- Seldom biopsied; poorly described in the literature

12.23 Yersiniosis

There are three species of the Gram-negative bacillus *Yersinia* (see below). All are zoonotic, affecting humans secondarily. Diagnosis is generally made *serologically* or by *cultures*, rather than by skin biopsy. PCR or DNA microarray to check for multiple organisms is available.

Variations

1. Plague: rare infection (still present in some undeveloped countries) occurs via primary inoculation or inhalation of *Yersinia pestis*, after contact with wild rodents and their fleas, resulting in pneumonia (pneumonic plague), or *fever*, *malaise*, *regional adenopathy* (bubonic plague), or septicemia, meningitis, pharyngitis, and shock. Pustules or carbuncles (1.89) may form at sites of bites or near buboes. Skin lesions from systemic infection may be macular erythema, *petechiae*, or *purpura* (1.120).

2. Yersiniosis: rare infection by *Y. enterocolitica* and *Y. pseudotuberculosis* occurs after contact with various animals, resulting in fever (1.45), *gastrointestinal disease* (1.49), and reactive *polyarthritis* (1.7). Red nodules (1.92) develop on the trunk or legs in 30% of patients, resembling *erythema nodosum* (16.1):

   a. Histology varies depending upon type of lesion biopsied.

   b. Microthrombi (1.137) and hemorrhage (1.40) are common.

CHAPTER 13

Fungal Diseases

13.1 Dermatophytosis (tinea)

(see Fig. 13.1A–F)

Very common superficial cutaneous infection by one of the three genera: *Microsporum*, *Epidermophyton*, and *Trichophyton*. Scaly, erythematous plaques, often *annular* (1.5, hence sometimes called "ringworm"), sometimes pustular, rarely vesicular (1.147). *KOH prep* shows branching septate hyphae without budding yeast, which may obviate the need for biopsy.

P
- Neutrophils sometimes in the stratum corneum, parakeratosis often
- Compact orthokeratosis rather than the normal basket-weave pattern may be a valuable clue of tinea in some locations
- Sandwich sign sometimes present: orthokeratosis or parakeratosis (1.104) alternated in layers with basket-weave stratum corneum, often a clue for the presence of hyphae
- Spongiosis (1.132) or intraepidermal vesicles (1.147) sometimes
- Psoriasiform epidermis sometimes (1.119)
- Folliculitis (10.2) sometimes
- *Variable inflammatory response*: skin may appear "normal" with H&E stains, or perivascular or diffuse mixed infiltrate of lymphocytes, histiocytes, neutrophils, or eosinophils
- *Fungal hyphae (2–4 microns in diameter) in stratum corneum or in follicles* sometimes visible with H&E, but best seen with PAS or GMS stains

Variations

1. Tinea capitis: mostly *children*, by definition on the *scalp* (1.124), often associated with adenopathy as a clue, alopecia (1.4) which eventually can scar, black-dot broken stubble of hairs. It may resemble seborrheic dermatitis (2.1) or folliculitis (10.2). Fungal spores may be large-spore (5–8 microns) endothrix within the hair shaft, large-spore ectothrix on the surface of the hair, or small-spore ectothrix (2–5 microns). Hyphae may not be present in the stratum corneum.
2. Tinea favosa (favus): variant of tinea capitis, mostly in Europe, Asia, and Africa, most commonly caused by *T. schoenleinii*, in which prominent heaped-up crusts called *scutula* appear.
3. Tinea corporis: more in adult men, involvement of the *body* in locations other than the sites seen in the other specific variants listed.
4. Tinea barbae: tinea of the *beard*, more in adult men, resembles bacterial folliculitis (10.2).
5. Tinea faciei: tinea of the *face* (1.44), often resembles many other facial rashes.
6. Tinea cruris: tinea of the *groin* (1.55) and medial thighs.
7. Tinea pedis: tinea of the *feet* (1.48), resembles eczema (2.1) and contact dermatitis (2.2).
8. Tinea manuum: tinea of the *hands*, especially the *palms* (1.100), often unilateral with bilateral tinea pedis (one hand–two feet syndrome), resembles eczema (2.1) and contact dermatitis (2.2).
9. Tinea unguium (tinea unguis, onychomycosis): tinea of the *nails* (1.85), often whitish, thickened, deformed. Biopsy of the subungual debris has a higher yield for finding fungus than the actual nail plate,[119] and sampling more deeply or proximally is also more helpful than the most distal edge.
10. Majocchi's granuloma (not to be confused with Majocchi's disease, 4.8): Nodules (1.92) associated with granulomatous inflammation around *ruptured follicles*, especially legs (1.67) of women.
11. Kerion: *boggy inflammatory pustular plaque* associated with exuberant inflammatory host reaction to the fungus, more common in zoophilic species such as *Microsporum canis*, in any of the above locations, especially scalp.
12. Tinea incognito: tinea that is difficult to recognize because the clinical morphology has been altered by topical corticosteroid treatment.

©2012 Elsevier Ltd, Inc, BV
DOI: 10.1016/B978-0-323-06658-7.00013-0

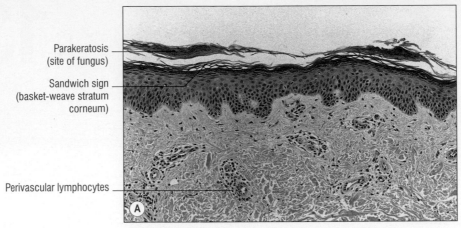

Parakeratosis (site of fungus)

Sandwich sign (basket-weave stratum corneum)

Perivascular lymphocytes

Fig. 13.1 A Tinea (sandwich sign).

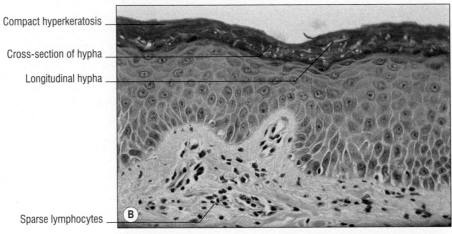

Compact hyperkeratosis

Cross-section of hypha

Longitudinal hypha

Sparse lymphocytes

Fig. 13.1 B Tinea.

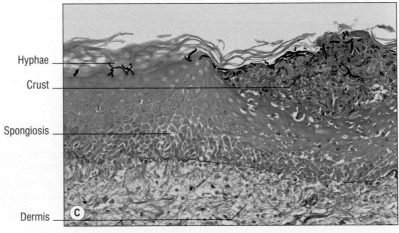

Hyphae

Crust

Spongiosis

Dermis

Fig. 13.1 C Tinea (GMS stain).

Differential diagnosis

1. Tinea versicolor (13.2), candidiasis (13.4), dermatomycosis (13.3, infection of stratum corneum, hair, or nails, by fungi other than true tinea, tinea versicolor, or *Candida*).
2. Normal-appearing skin (1.94).
3. Other diseases with neutrophils in the stratum corneum (1.89).

13.2 Tinea versicolor (TV, pityriasis versicolor)

(see Fig. 13.2A–C)

Very common infection due to a fungus which is usually normal follicular flora in the yeast form, but is pathologic in the hyphal state in the stratum corneum. Our friends in microbiology now prefer the single species name *Malassezia furfur* for the fungus previously thought to be two species:

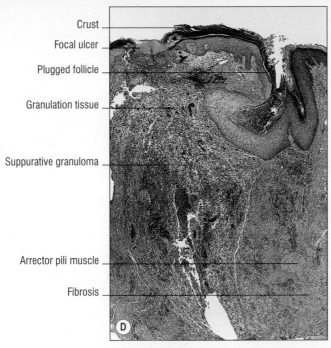

Crust
Focal ulcer
Plugged follicle
Granulation tissue

Suppurative granuloma

Arrector pili muscle
Fibrosis

Fig. 13.1 D Tinea folliculitis (Majocchi granuloma).

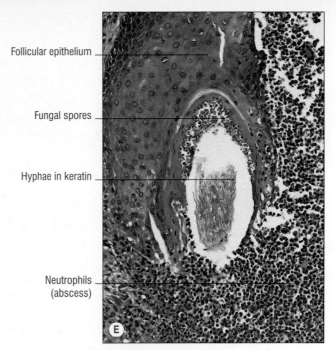

Follicular epithelium

Fungal spores

Hyphae in keratin

Neutrophils (abscess)

Fig. 13.1 E Tinea capitis.

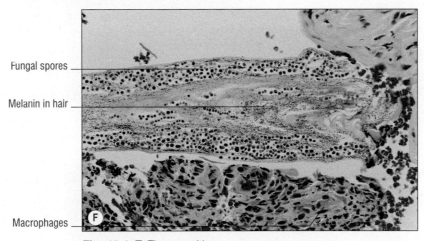

Fungal spores

Melanin in hair

Macrophages

Fig. 13.1 F Tinea capitis.

Pityrosporum orbiculare (rounded yeast) and *P. ovale* (more oval). This fungus does not grow in routine fungal cultures; special techniques are needed, so it is not cultured for practical purposes. Some clinicians prefer the name *pityriasis versicolor*, because it is not one of the three genera of true tinea (13.1). Young adults develop *hypopigmented* (1.150) or *brownish–red* (1.18), *slightly scaly patches* (hence the name "versicolor"). Most common on the *trunk* (1.141). More common in warmest seasons, and more common in warmer climates. KOH prep shows *"chopped spaghetti hyphae and meatball spores"*.

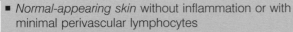

- *Normal-appearing skin* without inflammation or with minimal perivascular lymphocytes
- *Hyphae and budding yeast* from 2–4 microns *in stratum corneum* or in follicles; more readily seen with H&E stain than dermatophytes (13.1), but are best seen with PAS or GMS stains

Variation

1. *Malassezia folliculitis* (formerly *Pityrosporum folliculitis*) is a controversial entity since *Pityrosporum* is normal flora in follicles. It is identical to folliculitis of other causes (10.2), but numerous budding yeast without hyphae are present. The clinician may be interested in the presence of *Malassezia* in the follicles in cases of refractory folliculitis prior to attempting systemic antifungal therapy in those cases in which antibiotics directed at bacterial folliculitis failed.

Differential diagnosis

1. Normal-appearing skin (1.94).
2. Dermatophytosis (13.1) and candidiasis (13.4).

13.3 Tinea nigra

(see Fig. 13.3)
Rare *brown* (1.18) *macules of the palms or soles* (1.100), mostly in *warm climates*, occasionally confused clinically for

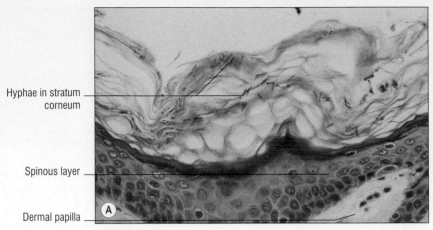

Hyphae in stratum corneum

Spinous layer

Dermal papilla

Fig. 13.2 A Tinea versicolor.

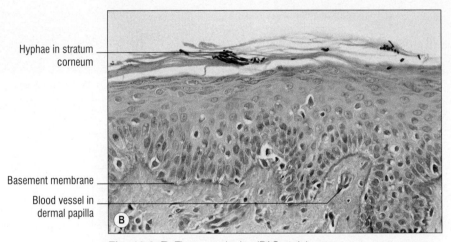

Hyphae in stratum corneum

Basement membrane

Blood vessel in dermal papilla

Fig. 13.2 B Tinea versicolor (PAS stain).

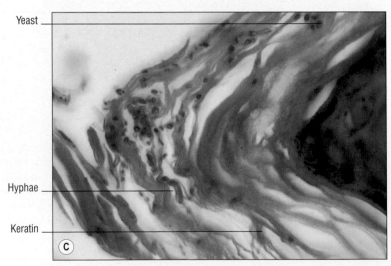

Yeast

Hyphae

Keratin

Fig. 13.2 C Tinea versicolor.

melanoma. Microbiologists have vacillated tremendously on the name for this fungus, changing the name at least three times in my career, so that at this moment the culprit is known as *Horteae* (formerly *Phaeoannellomyces, Exophiala* or *Cladosporium*) *werneckii*, which can be found with KOH prep or cultured.

- Skin may look normal with H&E stain at scanning magnification (1.94)
- *Brown septate hyphae in stratum corneum* can be seen with H&E stain

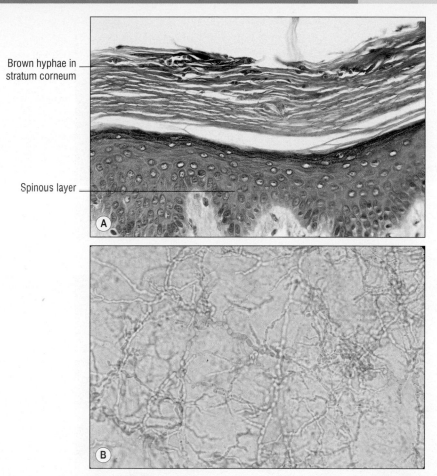

Brown hyphae in stratum corneum

Spinous layer

A

B

Fig. 13.3 Tinea nigra.

13.4 Candidiasis (moniliasis, candidosis)

(see Fig. 13.4A–C)

Some *Candida* (formerly *Monilia*) species, especially *Candida albicans*, are normal flora in yeast form in the mouth, gastrointestinal tract, and vagina. In some pathological situations, *Candida* shifts toward combined hyphal (pseudohyphal) and yeast forms, which causes *bright red plaques* or *papulopustules* in *moist areas* such as the *axilla* (1.10), *groin* (1.55), or *occluded areas*. *Candida* less commonly infects nail plates (1.85) than tinea. *Chronic paronychia* (infection around the nails) is commonly due to *Candida*, while acute paronychia is more likely due to *Staphylococcus* (12.3). Overgrowth of *Candida* in mucous membranes causes white maceration. This occurs in the mouth (1.82, *thrush*), especially on the *tongue* (1.139), on *uncircumcised glans penis (Candida balanitis*, 1.107), or in the vagina (*Candida vaginitis*). *Perleche* (2.2) of the angles of the lips (1.74) is sometimes due to *Candida*. *Candida* can be associated with antibiotic therapy, diabetes mellitus (1.26), topical corticosteroid therapy, HIV infection (14.12), or other conditions of immunosuppression. *Candida* grows easily in routine fungal cultures, and can be seen on KOH preps.

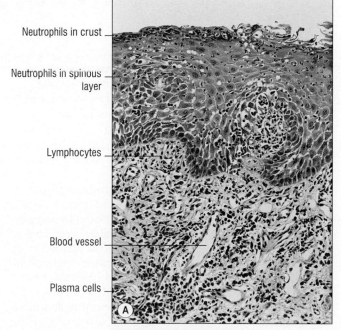

Neutrophils in crust

Neutrophils in spinous layer

Lymphocytes

Blood vessel

Plasma cells

A

Fig. 13.4 A Candidiasis (low mag.).

P
- Neutrophils, parakeratosis, and crusting common in the stratum corneum
- *Pseudohyphae and budding yeast in the stratum corneum (3–7 microns)*, which can sometimes be seen with H&E, but are more easily seen with PAS or GMS stains
- Perivascular lymphocytes and neutrophils in the dermis

Variations

1. Disseminated systemic candidiasis: *purpuric papules or nodules* (1.120) associated with candidal sepsis, immunosuppression, and *dermal budding yeast* more than pseudohyphae, sometimes with very little inflammatory reaction.

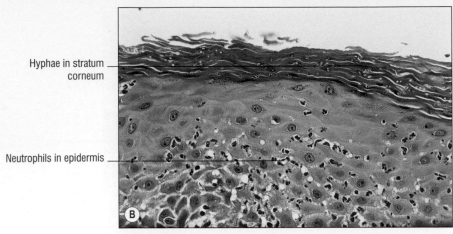

Hyphae in stratum corneum

Neutrophils in epidermis

Fig. 13.4 B Candidiasis (high mag.).

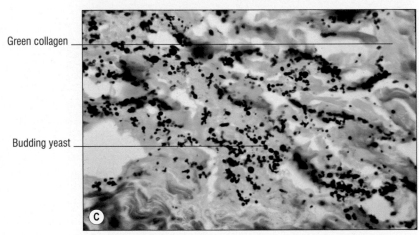

Green collagen

Budding yeast

Fig 13.4 C Disseminated candidiasis, seen in the dermis with GMS stain.

2. Chronic mucocutaneous candidiasis (CMC): genetically inherited group of heterogeneous immunologic predispositions to persistent mouth, skin, and nail candidiasis. Some patients also have increased infection by tinea, other infections, or endocrinopathies.

3. Median rhomboid glossitis: diamond-shaped eroded area on the dorsum of the tongue (1.139), which may be due to a developmental abnormality of the tongue, but likely is due to *Candida*.

4. Granuloma gluteale (granuloma gluteale infantum, or adultorum): solitary or multiple red–brown papules or nodules in groin or gluteal area related to irritant contact dermatitis from urine or *Candida*. Epithelial hyperplasia with mixed dermal perivascular infiltrate of lymphocytes, plasma cells, histiocytes, neutrophils, and/or eosinophils, sometimes with intraepidermal microabscesses. Not really a histologic granuloma. Yeast and hyphae are not always present in stratum corneum.

Differential diagnosis

1. Intertrigo (2.2), contact dermatitis (2.2), erythrasma (12.5), and acneiform eruptions (1.3).

2. Tinea (13.1) has hyphae without budding yeast, can be cultured, and is more often annular. *Candida* pseudohyphae are more likely to be oriented vertically, as opposed to horizontally in true tinea.

3. Tinea versicolor (13.2) does have budding yeast, but does not grow in routine culture, and is much different clinically.

4. Other diseases with neutrophils in the stratum corneum (1.89).

13.5 Cryptococcosis

(see Fig. 13.5A–C)

Uncommon infection by *Cryptococcus neoformans*, usually in immunosuppressed patients, often causing purulent or necrotic nodules or plaques on the skin, nearly always with systemic infection at other sites, especially the central nervous system. There are two major histologic patterns that may occur together in different parts of the same lesion:

1. Gelatinous pattern:
   a. Epidermis not very remarkable.
   b. *Budding yeast* (5–20 microns) are numerous in the dermis, staining faintly ("cryptically") with H&E, or better with GMS.
   c. *Prominent capsule* around organisms that does not stain with H&E, giving the *dermis a vacuolated gelatinous appearance*. The capsule contains mucin, staining with mucicarmine. Alcian blue can be used along with PAS, with Alcian blue staining the capsule, and PAS staining the central part of the yeast red.
   d. Very little inflammatory response.

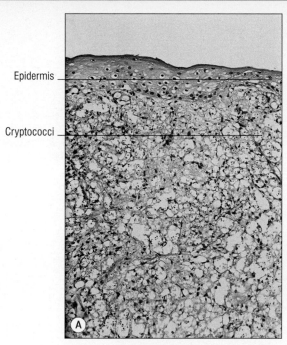

Fig. 13.5 A Cryptococcosis (low mag.).

Epidermis

Cryptococci

2. Granulomatous pattern:
   a. Often ulcerated with pseudoepitheliomatous hyperplasia (1.117).
   b. Yeast are smaller (2–10 microns) and less numerous; they are free in tissue or within histiocytes or giant cells.
   c. Dense mixed dermal *granulomatous infiltrate* of many neutrophils, histiocytes, giant cells, and plasma cells.

Differential diagnosis

1. The gelatinous reaction may resemble lesions with clear cells (1.22).
2. The small organisms in the granulomatous pattern (1.51) may resemble histoplasmosis (13.9).

13.6 Coccidioidomycosis

(see Fig. 13.6A–D)

Coccidioides immitis most commonly causes lung infections in endemic arid areas in the south-western US. A febrile illness sometimes called "valley fever" is usually self-limited, and asymptomatic infections also occur. Red skin nodules, sometimes verrucous (1.146), appear in the minority of patients

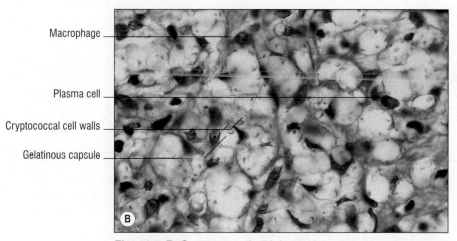

Macrophage

Plasma cell

Cryptococcal cell walls

Gelatinous capsule

Fig. 13.5 B Cryptococcosis (high mag.).

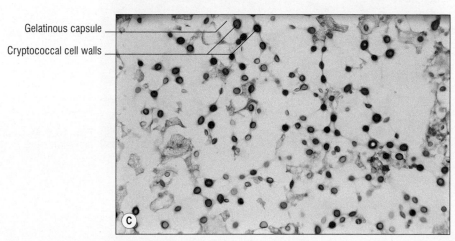

Gelatinous capsule

Cryptococcal cell walls

Fig. 13.5 C Cryptococcosis (PAS stain).

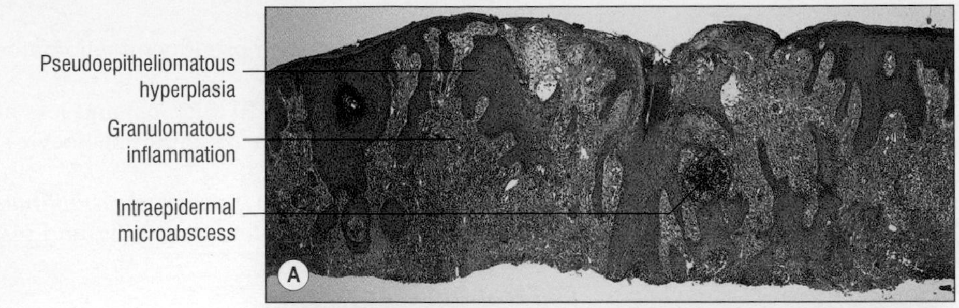

Pseudoepitheliomatous hyperplasia

Granulomatous inflammation

Intraepidermal microabscess

Fig. 13.6 A Coccidioidomycosis (low mag.).

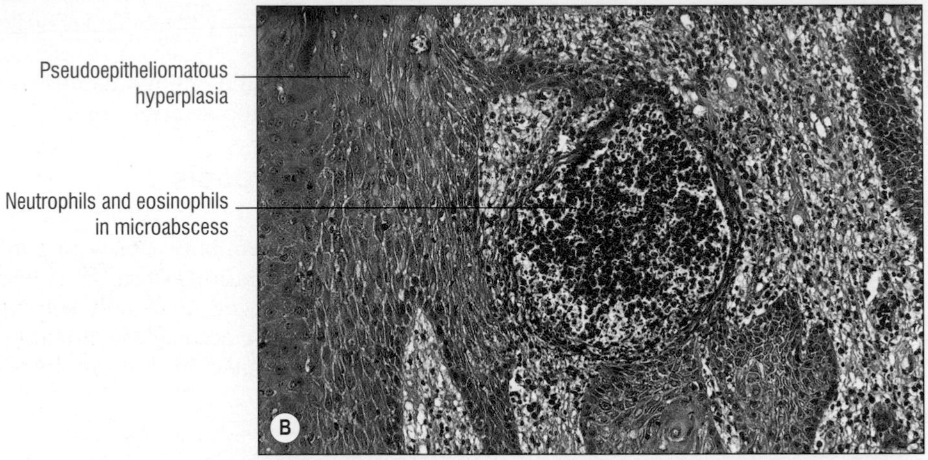

Pseudoepitheliomatous hyperplasia

Neutrophils and eosinophils in microabscess

Fig. 13.6 B Coccidioidomycosis (high mag.).

Neutrophils and nuclear dust

Lymphocyte

Large fungal spore in giant cell

Plasma cell

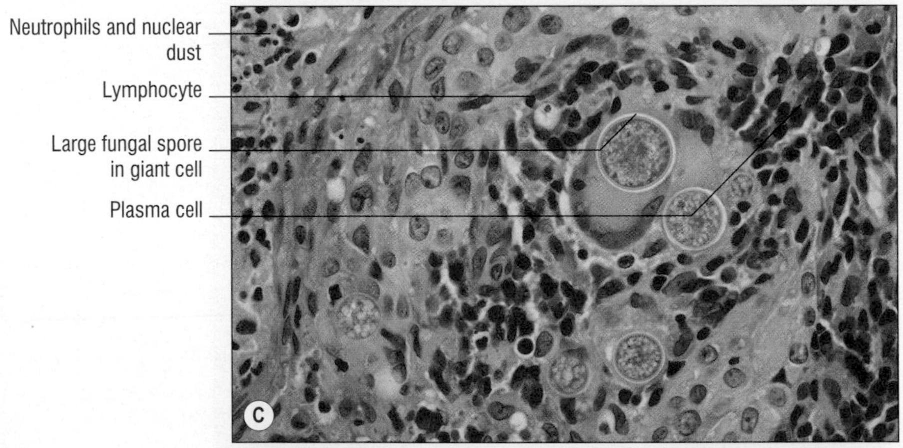

Fig. 13.6 C Coccidioidomycosis (high mag.).

Eosinophil

Neutrophil

Endospores within large spore

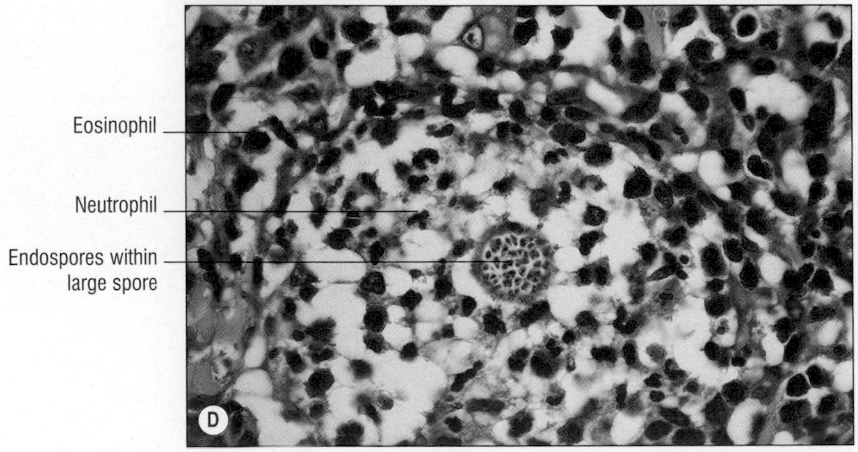

Fig. 13.6 D Coccidioidomycosis (high mag.).

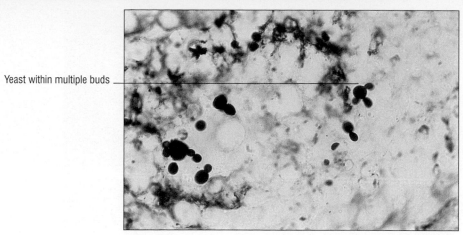

Yeast within multiple buds

Fig. 13.7 South American blastomycosis (GMS stain).

with disseminated infection, which is more common in blacks and Filipinos, more common on the face. Infection by primary inoculation is very rare. The dimorphic organism is dangerous to culture, because airborne arthrospores are very infectious.

- *Pseudoepitheliomatous hyperplasia* in older lesions, sometimes intraepidermal neutrophilic microabscesses
- Diffuse *suppurative granulomatous* dermal infiltrate of neutrophils, lymphocytes, histiocytes, plasma cells (and multinucleated giant cells in older lesions), and often *many eosinophils*. Sometimes caseation
- *Large thick-walled spores* measuring 10–80 microns with a granular cytoplasm or containing 2–10-micron *endospores*. Often visible with H&E, but best seen with PAS or GMS stains

Differential diagnosis

1. Pseudoepitheliomatous hyperplasia (1.117).
2. Neutrophils in the dermis (1.89).
3. Granulomas (1.51).
4. The large spores with endospores may resemble myospherulosis (collections of erythrocytes altered by endogenous or exogenous lipids) or rhinosporidiosis (13.15).

13.7 South American blastomycosis (paracoccidioidomycosis)

(see Fig. 13.7)
Paracoccidioides brasiliensis, a dimorphic fungus in culture, causes *lung* infection or traumatic infection, followed by regional lymphadenopathy and systemic infection, mucocutaneous ulcerations and *verrucous plaques* (1.146).

- Pseudoepitheliomatous hyperplasia; sometimes intraepidermal neutrophilic microabscesses
- Diffuse mixed dermal infiltrate of neutrophils (often abscesses), lymphocytes, histiocytes, plasma cells, and multinucleated giant cells
- Spores 5–20 microns. The diagnostic organisms are up to 60 microns and have multiple buds resembling a "marine pilot's wheel," but may be difficult to find even with PAS or GMS stains

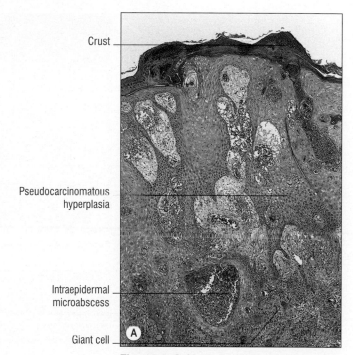

Crust

Pseudocarcinomatous hyperplasia

Intraepidermal microabscess

Giant cell

Fig. 13.8 A North American blastomycosis (low mag.).

Differential diagnosis

1. Other diseases with pseudoepitheliomatous hyperplasia (1.117), neutrophils in the dermis (1.89), or granulomas (1.51).

13.8 North American blastomycosis

(see Fig. 13.8A–D)
Blastomyces dermatitidis, a dimorphic fungus, mainly infects the lungs in residents of states bordering the Ohio and Mississippi rivers, and in the south-eastern US. The pulmonary infection usually clears, but dissemination can spread to bone (1.16), genitourinary tract, brain, and skin. Skin lesions are usually *crusted verrucous plaques*, with annular pustular borders (1.146) or ulcers (1.142). Primary inoculation into the skin, with regional adenopathy, but without systemic disease, is very rare.

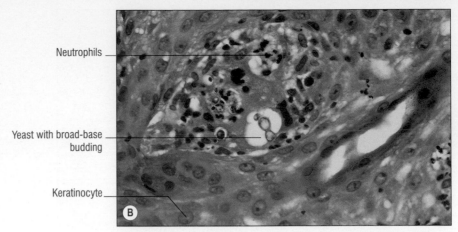

Neutrophils

Yeast with broad-base budding

Keratinocyte

Fig. 13.8 B North American blastomycosis (high mag.).

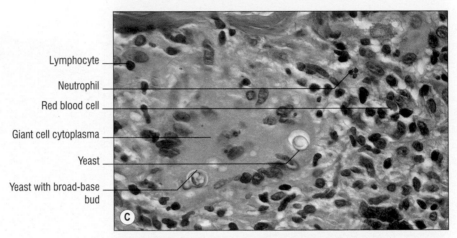

Lymphocyte

Neutrophil

Red blood cell

Giant cell cytoplasma

Yeast

Yeast with broad-base bud

Fig. 13.8 C North American blastomycosis (high mag.).

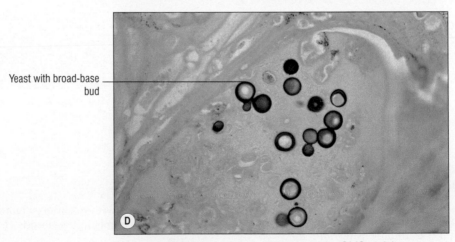

Yeast with broad-base bud

Fig. 13.8 D North American blastomycosis (GMS stain).

P
- Pseudoepitheliomatous hyperplasia; sometimes intraepidermal neutrophilic microabscesses
- Diffuse mixed infiltrate of neutrophils (often abscesses), lymphocytes, histiocytes, plasma cells, and multinucleated giant cells; no caseation
- Thick-walled spores 8–15 microns, sometimes with a characteristic broad-based bud, either within giant cells or free in the tissue. Often visible with H&E, but seen best with PAS or GMS stains

Differential diagnosis

1. Other diseases with pseudoepitheliomatous hyperplasia (1.117), neutrophils in the dermis (1.89), or granulomas (1.51).

13.9 Histoplasmosis

(see Fig. 13.9A–D)

Histoplasma capsulatum, a dimorphic soil fungus, is found worldwide, but is especially common in the central eastern

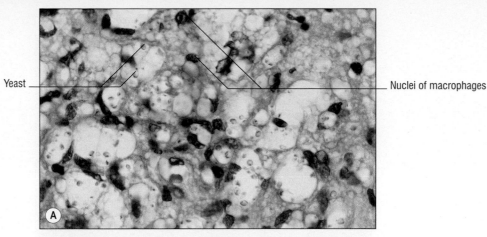

Yeast ———— Nuclei of macrophages

Fig. 13.9 A Histoplasmosis.

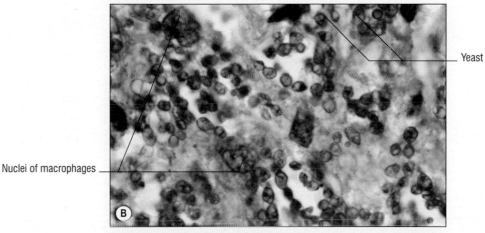

Nuclei of macrophages ———— Yeast

Fig. 13.9 B Histoplasmosis (PAS stain).

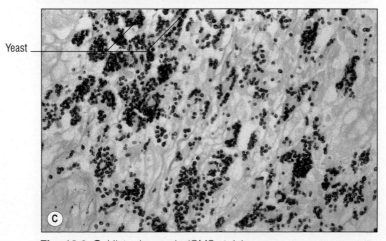

Yeast ————

Fig. 13.9 C Histoplasmosis (GMS stain).

US. It usually initially infects the *lungs*, is often asymptomatic, and usually spontaneously resolves. In exceptional cases, systemic dissemination occurs, especially in immunosuppressed patients. *Skin lesions vary greatly in morphology*, and usually are papules or nodules, plaques, or ulcers. Some patients develop mouth (1.82) ulcers without internal dissemination. Primary inoculation into the skin, with regional adenopathy, but without systemic disease, is very rare. Urine antigen test available.

- Epidermis or mucosa often ulcerated
- *Diffuse mixed dermal infiltrate* of neutrophils, lymphocytes, histiocytes, and a few giant cells; necrosis is common (1.88)
- Sparse leukocytoclastic vasculitis (4.1) infiltrate in some patients with AIDS, instead of the diffuse infiltrate
- Numerous *small 2–4-micron spores* surrounded by a *clear space* (pseudocapsule) can be seen within histiocytes and giant cells with H&E stains. They are seen more readily with PAS, GMS, Giemsa, or Gram stains

P

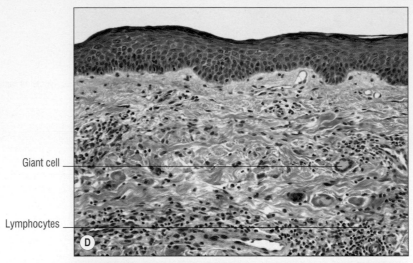

Giant cell

Lymphocytes

Fig. 13.9 D Histoplasmosis (medium power).

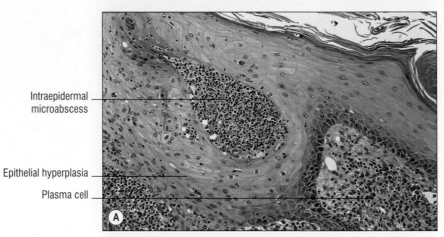

Intraepidermal microabscess

Epithelial hyperplasia

Plasma cell

Fig. 13.10 A Chromomycosis (low mag.)

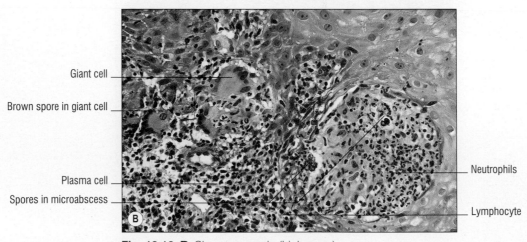

Giant cell

Brown spore in giant cell

Plasma cell

Spores in microabscess

Neutrophils

Lymphocyte

Fig. 13.10 B Chromomycosis (high mag.)

Variation

1. African histoplasmosis: *Histoplasma capsulatum* var. *duboisii*: larger yeast (8–15 microns).

Differential diagnosis

1. Small organisms of similar size are seen within histiocytes in rhinoscleroma (12.9), granuloma inguinale (12.8), leishmaniasis (15.1), penicilliosis (13.19), and granulomatous cryptococcosis (13.5).

2. Other diseases with neutrophils in the dermis (1.89) or granulomas (1.51).

13.10 Chromomycosis (chromoblastomycosis)

(see Fig. 13.10A–D)

Phialophora, *Fonsecaea*, and *Cladosporium* species cause *verrucous plaques* (1.146) at sites of *primary inoculation*, sometimes

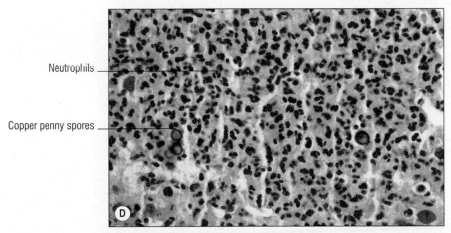

Cytoplasm of giant cell

Copper penny spores

Macrophage

Fig. 13.10 C Chromomycosis (high mag.).

Neutrophils

Copper penny spores

Fig. 13.10 D Chromomycosis (high mag.).

with slow local dissemination, but systemic infection is rare. Lesions are rarely annular (1.5).

- Pseudoepitheliomatous hyperplasia; sometimes intraepidermal neutrophilic microabscesses
- Diffuse mixed dermal infiltrate of neutrophils (often abscesses), lymphocytes, histiocytes, plasma cells, and multinucleated giant cells; no caseation
- Clusters or chains of brown spores (Medlar bodies, "copper pennies") of 6–12 microns within histiocytes in microabscesses, as well as free within the tissue. Spores reproduce by fission instead of budding

Differential diagnosis

1. Other diseases with pseudoepitheliomatous hyperplasia (1.117), neutrophils in the dermis (1.89), or granulomas (1.51).
2. Pheohyphomycosis (13.17): brown hyphae are seen in the dermis and subcutaneous tissue instead of copper penny spores.
3. Tinea nigra (13.3): brown hyphae are limited to the stratum corneum.

13.11 Sporotrichosis

(see Fig. 13.11A–C)

Sporotrichum schenckii produces *nodules and pustules*, especially on *hands, fingers* (1.56), and forearms, after primary inoculation, especially from *rose thorns* or sphagnum moss.

Nodules may spread in a *linear pattern* up the lymphatics, rarely disseminating into joints or systemically.

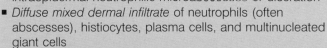

- *Pseudoepitheliomatous hyperplasia*; often with intraepidermal neutrophilic microabscesses or ulceration
- *Diffuse mixed dermal infiltrate* of neutrophils (often abscesses), histiocytes, plasma cells, and multinucleated giant cells
- *Round, oval,* or *cigar-shaped spores range of 3–8 microns* but are often difficult to find, even with PAS and GMS stains
- Rarely, eosinophilic star-like deposits around the yeast (asteroid bodies), not to be confused with the intracytoplasmic asteroid bodies sometimes seen with sarcoidosis (7.5)

Differential diagnosis

1. Other sporotrichoid lesions (1.133).
2. Other diseases with pseudoepitheliomatous hyperplasia (1.117), neutrophils in the dermis (1.89), or granulomas (1.51).

13.12 Zygomycosis (phycomycosis, mucormycosis)

(see Fig. 13.12A,B)

Infection usually presents as an indurated, often necrotic, plaque resembling ecthyma gangrenosum (12.17), associated

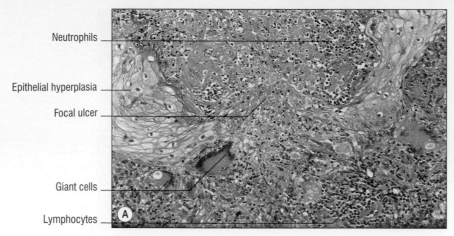

Neutrophils

Epithelial hyperplasia

Focal ulcer

Giant cells

Lymphocytes

Fig. 13.11 A Sporotrichosis (low mag.).

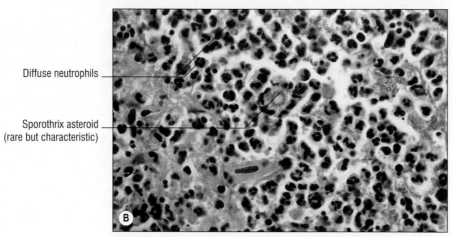

Diffuse neutrophils

Sporothrix asteroid
(rare but characteristic)

Fig. 13.11 B Sporotrichosis (medium mag.).

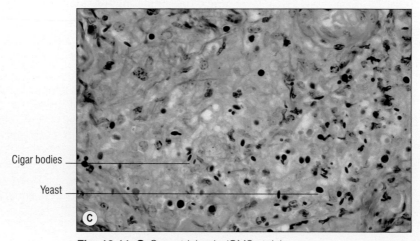

Cigar bodies

Yeast

Fig. 13.11 C Sporotrichosis (GMS stain).

with diabetes, burns, and immunosuppression. There are different forms: rhinocerebral, primary cutaneous, pulmonary, gastrointestinal, and disseminated. Infection usually by one of the three genera: *Rhizopus*, *Mucor*, or *Absidia*.

Variation

1. Subcutaneous phycomycosis: deep infection by a variety of other non-septate fungi.

- Epidermis often ulcerated
- Granulation tissue, thrombi, *necrosis*
- *Sparse inflammation in many cases*, or neutrophilic abscesses may be present
- *Non-septate* (coenocytic), *large hyphae* (diameter up to 30 microns) with *right-angled branching* are seen with H&E, but are best seen with PAS or GMS stains.

Differential diagnosis

1. Other diseases with necrosis of dermis (1.88).
2. Other fungi generally appear as yeast or septate hyphae with smaller diameter and no right-angle branching.

13.13 Aspergillosis

(see Fig. 13.13A–D)

Aspergillus species infects the skin most commonly in immunosuppressed patients, often through *hematogenous spread.* *Plaques are erythematous or necrotic.*

Differential diagnosis

1. Other diseases with necrosis of dermis (1.88).

> - *Diffuse mixed dermal infiltrate* of neutrophils, lymphocytes, histiocytes, or multinucleated giant cells. Often there is a *predominance of dermal necrosis* with very little inflammation
> - Numerous septate hyphae (diameters of 2–4 microns) with *branching at acute angles of 45°–60°*, in the dermis and *often in blood vessels*
> - An immunostain for *Aspergillus* is available but it might not be specific versus other fungi.

13.14 Mycetoma (madura foot, maduromycosis)

(see Fig. 13.14)

Mycetoma usually presents as *draining sinus tracts, nodules, ulceration, and fibrosis* of the skin, subcutaneous tissue, usually on the foot (1.48), often eventually resulting in *massive enlargement and bony deformity.* It is due to primary inoculation of a wide variety of bacteria (then called *Actinomycetoma*, due to *Nocardia, Actinomyces, Actinomadura, Streptomyces,* and other bacteria, 12.16, 12.17), or true fungi (then called *Eumycetoma*, due to many different organisms, most notably *Pseudoallescheria boydii, Phialophora verrucosa, Aspergillus, Curvularia,* and *Madurella*).

> - *Abscesses of neutrophils, mixed infiltrate*, granulomatous inflammation, and/or granulation tissue, with fibrosis in older lesions
> - *Granules* (also known as sclerotia, large colonies of bacteria or fungi, usually from 0.5 mm to 3 mm, large enough to be seen grossly
> - Bacteria granules (sulfur granules) tend to be whitish to yellowish, and filaments within or radiating from the granules tend to be less than 1 micron thick. By contrast, true fungi tend to have brown or black granules with thicker hyphae (diameter about 5 microns)

Differential diagnosis

1. Actinomycosis (12.16) and botryomycosis (12.16) have similar granules, but the clinical presentation is different.

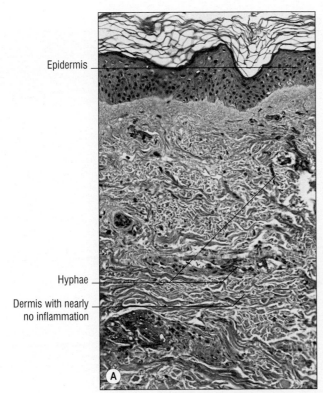

Epidermis

Hyphae

Dermis with nearly no inflammation

A

Fig. 13.12 A *Rhizopus* infection (low power).

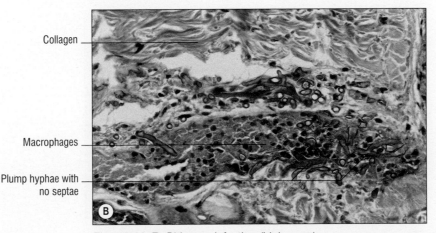

Collagen

Macrophages

Plump hyphae with no septae

B

Fig. 13.12 B *Rhizopus* infection (high mag.).

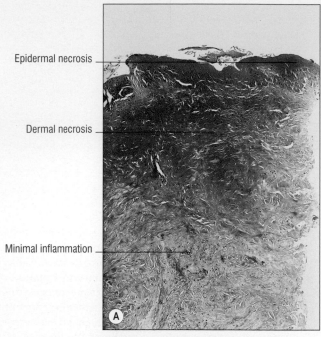

Fig. 13.13 A Aspergillosis (low mag.).

Epidermal necrosis

Dermal necrosis

Minimal inflammation

2. Chromomycosis (13.10): verrucous plaque, brown copper penny spores, but no granules.
3. Pheohyphomycosis (13.17) and hyalohyphomycosis (13.18): subcutaneous nodules or cysts, often more demarcated and less extensive, without granules.
4. Other diseases with diffuse neutrophils (1.89), granulomas (1.51), or ulcers (1.142).

13.15 Rhinosporidiosis
(see Fig. 13.15)

Red, friable, often pedunculated (1.106) *nodule*, most common around *nose* (1.95) or *eye* (1.41) after traumatic inoculation with *Rhinosporidium seeberi*. It is mainly found in India and South America. The organism does not grow in routine culture.

- *Polypoid* lesions of *granulation tissue* with mixed inflammatory infiltrate
- Characteristic numerous *huge sporangia* (up to 500 microns) containing endospores

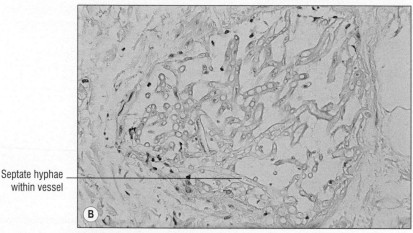

Septate hyphae within vessel

Fig. 13.13 B Aspergillosis (high mag.).

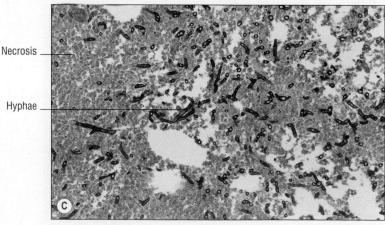

Necrosis

Hyphae

Fig. 13.13 C Aspergillosis (high mag.).

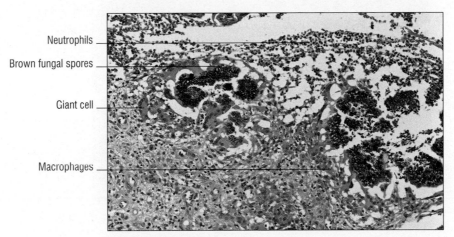

Septate hyphae

Fig. 13.13 D Aspergillosis (high mag., GMS stain).

Neutrophils

Brown fungal spores

Giant cell

Macrophages

Fig. 13.14 Mycetoma.

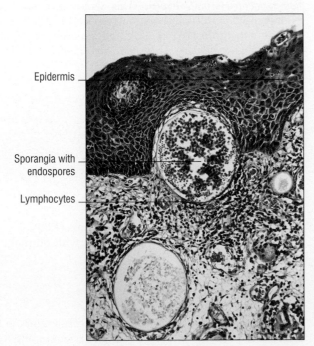

Epidermis

Sporangia with endospores

Lymphocytes

Fig. 13.15 Rhinosporidiosis.

Differential diagnosis

1. The spores and endospores of coccidioidomycosis (13.6) are much smaller.

13.16 **Lobomycosis (Lobo's disease, lacaziosis, keloidal blastomycosis)**

(see Fig. 13.16)

Rare infection by *Lacazia loboi* (formerly *Loboa loboi*, and before that, *Paracoccidioides loboi*, another example of constant name changing to increase microbiologist employment), in Central or South America, producing chronic hyperpigmented *keloidal nodules* (27.2) on exposed areas such as the ears, elbows, or knees. It does not grow in routine culture.

- *Granulomatous* inflammation (1.51), with multinucleated giant cells, plasma cells, and lymphocytes
- Prominent *fibrosis*
- Spores are uniform in size (6–12 microns), easily seen with H&E, and form a "*string of pearls*" chain

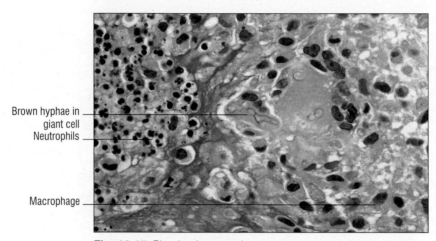

"String of pearls" spores

Fig. 13.16 Lobomycosis (GMS stain).

Brown hyphae in
giant cell
Neutrophils

Macrophage

Fig. 13.17 Pheohyphomycosis.

13.17 Pheohyphomycosis

(see Fig. 13.17)
This is defined as infection of the dermis or soft tissue by *pigmented hyphae*. Sometimes tinea nigra (13.3) and black piedra (12.5) are considered to be superficial forms of pheohyphomycosis, but the term is more commonly used for deeper infections. Skin lesions may be deep nodules (1.135), abscesses, or verrucous plaques (1.146). Many different organisms have been implicated, especially *Alternaria, Bipolaris, Curvularia, Exophiala, Exserohilum,* and *Phialophora*.

- Brown hyphae (*dematiacious hyphae*) found in the dermis or subcutaneous tissue
- Variable mixed inflammatory reaction, *suppurative granulomatous* often, fibrosis often
- Walled-off cystic space (*pheomycotic cyst*) sometimes
- Foreign body, such as wood splinter, may be present (7.6)

Differential diagnosis

1. Other infections by dematiaceous fungi include dermatomycosis (13.1), tinea nigra (superficial pheohyphomycosis, 13.3), chromomycosis (13.10), and mycetoma (13.14).
2. Other granulomas (1.51) or diseases with dermal neutrophils (1.89).

13.18 Hyalohyphomycosis

This is defined as infection of the dermis or soft tissue by *non-pigmented septate hyphae*. This would exclude pheohyphomycosis (13.17) and zygomycosis (13.12), but would include aspergillosis (13.13). A hodge-podge of organisms, including *Acremonium, Fusarium,* and *Penicillium* has been implicated.

- *Necrosis* often prominent (1.88)
- Inflammation may be sparse, or suppurative and granulomatous
- *Non-pigmented hyalinized septate hyphae* often visible with H&E, better seen with PAS or GMS stains

Differential diagnosis

1. Other diseases with necrosis of dermis (1.88).
2. Other granulomas (1.51) or diseases with dermal neutrophils (1.89).

13.19 Penicilliosis

(see Fig. 13.19A,B)
Infection of the lung by *Penicillium marneffei*, mainly in *Southeast Asia* in patients with *AIDS* (14.12), disseminating to other organs later. Acneiform papules (1.3) resemble molluscum

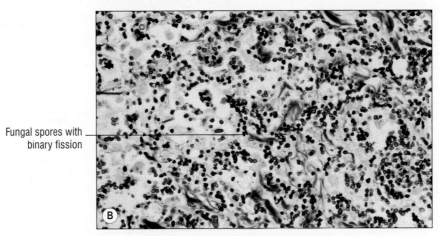

Macrophage

Fungal spores

Fig. 13.19 A Penicilliosis.

Fungal spores with binary fission

Fig. 13.19 B Penicilliosis (GMS stain).

contagiosum (14.4) clinically. The fungus is dimorphic in culture, unlike other members of the *Penicillium* genus. It appears in yeast form in vivo.

- Diffuse suppurative granulomatous inflammation
- Necrosis prominent with sparse inflammation in patients with poor immunity (1.88)
- Yeast with diameter of 3 microns in histiocytes, up to 8 microns when extracellular, dividing by binary fission without buds, appearing elongated and septate
- Positive staining of yeast with PAS and GMS, but not with mucicarmine

Differential diagnosis

1. Histoplasmosis (13.9): also seen with AIDS, uniformly smaller yeast (2–4 microns), instead of small intracellular and larger extracellular yeast, more rounded instead of elongated, and budding with a narrow base instead of dividing by binary fission.
2. Cryptococcosis (13.5): also common with AIDS, but more rounded 5–20-micron yeast that buds, often gelatinous appearance of biopsy, mucin in capsule.
3. Other granulomas (1.51) or diseases with dermal neutrophils (1.89).

CHAPTER 14

Viral, Rickettsial, and Chlamydial Diseases

14.1 Human papillomavirus infection (HPV, viral wart, verruca vulgaris)

(see Fig. 14.1A–H)

Verrucous papules (1.146) due to infection with HPV, of which there are more than 60 subtypes. Warts often bend the dermatoglyphic lines and may have black dots representing thrombosed capillaries in dermal papillae (so-called "seeds" in a "seed wart").

P
- *Hyperkeratosis* (1.61), *papillomatosis*, hypergranulosis (1.60)
- *Columns of parakeratosis* (1.104), especially over projecting dermal papillae
- Vacuolated superficial keratinocytes with pyknotic raisin-like nuclei (*koilocytes*)
- Bete ridges often slope inward at borders of lesion (*arborization*), sometimes giving the lesion a spread-fingers appearance
- *Dilated capillaries* in dermal papillae
- Perivascular lymphocytes (1.109)

Variations

1. Verruca vulgaris (VV): the common wart, commonly HPV-2, most common on acral skin of the *hands and fingers* (1.56).
2. Plantar wart: located on *plantar* aspect of the foot (1.48), commonly HPV-1, less papillomatosis, more hypergranulosis.
3. Myrmecia wart: "*anthill wart*" (Myrmicinae is the subfamily name for fire ants) with *tremendous mounds of hypergranulosis* and koilocytes resembling specks of dirt of an anthill, HPV-1, mostly on soles and toes.
4. Filiform wart: more extreme delicate papillomatosis, more on the face.
5. Verruca plana (flat wart): children or young adults, often face, legs (spread by shaving), commonly HPV-3, often multiple, *papules less than 4 mm in diameter with flat-topped* smoother surface, may be subtle, minimal papillomatosis and no parakeratosis.

6. Condyloma acuminatum (venereal wart): *genital warts*, commonly HPV-6 or 11, and less often 16 or 18 which may evolve to Bowen's disease or bowenoid papulosis, less hyperkeratosis, more massive acanthosis, and more gentle papillomatosis instead of pointed projections (condyloma means "fist" or "knuckle").
7. Condyloma acuminatum after podophyllin application: a pseudomalignancy (1.118), many mitoses *arrested in metaphase*, which may resemble squamous cell carcinoma or bowenoid papulosis.
8. Epidermodysplasia verruciformis (EDV): familial cellular immunity defect, warts become confluent, mostly HPV-5 or 8 and less commonly other types, may clinically resemble pityriasis rosea (2.4), often *bubbly bluish cytoplasm* in keratinocytes, sometimes *cytologic atypia* (hyperchromatic pleomorphic cells), may evolve to squamous cell carcinoma.
9. Bowenoid papulosis (18.10): condyloma acuminatum in which bowenoid changes are found, often *multiple* and *more brownish papules*, usually due to HPV-16, 18, or certain other types, may actually be a squamous cell carcinoma in situ, but is not usually aggressive.
10. Pruritic vulvar squamous papillomatosis: *small, itchy, subtle papules of the labia minora* (1.149), which may appear normal, with variable koilocytic changes, lichenification, submucosal edema, and perivascular lymphocytes, polymerase chain reaction (PCR) may be needed to find HPV, which may not be the cause in all cases.
11. Focal epithelial hyperplasia (Heck's disease): HPV-13 or 32 produces *multiple papules on the mucosal lip* (1.74) or elsewhere in the mouth (1.82), often familial in patients with *native American heritage*.

©2012 Elsevier Ltd, Inc, BV
DOI: 10.1016/B978-0-323-06658-7.00014-2

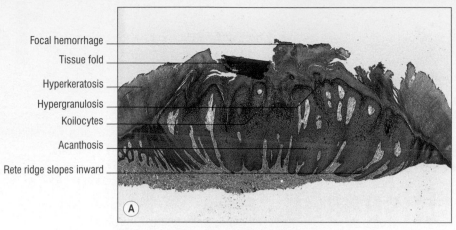

Focal hemorrhage
Tissue fold
Hyperkeratosis
Hypergranulosis
Koilocytes
Acanthosis
Rete ridge slopes inward

Fig. 14.1 A Verruca vulgaris (low mag.).

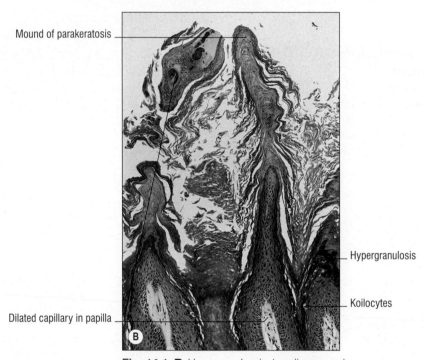

Mound of parakeratosis

Hypergranulosis

Koilocytes

Dilated capillary in papilla

Fig. 14.1 B Verruca vulgaris (medium mag.).

Differential diagnosis

1. Other papillomas (1.102) do not have koilocytes, but this may be confused with other causes of epidermal vacuolization (1.144). Electron microscopy, immunoperoxidase staining, or molecular genetic techniques may be needed if proof of HPV is desired.
2. Verrucous carcinoma (18.11) is more massive, and bowenoid papulosis (18.10) has more mitoses and cytologic atypia.
3. Other causes of keratinocyte vacuolization (1.144).

14.2 Herpes simplex (herpes type 1 and 2) and varicella zoster (herpes type 3)

(see Fig. 14.2A–D)
These two herpes viruses are common, and present as painful *grouped vesicles* on an erythematous base, later becoming crusted or ulcerated (1.142). The virus then becomes latent in the nerve ganglion cells. Herpes simplex most commonly occurs on *the penis* (1.107), *vulva* (1.149), *buttock, lip* (1.74), *or face* (1.44). Severe extensive primary involvement of the mouth is *herpetic gingivostomatitis*. Dissemination in eczema patients is called *eczema herpeticum* (*Kaposi varicelliform eruption*). Involvement of the finger is *herpetic whitlow*. Recurrences in the same location are common. *Varicella* (*chickenpox*) is spread through the respiratory route, and presents in childhood as an acute febrile illness with pharyngitis, vesicles in the mouth, and generalized vesicles, beginning centrally, and spreading peripherally. The virus then typically remains dormant for years or forever. A single recurrence may occur many years later as *shingles* (*zoster*), with *unilateral vesicles in a dermatome*, often purpuric (1.120), most common on the *trunk or face*. Subsequent recurrences are very rare unless there is immunosuppression. A vaccine for varicella zoster is now widely available. The diagnosis of both types of herpes virus is usually made clinically, or with *cultures, fluorescent antibody smears*, or *Tzanck smears*.

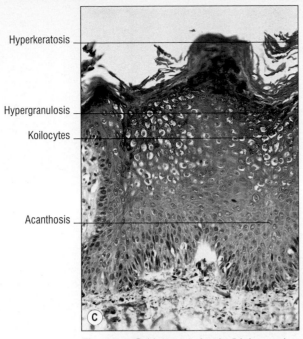

Hyperkeratosis

Hypergranulosis

Koilocytes

Acanthosis

Fig. 14.1 C Verruca vulgaris (high mag.).

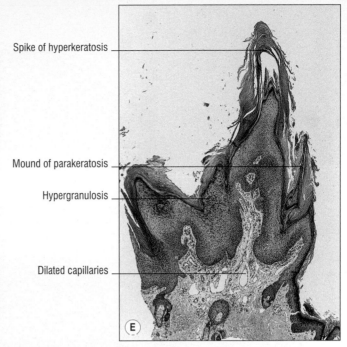

Spike of hyperkeratosis

Mound of parakeratosis

Hypergranulosis

Dilated capillaries

Fig. 14.1 E Filiform wart.

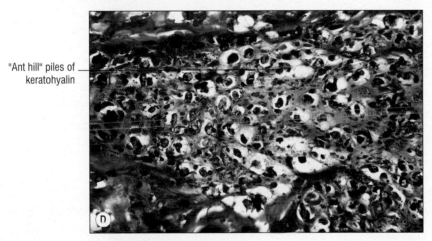

"Ant hill" piles of keratohyalin

Fig. 14.1 D Myrmecia wart.

P
- The two viruses cannot be distinguished with routine H&E staining
- *Intraepidermal vesicle* or ulceration
- *Epidermal necrosis* and *ballooning degeneration*: herpetic cytopathic changes are enlarged and pale keratinocytes, with *steel-gray nuclei*, *margination of chromatin* at the edge of the nucleus, sometimes with *pink intranuclear inclusions* surrounded by an artifactual cleft (Cowdry type A inclusions, Lipschutz bodies), *acantholysis*, or multinucleated keratinocyte formation
- Extravasated erythrocytes often (1.40)
- Perivascular or diffuse lymphocytes or neutrophils, sometimes with changes of leukocytoclastic vasculitis (4.1)

Differential diagnosis

1. Ballooning degeneration to a lesser degree can sometimes be seen in smallpox or vaccinia (14.3) and orf or milker's nodule (14.5), but multinucleated

keratinocytes are rarely seen, and inclusion bodies, if found, are more likely to be intracytoplasmic.
2. Other acantholytic diseases (1.2) or those with necrotic keratinocytes (1.86).
3. Other diseases with intraepidermal vesicles (1.147, Chapter 5).
4. Other genital ulcers (12.13).

14.3 Smallpox and vaccinia

(see Fig. 14.3)

Smallpox (variola), a deadly disease, has been eradicated due to vaccination with the vaccinia virus (mutant of cowpox). Rare disseminated skin infections are seen with the vaccinia virus in patients with eczema (*eczema vaccinatum*). Patients with immunodeficiency may also develop dissemination, or the vaccination site may fail to heal. Routine vaccination has now been largely discontinued, except in military personnel, due to the potential use of smallpox in biological warfare.

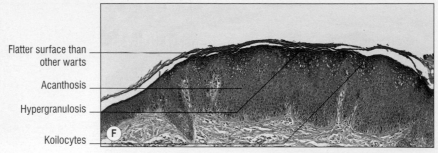

Flatter surface than other warts

Acanthosis

Hypergranulosis

Koilocytes

Fig. 14.1 F Verruca plana.

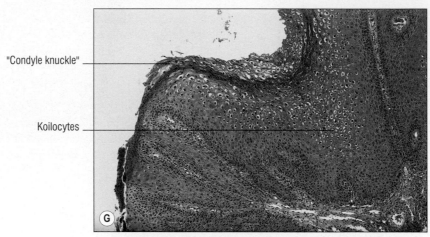

"Condyle knuckle"

Koilocytes

Fig. 14.1 G Condyloma acuminatum.

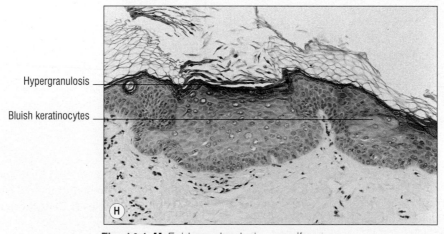

Hypergranulosis

Bluish keratinocytes

Fig. 14.1 H Epidermodysplasia verruciformis.

P
- *Intraepidermal vesicles* (1.147) with few balloon cells (usually not multinucleated) and *inclusion bodies* that are primarily *intracytoplasmic* (Guarnieri bodies)
- Mixed diffuse dermal infiltrate of lymphocytes and neutrophils

Differential diagnosis

1. Herpes simplex and varicella zoster (14.2) exhibit more multinucleated giant cells and the inclusion bodies are intranuclear.

14.4 Molluscum contagiosum

(see Fig. 14.4A,B)

Very common *white* (1.150) *umbilicated papules*, common on *penis* (1.107), *vulva* (1.149), or *groin* (1.55) as a sexually transmitted disease. Children acquire infection from close contact or swimming pools, with lesions on the *eyelids, face, trunk,* and *axilla*. It is a poxvirus. The diagnosis is usually made clinically, but inflamed red lesions are more difficult to recognize, and are more likely to be biopsied, especially when large or solitary. Widespread lesions can occur with atopic dermatitis, immunosuppressive therapy, or HIV infection. Usually infection is self-limited, resolving in 6 months to years.

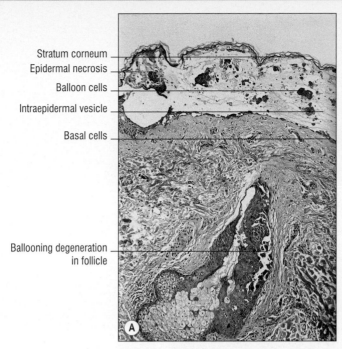

Stratum corneum
Epidermal necrosis
Balloon cells
Intraepidermal vesicle
Basal cells

Ballooning degeneration
in follicle

Fig. 14.2 A Herpes virus infection (low mag.).

- Epidermal hyperplasia producing a *crater* filled with molluscum bodies (Henderson–Patterson bodies) that are huge, up to 35 microns, eosinophilic to *basophilic intracytoplasmic inclusions* that push the nucleus and numerous keratohyaline granules aside
- Intact lesions show little or no inflammation, while ruptured lesions exhibit a dense mixed inflammatory response consisting of mononuclear cells, neutrophils, and multinucleated giant cells

Differential diagnosis

1. The diagnosis is obvious once molluscum bodies are identified, but they may be sparse in some densely inflamed lesions. Rarely they might be confused with warts (14.1).

14.5 Orf and milker's nodule (collectively called farmyard pox)

(see Fig. 14.5A,B)

These two parapox viruses cause *hemorrhagic crusted blisters*, pustules, or plaques on the *fingers and hands* (1.56). The H&E

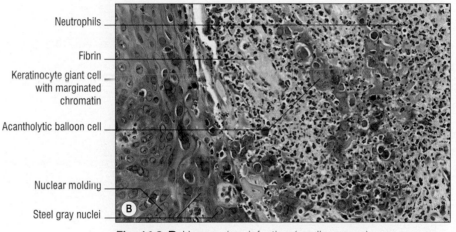

Neutrophils
Fibrin
Keratinocyte giant cell
with marginated
chromatin
Acantholytic balloon cell

Nuclear molding
Steel gray nuclei

Fig. 14.2 B Herpes virus infection (medium mag.).

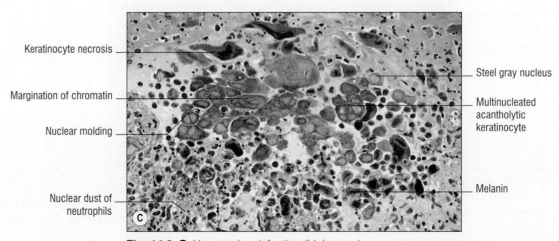

Keratinocyte necrosis
Margination of chromatin
Nuclear molding
Nuclear dust of
neutrophils

Steel gray nucleus
Multinucleated
acantholytic
keratinocyte
Melanin

Fig. 14.2 C Herpes virus infection (high mag.).

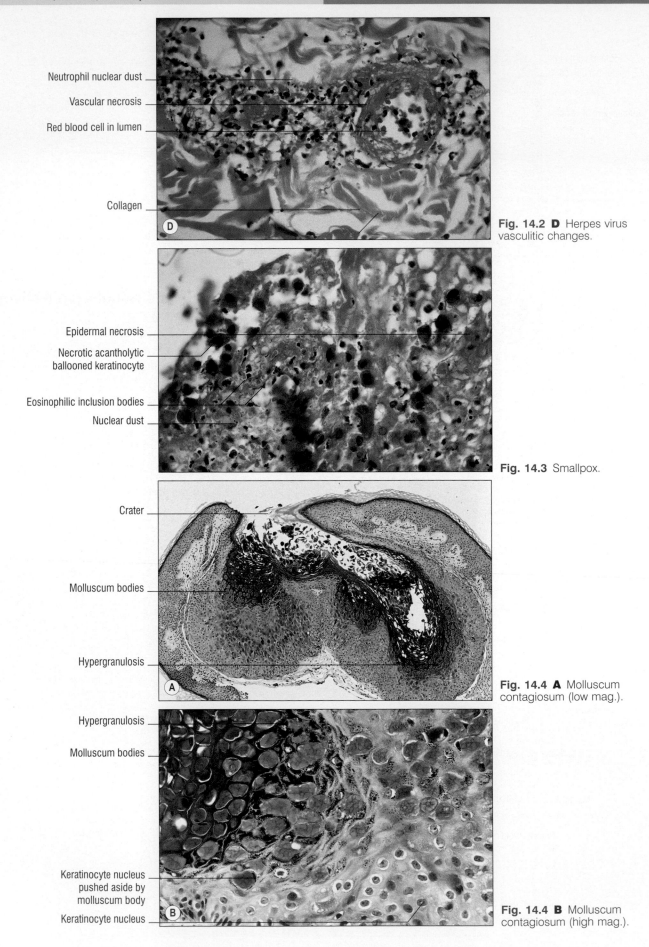

Neutrophil nuclear dust

Vascular necrosis

Red blood cell in lumen

Collagen

Fig. 14.2 D Herpes virus vasculitic changes.

Epidermal necrosis

Necrotic acantholytic ballooned keratinocyte

Eosinophilic inclusion bodies

Nuclear dust

Fig. 14.3 Smallpox.

Crater

Molluscum bodies

Hypergranulosis

Fig. 14.4 A Molluscum contagiosum (low mag.).

Hypergranulosis

Molluscum bodies

Keratinocyte nucleus pushed aside by molluscum body

Keratinocyte nucleus

Fig. 14.4 B Molluscum contagiosum (high mag.).

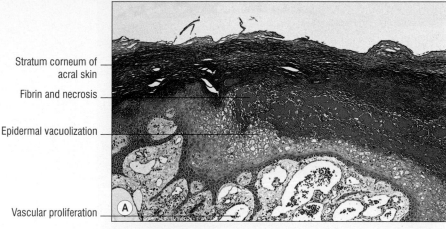

Stratum corneum of acral skin

Fibrin and necrosis

Epidermal vacuolization

Vascular proliferation

Fig. 14.5 A Orf.

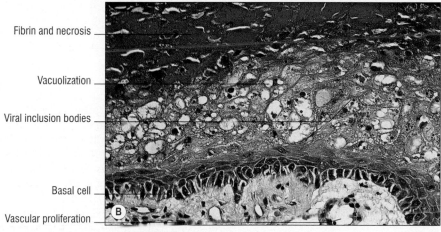

Fibrin and necrosis

Vacuolization

Viral inclusion bodies

Basal cell

Vascular proliferation

Fig. 14.5 B Orf.

and electron microscopic findings of orf and milker's nodule are identical, so they are distinguished by history. Orf (ecthyma contagiosum) is acquired from handling infected *sheep* (especially scabby mouth in lambs), and milker's nodules from *cows* (especially the udders). The virus can live on fenceposts or soil for at least 6 months, so there may not be an obvious exposure to animals. Lesions resolve in about 6 weeks. The viruses do not grow in routine culture.

- Histology varies greatly depending on the age of the lesion
- *Vacuolated superficial epidermis* (1.144) with *inclusion bodies* that are predominantly *intracytoplasmic*, occasionally intranuclear
- *Epidermal necrosis*, often with extremely *delicate finger-like projections* into the dermis
- *Dense, diffuse, mixed inflammatory infiltrate* in the dermis
- Dermal edema (1.30), extravasated erythrocytes (1.40), dilated blood vessels

Differential diagnosis

1. Pyogenic granuloma (25.3), Sweet's syndrome (3.7), herpetic whitlow (14.2), erythema multiforme (3.2), sporotrichosis (13.11), atypical mycobacterial infection

(12.11), and squamous cell carcinoma (18.11) can cause clinical confusion.
2. Lesions with impressive, delicate, finger-like epithelial projections are characteristic, but other lesions may be confused with vaccinia (14.3), papillomavirus infections (14.1), herpes virus infections (14.2), or other diseases with epidermal necrosis (1.87).

14.6 Coxsackie virus infection

Infections by these viruses can cause morbilliform eruptions (1.81), pneumonia, meningoencephalitis, or myocarditis. Most infections are harmless and self-limited. *Hand–foot–mouth disease* (usually Coxsackie virus type A-16) causes fever and constitutional symptoms with *small oval vesiculopustules* along *creases of palms and soles* (1.100), and in the *mouth* (1.82). Viral culture may be positive from stool (less often from vesicles). PCR has been used.

- Intraepidermal multiloculated vesicles or pustules
- Epidermal necrosis (1.87) or ballooning degeneration (1.147) without inclusion bodies or multinucleated keratinocytes
- Papillary dermal edema, sometimes resulting in subepidermal blisters (1.30)
- Perivascular lymphocytes (1.109) or neutrophils

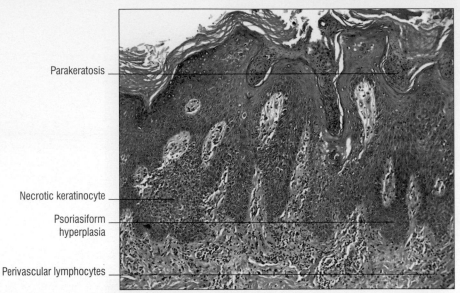

Parakeratosis

Necrotic keratinocyte

Psoriasiform hyperplasia

Perivascular lymphocytes

Fig. 14.7 Necrolytic acral erythema. A psoriasiform eruption with necrotic keratinocytes seen with hepatitis C.

Variation

1. Herpangina: constitutional symptoms, *soft palate ulcers in children*.

14.7 Viral exanthems

(see Fig. 14.7)
Many different viruses cause common morbilliform eruptions, which cannot be covered in detail in this book. The skin biopsy is usually non-specific, and the diagnosis often rests upon the clinical findings, viral cultures, or serologic testing.

- Epidermis normal or with focal parakeratosis or *focal spongiosis*
- Mild ballooning degeneration or multinucleated keratinocytes rarely (not as prominent as seen with herpes viruses, 14.2) or focal keratinocyte necrosis (1.87)
- *Perivascular or interface lymphocytes*

Variations

1. Measles (First disease, rubeola): high fever, *cough, coryza,* conjunctivitis, *Koplik's spots* on buccal mucosa, morbilliform *rash more prone to become confluent*. Besides having the changes listed above, it may resemble erythema multiforme (3.2).
2. Scarlet fever (Second disease, 12.2): caused by *Streptococcus*, not a virus.
3. Rubella (Third disease, German measles): *mild fever,* less constitutional symptoms, posterior neck and *post-auricular adenopathy* before the morbilliform eruption starts on face and centrally, clears rapidly in 2–3 days, *petechiae on soft palate* (Forchheimer's sign, 1.98), keratinocytic multinucleated giant cells occur rarely but are usually limited to lymph nodes or other internal organs. Congenital rubella syndrome can occur if mother is infected in first trimester.
4. Duke's disease (Fourth disease): no longer considered to be a real entity.
5. Erythema infectiosum (Fifth disease): due to parvovirus B19, malar erythema (*slapped cheek*), followed by morbilliform eruption with *reticulated pattern* (1.123) on extremities, very few symptoms. Usually harmless, but bone marrow aplasia, hemolytic anemia, or miscarriage can occur. Parvovirus may also be a cause of the *purpuric glove and sock syndrome* (1.120).
6. Roseola (Sixth disease, exanthem subitum): due to herpes type 6 or 7, *high fever*, then *morbilliform rash after fever abates*, mostly infants *under age 2 years*.
7. Herpes type 6: this virus has been implicated in most cases of roseola, Rosai–Dorfman disease (17.13), and a mononucleosis-like disease (14.8).
8. Herpes type 7: low-titer antibodies to this virus are found in 70% of the population, and it has been implicated in pityriasis rosea (2.4), and 30% of cases of roseola.
9. Herpes type 8: low-titer antibodies found in 5–25% of the US population. Has been implicated in all forms of Kaposi sarcoma (25.9).
10. Hepatitis A: acute hepatitis due to fecally contaminated food or water, influenza-like illness, and sometimes a morbilliform rash, self-limited, with permanent immunity.
11. Hepatitis B: acute hepatitis or asymptomatic infection transmitted sexually or by contaminated blood, resulting in 5% chronic carrier state. Associated with Gianotti–Crosti syndrome, vasculitis (4.1), polyarteritis nodosa (4.4), erythema multiforme (3.2), and cryoglobulinemia (4.9). Immunization is available.
12. Hepatitis C: most initial infections are asymptomatic, mostly transmitted by contaminated blood, chronic hepatitis in 70%, sometimes resulting in cirrhosis or hepatocellular carcinoma. Associated with a wide variety of skin lesions, including porphyria cutanea tarda (8.1), lichen planus (2.11), vasculitis (4.1), cryoglobulinemia (4.9), urticaria (3.1), erythema multiforme (3.2), and erythema nodosum (16.1).

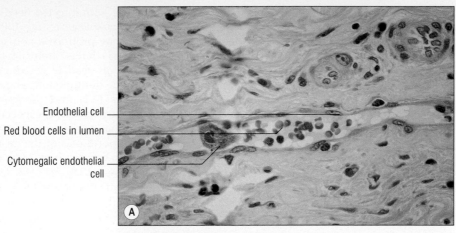

Fig. 14.9 A Cytomegalovirus infection.

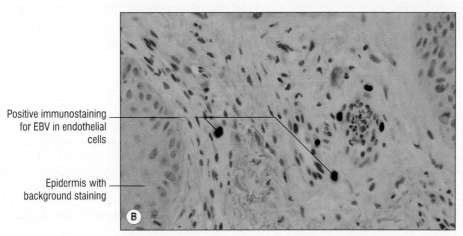

Fig. 14.9 B Cytomegalovirus infection (immunostaining).

Differential diagnosis

1. Morbilliform eruptions (1.81).
2. Diseases with perivascular dermatitis (1.109) or interface dermatitis (1.64).
3. Diseases with spongiosis (1.132).

14.8 Epstein–Barr virus infection (EBV, herpes type 4)

EBV causes a wide variety of illnesses, including oral ulcers (1.82).

Variations

1. Mononucleosis: fever (1.45), pharyngitis, headache, lymphadenopathy, hepatosplenomegaly, morbilliform eruption (1.81), histology like other viral exanthems (14.7).
2. Oral hairy leukoplakia: white corrugated protrusions on the *lateral aspects* of the *tongue* (1.139) in patients with *HIV virus* infection (14.12). Biopsy has irregular keratin projections, parakeratosis, acanthosis, and groups of pale epithelial cells (1.99).
3. Gianotti–Crosti syndrome (14.11).
4. Kikuchi's syndrome (24.14).

14.9 Cytomegalovirus infection (CMV, herpes type 5)

(see Fig. 14.9A,B)

CMV is widely prevalent in its latent state in the general population, and mainly reactivates when there is immuno-suppression. Fever occurs along with infection of many internal organs, especially causing pneumonitis, hepatitis (1.75), encephalitis, chorioretinitis (1.41), and gastroenteritis (1.49). A wide variety of skin manifestations include blueberry muffin babies (*dermal hematopoiesis*, 24.19), *ulcers* (especially *perianal* 1.108 and mouth 1.82), *mononucleosis-like syndrome* (14.8, especially after ampicillin), *morbilliform eruption* (1.81), urticaria, purpura (1.120), bullae (1.147), or verrucous lesions (1.146). Serologic testing is widely available. The virus can be cultured from urine, blood, or tissue. The specific cytomegalic cells described below are more likely to be found in the ulcers rather than in the more non-specific rashes.

- Epidermis normal, verrucous or ulcerated
- Vascular dilation with large *cytomegalic endothelial cells*
- *Intranuclear and intracytoplasmic inclusion bodies* (halo around intranuclear inclusions forming an "owl's eye" appearance)
- Variable perivascular lymphocytes or neutrophils (1.109)

- Positive CMV immunostain (readily available commercially, does not cross-react with other herpes viruses or HPV)
- Viral particles indistinguishable from other herpes viruses by electron microscopy

14.10 Kawasaki's disease

Uncommon childhood illness presumed to be viral or bacterial toxin related, but specific etiology is unknown. *Polymorphous*, often urticarial exanthem (1.81), *red or fissured lips*, *pharyngitis*, *strawberry tongue* (1.139), *acral erythema* and edema with *subsequent desquamation, conjunctivitis* (1.43), *cervical lymphadenopathy*, fever for more than 5 days, *coronary artery aneurysms* (20% incidence if untreated). Diagnosis is primarily clinical, after excluding other possible infections.

- *Arteritis* (like polyarteritis, 4.4) *in the heart* (leading to thrombosis or aneurysm), but not in the skin
- Non-specific perivascular (1.109) lymphocytes (not neutrophils) in biopsies from the rash

14.11 Gianotti–Crosti syndrome (papular acrodermatitis of childhood)

Uncommon, syndrome of *children*, due to a variety of viruses (especially hepatitis B, Epstein–Barr, Coxsackie, and others), *papulovesicles on the face* (1.44), *extremities* (1.6), and buttock, with *relative sparing of the trunk* (unlike most other viral exanthems), mild constitutional symptoms, sometimes lymphadenopathy, *self-limited* in a few weeks or several months.

- Focal parakeratosis, sometimes crusting (1.104)
- *Focal spongiosis*, acanthosis, *dyskeratosis* (1.27)
- Papillary dermal edema often (1.30)
- *Perivascular lymphocytes*, rare eosinophils
- Extravasated red blood cells sometimes (1.40)

Variation

1. Papulovesicular acrolocated syndrome: "splitters" use this term for cases other than those due to hepatitis B, reserving the term Gianotti–Crosti only for those due to hepatitis B, which is rare in the US ("lumpers" are winning nowadays).

Differential diagnosis

Gianotti–Crosti syndrome is mainly a clinical diagnosis, since viral testing is usually not done.
1. Other red papular diseases (1.122) or morbilliform eruptions (1.81).
2. Atopic dermatitis (2.1): far more common, also often on face and extremities, less acute onset, more scaly, more chronic.
3. Other spongiotic diseases (1.132), perivascular dermatitis (1.109).

14.12 Human immunodeficiency virus (HIV) infection

Common, worldwide epidemic infection with HIV-1 virus (formerly called HTLV-3, not to be confused with HTLV-1, 24.1), or with HIV-2 virus endemic in Africa, spread by venereal contact, drug abuse with infected needles, or blood transfusions. Diagnosed with *serologic testing*. Initial infection may be asymptomatic, or may produce a non-specific fever or morbilliform eruption (1.81) that is rarely biopsied, or lymphadenopathy, may eventually lead to a reduction in CD4 lymphocytes and acquired immunodeficiency syndrome (*AIDS*). *Seborrheic dermatitis* (2.1) and *psoriasis* (2.8) may become severe. Prone to many *infections*, especially bacillary angiomatosis (12.15), candidiasis (13.4), cryptococcosis (13.5), penicilliosis (13.19), cryptosporidiosis of the gastrointestinal tract, cytomegalovirus (14.9), herpes virus (14.2), hairy leukoplakia (14.8), histoplasmosis (13.9), *Mycobacterium avium* complex (12.11), pneumocystis pneumonia (15.12), toxoplasmosis (15.15), and warts (14.1). Lymphoma or *Kaposi sarcoma* (25.9) may develop.

Variations

1. HIV lipodystrophy (16.11).
2. Interface dermatitis of HIV infection (1.64).

14.13 Rickettsial diseases

Rare to uncommon arthropod-borne infections by these obligate intracellular virus-like coccobacilli are *usually diagnosed serologically* rather than by biopsy. *Rocky Mountain spotted fever* (*RMSF*) is an acute illness due to tick-borne *Rickettsia rickettsii*, mainly found in the US. Patients are *acutely ill with fever* and a morbilliform rash that begins in acral locations and later becomes generalized and *petechial*, possibly resulting in death unless there is early treatment. Other *tick-borne spotted fevers* include African (*R. conorii*), Siberian (*R. siberica*), and Queensland (*R. australis*). There is often an initial necrotic bite site known as a *tache noire* (black spot). Mouse mite-borne *rickettsialpox* (*R. akari*) begins with a papule or vesicle at the bite site, later becoming more generalized and vesicular or morbilliform, resembling varicella (14.2) without oral lesions. The typhus group includes mite-borne *scrub typhus* of south-east Asia (*Orientia tsutsugamushi*, formerly *R. tsutsugamushi*), worldwide human body louse-borne *epidemic typhus* (*R. prowazekii*), and worldwide urban rat flea-borne *endemic* (*murine*) *typhus* (*R. typhi*, formerly *R. mooseri*). Like most of the spotted fevers, patients develop a papule or black eschar at the site of the bite in some of these diseases, with subsequent febrile influenza-like illness with morbilliform eruptions in all of them. Q fever (*Coxiella burnettii*) has no skin lesions.

- Epidermal necrosis (1.87) or spongiosis (1.132) at initial bite site
- Dermal edema (1.30), or subepidermal blister (1.147) in rickettsialpox, which may appear to be intraepidermal after re-epithelialization
- *Vasculitis* (1.145) with predominance of lymphocytes and histiocytes, although some cases are neutrophilic
- Extravasated erythrocytes (1.40) and thrombi (1.137) often
- Organisms are difficult to demonstrate by special stains such as Giemsa, but *direct immunofluorescence and immunoenzyme antibodies* demonstrating the organisms in frozen sections are available

Differential diagnosis

1. Ehrlichiosis: tick-borne infection due to *Ehrlichia* species presents similar to RMSF as headache, fever, myalgia, leukopenia, thrombocytopenia, and elevated liver enzymes, but maculopapular or petechial rash in only 20% of patients. Biopsies have not been well described.

2. Other morbilliform (1.81), or petechial (1.120), febrile (1.45) eruptions.

3. Other causes of vasculitis (1.145) or perivascular dermatitis (1.109).

14.14 Lymphogranuloma venereum (LGV)

Rare venereal infection with *Chlamydia trachomatis* (types L1, L2, and L3), which is difficult to culture. The readily available chlamydia group antigen complement-fixation *serologic test* is often used to make the diagnosis, but it cross-reacts with the far more common epidemic *Chlamydia trachomatis* serotypes D–K that cause non-specific urethritis and salpingitis. A more specific direct immunofluorescence antibody is available. *Unimpressive 2–3-mm papules or erosions* occur on the *penis* (1.107) or *vulva* (1.149), which are usually not biopsied. Subsequent severe inguinal lymphadenopathy (*buboes*) may result in the *"groove sign"* when lymph nodes on both sides of Poupart's ligament are enlarged, mainly in men. Lymph nodes have stellate abscesses with histiocytes and plasma cells. Elephantiasis and vegetating ulcers (*esthiomene*, Greek for "eating away") like those of granuloma inguinale (12.8) may occur in both men and women. Rectovaginal fistulas may appear.

- Epidermis normal or ulcerated (1.142)
- *Diffuse mixed infiltrate* of neutrophils, lymphocytes, histiocytes, *plasma cells* (1.111), and sometimes multinucleated giant cells (1.84)
- Although abscesses may be seen in the skin, stellate abscesses are usually seen only in the lymph nodes, later becoming granulomatous
- Organisms rarely demonstrated with Giemsa stain in histiocytes (Gamma–Favre bodies)

Differential diagnosis

1. Other genital ulcers (12.13).

14.15 Psittacosis

Infection by *Chlamydophila psittaci* (formerly *Chlamydia psittaci*), also known as *ornithosis*, primarily affects *parrots* (psittacines) and other birds, and is only rarely transmitted to humans by the respiratory route. Fever, *pneumonitis*, and systemic illness may be mild or serious. Skin lesions consist of red macules (*Horder's spots*) similar to the rose spots of typhoid fever, or lesions resembling urticaria (3.1), erythema multiforme (3.2), erythema nodosum, or purpura of disseminated intravascular coagulation (4.14). The diagnosis is primarily confirmed serologically. Skin biopsies are rarely performed, with histology depending upon the type of lesion biopsied.

CHAPTER 15

Parasitic Diseases

This chapter covers most of the more important parasites, or those with more specific pathologic findings in the skin. Many others are omitted because they either mostly involve deeper tissue, they produce non-specific findings in the skin unless the parasite is identifiable, or because they are more obscure.

15.1 Leishmaniasis

(see Fig. 15.1A–E)
Infection of the skin by protozoa of *Leishmania* and *Viannia* species, with red plaques, nodules, or ulcers (1.142) at the site on exposed areas of the body (often face, 1.44) of the bite of the vectors, *Phlebotomus* (mostly Old World) or *Lutzomyia* (mostly New World) sand flies. Culture possible but difficult with the Nicolle–Novy–MacNeal (NNN) media.

P
- Epidermis normal, atrophic, hyperplastic, or ulcerated
- Diffuse mixed *granulomatous* dermal infiltrate of lymphocytes, histiocytes, *plasma cells*, neutrophils, and multinucleated giant cells; occasional caseation necrosis
- Fibrosis in some older lesions
- *Amastigote organisms* are usually present within histiocytes and are visible with H&E stains, but are best seen with the *Giemsa stain*. Sometimes they marginate around the edge of a clear space in the tissue like flashing lights around the edge of a sign (marquee sign). They measure 2–3 microns, with a 1-micron round nucleus and a smaller rod-shaped paranucleus (*kinetoplast*). Sometimes they can be seen on a Tzanck smear.

Differential diagnosis

1. Other granulomas (1.51).
2. Other diseases with "parasitized histiocytes" with small organisms of 2–3 microns include rhinoscleroma (12.9) and histoplasmosis (13.9). Granuloma inguinale (12.8) generally is limited to the genital region. Cultures, polymerase chain reaction (PCR), and other techniques may be needed. Topical aluminum chloride particles are negative with special stains (7.6). Malakoplakia (12.21) has macrophages containing 5–15-micron granules that stain positive with PAS, von Kossa, and Perl's stains, but is most common in the groin and perianal areas.

15.2 Protothecosis

(see Fig. 15.2A,B)
Nodule, plaque, or ulcer due to very rare infection by *Prototheca* species, an achloric alga, usually in immunosuppressed patients.

P
- Epidermis ulcerated or hyperplastic
- Mixed diffuse infiltrate of neutrophils, lymphocytes, histiocytes, and multinucleated giant cells
- Dermal necrosis common (1.88)
- Organisms sometimes visible with H&E, but best seen with PAS, GMS, or acid mucopolysaccharide stains. *Characteristic numerous septations* within some organisms (sporangia or morula forms). Size varies greatly from 2 to 11 microns

Differential diagnosis

1. Other granulomas (1.51), other diseases with neutrophils (1.89).

15.3 Cysticercosis

(see Fig. 15.3A,B)
The most commonly encountered tapeworm (phylum Cestoda) is the pork tapeworm, *Taenia solium*. There is a nodule at site of encysted worm.

P
- Larva (*cysticercus*, 6–18 mm long) has secretory tegument surrounded by a unilocular cystic cavity and fibrosis in subcutaneous tissue, usually in subcutaneous or deeper soft tissue, often pale and necrotic
- *Scolex* (mouth) is important to find on deeper levels, with sucking grooves known as bothria. This particular tapeworm has *hooklets* and *two pairs of sucker cups*.
- *Calcareous bodies* (purplish oval calcified fecal concretions, 1.19) common, not specific to this worm
- *Very little inflammation* is present until larva dies; then mixed inflammatory infiltrate of neutrophils, lymphocytes, histiocytes (1.51), and eosinophils (1.36) may occur, sometimes with calcification

©2012 Elsevier Ltd, Inc, BV
DOI: 10.1016/B978-0-323-06658-7.00015-4

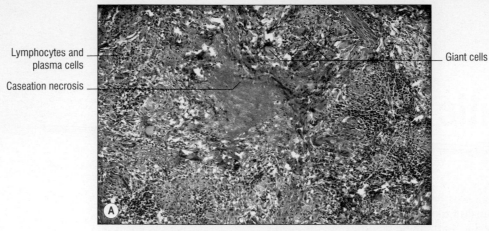

Lymphocytes and plasma cells

Caseation necrosis

Giant cells

Fig. 15.1 A Leishmaniasis (medium mag.).

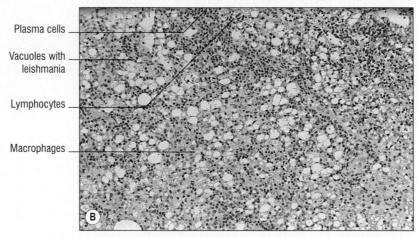

Plasma cells

Vacuoles with leishmania

Lymphocytes

Macrophages

Fig. 15.1 B Leishmaniasis (medium mag.).

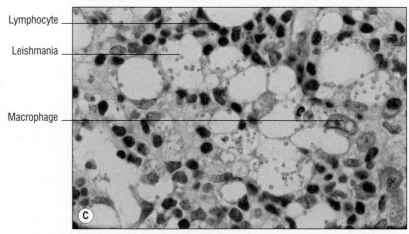

Lymphocyte

Leishmania

Macrophage

Fig. 15.1 C Leishmaniasis (high mag.).

Differential diagnosis

1. Coenuriasis is due to the dog tapeworm *Taenia multiceps*. It has multiple scolices.
2. Sparganosis is due to the tapeworm *Spirometra* species. Infection occurs from eating uncooked frogs or fish, or application of a poultice. It produces a multilocular cyst with subtegumental cells and a secretory tegument, but no scolex.

15.4 Dirofilariasis

(see Fig. 15.4)

Nodule at site of a roundworm (phylum Nematoda) of the genus *Dirofilaria*, transmitted by mosquitoes.

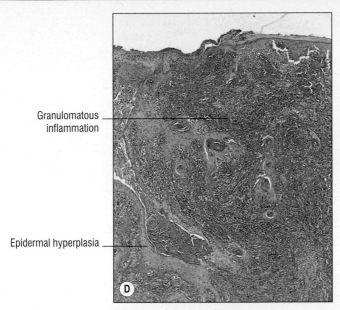

Granulomatous inflammation

Epidermal hyperplasia

Fig.15.1 D Pseudocarcinomatous hyperplasia and granulomatous inflammation in leishmaniasis.

Dirofilaria immitis often causes "heartworm" in dogs, rarely infecting man.

■ *Tightly-coiled solitary worm* with a *thick cuticle*, considerable muscle, and a diameter of 125–250 microns, usually in the subcutaneous tissues
■ Mixed inflammatory infiltrate of lymphocytes, histiocytes (1.51), plasma cells, eosinophils (1.36), and multinucleated giant cells

Differential diagnosis

Details of other roundworms (Nematoda) are beyond the scope of this book.

1. Gnathostomiasis caused by eating raw fish with the worm *Gnathostoma spinigerum* classically presents as migratory erythematous, edematous dermal or subcutaneous plaques, with numerous eosinophils. Worms 0.4–4 mm in diameter are rarely found.
2. Trichinosis (*Trichinella spiralis* and other species) most commonly due to eating raw pork, presents as myalgia

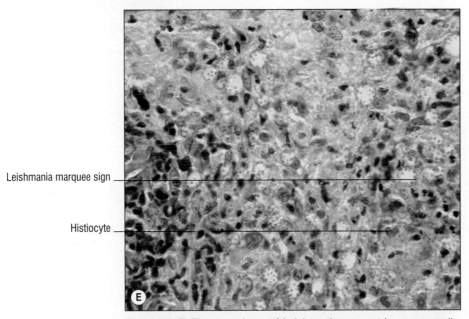

Leishmania marquee sign

Histiocyte

Fig. 15.1 E The organisms of *Leishmania* may not be more easily seen with this Giemsa stain compared with H&E.

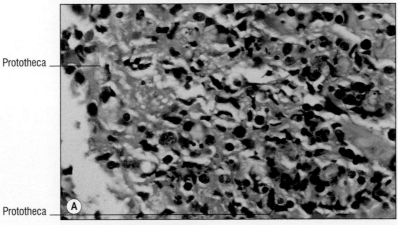

Prototheca

Prototheca

Fig. 15.2 A Protothecosis.

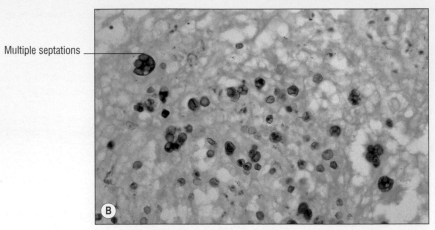

Multiple septations

Fig. 15.2 B Protot</br>hecosis (GMS stain).

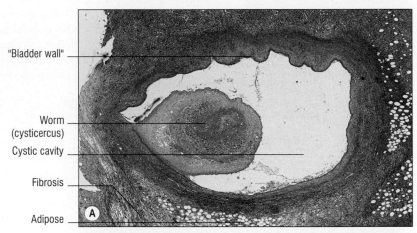

"Bladder wall"

Worm (cysticercus)

Cystic cavity

Fibrosis

Adipose

Fig. 15.3 A Cysticercosis.

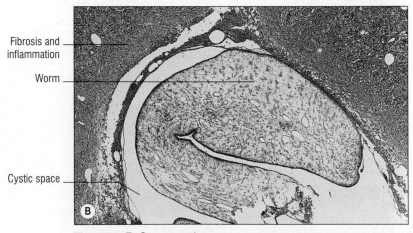

Fibrosis and inflammation

Worm

Cystic space

Fig. 15.3 B Sparganosis.

with other systemic symptoms from infection of the muscle by the worms.

15.5 Onchocerciasis

(see Fig. 15.5)

Exfoliative erythroderma (1.39) if microfilariae of the filarial roundworm *Onchocerca volvulus* infest the dermis after transmission by the *Simulium* black fly vector. *Nodule (onchocercoma)* at site of mature worms.

- Onchocercoma: *adult worms* (100–500 microns in diameter) live in orgies within *nodules in the subcutaneous tissue*, surrounded by *dense fibrosis* (1.125) or multinucleated giant cells (1.51). Female worms have paired uteri
- Dermatitis: *microfilariae* (5–9 microns in diameter) are found either within adult female worms or migrating freely in the *dermis*

15.6 Cutaneous larval migrans

Serpiginous (1.127) red plaques at site of migrating round-worms of *Ancylostoma*, *Necator*, or other non-human hook-worms. Most common on the *feet* (1.48), *buttock*, genitals, and hands.

P
- Scale crust, spongiosis (1.132), or intraepidermal vesicle containing eosinophils (1.147)
- Dermal edema (1.30)
- Perivascular lymphocytes, histiocytes, and many eosinophils (1.36)
- Larva (about 0.5 mm thick and up to 10 mm long) difficult to find, usually in deeper epidermis

15.7 Arthropod bites and stings (arthropod assaults)

(see Fig. 15.7A–D)
Red papules, nodules, vesicles, or pustules at site of bites or stings. Pathology varies greatly.

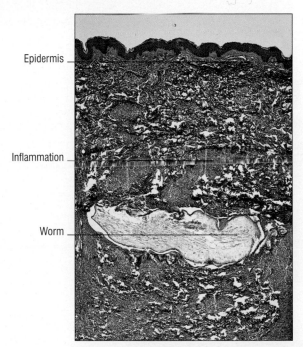

Epidermis

Inflammation

Worm

Fig. 15.4 Dirofilariasis.

- Epidermis may have scale crust, epidermal necrosis (1.87), or epidermal hyperplasia (1.61)
- *Spongiosis* or intraepidermal vesicle (1.147) often
- Dermal edema (1.30) often, sometimes subepidermal vesicle
- *Perivascular* (usually *superficial and deep*) neutrophils, lymphocytes (sometimes atypical or CD30+), or *eosinophils*; older lesions show diffuse or nodular inflammation (1.91) similar to lymphocytoma cutis (24.14)
- Endothelial swelling often

Variations

1. Maculae ceruleae are bluish macules (1.14) due to dermal hemorrhage at sites of bites from pediculosis.
2. Fire ant stings (*Solenopsis invicta*) tend to be more pustular (1.89) with neutrophils.
3. Papular urticaria: red papules, mostly in children, thought to be hypersensitivity to arthropod bites, unlike generic urticaria (3.1).
4. Ticks (*Ixodoidea*) may be found attached to the skin with eosinophilic cement around the pigmented mouthparts. Ticks have a thick chitinous skeleton and plenty of skeletal muscle. *Dermacentor* is a larger tick that prefers to attach on the legs. *Amblyomma americanum* (Lone Star tick, with white dot on adult females) prefers to attach to the head or neck. Deer tick, *Ixodes scapularis*, prefers to attach to the trunk or scapula area.

Differential diagnosis

1. Seabather's eruption: very pruritic (1.114) papules under bathing suits, after swimming in salt water, most likely from cnidarian (coelenterate) larvae, such as *Linuche unguiculata*. Histology like arthropod bites except neutrophils more likely to be present along with lymphocytes and eosinophils. Do not confuse with swimmer's itch, due to freshwater schistosomes (15.16).
2. Marine animal stings, such as jellyfish and Portuguese man-of-war, may show nematocysts on the stratum corneum with refractile tubular threads in the spinous layer of the epidermis. Sea urchins (*Echinodermata*) produce a granulomatous reaction (15.1) to fragments of spines.

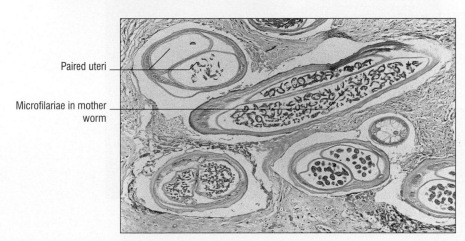

Paired uteri

Microfilariae in mother worm

Fig. 15.5 Onchocerciasis.

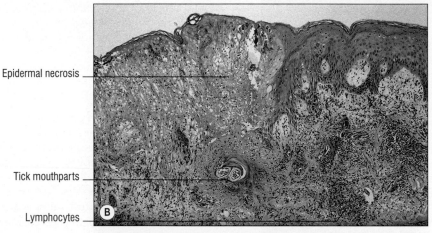

Intraepidermal vesicle

Edema

Perivascular lymphocytes and eosinophils

Fig. 15.7 A Arthropod bite (acute).

3. Animal bites: various degrees of mixed inflammation, ulceration (1.142), and necrosis (1.87) are found, with deep infection occurring later in some cases (12.3).
4. Although not all arthropod bites contain eosinophils, other diseases with eosinophils (1.36) or spongiosis (1.132) should be considered.

15.8 Demodicosis

(see Fig. 15.8A,B)

Demodex mites are common enough to be considered normal fauna of the pilosebaceous units, and therefore often not mentioned in pathology reports. They usually cause no disease, but have been implicated in demodectic acne rosacea (10.1), blepharitis (1.43), perioral dermatitis, and demodectic folliculitis (10.2). Usually there are papules or pustules, but the term pityriasis folliculorum has been used when there is a scaly sandpaper-like appearance to the skin.

- *Demodex folliculorum* (100–400 microns) is usually *found within hair follicles*. It is *elongated*, almost worm-like, has eight legs, and the mouthparts are usually found aimed downward into the follicle, while the caudal tail end points outward

P

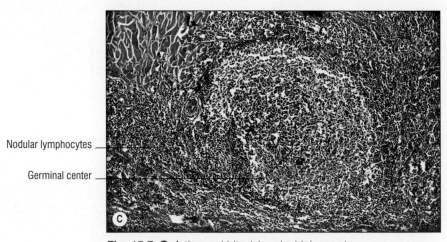

Epidermal necrosis

Tick mouthparts

Lymphocytes

Fig. 15.7 B Arthropod bite (chronic, low mag.).

Nodular lymphocytes

Germinal center

Fig. 15.7 C Arthropod bite (chronic, high mag.).

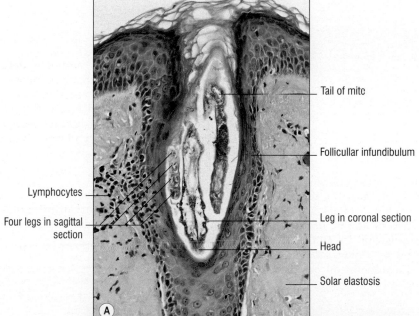

Exoskeleton
Leg
Skeletal muscle

Fig. 15.7 D Tick.

Tail of mite

Follicullar infundibulum

Lymphocytes

Four legs in sagittal section

Leg in coronal section

Head

Solar elastosis

Fig. 15.8 A Demodicosis.

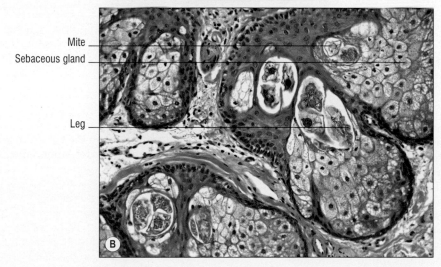

Mite
Sebaceous gland

Leg

Fig. 15.8 B Many *Demodex* mites in the pilosebaceous glands.

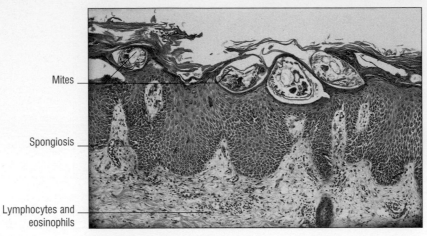

Mites

Spongiosis

Lymphocytes and
eosinophils

Fig. 15.9 Scabies.

- *Demodex brevis* is slightly smaller (hence, "brevis") and is usually found *within the sebaceous glands*
- Variable inflammatory reaction. Most often few lymphocytes in the pilosebaceous unit. Sometimes suppurative or granulomatous inflammation

15.9 Scabies

(see Fig. 15.9)

Common, *extremely pruritic* (1.114), sparse, occasionally extensive papules, vesicles, pustules, or burrows, especially in *axilla* (1.10), *nipples* (1.90), groin (1.55), genitals (1.107, 1.149), trunk, extremities, and *finger webs* of adults, including face and scalp in infants, due to burrowing by *Sarcoptes scabiei* mites. Mites can often be found by doing scrapings from lesions mounted on a slide with mineral oil or potassium hydroxide without doing a biopsy.

- *Eggs or mites* (200–400 microns), or *scybala* (brown feces) are present in the *subcorneal* zone
- Sometimes spongiosis (1.132) or epidermal hyperplasia (1.61)
- Perivascular (1.109) or moderately diffuse dermal lymphocytes and *eosinophils*

Variations

1. Crusted "Norwegian" scabies: more severe thicker plaques, localized or extensive, often in debilitated, retarded, or immunosuppressed patient without urge to scratch, numerous mites present within hyperkeratotic plaques, may be confused with other papulosquamous (1.103) or verrucous lesions (1.146), especially palmoplantar keratoderma (2.15).
2. Nodular scabies: prurigo-like red nodules, especially of the scrotum and penis (1.107), associated with chronic scratching, usually with no mites found within these lesions, may be confused with other nodules in childhood (1.93).

Differential diagnosis

1. Other diseases with eosinophils (1.36), or severe pruritus (1.114).
2. Folliculitis (10.2) resembles it clinically.

3. Eczema (1.29).
4. Grover's disease (5.6).
5. Prurigo nodularis (2.3) and neurodermatitis (2.1). Scabies is easily missed, since mites can be sparse, but also frequently overdiagnosed. Some patients with Morgellon's disease (debated entity) are convinced they have parasites or fibers in their skin. Delusions of parasitosis (Ekbom's syndrome) is also a common problem.

15.10 Myiasis

Infestation of the skin by larvae (maggots) of several different species of flies of the order Diptera, phylum Arthropoda, class Insecta.

- *Maggots* found in dermis or subcutaneous tissue with characteristics depending upon the species. Many have a thick corrugated skeletal wall.
- *Dermatobia hominis* is a more commonly encountered maggot in Central America (especially Belize) with undulating chitinous walls and black spines (setae)
- Diffuse mixed infiltrate (1.91) of lymphocytes, histiocytes, and eosinophils (1.36)

15.11 Tungiasis

(see Fig. 15.11)

Nodule or papule, usually on the toe, from burrowing by the sand flea *Tunga penetrans* (order Siphonaptera).

- Hyperkeratosis, acanthosis, crusting
- *Female flea beneath the stratum corneum* may reach 5 mm in diameter when female becomes swollen with eggs. Skeletal muscle and red hollow tubules present
- Mixed inflammatory infiltrate, sometimes abscess formation

15.12 Pneumocystosis

Pneumocystis jirovecii (formerly *P. carinii*), now thought to be a fungus resembling a protozoan, most commonly causes *lung infections* in immunosuppressed patients known as PCP (pneumocystis pneumonia, formerly standing for

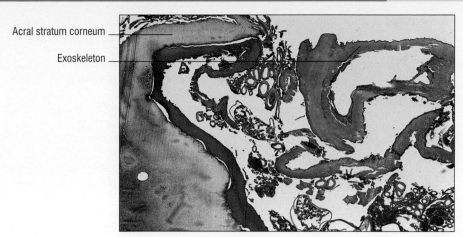

Acral stratum corneum

Exoskeleton

Fig. 15.11 Tungiasis.

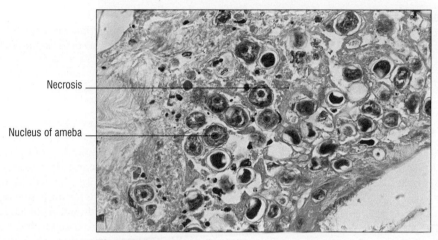

Necrosis

Nucleus of ameba

Fig. 15.13 Amebiasis.

pneumocystis carinii pneumonia). Very rare skin infection associated with *AIDS* (14.12), presents as *pedunculated* (1.106), friable, *necrotic papules or nodules*, especially of the *ear canal* (1.28).

> **P**
> - Foamy stroma with H&E stain (1.46)
> - Round, *no-budding 5–10-micron cysts* (teacup in saucer appearance) in the dermis or subcutaneous tissue are best *stained with GMS*

15.13 Amebiasis

(see Fig. 15.13)
Painful *ulcers* (1.142), fistulas, or nodules are most common in the *perianal* (1.108), buttock, or *genital area* (1.107, 1.149). *Entamoeba histolytica, Naegleria, Acanthamoeba* (most common one found in skin), or other amebas are the culprits. *Balamuthia mandrillis* commonly affects the CNS, but skin nodules or plaques can be present at sites of inoculation, especially around the nose. Immunofluorescence or PCR can be used for diagnosis.

Differential diagnosis

1. Syphilis (12.13), lymphogranuloma venereum (14.14), chancroid (12.7), condyloma acuminatum (14.1), and squamous cell carcinoma (18.11).

2. Other granulomas (1.51) or diseases with pseudoepitheliomatous hyperplasia (1.116).

> **P**
> - Ulceration or pseudoepitheliomatous hyperplasia
> - Granulation tissue, dermal edema (1.30), necrosis (1.88), fibrosis
> - Mixed diffuse inflammation, may be granulomatous
> - Trophozoites resembling epithelioid histiocytes (1.38), 15–40 microns, with a bubbly or granular cytoplasm and single nucleus that has marginated chromatin may be seen with H&E, but are more easily seen with PAS
> - Erythrophagocytosis by trophozoites sometimes
> - Some species can be cultured. Others can be identified by immunofluorescence or PCR

15.14 Trypanosomiasis

A. African trypanosomiasis (sleeping sickness)

Trypanosoma brucei gambiense and *T. brucei rhodesiense* are protozoans that are spread by bite of the *Glossina* tsetse fly. A 2–5-cm *chancre* develops at the site, with regional *lymphadenopathy*. Prominent posterior cervical lymphadenopathy is *Winterbottom's sign*. Later, edema of the hands, feet, and face, and an *annular* (1.5), urticarial, *petechial* (1.120) or *morbilliform rash* develops. Finally, lethargy, coma, and death may occur.

The trypanosomes are usually demonstrated in the blood or lymph nodes by smears or cultures.

B. American trypanosomiasis (Chagas disease)

T. cruzi is transmitted by the bites of the reduviid bug (assassin bug of the family Triatomidae). The bite becomes edematous or nodular (*chagoma*), sometimes resulting in fat destruction (*lipochagoma*). Regional *lymphadenopathy* is common. *Romana's sign* (oculoglandular syndrome, 12.6, 12.15) is unilateral eyelid edema (1.43). Later *high fever*, constitutional symptoms, *myocarditis, meningoencephalitis*, hepatosplenomegaly, megacolon, and a morbilliform eruption may occur. The trypanosomes are usually demonstrated in the blood or lymph nodes by smears or cultures. Diagnosis may be made serologically or by PCR.

- Ulceration (1.142) or epithelial hyperplasia (1.61)
- Mixed inflammation: histiocytes (1.76), *plasma cells*, and lymphocytes
- *Trypanosomes have a nucleus and kinetoplast that is Giemsa stain positive*

Differential diagnosis

1. Other diseases with parasitized macrophages (12.8), especially leishmaniasis (15.1).
2. Other diseases with plasma cells (1.111), especially syphilis (12.13).

15.15 Toxoplasmosis

Toxoplasma gondii is a protozoan for which *cats* are the usual definitive host. Humans usually become infected by ingesting oocyts, and less often by eating uncooked meat of infected animals. Infection can be congenital (one of the *TORCH congenital infections*, which includes toxoplasmosis, "other," rubella (14.7), cytomegalovirus (14.9), and herpes virus (14.2)) or *acquired* most often in the setting of HIV infection (14.12) or other *immunosuppression*. It can cause fever (1.45), lymphadenopathy, ocular disease (1.41), and disseminated disease that includes encephalitis. Skin lesions occur in less than 10% of patients with dissemination, and are rarely biopsied. A wide variety of morphologies have been reported:

morbilliform (1.81), purpuric (1.120), urticarial, nodular (1.92), and others.

- Pseudoepitheliomatous hyperplasia (1.116) or epidermal necrosis (1.87) sometimes
- *Perivascular* (1.109) or interface (1.64) *lymphocytes and macrophages*
- Dermal necrosis (1.88) and extravasated erythrocytes sometimes (1.40)
- *Trophozoites* (2–8 microns), or *cysts* (8–30 microns) containing numerous smaller bradyzoites are found in macrophages or free in the dermis in half of the cases, some forms are PAS positive
- Immunostains, serology, and PCR detection is available

Differential diagnosis

1. Leishmaniasis (15.1), trypanosomiasis (15.14), histoplasmosis (13.9), and cytomegalovirus infection (14.9).

15.16 Schistosomiasis

(see Fig 15.16A,B)

Schistosoma mansoni (Caribbean, South America), *S. haematobium* (Middle East, Africa), and *S. japonicum* (south-east Asia, no egg spine) are flukes (trematodes) of the flatworm phylum Platyhelminthes, whose cercarial larvae develop in aquatic snails. The cercaria burrow into human skin, producing red pruritic papules (similar to swimmer's itch described below), later migrating to veins. Adult worms of *S. mansoni* live in the portal and mesenteric veins, discharging eggs with lateral spines into the stools. *S. japonicum* develops in veins of the small intestine, passing eggs with no spine into the stools. *S. haematobium* develops in the pelvic and bladder veins, passing eggs with apical spines into urine. Migration of eggs to veins of the *genital or perianal regions* (1.108) produce *verrucous nodules* (1.92) or *ulcers* (1.142).

- *Granulomas* (1.51) and *neutrophils* (1.89) around *eggs (up to 120 microns long*, some are PAS or AFB stain positive)
- Egg spine positions determine species (but so does geographic origin of case)
- Adult worms (15–25 mm long) rarely seen in blood vessels

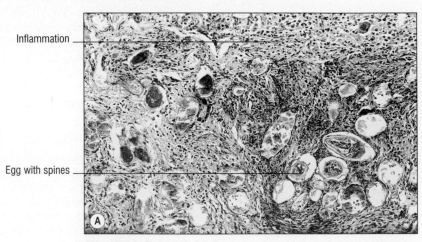

Fig. 15.16 A Schistosomiasis

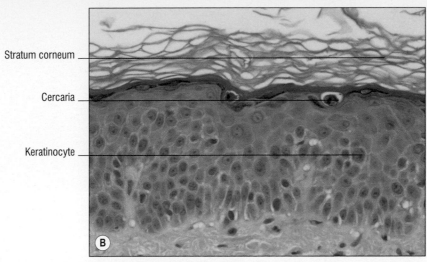

Stratum corneum

Cercaria

Keratinocyte

Fig. 15.16 B Swimmer's itch.

Variation

1. Swimmer's itch: red pruritic papules due to freshwater non-human cercarial larvae of schistosomes, typically found in exposed areas of skin as opposed to the clothed areas of skin in seabather's eruption (15.7). Self-limited within a few days, since organisms die in the improper host. Biopsy is rarely performed, but has dermal edema, and sparse perivascular eosinophils and neutrophils.

CHAPTER 16

Panniculitis

Panniculitis is inflammation in the subcutaneous fat. The classification of panniculitis is unsatisfactory, as there is considerable overlap between the clinical and histologic features of these diseases. Although many authors categorize a panniculitis as a "septal" panniculitis if it involves primarily the septae between fat lobules, and "lobular" if it involves primarily the fat lobule itself, this has limited utility because only one disease can be consistently classified as septal (erythema nodosum, 16.1), while all of the others are either lobular or show mixed features. Because the histology changes greatly with the evolution of the lesions, and it is often difficult to assign an inflammatory disease of the fat to one of the specific entities described below, the pathologist must sometimes sign out a case as "panniculitis, unclassified type". Panniculitis also occurs in the following diseases that are discussed in other chapters (1.101):

1. Lupus panniculitis (17.6)
2. Foreign body panniculitis (7.6)
3. Infectious panniculitis (Chapters 12 and 13)
4. Scleroderma (9.3)
5. Lymphoma or leukemia (Chapter 24)
6. Necrobiosis lipoidica, deep granuloma annulare, and rheumatoid nodules (7.1 to 7.3)
7. Sarcoidosis (7.5)
8. Cytophagic histiocytic panniculitis (24.4)

16.1 Erythema nodosum (EN)

(see Fig. 16.1A–C)
Common *painful* (1.96) *red nodules of the shins* (1.67) in young adults, most commonly a reaction to birth control pills, other drugs (3.5), streptococcal pharyngitis, inflammatory bowel disease, sarcoidosis (7.5), yersiniosis (12.23), or coccidioidomycosis (13.6).

- *Septal panniculitis* of lymphocytes, histiocytes, neutrophils, and/or eosinophils. Multinucleated giant cells (1.51) in older lesions, without caseation
- Septal fibrosis in older lesions
- Mild fat necrosis sometimes, with foamy histiocytes

Variation

1. Chronic EN (subacute nodular migratory panniculitis of Vilanova and Pinol Aguade): term used for older, more chronic, often granulomatous or fibrotic lesions now thought to be part of the EN spectrum.

Differential diagnosis

1. Infection-related panniculitis (16.6).
2. Most other forms of panniculitis (1.101) are lobular rather than septal.

16.2 Weber–Christian disease (relapsing febrile nodular non-suppurative panniculitis)

(see Fig. 16.2)
Acute onset of *red nodules, usually on the legs*, sometimes associated with febrile episodes (1.45).

- Lobular panniculitis
- Numerous *neutrophils* (1.89) in early lesions, followed by *numerous foamy histiocytes* and fat necrosis
- Fibrosis in the oldest lesions

Differential diagnosis

1. It is generally agreed that Weber–Christian disease is not a distinct entity, as foamy histiocytes can be seen in many of the other diseases with panniculitis (1.46).
2. Infection-related panniculitis (16.6)
3. Other forms of panniculitis (1.101), especially alpha-1 antitrypsin deficiency (16.10).

16.3 Cold panniculitis

Uncommon red nodules due to *local cold exposure*, such as from eating ice, more common in *children*.

- Lobular panniculitis of neutrophils, lymphocytes, and histiocytes
- *Cystic spaces in subcutaneous fat* due to ruptured fat cells

©2012 Elsevier Ltd, Inc, BV
DOI: 10.1016/B978-0-323-06658-7.00016-6

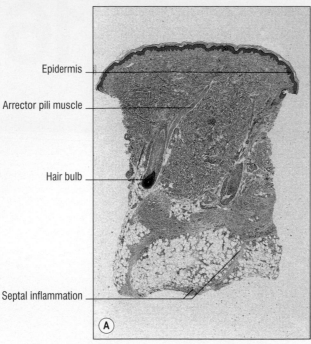

Epidermis

Arrector pili muscle

Hair bulb

Septal inflammation

Ⓐ

Fig. 16.1 A Erythema nodosum (low mag.).

Differential diagnosis

1. Other forms of panniculitis (1.101).

16.4 Sclerema neonatorum

Very rare extensive plaques of indurated, *sclerotic skin* (1.125) in *neonates*, which may be fatal. Do not confuse the name sclerema with scleroderma (9.3) or scleredema (8.12).

- *Needle-shaped clefts* (1.23) within fat cells and foamy histiocytes
- Mild fat necrosis surrounded by sparse or absent granulomatous infiltrate of lymphocytes, histiocytes, and multinucleated giant cells
- Prominent sclerosis or fibrosis (1.125)

Differential diagnosis

1. Although subcutaneous fat necrosis of the newborn (16.5) exhibits similar needle-shaped clefts, it is a milder disease, is more localized, and usually has more inflammation, more calcification, and less fibrosis.

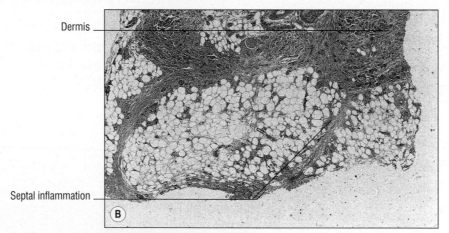

Dermis

Septal inflammation

Ⓑ

Fig. 16.1 B Erythema nodosum (medium mag.).

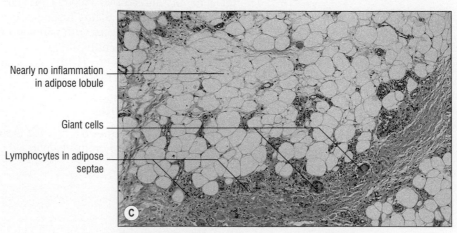

Nearly no inflammation in adipose lobule

Giant cells

Lymphocytes in adipose septae

Ⓒ

Fig. 16.1 C Erythema nodosum (high mag.).

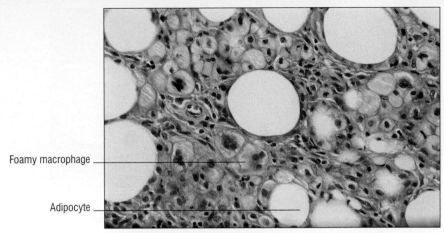

Foamy macrophage ———

Adipocyte ———

Fig. 16.2 "Weber–Christian disease".

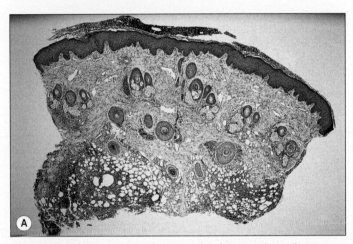

A

Fig. 16.5 A Subcutaneous fat necrosis of the newborn (low mag.).

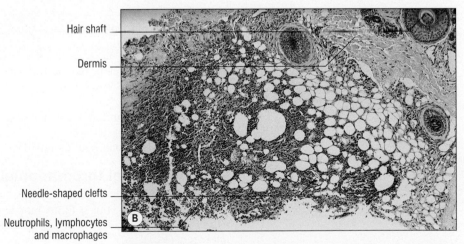

Hair shaft ———

Dermis ———

Needle-shaped clefts ———

Neutrophils, lymphocytes and macrophages ———

B

Fig. 16.5 B Subcutaneous fat necrosis of the newborn (medium mag.).

16.5 Subcutaneous fat necrosis of the newborn

(see Fig. 16.5A–C)
Uncommon, localized, *indurated subcutaneous nodules in the newborn*, of unknown cause, usually self-limited, sometimes associated with hypercalcemia.

- *Needle-shaped clefts* (1.23) within fat cells, and foamy histiocytes
- Fat necrosis and *granulomatous infiltrate* of lymphocytes, histiocytes, and multinucleated giant cells
- *Calcification* common (1.19)

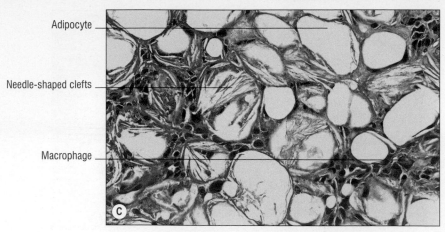

Adipocyte

Needle-shaped clefts

Macrophage

Fig. 16.5 C Subcutaneous fat necrosis of the newborn (high mag.).

Differential diagnosis

1. Sclerema neonatorum (16.4) and post-steroid panniculitis (after rapid discontinuation of corticosteroids in children) also has needle-shaped clefts.
2. Other forms of panniculitis (1.101) may be considered if the needle-shaped clefts are not apparent, but in infants this is the most common type of panniculitis.
3. Other diseases with granulomas (1.51).

16.6 Erythema induratum (nodular vasculitis)

(see Fig. 16.6A–C)
Uncommon *red nodules of the calf*, sometimes representing a tuberculid (Bazin's disease, 12.10), but usually idiopathic.

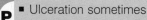

P
- Ulceration sometimes
- *Lobular granulomatous panniculitis* with mixed infiltrate of lymphocytes, histiocytes, plasma cells, and multinucleated giant cells
- Caseation necrosis sometimes
- *Vasculitis in the fat* often involving arteries or small veins
- Fibrosis in older lesions

Variation

1. Lipogranulomatosis subcutanea of Rothmann–Makai: a garbage dump category for unclassifiable idiopathic non-caseating granulomatous panniculitis with fat necrosis that does not seem to fit any specific entity in this chapter.

Differential diagnosis

1. Erythema nodosum is more common, usually found on the anterior legs instead of posterior, is more septal, usually less granulomatous, and is usually without vasculitis.
2. Other granulomatous diseases (1.51).
3. Other causes of vasculitis (1.145), especially polyarteritis nodosa (4.4).
4. Infection-related panniculitis: also consider infection, and contemplate doing special stains or cultures, when

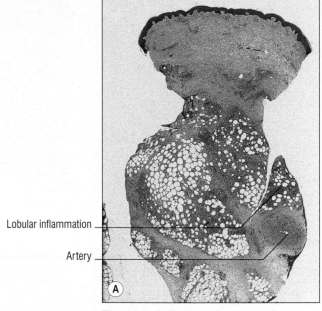

Lobular inflammation

Artery

Fig. 16.6 A Erythema induratum (low mag.).

neutrophils, granulomas, or necrosis are seen with panniculitis.
5. Other forms of panniculitis (1.101).

16.7 Superficial thrombophlebitis

(see Fig. 16.7A,B)
Somewhat common, but seldom biopsied, inflammation of veins, usually of the *legs* (1.67), sometimes with a *chord-like thickening* (1.21).

- *Mixed infiltrate* of neutrophils, lymphocytes, histiocytes, or multinucleated giant cells *within and surrounding a vein* in the deep dermis or subcutaneous fat
- Thrombosis frequent (1.137)

P

Variations

1. Trousseau's syndrome (4.16): thrombophlebitis associated with *internal malignancy* (1.105).

Fat necrosis

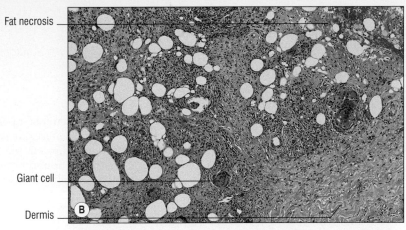

Giant cell

Dermis

Fig. 16.6 B Erythema induratum (medium mag.).

Fibrosis

Vasculitis

Granuloma
(macrophages)

Giant cell

Adipose

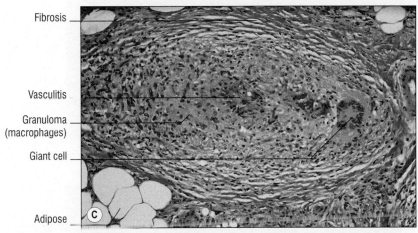

Fig. 16.6 C Erythema induratum (high mag., in a patient with tuberculosis).

Fibrosis

Occluded inflamed vein

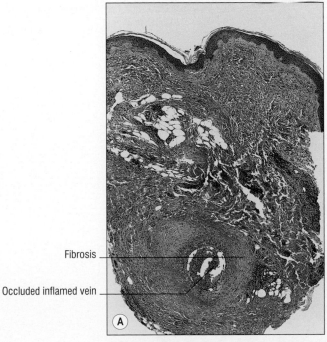

Fig. 16.7 A Superficial thrombophlebitis (low mag.).

2. Mondor's disease (4.16): thrombophlebitis presenting as a chord-like thickening on the chest, either idiopathic or associated with trauma or *rheumatologic disease*.

Differential diagnosis

1. Arteritis (4.4) involves an artery rather than a vein, and the Verhoeff van-Gieson stain may be helpful in identifying the internal elastic lamina usually found in arteries.
2. Other forms of panniculitis (1.101).

16.8 Pancreatic panniculitis

(see Fig. 16.8)

Rare, *tender red nodules* on the shins, thighs or buttocks, sometimes fluctuant, associated with enzyme release (trypsin, amylase, lipase) from *pancreatitis* (often with abdominal pain) or *pancreatic carcinoma* (abdominal pain may be absent), and ankle arthralgia.

- *Mixed lobular panniculitis* with lymphocytes, foamy histiocytes, and multinucleated giant cells
- Fat necrosis with "*ghost-like*" *fat cells and basophilic deposits* of calcium salts of fatty acids

Differential diagnosis

1. Other forms of panniculitis (1.101) or conditions with bluish material with H&E stain (1.15).

16.9 Lipodermatosclerosis (hypodermitis sclerodermiformis, sclerosing panniculitis)

(see Fig. 16.9)

Uncommon, extremely bound-down *indurated skin* and subcutaneous tissue of the *lower legs* (1.67), usually associated with *chronic stasis*. "Hypoderm" in old terminology is the subcutaneous fat, so it is inflamed (-itis) and scleroderma-like (sclerodermiformis).

- Epidermal or dermal changes similar to stasis dermatitis (2.1)
- *Fat necrosis*, *sclerosis*, *foamy macrophages*, lymphocytes, in a diffuse or *lobular pattern*

Variation

1. Lipomembranous panniculitis: a peculiar form of fat necrosis is seen, with an *arabesque pattern* of PAS-positive necrotic membranes in the fat, resembling parasite intestinal walls, found not only with stasis, but also with other peripheral vascular diseases,

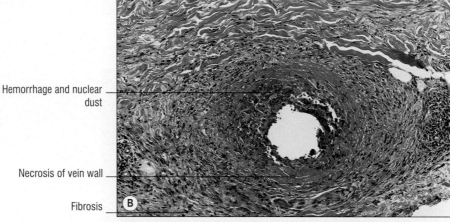

Hemorrhage and nuclear dust

Necrosis of vein wall

Fibrosis

B

Fig. 16.7 B Superficial thrombophlebitis (high mag.).

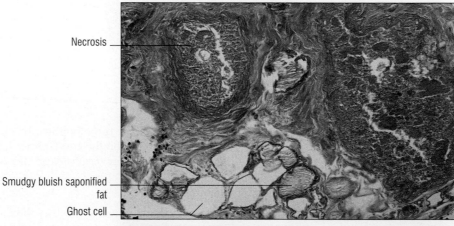

Necrosis

Smudgy bluish saponified fat

Ghost cell

Fig. 16.8 Pancreatic fat necrosis.

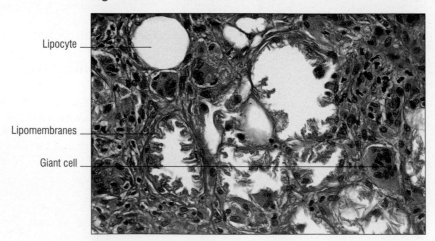

Lipocyte

Lipomembranes

Giant cell

Fig. 16.9 Lipomembranous panniculitis.

autoimmune rheumatologic diseases, and infection with mycobacteria. It sometimes is granulomatous (1.51).

Differential diagnosis

1. Infection-related panniculitis (16.6).
2. Other diseases with scars, sclerosis, or fibrosis (1.125), or panniculitis (1.101).

16.10 Alpha-1 antitrypsin deficiency panniculitis

Rare, *draining ulcerated nodules* (1.142) or cellulitis-like plaques, on trunk or proximal extremities, sometimes at sites of trauma, sometimes familial. *Alpha-1 antitrypsin deficiency* leads to proteolytic activity that may result in *emphysema*, hepatitis, cirrhosis, or angioedema.

- *Lobular panniculitis with neutrophils* and lymphocytes (sometimes mixed with septal pattern)
- *Fat necrosis* with foamy macrophages (1.76)
- *Cystic spaces* may occur in dissolved fat lobules
- Necrosis and inflammation may spill over into the dermis, resulting in necrosis draining through *ulcers*
- Fibrosis in late lesions

Differential diagnosis

1. Since the histologic features are not specific, and other forms of panniculitis (1.101) can be similar, the diagnosis mainly rests upon the markedly decreased serum alpha-1 antitrypsin level.

2. Weber–Christian disease (16.2): some previously reported cases might be this disorder.
3. Infection-related panniculitis (16.6) and other disorders with neutrophils (1.89).

16.11 Lipodystrophy

Also known as *lipoatrophy*, this is a confusing hodge-podge of diseases with localized or generalized loss of fat with depressed sunken skin in those areas. Lipodystrophy can occur as an end result of morphea, scleroderma, and many forms of panniculitis, but this designation is usually reserved for a group of diseases associated with *diabetes mellitus* (1.26), *hypertriglyceridemia, C3 deficiency*, or *glomerulonephritis*.

- Early lesions may show the *inflammatory pattern* in the fat: fat necrosis with foamy lipophages (1.76), plasma cells (1.111), and lymphocytes, with relatively normal lipocytes and blood vessels
- Other early lesions may show the *involutional pattern* in the fat: small lipocytes, hyalinization (1.35), myxoid changes (1.83), and increased numbers of small blood vessels
- Late lesions have a profound decrease or absence of fat

Variation

1. HIV lipodystrophy (14.12): sunken facies and fat loss in other areas, buffalo hump, hyperlipidemia, diabetes mellitus, related to proteinase inhibitor drug therapy.

Differential diagnosis

1. Other forms of panniculitis (1.101).

Other Non-neoplastic Diseases

17.1 Acrodermatitis enteropathica

Rare autosomal recessive disorder due to a *defect in zinc absorption* (mutation in intestinal zinc-specific transporter SCL39A4). Decreased zinc levels can be documented in the serum. Infants develop *perioral* (1.82), *groin* (1.55), *perianal* (1.108), *scalp* (1.124), and *acral eczematous plaques* (1.29), with *diarrhea* (1.49), *alopecia* (1.4), glossitis (1.139), and secondary infection with bacteria and *Candida* (13.4).

P
- *Scale crust often*, with confluent parakeratosis (1.104), fibrin, and neutrophils in the stratum corneum (1.89), and sometimes bacteria and *Candida*
- Hypogranulosis (1.63)
- *Psoriasiform hyperplasia*, spongiosis (1.132), sometimes intraepidermal vesicles
- *Pale* (1.99) or dyskeratotic epidermis (1.27)
- Perivascular lymphocytes (1.109)

Differential diagnosis

1. Other diseases with psoriasiform dermatitis (1.119), especially eczema and other nutritional deficiencies (2.1).

17.2 Vitiligo

(see Fig. 17.2)
Common *autoimmune depigmentation* of skin, especially around the *eyes, mouth, genitals, and hands*. Associated with other autoimmune diseases, especially thyroid disease (1.138).

P
- *Decreased or absent melanin and melanocytes* in basal layer in well-developed lesions. This may be difficult to appreciate with H&E staining. Special stains for melanin may be needed
- Perivascular lymphocytes (1.109) only in early lesions

Variation

1. Vogt–Koyanagi–Harada syndrome: aseptic meningitis, followed by uveitis (1.41) and dysacousia (a type of hearing impairment). Vitiligo and alopecia areata (10.9) are common.

Differential diagnosis

1. Post-inflammatory hypopigmentation: decreased melanin in basal layer, but melanocytes are present.
2. Albinism (11.9): present since birth, melanin absent from basal layer, but melanocytes are present.
3. Piebaldism (11.9): present since birth, white forelock.
4. Many other diseases may produce hypopigmentation (1.150).

17.3 Graft-versus-host disease (GVH, GVHD)

(see Fig. 17.3A–C)
Somewhat common disorder in *bone marrow transplant* patients, in which immunocompetent lymphocytes in the transplant attack the host. Less common in other forms of transplantation, blood transfusions. Human herpesvirus (HHV)6, HHV7, cytomegalovirus, Epstein–Barr virus, or parvovirus may play a role, especially in autologous GVH. Congenital GVH occurs when maternal lymphocytes cross the placenta and react against an immunodeficient fetus. *Scaly erythematous patches* or plaques (often initially on acral skin), later elsewhere, commonly between days 10 and 21 after bone marrow transplant. Involvement of (1) skin, (2) gastrointestinal tract with *diarrhea* (1.49), and (3) *liver* with elevated liver function tests (1.75). Severity of GVH is sometimes graded as below.

P
- Epidermal atrophy sometimes (1.9)
- Mild spongiosis sometimes (1.132)
- Grade 1: liquefaction degeneration (vacuolar alteration) of the basal layer
- Grade 2: dyskeratotic or necrotic keratinocytes, sometimes with adjacent lymphocytes ("satellite cell necrosis"), sparse perivascular or interface dermatitis, melanin incontinence (1.79) sometimes
- Grade 3: subepidermal microvesicle
- Grade 4: frank subepidermal blister (1.147), complete epidermal necrosis in severe cases

©2012 Elsevier Ltd, Inc, BV
DOI: 10.1016/B978-0-323-06658-7.00017-8

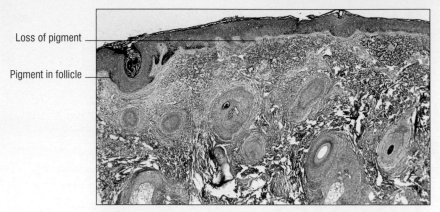

Loss of pigment

Pigment in follicle

Fig. 17.2 Vitiligo. The Fontana melanin stain shows repigmentation near follicle, compared to adjacent epidermis.

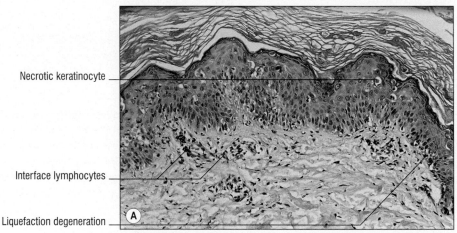

Necrotic keratinocyte

Interface lymphocytes

Liquefaction degeneration

Fig. 17.3 A Graft-versus-host disease (acute).

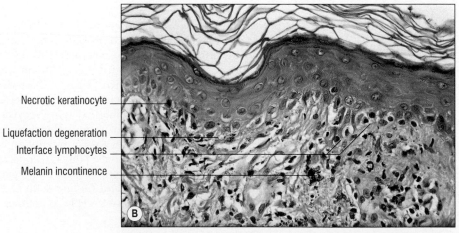

Necrotic keratinocyte

Liquefaction degeneration

Interface lymphocytes

Melanin incontinence

Fig. 17.3 B Graft-versus-host disease (chronic lichenoid).

Variations

1. Chronic GVH: as opposed to changes of acute GVH described above, usually chronic GVH is defined as the eruption *more than 100 days post-transplant*. It is more likely to be *lichenoid* (1.72), with more poikiloderma (1.112) and *sclerosis* (1.125) later.
2. Follicular GVH: clinically and histologically primarily around follicles.
3. Bullous GVH: appears similar to toxic epidermal necrolysis (3.2).

4. Autologous GVH and eruption of lymphocyte recovery: patients with transplants from their own marrow (autologous) theoretically should not develop a true graft versus their own host tissue. These patients, and those with the eruption of lymphocyte recovery, are thought to have a complex imbalance of immunologic factors and a response to various cytokines. The eruption of lymphocyte recovery presents as macular erythema at about the same time as acute GVH, accompanied by fever at about the time the peripheral

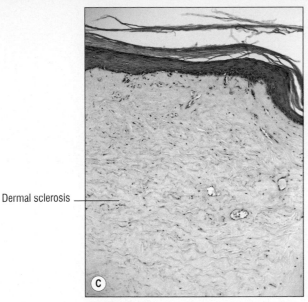

Dermal sclerosis

Fig. 17.3 C Sclerodermoid graft-versus-host disease.

white blood cell count is recovering as the graft takes. The histology is similar to acute GVH.

Differential diagnosis

1. Acute GVH is nearly identical with erythema multiforme (3.2), but the infiltrate tends to be sparser in GVH, and the clinical features are different.
2. Other diseases with interface dermatitis (1.64).
3. Other diseases with dyskeratotic or necrotic keratinocytes (1.27, 1.87).
4. Drug eruption, common in these same patients, may be nearly impossible to distinguish (3.5). Eosinophils are not reliable in helping to tell the difference.

17.4 Aplasia cutis congenita

Rare, localized absence of skin *at birth*, most commonly presenting as an *ulcer* (1.142) on the vertex of the *scalp* (1.124), typically 1–3 cm. A ring of long hair sometimes surrounds the defect (*hair collar sign*), which can also be seen with heterotopic meningeal tissue (26.6). Eventually it heals as an area of scarring alopecia (1.4). Sometimes there are associated malformations, such as a skull defect.

> **P**
> - Epidermal atrophy (1.9) with superficial or deep ulcer
> - Dermal atrophy (1.8), fibrosis with absent adnexa
> - Lymphocytes and neutrophils associated with ulcer

Differential diagnosis

1. So-called congenital absence of skin (Bart's syndrome) is now considered to be a form of epidermolysis bullosa (6.6).
2. Injury from forceps, amniocentesis, or other iatrogenic cause.

17.5 Polymorphous light eruption (PMLE)

(see Fig. 17.5A,B)

Uncommon familial "allergy" to sunlight, onset after puberty, with various clinical morphologies of lesions (polymorphous) that tend to be of a consistent form in a given individual: macular erythema, papules, vesicles, or plaques. Worse in the spring, improves later in summer and winter as patient "hardens" to sunlight exposure. Positive phototesting (usually to ultraviolet A).

> **P**
> - Variable histology depending upon the type of lesion
> - Spongiosis (1.132) or intraepidermal vesicles sometimes (1.147)
> - Necrotic keratinocytes sometimes (1.87)
> - Usually no liquefaction degeneration of the basal layer
> - Superficial dermal edema or subepidermal vesicle sometimes (1.147)
> - *Superficial and deep perivascular* (1.109) or nodular *lymphocytes* (1.91, usually spares follicles)
> - Negative direct immunofluorescence for immunoglobulin and complement deposition

Variations

1. Actinic prurigo (Hutchinson's summer prurigo): more in native Americans, onset earlier in childhood than other forms of PMLE, pruritic eczematous papules and plaques may become lichenified, sometimes with cheilitis. Early lesions have spongiotic dermatitis (1.132), older ones are like prurigo nodularis (2.3).
2. Hydroa vacciniforme: necrotic spongiotic intraepidermal vesicles (vaccinia-like), with epidermal and dermal necrosis (1.88), sometimes with dermal hemorrhage (1.40) and thrombosis (1.137), healing with scars, beginning in childhood.
3. Hydroa aestivale: milder form of hydroa vacciniforme, without scarring, questionable as a distinct entity.

Differential diagnosis

1. PMLE is predominantly a clinical diagnosis made after all other causes of a photodermatitis have been excluded (1.110), especially lupus erythematosus (17.6), porphyria (8.1), photocontact (2.2), and photodrug eruptions (3.5). Lupus erythematosus has other clinical and laboratory features in its systemic form, liquefaction degeneration of the basal layer, thickening of the basement membrane, periadnexal inflammation, and dermal mucin.

17.6 Lupus erythematosus (LE)

(see Fig. 17.6A–O)

Somewhat common *autoimmune disorder* (associated with HLA-DR2 and DR3), eight times more common in *females*, especially age 30–40 years old. LE is in the "miscellaneous" chapter because the clinical lesions vary from being papulosquamous plaques (1.103), reactive erythema (Chapter 3), vasculitis (Chapter 4), subepidermal vesicles with neutrophils (1.147), and can overlap with other rheumatologic disorders such as dermatomyositis (17.7) and scleroderma (9.3). The American College of Rheumatology requires the presence of

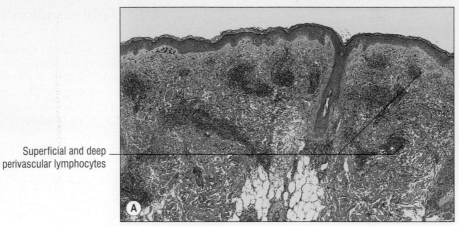

Superficial and deep
perivascular lymphocytes

Fig. 17.5 A Polymorphous light eruption.

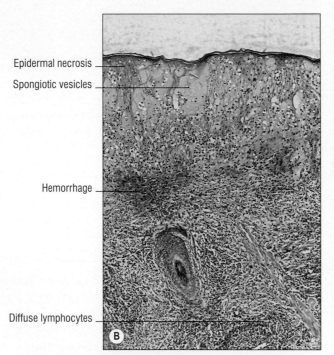

Epidermal necrosis

Spongiotic vesicles

Hemorrhage

Diffuse lymphocytes

Fig. 17.5 B Hydroa vacciniforme.

- Hyperkeratosis sometimes
- *Follicular plugging* (1.47)
- *Epidermal atrophy* (1.9) or hyperplasia (1.61)
- Colloid bodies sometimes in basilar epidermis or papillary dermis (1.27)
- *Liquefaction degeneration* of the basal layer (1.64)
- *Melanin incontinence* (1.79)
- *Thickened basement membrane* (PAS staining may help to demonstrate this)
- Increased *mucin* (1.83) in the dermis (sometimes seen with H&E, but best seen with Alcian blue or colloidal iron stains)
- Perivascular and *periadnexal*, sometimes lichenoid, lymphocytes, with occasional plasma cells (1.111), but no eosinophils
- *Immunofluorescence* (lupus band test) reveals granular deposits of IgM, IgG, and complement at the dermal–epidermal junction. Positive staining in both normal and lesional skin correlates with antibodies to double-stranded DNA and more severe systemic LE (SLE). Normal skin is negative and lesional skin is positive in patients with subacute cutaneous LE or chronic cutaneous LE

four of *eleven criteria* for the diagnosis of systemic lupus erythematosus (SLE):

1. Malar rash (usually macular erythema "butterfly rash" over the cheeks).
2. Discoid rash (see below).
3. Photosensitivity.
4. Oral ulcers.
5. Arthritis.
6. Serositis (pleuritis or pericarditis).
7. Renal disorder (proteinuria or cellular casts).
8. Neurologic disorder (seizures or psychosis).
9. Hematologic disorder (hemolytic anemia, leukopenia, lymphopenia, or thrombocytopenia).
10. Immunologic disorder (anti-dsDNA, anti-Sm, or antiphospholipid antibodies).
11. Antinuclear antibody (ANA) in significant titers.

Variations

1. Discoid LE (chronic cutaneous LE, DLE, CCLE): *thicker, scaly*, often *disc-shaped*, somewhat annular (1.5) *crusted plaques*, sometimes with *"carpet-tack" follicular plugs*, usually on exposed skin (especially face, and concha of ears), may cause *scarring*, especially scarring alopecia (1.4), no *systemic disease in 90%* of these patients (so diagnosis depends mostly upon the skin biopsy instead of upon the eleven criteria enumerated previously), *more epidermal hyperplasia* (1.61, 1.134), prominent follicular plugging, and more prominent, *deeper lymphocytic infiltrate* than average in SLE.
2. Subacute cutaneous lupus erythematosus (SCLE): usually positive for *Ro (SSA) antibody*, sometimes La (SSB) antibody, sometimes negative ANA, more photosensitivity more HLA-B8 or DR3 haplotype, more

psoriasiform (1.119) or *annular* (1.5) lesions, better prognosis than SLE, less chance of kidney disease, histology similar to SLE.

3. Lupus profundus (lupus panniculitis): the above epidermal and dermal changes may or may not be present. There is a *lobular panniculitis* (1.101), often with *nodular* aggregates of mostly *lymphocytes* (mostly *CD4+ with B-cell nodules*), *plasma cells*, *fat necrosis* may be impressive, fibrosis, or calcification. It may be difficult to distinguish from subcutaneous T-cell lymphoma (24.3), which may actually overlap. The latter has mostly CD8+ T lymphocytes, which often rim the adipocytes, without B-cell nodules or plasma cells, often with karyophagocytosis.

4. Bullous LE: blisters usually indicate more severe systemic disease, antibodies to type VII collagen in

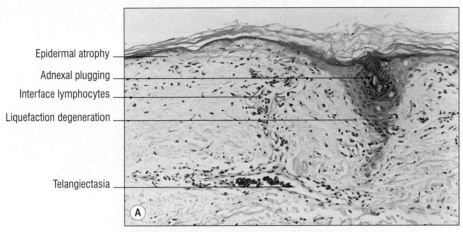

Epidermal atrophy
Adnexal plugging
Interface lymphocytes
Liquefaction degeneration

Telangiectasia

Fig. 17.6 A Lupus erythematosus.

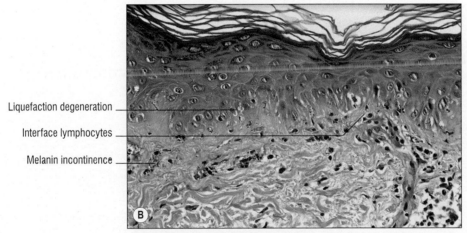

Liquefaction degeneration
Interface lymphocytes
Melanin incontinence

Fig. 17.6 B Lupus erythematosus.

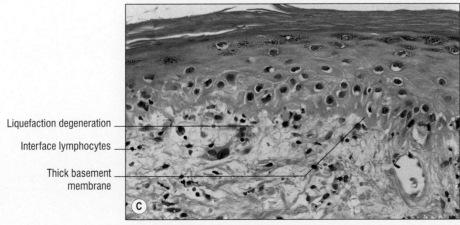

Liquefaction degeneration
Interface lymphocytes
Thick basement membrane

Fig. 17.6 C Lupus erythematosus.

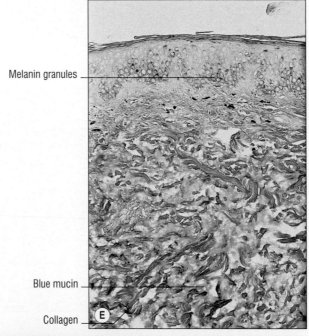

Collagen

Perivascular lymphocytes

Bluish mucin

Fig. 17.6 D Lupus erythematosus.

Melanin granules

Blue mucin

Collagen

Fig. 17.6 E Lupus erythematosus (colloidal iron stain for mucin).

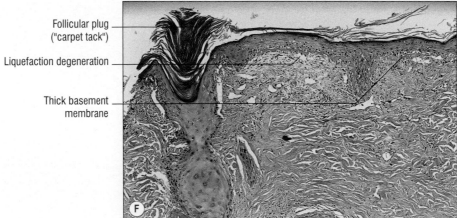

Follicular plug ("carpet tack")

Liquefaction degeneration

Thick basement membrane

Fig. 17.6 F Discoid lupus erythematosus (low mag.).

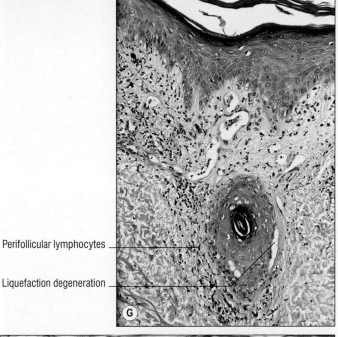

Perifollicular lymphocytes

Liquefaction degeneration

Fig. 17.6 G Discoid lupus erythematosus (medium mag.).

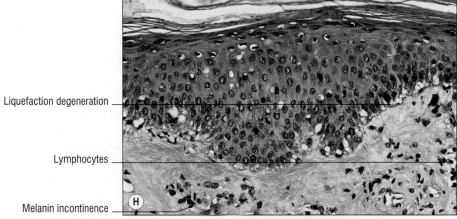

Liquefaction degeneration

Lymphocytes

Melanin incontinence

Fig. 17.6 H Discoid lupus erythematosus (high mag).

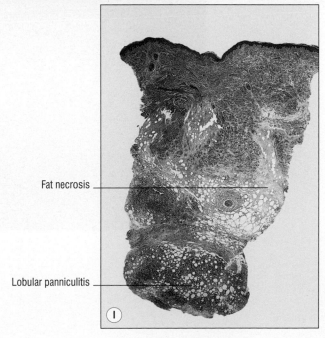

Fat necrosis

Lobular panniculitis

Fig. 17.6 I Lupus panniculitis (low mag.).

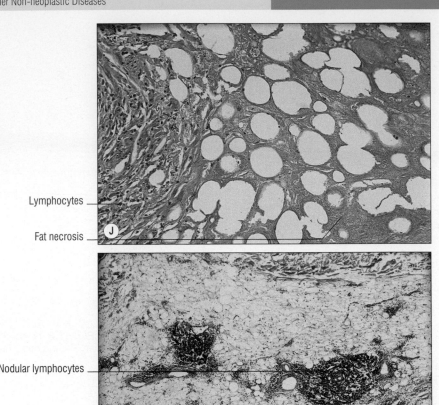

Lymphocytes

Fat necrosis

Fig. 17.6 J Lupus panniculitis (medium mag.).

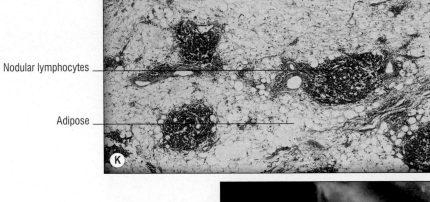

Nodular lymphocytes

Adipose

Fig. 17.6 K Lupus panniculitis (medium mag.).

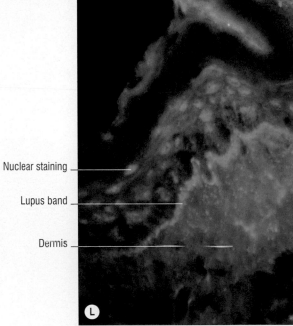

Nuclear staining

Lupus band

Dermis

Fig. 17.6 L Mixed connective tissue disease (IgG immunofluorescence).

Epidermal necrosis

Epidermal atrophy

Liquefaction degeneration

Necrotic keratinocyte

Perivascular lymphocytes

Fig. 17.6 M Rowell syndrome.

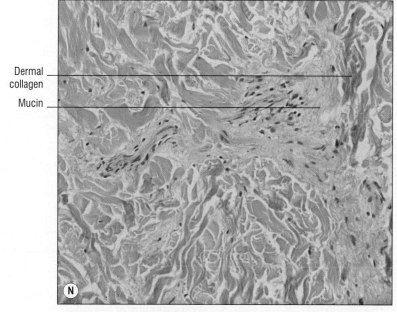

Dermal collagen

Mucin

Fig. 17.6 N Dermal mucinosis in tumid lupus erythematosus, without epidermal changes.

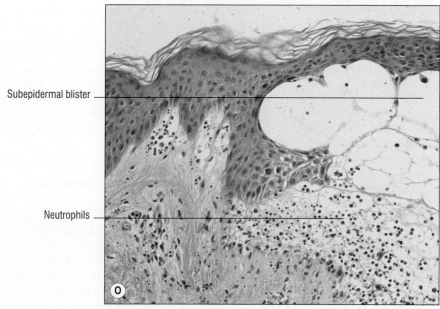

Subepidermal blister

Neutrophils

Fig. 17.6 O Bullous lupus erythematosus.

some cases may indicate some overlap with EBA (6.6), *subepidermal blister* (1.147) containing mainly *neutrophils* (1.89) instead of lymphocytes, often more mucin in the dermis.

5. Mixed connective tissue disease (MCTD, Sharp's syndrome): high titer of *antibodies to ribonuclear protein* (RNP), clinical overlap with scleroderma and dermatomyositis, histology as in SLE, immunofluorescence more likely to show speckled epidermal *nuclear staining* in addition to the lupus band at the dermal–epidermal junction.

6. Jessner's lymphocytic infiltrate: this is a poorly defined entity of non-scaly facial red macules or plaques with diffuse dermal lymphocytes. Most patients probably have LE, PMLE (17.5), or lymphocytoma cutis (24.14).

7. Lupus anticoagulant syndrome: antiphospholipid or anticardiolipin antibodies, livedo reticularis (3.10), and vascular occlusive episodes may occur.

8. Drug-induced LE (3.5): ANA positive, antihistone antibody may be positive (usually negative in non-drug-induced SLE), negative anti-dsDNA, anti-Sm, and anti-Ro.

9. Sjögren's syndrome: dry eyes (keratoconjunctivitis sicca) and dry mouth (decreased salivary secretion), inflammation in salivary gland biopsy, usually positive for *Ro (SSA) antibody*, sometimes La (SSB) antibody, associated with other rheumatologic diseases.

10. Neonatal LE: rash (often annular or raccoon-face erythema around eyes) starts a few weeks post-partum, usually resolves in 6 months, due to transplacental antibody transfer from mother, usually positive for *Ro (SSA) antibody*, sometimes La (SSB) antibody, 50% incidence of congenital heart block, which may cause death.

11. Hereditary complement deficiencies: especially the most common C2 deficiency, may have SLE lesions.

12. Rowell syndrome: LE with necrotic keratinocytes, having an erythema multiforme appearance (3.2). Often Ro antibody positive.

13. Tumid LE: urticarial-appearing lesions without epidermal changes or significant liquefaction degeneration of the basal layer, with perivascular or nodular lymphocytic inflammation, sometimes with considerable dermal mucin.

14. Chilblain LE: lesions resembling cold injury of chilblains (perniosis, 3.12), especially finger and toe erythematous plaques.

Differential diagnosis

1. Other diseases that clinically present as a photodermatitis (1.110). More likely to have necrotic keratinocytes, spongiosis and eosinophils, compared to LE.

2. Other diseases with interface dermatitis (1.64), especially dermatomyositis (17.7), or lichenoid dermatitis (1.72). Of the lichenoid rashes, lichen planus (2.11) and lichenoid drug eruption (3.5) most commonly resemble LE. CD123 cells are more common in the dermis around vessels with LE than for dermatomyositis or polymorphous light eruption, though this is not yet routinely performed. In dermatomyositis, smaller numbers of CD123 cells are found in the papillary dermis.

3. Other diseases with follicular plugging (1.47).
4. Other diseases with mucin in the dermis (1.83).

17.7 Dermatomyositis

(see Fig. 17.7A,B)
Uncommon rheumatologic disease with *diffuse red rash of the trunk* (often with poikiloderma, 1.112), edematous purplish (1.149) *heliotrope eyelids*, periungual telangiectasias, *proximal muscle weakness, EMG abnormalities, myositis on muscle biopsy,* and *elevated muscle enzymes such as CPK and aldolase*. ANA is positive in 50% of patients. Associated with internal malignancy (1.105) in 30% of adults, especially of the ovary, breast, lung and colon. The childhood form is more likely to calcify and is not associated with malignancy.

- Epidermis atrophic or normal
- *Liquefaction degeneration* of the basal layer
- Thickened basement membrane sometimes
- Dermal edema (1.30)
- Dermal mucin (1.83, best seen with Alcian blue or colloidal iron stains)
- *Sparse* perivascular or *interface lymphocytes*
- Sometimes dermal or subcutaneous calcification (1.19)
- Direct immunofluorescence usually negative

P

Variations

1. Amyopathic dermatomyositis (dermatomyositis sine myositis, clinically amyopathic dermatomyositis): same rash, no muscle involvement, same histology.
2. Drug-induced dermatomyositis (3.5).

Differential diagnosis

1. LE (17.6) cannot be distinguished from dermatomyositis without clinical information[161] and laboratory blood tests. LE usually has more inflammation, while dermatomyositis is subtle. Positive routine direct immunofluorescence (IgG, IgM, or C3 along dermal–epidermal junction) is seen in LE, with negative immunofluorescence in dermatomyositis, though this really is not a practical way of distinguishing them. It has been reported that dermatomyositis may have C5b-C9 around vessels and the dermal–epidermal junction, in contrast to LE, though this is not routinely done.
2. Other diseases with interface dermatitis (1.64).

17.8 Relapsing polychondritis

(see Fig. 17.8)
Rheumatologic disorder with relapsing *diffuse painful erythema of ear* (1.28), *sparing earlobe*, associated with antibodies to type II collagen in cartilage (not generally tested clinically, because is specific to this disease). Damage to ear, bronchial, or nose cartilage may result in ear deformity, floppy ears, airway collapse, or saddle nose (1.95). Other manifestations include arthritis (1.7), ocular inflammation (1.41), and cardiac valvular disease (1.57).

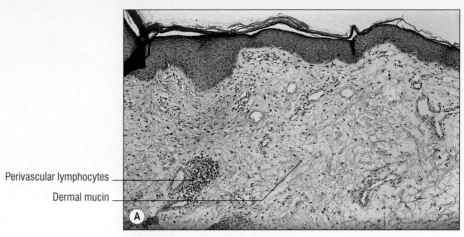

Perivascular lymphocytes
Dermal mucin

Fig. 17.7 A Dermatomyositis (low mag.).

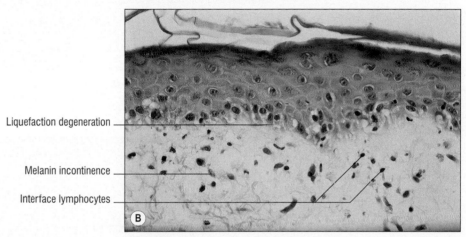

Liquefaction degeneration

Melanin incontinence

Interface lymphocytes

Fig. 17.7 B Dermatomyositis (high mag.).

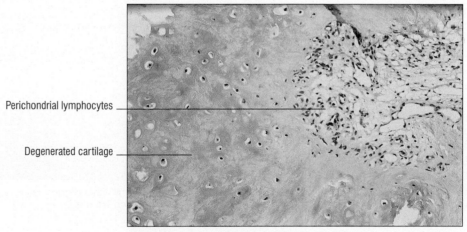

Perichondrial lymphocytes

Degenerated cartilage

Fig. 17.8 Relapsing polychondritis.

P
- *Perichondrial inflammation* (neutrophils, lymphocytes, or plasma cells)
- *Degeneration of cartilage* with loss of chondroitin sulfate (decreased basophilia) and vacuolization of chondrocytes
- *Perichondrial fibrosis* in older lesions

Differential diagnosis

1. Cellulitis (12.3): lacks the other systemic findings, more neutrophils, positive stains or cultures sometimes, response to antibiotics.
2. Chondrodermatitis (17.9) or trauma to ear.
3. Contact dermatitis (2.2): more scale or clinical microvesiculation, spongiosis.

17.9 **Chondrodermatitis nodularis chronica helicis (CNCH, CNH)**

(*see Fig. 17.9A,B*)

Solitary painful nodule (1.97) of the ear helix (1.28), often related to actinic damage or cold injury.

- *Hyperplasia of epidermis* (1.61), often with focal ulceration
- *Granulation tissue*, fibrosis, *solar elastosis*, and mixed inflammatory infiltrate (lymphocytes, neutrophils, plasma cells) between ulcer and underlying cartilage
- *Degeneration of cartilage*, often blending with fibrosis, sometimes with transepidermal elimination

Differential diagnosis

1. Weathering nodules of the ears (9.1).
2. Relapsing polychondritis (17.8).
3. Pseudocyst of the auricle (19.13).
4. Squamous cell carcinoma (18.11).

17.10 **Other pigmentary anomalies**

Most of these hyperpigmented (1.18) or hypopigmented (1.150) disorders are diagnosed clinically, and the histopathology is often not specific, and is often not done. Fontana melanin stain may be done to assess prevalence of melanin, but melanocytes themselves are difficult to quantify, even with S-100 staining or electron microscopy. Most of them show increased or decreased melanin at the basal layer, with or without melanin incontinence (1.79).

Variations

1. Idiopathic guttate hypomelanosis: *small drop-like white macules*, usually on the *undamaged* forearms (1.6) and legs (1.67), with decreased melanocytes and melanin, epidermal atrophy (1.9).
2. Nevus depigmentosus (achromic nevus): localized *congenital depigmented patch*, usually *solitary* and persistent, no associated abnormalities, normal or somewhat reduced number of melanocytes with short dendrites, unlike piebaldism (11.9), in which melanocytes are largely absent.
3. Nevus anemicus: congenital *solitary pale area of skin*, with extension possible by blanching of the border with diascopy especially on the upper trunk, due to *blood vessel increased sensitivity to catecholamines*, There is no melanocyte or melanin abnormality, and biopsies look normal.
4. Melasma (chloasma): *hormone or pregnancy-induced hyperpigmentation of the face* (1.44), mostly females, with increased basal layer melanin.
5. Riehl's melanosis: *brown–gray* (1.54) pigmentation with rapid onset on the *face*, with perifollicular hyperpigmentation in the periphery, a questionable entity possibly related to cosmetic allergy. Biopsy has lymphocytic perivascular (1.109) or interface (1.64) dermatitis with melanin incontinence.
6. Poikiloderma of Civatte: mottled pigmentation (1.112) and telangiectasia on the cheeks and neck of women,

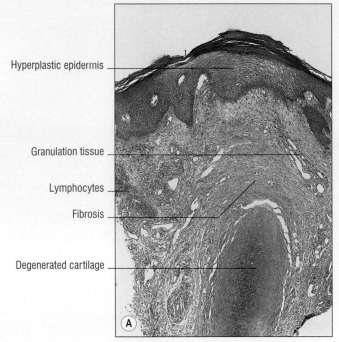

Fig. 17.9 A Chondrodermatitis nodularis helicis (low mag.).

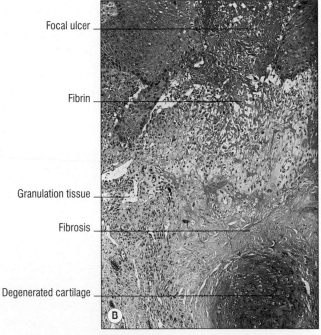

Fig. 17.9 B Chondrodermatitis nodularis helicis (medium mag.).

probably related to photocontact dermatitis from cosmetics or perfumes.

7. Addison's disease: *adrenal insufficiency* with *diffuse hyperpigmentation* of skin and oral mucosa, increased basal layer melanin, sometimes melanin incontinence.
8. Cronkite–Canada syndrome: diffuse hyperpigmentation (1.18), alopecia (1.4), *GI polyps*, and enteropathy (1.43).
9. Diabetic dermopathy (pigmented pretibial patches): *atrophic pigmented macules* on the *anterior legs* (1.67) of *diabetics* (1.26), perhaps related to trauma, seldom

biopsied, *dermal hemosiderin* (1.58), papillary dermal blood vessels increased, sparse perivascular lymphocytes.

10. Dowling–Degos disease (DDD, reticulate pigmented dermatosis of the flexures, reticulate acropigmentation of Kitamura): autosomal dominant, mutation in keratin-5 gene, *reticulated* (1.123) *hyperpigmentation* of axilla (1.10), groin (1.55), inframammary area, and antecubital fossa (1.6) beginning in adulthood. Biopsy has delicate, elongated, hyperpigmented rete ridges, resembling a reticulated seborrheic keratosis (18.2).

11. Post-inflammatory hypopigmentation: decreased pigment of skin following a previous inflammatory rash, *decreased melanin at basal layer*, sometimes with mild melanin incontinence.

12. Post-inflammatory hyperpigmentation (PIH, don't confuse with pseudoepitheliomatous hyperplasia (PEH), 1.116): increased pigment of skin following a previous inflammatory rash, increased or normal amount of melanin at the basal layer, often with *prominent melanin incontinence*. Collectively can be called post-inflammatory pigmentary alteration (PIPA) when there is a combination of hyper- and hypopigmentation (see also poikiloderma, 1.112).

17.11 Other mouth lesions

Variations

1. Aphthous ulcers (aphthosis, canker sore): common, idiopathic, solitary or multiple ulcers of the buccal and lip mucosa (1.74), ventral and lateral tongue (1.139), and soft palate (1.98). *Minor aphthae* are smaller than 1 cm and heal in 1–2 weeks. *Major aphthae* (Sutton's disease, periadenitis mucosae necrotic recurrens) are larger and may take months to heal. Prior to ulceration, there is spongiosis (1.132). Ulcers are coated with a prominent fibrinous gray membrane that contains neutrophils. Aphthae have nothing to do with herpes virus (14.2), despite widespread confusion to the contrary. Oral ulcers also appear in Behçet's syndrome (4.11). In immunosuppressed patients, cytomegalovirus (14.9) should be considered.

2. Necrotizing sialometaplasia: abrupt onset of a deep ulcer on the hard palate, spontaneously healing in 2–3 months. Biopsy shows necrosis of salivary glands and ducts with squamous metaplasia (1.116) resembling squamous cell carcinoma. It is a pseudomalignancy (1.118).

3. White sponge nevus: autosomal dominant, mutation of keratin 4 or 13 (mucosal keratins above the basal layer), onset at birth or childhood, extensive thickened, corrugated white plaques in the mouth, and sometimes of other mucosal surfaces. It does not become a squamous cell carcinoma. Biopsy shows epithelial hyperplasia and vacuolar swelling of keratinocytes, sparing the basal layer. Biopsy identical to pachyonychia congenita (2.15) and oral focal epithelial hyperplasia (14.1). Leukoedema of the oral mucosa also resembles white sponge nevus, but has an adult onset, a patchy instead of diffuse distribution, and exacerbations and remissions.

CHAPTER 18

Epithelial Neoplasms

18.1 Epidermal nevus (linear epidermal nevus)

(see Fig. 18.1A,B)
Somewhat common, *linear, warty plaque*, usually on the extremities, sometimes on trunk, *since birth* or early childhood, *persists* indefinitely. They may follow Blashko's lines, sometimes related to a post-zygotic somatic mosaicism for mutations in the FGFR3 gene or PIK3CA gene, which also has been found in families with seborrheic keratoses. It is a congenital hamartoma (nevus) of proliferating epidermis, while most other nevi are melanocytic (20.5).

P
- Hyperkeratosis, papillomatosis, acanthosis, sometimes hypergranulosis
- Epidermolytic hyperkeratosis rarely (11.1)
- Acantholytic dyskeratosis rarely (11.3)
- Perivascular lymphocytes often

Variations

1. Nevus comedonicus (acne nevus): numerous open comedones in the linear plaque, may resemble acne. Sometimes associated with craniosynostosis, syndactyly, and FGFR2 mutation. May be a mosaic Apert syndrome.
2. Epidermal nevus syndrome: associated with ocular, skeletal, or neurological disease. Usually these are larger epidermal nevi. Similar to nevus sebaceus syndrome (21.2).
3. Linear porokeratosis: cornoid lamellae (18.4).
4. Linear basal cell nevus: identical to basal cell carcinoma (BCC), but starts in childhood and is linear.
5. Nevus unius lateris: extensive unilateral plaque with abrupt midline demarcation, usually on the trunk.
6. Systematized epidermal nevus (ichthyosis hystrix): literally "fish-porcupine", term used when there is extensive involvement, usually on the trunk, often with a marble-cake whorled appearance. Whorling also occurs in incontinentia pigmenti (11.6), and hypomelanosis of Ito (11.7), but those conditions are more macular. May closely resemble some forms of ichthyosis (11.1).
7. Inflammatory linear verrucous epidermal nevus (ILVEN): more erythematous, more psoriasiform (1.119), and more lymphocytic inflammation. Parakeratosis with hypogranulosis often alternates with orthokeratosis and a prominent granular layer.
8. Epidermolytic epidermal nevus: epidermolytic hyperkeratosis (11.1) occurs (keratin 1 and 10 defect).
9. Nevus sebaceus (21.2): the ultimate "lumper" considers nevus sebaceus to be a variant of epidermal nevus that occurs more on the head and neck, usually near the scalp, that has proliferating sebaceous and apocrine glands in addition to the papillomatous epidermis. With this concept, the other epidermal nevi without the sebaceous or apocrine gland components would be "keratinocytic epidermal nevi".
10. Pigmented hairy epidermal nevus: see Becker's nevus, 20.3.

Differential diagnosis

1. Other papillomatous diseases (1.102) or linear diseases (1.73). Clinical information may be needed to make the distinction in some cases.
2. Seborrheic keratosis (18.2): may appear histologically identical, but usually is not linear and almost always starts after age 30 years old.
3. Lichen striatus (2.5): usually not present at birth, less hyperkeratosis and acanthosis, more spongiosis, more dyskeratosis, more lichenoid inflammation, resolves spontaneously.

18.2 Seborrheic keratosis (SK)

(see Fig. 18.2A–G)
Very common *stuck-on brown papules or plaques* (aging barnacles) anywhere on the skin except palms and soles of patients over 30 years old. May look greasy, and common in areas with sebaceous glands (trunk and face), hence the name "seborrheic", but they have nothing to do with sebaceous glands. Keratosis is a lesion with hyperkeratosis, since the suffix -osis means condition or disorder of.

©2012 Elsevier Ltd, Inc, BV
DOI: 10.1016/B978-0-323-06658-7.00018 X

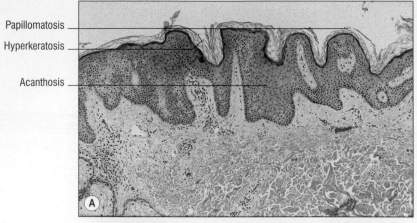

Papillomatosis
Hyperkeratosis

Acanthosis

Fig. 18.1 A Epidermal nevus.

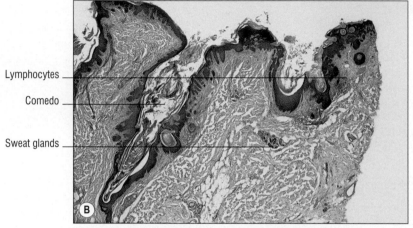

Lymphocytes

Comedo

Sweat glands

Fig. 18.1 B Nevus comedonicus.

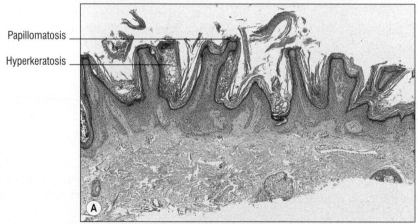

Papillomatosis

Hyperkeratosis

Fig. 18.2 A Seborrheic keratosis (hyperkeratotic).

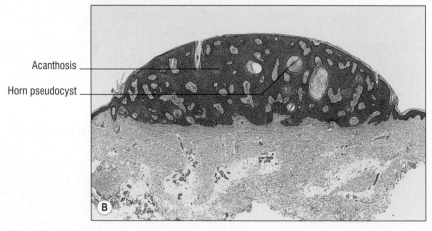

Acanthosis

Horn pseudocyst

Fig. 18.2 B Seborrheic keratosis (acanthotic).

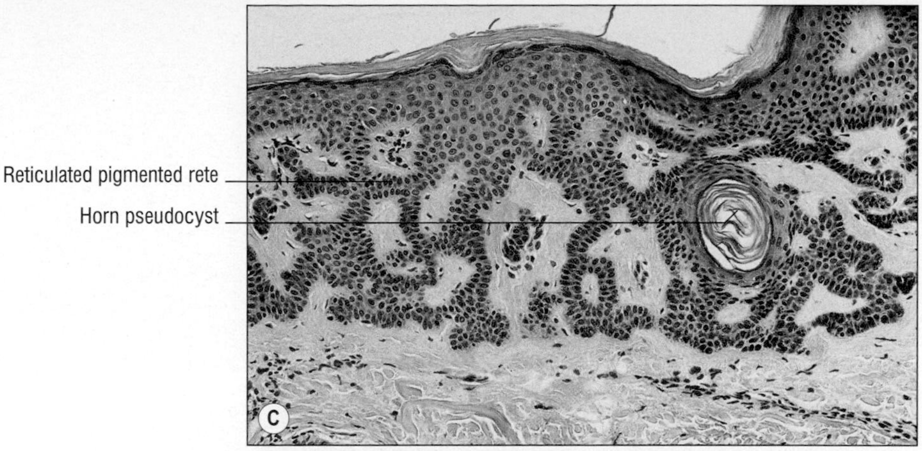

Reticulated pigmented rete

Horn pseudocyst

Fig. 18.2 C Seborrheic keratosis (reticulated).

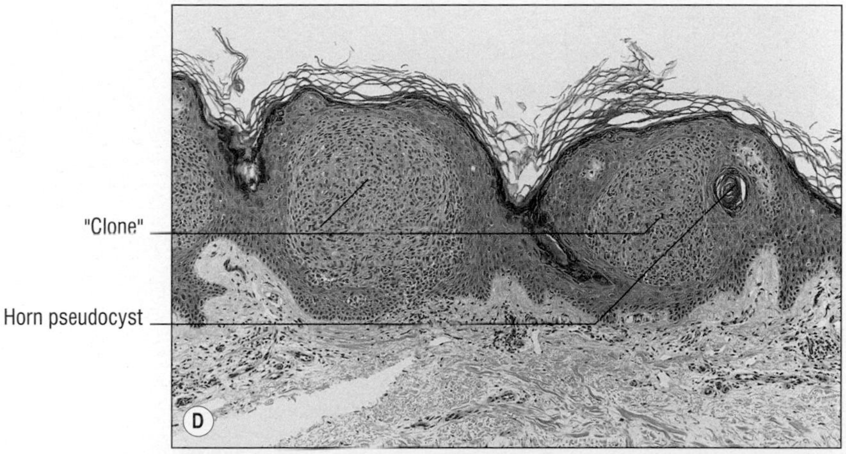

"Clone"

Horn pseudocyst

Fig. 18.2 D Seborrheic keratosis (clonal).

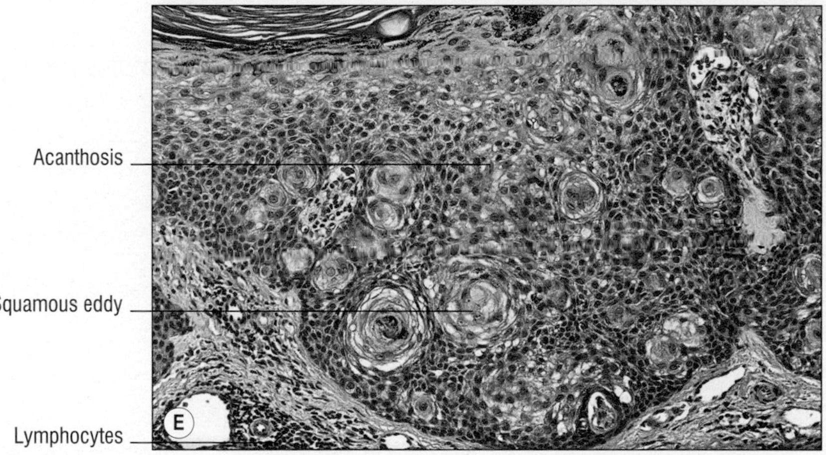

Acanthosis

Squamous eddy

Lymphocytes

Fig. 18.2 E Irritated seborrheic keratosis.

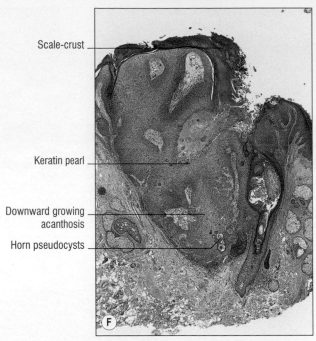

Scale-crust

Keratin pearl

Downward growing acanthosis

Horn pseudocysts

Fig. 18.2 F Inverted follicular keratosis.

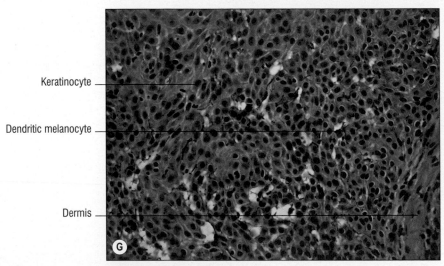

Keratinocyte

Dendritic melanocyte

Dermis

Fig. 18.2 G Melanoacanthoma.

P
- *Epidermal proliferation* (variable combinations of hyperkeratosis, papillomatosis, acanthosis)
- Keratinocytes often appear basaloid
- Often *horn pseudocysts* (are called "pseudo" because they connect to surface, and represent papillomatosis)
- Often abundant *melanin* in basal layer or throughout epidermis
- Sharp demarcation "*string sign*" of base of epidermal proliferation

Variations

1. Stucco keratosis (keratosis alba): *white*, more on lower legs of old patients, *church-spire* rete ridges, fewer horn cysts, and less melanin, similar to acrokeratosis verruciformis (18.3).
2. Hyperkeratotic SK: *more hyperkeratosis*, *more papillomatosis*, less melanin, fewer horn cysts.

3. Acanthotic SK: *smooth*, *less warty surface*, more likely to resemble a nevus clinically, more acanthosis, more melanin, less hyperkeratosis, less papillomatosis.
4. Adenoid (reticulated) SK: more on sun-exposed skin, thin, anastomosing *net-like* strands of epithelium (unfortunately called "adenoid" because dermal papillae as sectioned may vaguely resemble glands), may be related to, or arise from, a solar lentigo.
5. Macular SK (incipient SK): brown *macule*, more on *sun-exposed* skin, may arise in a solar lentigo, may eventually become a reticulated SK. Solar lentigo (20.4) has been considered to be associated with, or evolve into, macular SK, but macular SK has more compact stratum corneum, more acanthosis, and occasional early horn pseudocysts, compared with solar lentigo.
6. Large cell acanthoma: deemed by "splitters" to be a separate entity because of its large keratinocytes. Probably most cases are solar lentigo as it evolves into

macular SK (see above). Some cases might be Bowen's disease.

7. Dermatosis papulosa nigra: *multiple tag-like black papules* on *face* (1.44) of *black patients*, often numerous, smaller size, more melanin, less basaloid cells.

8. Melanoacanthoma: extremely *heavily pigmented acanthotic type* of SK, may have increased dendritic melanocytes throughout epidermis.

9. Irritated or inflamed seborrheic keratosis (ISK): redness or crusting often present clinically. The "splitters" distinguish inflamed seborrheic keratosis (which just has inflammation) from irritated seborrheic keratosis, which has crusting, *squamous eddies* or pearls (1.134), sometimes spongiosis (1.132), sometimes acantholysis (1.2), often mild or moderate atypia, *inflammation*, may resemble squamous cell carcinoma (SCC, 18.11).

10. Borst–Jadassohn (clonal) SK: a variant of irritated SK (1.37) with discrete keratinocyte nests that appear different and demarcated from their neighbors, either because they are pale, dyskeratotic, or whorled.

11. Inverted follicular keratosis (IFK): irritated SK that *grows downward* along a follicle, with fewer clear cells than a trichilemmoma (22.5).

12. Tumor of the follicular infundibulum (22.5) might be considered a variant of SK by the "lumpers".

13. Lichenoid keratosis (18.8).

Differential diagnosis

1. Actinic keratosis (18.8): limited to sun-damaged areas, atypical keratinocytes and inflamed even when not "irritated", usually no string sign, no horn pseudocysts, usually no pigment.

2. Verruca vulgaris (14.1): mounds of parakeratosis, hypergranulosis, koilocytosis, and dilated vessels in papillae.

3. Other diseases with papillomatosis (1.102).

4. Other diseases with basaloid cells (1.11).

5. Other diseases with horn cysts (1.59).

18.3 Acrokeratosis verruciformis (AKV)

(see Fig. 18.3)
Rare, small warty papules on the dorsum of acral forearms, hands, and feet (1.56), genetically inherited, often associated

with Darier's disease (11.3), and related to the same ATP2A2 gene mutation.

- Orthokeratosis, hypergranulosis (1.60), acanthosis (1.61)
- Papillomatosis, often resembling *church spires*

Differential diagnosis

1. Viral warts (14.1): koilocytosis, mounds of parakeratosis, dilated blood vessels in the dermal papillae.

2. Other diseases with papillomatosis (1.102): differentiation from hyperkeratotic seborrheic keratosis or stucco keratosis (18.2) is impossible without clinical information.

18.4 Porokeratosis

(see Fig. 18.4A–C)
Uncommon *annular* (1.5) hyperkeratotic papule or plaque with a *thread-like elevated border*. It is a misnomer, as porokeratosis has nothing to do with pores of sweat glands. Some forms of porokeratosis can develop SCC.

- *Cornoid lamella* (a column of parakeratosis under which there is hypogranulosis and keratinocytes with dyskeratosis or pale staining) corresponding to the annular ridge seen clinically. Usually on a transverse section there is a cornoid lamella at both two-dimensional edges of the specimen, with the superficial surface of column slanting toward the inside of the lesion, but multiple haphazard cornoid lamellae may be present in the same biopsy
- Epidermis in central part of lesion may be normal, hyperplastic, or atrophic (1.9)
- Perivascular (1.109) or lichenoid (1.72) lymphocytes, sometimes localized beneath cornoid lamella

Variations

1. Superficial disseminated porokeratosis: numerous lesions, not apparently related to the sun.

2. Disseminated superficial actinic porokeratosis (DSAP): associated with SART3 gene mutations, numerous lesions, questionable relationship to the sun, most

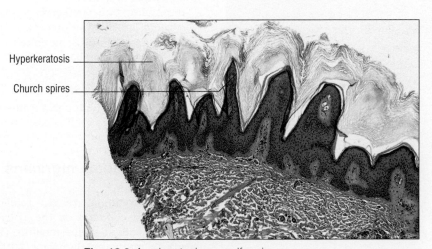

Fig. 18.3 Acrokeratosis verruciformis.

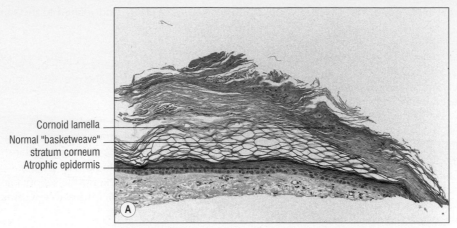

Fig. 18.4 A Porokeratosis (disseminated superficial actinic porokeratosis).

Cornoid lamella
Normal "basketweave" stratum corneum
Atrophic epidermis

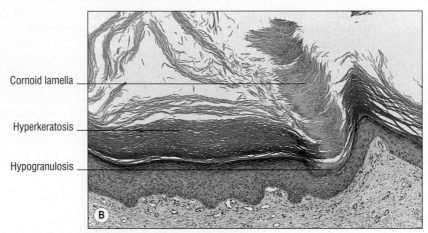

Cornoid lamella
Hyperkeratosis
Hypogranulosis

Fig. 18.4 B Porokeratosis.

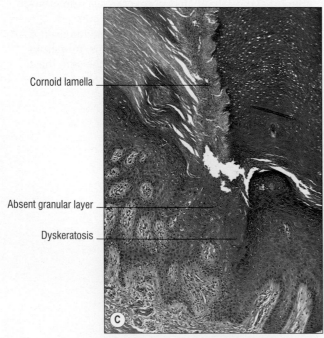

Cornoid lamella
Absent granular layer
Dyskeratosis

Fig. 18.4 C Porokeratosis of Mibelli.

common on the legs (1.67), cornoid lamella may be subtle and easily missed.

3. Porokeratosis of Mibelli: solitary, larger variant, more hyperkeratotic, prominent cornoid lamella.
4. Porokeratosis punctata palmaris et plantaris: discrete small foci of hyperkeratosis of palms and soles, resembling punctate keratoderma (2.15), except that cornoid lamellae are present.
5. Linear porokeratosis: an epidermal nevus variant (18.1) with cornoid lamellae.

Differential diagnosis

1. Other diseases with parakeratosis (1.104) or hyperplasia of epidermis (1.61). It is easy to miss this diagnosis if the cornoid lamella is not recognized.

18.5 Acanthosis nigricans

(see Fig. 18.5)

Somewhat common, *velvety papillomatous hyperpigmented plaques*, most common on the *axilla* (1.10) and *neck* (1.86), associated with diabetes mellitus (1.26), endocrinopathies, obesity, or internal malignancy (1.105). It is not a neoplasm, but is included in this chapter because of its resemblance to seborrheic keratosis histologically.

- Hyperkeratosis, *papillomatosis*
- Acanthosis minimal or absent (a misnomer)
- *Basal layer hyperpigmentation* often

Variations

1. Confluent and reticulated papillomatosis of Gougerot and Carteaud: more generalized on the trunk, more reticulated (1.123), more stuck-on scale and less velvety, *Pityrosporum* often present, may respond to minocycline.
2. Pseudoacanthosis nigricans: only "splitters" make the distinction, associated with obesity, resolves with weight loss.
3. Malignant acanthosis nigricans: associated with internal malignancy.
4. Tripe palm (acanthosis palmaris): velvety changes of the palms associated with internal malignancy (1.105).

Differential diagnosis

1. Other diseases with papillomatosis (1.102), especially epidermal nevus (18.1), seborrheic keratosis (18.2), Dowling–Degos disease (17.10) and verruca vulgaris (14.1), are completely different clinically.

18.6 Clear cell acanthoma (pale cell acanthoma)

(see Fig. 18.6A,B)

Uncommon *red papule* or plaque, usually on the *leg* (1.67). Considered by a few "lumpers" to be a clear cell variant of irritated seborrheic keratosis (18.2). The suffix -oma means tumor, so this is a tumor with acanthosis.

- *Scale-crust* on surface of epidermis often **P**
- Neutrophils in epidermis, often with *microabscesses in stratum corneum* (1.89)
- *Psoriasiform* proliferation of *pale* ("*clear*") *keratinocytes, with sharp demarcation* from normal epidermis. The glycogen in the pale cells is PAS-positive, diastase labile
- Perivascular lymphocytes
- Dilated blood vessels in edematous pale dermal papillae

Differential diagnosis

1. Other lesions with clear cells (1.22), or a psoriasiform appearance (1.119). Trichilemmoma (22.5) is usually on the face and has a pushing, downward-growing lobule instead of a psoriasiform silhouette.
2. Bowen's disease (18.10): more atypia, dyskeratosis.

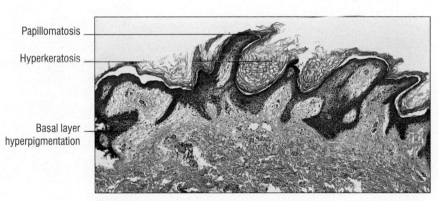

Papillomatosis

Hyperkeratosis

Basal layer hyperpigmentation

Fig. 18.5 Acanthosis nigricans.

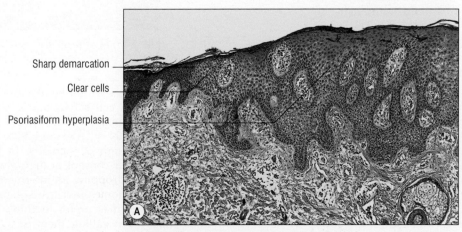

Sharp demarcation

Clear cells

Psoriasiform hyperplasia

Fig. 18.6 A Clear cell acanthoma (low mag.).

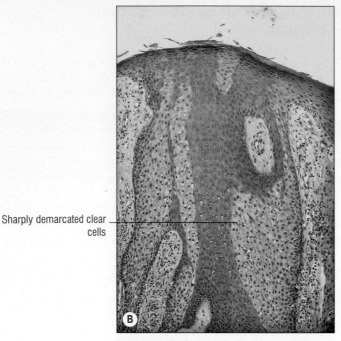

Sharply demarcated clear cells

Fig. 18.6 B Clear cell acanthoma (high mag.).

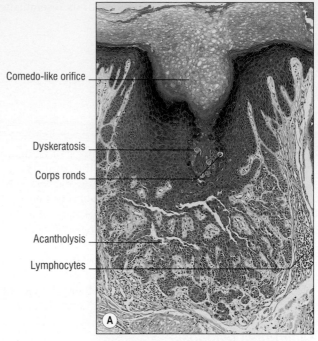

Comedo-like orifice

Dyskeratosis

Corps ronds

Acantholysis

Lymphocytes

Fig. 18.7 A Warty dyskeratoma (low mag.).

18.7 Warty dyskeratoma

(see Fig. 18.7A,B)
Uncommon *verrucous papule* (1.146) on sun-damaged skin of the *face* (1.44).

> **P** ▪ *Comedo-like invagination of epidermis* filled with hyperkeratosis, parakeratosis, and *acantholytic, dyskeratotic keratinocytes* (including corps ronds and grains)
> ▪ Dermal papillae lined by basal cells may project up into the invagination, resembling villi

Differential diagnosis

1. Other diseases with acantholytic dyskeratosis (1.2), especially Darier's disease (11.3) and transient acantholytic dermatosis (5.6) are much different clinically. Acantholytic actinic keratosis (18.8) and acantholytic SCC (18.11) have cytologic atypia.

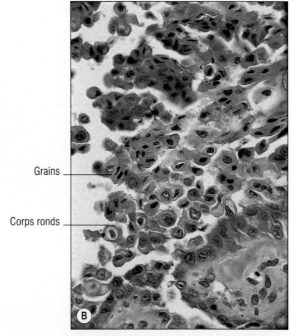

Grains

Corps ronds

Fig. 18.7 B Warty dyskeratoma (high mag.).

18.8 Actinic keratosis (AK, solar keratosis)

(see Fig. 18.8A–I)
A very common *precancerous* ill-defined *white–red papule* (sometimes macular, diffuse, multifocal, or subclinical), often multiple, in *sun-damaged areas* (1.110), more in older patients. Considered to be a low-grade dysplasia (defined as atypia of epithelium), or by some authorities to be a lesion on the road to an early low-grade carcinoma in situ (18.10), analogous to one of the lower grades of intraepithelial neoplasia seen in the cervix (CIN grade 1, 2 or 3, cervical intraepithelial neoplasia), vulva (VIN) or penis (PIN). In skin, it has been proposed to use keratinocytic intraepithelial neoplasia (KIN grade 1, 2, 3) wherein grade 1 would be like most AKs, and 3 would be like squamous cell carcinoma in situ (SCCIS, 18.10). This concept has not generally been adopted, so nowadays we basically have KIN 1 (AK) and KIN 2 (SCCIS) without an intermediate grade 2. Actually, in the cervix, pathologists have the similar concept of high-grade (3) and low-grade (1) lesions, also dropping an intermediate grade. Less than 1 in 100 AKs becomes invasive squamous carcinoma (18.11). Some authorities prefer to think of AKs as superficial carcinomas (even calling them SCC of the AK type), mainly to convince insurance companies of their

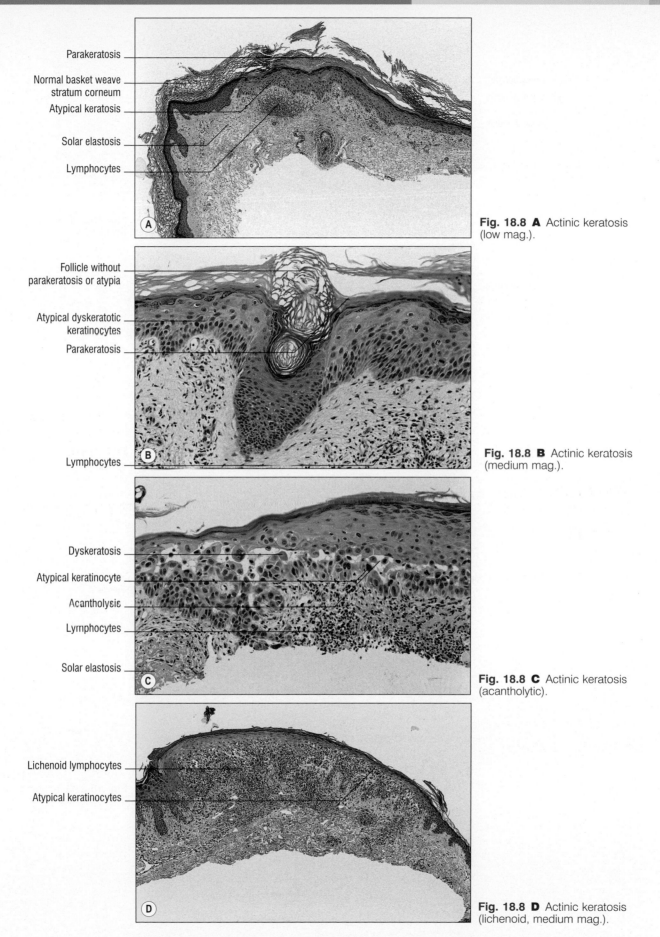

Parakeratosis

Normal basket weave
stratum corneum

Atypical keratosis

Solar elastosis

Lymphocytes

Fig. 18.8 A Actinic keratosis
(low mag.).

Follicle without
parakeratosis or atypia

Atypical dyskeratotic
keratinocytes

Parakeratosis

Lymphocytes

Fig. 18.8 B Actinic keratosis
(medium mag.).

Dyskeratosis

Atypical keratinocyte

Acantholysis

Lymphocytes

Solar elastosis

Fig. 18.8 C Actinic keratosis
(acantholytic).

Lichenoid lymphocytes

Atypical keratinocytes

Fig. 18.8 D Actinic keratosis
(lichenoid, medium mag.).

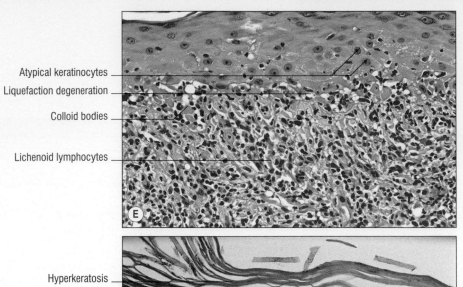

Atypical keratinocytes

Liquefaction degeneration

Colloid bodies

Lichenoid lymphocytes

E

Fig. 18.8 E Actinic keratosis (high mag.).

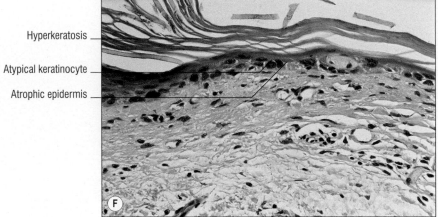

Hyperkeratosis

Atypical keratinocyte

Atrophic epidermis

F

Fig. 18.8 F Actinic keratosis (atrophic).

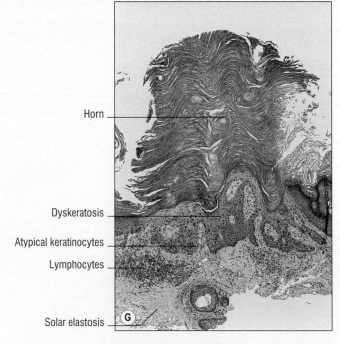

Horn

Dyskeratosis

Atypical keratinocytes

Lymphocytes

Solar elastosis

G

Fig. 18.8 G Actinic keratosis (hyperkeratotic).

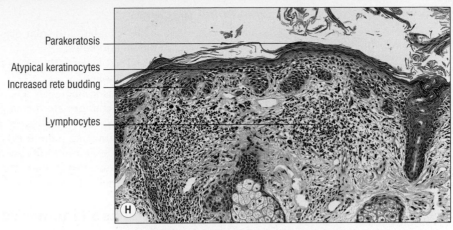

Parakeratosis
Atypical keratinocytes
Increased rete budding

Lymphocytes

Fig. 18.8 H Actinic keratosis (multiple "buds").

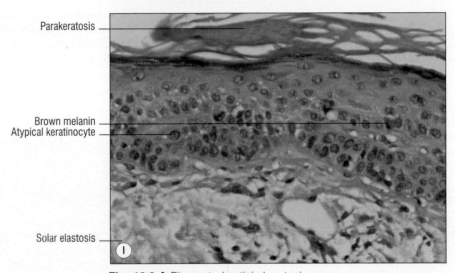

Parakeratosis

Brown melanin
Atypical keratinocyte

Solar elastosis

Fig. 18.8 I Pigmented actinic keratosis.

importance, as compared to keratoses with no malignant potential (18.2). Telling patients they are carcinomas seems to be a bit of an alarmist approach.

P

- Often hyperkeratosis, sometimes ulceration
- *Parakeratosis* (1.104), especially overlying atypical keratinocytes, often sparing epidermis over adnexa ("*alternating*" pink and blue hue in stratum corneum called the "flag sign")
- *Atypical keratinocytes*, sometimes subtle, often more atypical in deeper epithelium, with loss of orderly keratinocyte maturation, hyperchromatism, pleomorphism, increased mitoses, dyskeratosis (1.27), often sparing the epidermis above adnexa, and often *too many buds* into the papillary dermis
- Perivascular (1.109) or lichenoid lymphocytes, sometimes plasma cells (1.111)
- *Solar elastosis* in the dermis (9.1)

Variations

1. Hypertrophic AK (hyperkeratotic AK, HAK): prominent hyperkeratosis and acanthosis, may produce a cutaneous horn, (1.61), especially common on dorsum of hand (1.56).

2. Atrophic AK: epidermal atrophy (1.9), may resemble lupus erythematosus (17.6).

3. Acantholytic AK: focal acantholysis, resembling other acantholytic diseases (1.2).

4. Lichenoid AK: usually *more red* than average AK, *lichenoid* infiltrate in dermis; atypia may be minimal. Lichenoid keratosis (lichen planus-like keratosis, LPLK) is a less specific term than lichenoid actinic keratosis, used when it is unclear whether the lesion represents an inflamed AK, inflamed SK (18.2), or inflamed solar lentigo, resembling lichen planus (2.11) and other lichenoid diseases (1.72).

5. Pigmented AK:[162] brownish–red papule or plaque (1.18), increased melanin in the epidermis; may resemble seborrheic keratosis (18.2), solar lentigo (20.3), or lentigo maligna (20.11). Some patients with sun damage have several of these lesions coexisiting in the same vicinity, so beware of sampling problems.

6. Bowenoid AK: a nasty term to avoid since it is used so differently by various authorities. Some use it as a synonym for follicular AK (below). Others use it to mean that it is more of an advanced AK (either clinically a wider plaque or that it has only focal areas of full-thickness atypia in the epidermis). Still others have said that true Bowen's disease is on sun-protected skin (based upon the old days when it was often arsenic

induced), while bowenoid AK is used for SCCIS of sun-exposed skin.

7. Follicular AK (superficial spreading AK, AK with follicular involvement): more extension of atypical keratinocytes down the follicles (or less often down sweat ducts: "syringotropic"), not qualifying for true invasion of SCC, but rendering the lesion more refractory to superficial therapies such as cryotherapy or topical chemotherapy. In most cases, atypical kertinocytes spare adnexa in AKs, but this is an exception. Some books erroneously state that Bowen's disease (18.10) often has atypical cells extending down follicles, while AK cannot.

8. Actinic cheilitis: diffuse AK of lip (1.74, usually lower lip), often eroded.

9. Premalignant leukoplakia: whitish plaque (1.71) inside mouth (1.82), unrelated to sun, sometimes related to tobacco, or on lip as synonymous with actinic cheilitis.

Differential diagnosis

1. When cytologic atypia is minimal (a common occurrence), other papillomas may be considered (1.102), especially seborrheic keratosis (18.2) or verruca vulgaris (14.1). Seborrheic keratosis is more stuck-on, browner, more sharply demarcated at the base, not necessarily sun exposed, and has more atypia, more horn pseudocysts, and more melanin.

2. Superficial BCC (18.13): sometimes the crowding of basal cells can be subtle, and it can resemble an AK.

18.9 Arsenical keratosis

Rare nowadays, these *hyperkeratotic papules* appear mainly on the *palms or soles* (1.100), due to arsenic in medication or well water (sometimes due to contamination from spraying fields with arsenical pesticides). Associated with BCCs, Bowen's disease, SCCs, and internal malignancy (1.105), especially *gastrointestinal tract adenocarcinoma* (1.49).

P
- Hyperkeratosis, acanthosis
- Cytologic atypia of keratinocytes often, may represent SCCIS, similar to Bowen's disease (18.10)
- Variable perivascular lymphocytes in the dermis

Differential diagnosis

1. Actinic keratosis (18.8) is related to solar elastosis, almost never on palms and soles.
2. Seborrheic keratosis (18.2) lacks cytologic atypia, does not occur on palms and soles.
3. Verruca vulgaris (14.1) has koilocytosis and usually no atypia, unless bowenoid changes are developing.
4. Palmoplantar keratoderma (2.15), especially punctate keratoderma, keratosis punctata, palmar pits and palmar keratoses related to Darier's disease and nevoid BCC syndrome, may require clinical data to distinguish.
5. Other diseases with epithelial hyperplasia (1.61).

18.10 Bowen's disease (squamous cell carcinoma in situ)

(see Fig. 18.10A–C)
Common hyperkeratotic erythematous plaque, often crusted, on sun-exposed or covered skin. Formerly thought to be associated with internal malignancy in the era of a higher incidence of arsenic exposure (18.9).

P
- *Parakeratosis* (1.104, often confluent), hyperkeratosis, acanthosis
- *Atypical keratinocytes* with hyperchromatism, pleomorphism, increased atypical mitoses (sometimes bizarre), *dyskeratosis*, and loss of orderly maturation ("*wind-blown epidermis*") throughout the epidermis. The full-thickness epidermal atypia may produce the "*flip sign*", whereby the epidermis has lost its polarity to the point that the superficial epidermis resembles the deeper epidermis (so that if you flipped it upside down you barely could tell the difference), instead of the normal situation where the superficial portion has larger, more mature, more eosinophilic keratinocytes with a larger, less dense nucleus. Sometimes keratinocytes are pale or vacuolated (1.144)
- Perivascular or lichenoid infiltrate of lymphocytes or plasma cells

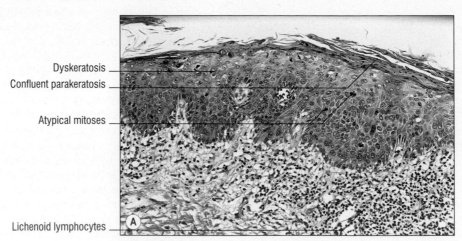

Dyskeratosis
Confluent parakeratosis

Atypical mitoses

Lichenoid lymphocytes

Fig. 18.10 A Bowen's disease (low mag.).

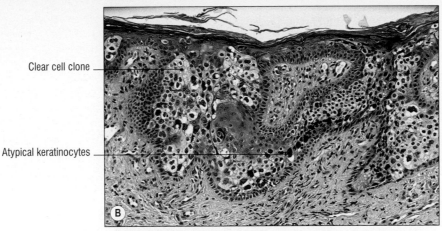

Fig. 18.10 B Bowen's disease (Borst–Jadassohn changes).

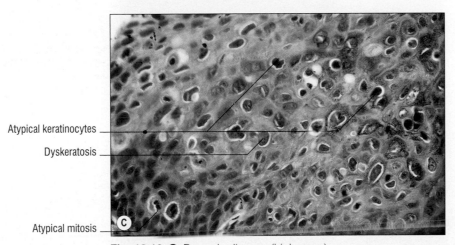

Fig. 18.10 C Bowen's disease (high mag.).

Variations

1. Erythroplasia of Queyrat: Bowen's disease on the glans penis.
2. Borst–Jadassohn changes (1.37) may occur in either Bowen's disease or in an irritated "clonal" SK (18.2).
3. Bowenoid papulosis: multiple verrucous papules in genital region, often more pigmented, with histology of Bowen's disease; related to papillomavirus (14.1) type 16 or 18 or other oncogenic strains.
4. Pigmented Bowen's disease: more melanin in lesion.

Differential diagnosis

1. Other papulosquamous plaques (1.103).
2. Actinic keratosis (18.8): papule instead of a plaque clinically in most cases, less severe atypia that does not involve full-thickness epidermis.
3. Seborrheic keratosis (18.2): clinical stuck-on appearance, string sign, more likely to be brown, more horn pseudocysts, less atypia even when irritated, and often more melanin.
4. Arsenical keratosis (18.9): rare, mostly palms and soles, arsenic exposure documented.
5. Diseases with pagetoid change or epidermotropism (1.37).
6. Psoriasiform lesions (1.119), especially psoriasis (2.8), lack the cytologic atypia.

18.11 Squamous cell carcinoma (SCC)

(see Fig. 18.11A–H)

The second most common type of skin cancer, may grow slowly or rapidly. Red papule, nodule, or plaque, often *hyperkeratotic or ulcerated* (1.142), mostly on *sun-damaged skin*, but less often in irradiated sites, burn scars, chronically infected sites, or associated with other dermatoses, such as lichen sclerosus, lichen planus, discoid lupus erythematosus, xeroderma pigmentosum, porokeratosis, and arsenical keratosis. Sun-exposed SCCs metastasize in less than 1% of cases, but the incidence is higher on the lip, in sun-covered areas and other situations mentioned above, and in neoplasms more than 10 mm thick.

- *Invasion of dermis by atypical keratinocytes* (hyperchromatic, pleomorphic cells, often epithelioid, with atypical mitoses)
- Sometimes squamous eddies or *keratin pearls* (1.27)
- Variable perivascular (1.109), lichenoid (1.72), or diffuse (1.91) lymphocytes (1.76) or plasma cells (1.111)
- Perineural invasion in some aggressive forms (more common than in BCC)

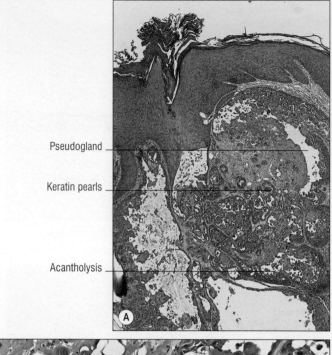

Pseudogland

Keratin pearls

Acantholysis

Fig. 18.11 A Squamous cell carcinoma (well differentiated, low mag.).

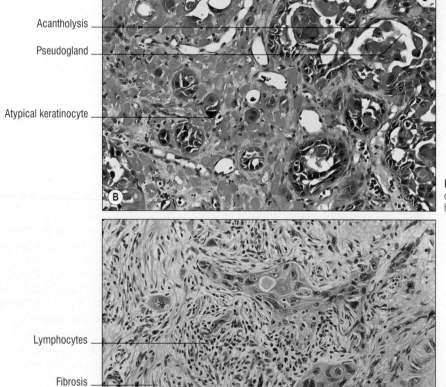

Acantholysis

Pseudogland

Atypical keratinocyte

Fig. 18.11 B Squamous cell carcinoma (well differentiated, high mag.).

Lymphocytes

Fibrosis

Atypical keratinocytes

Fig. 18.11 C Squamous cell carcinoma (infiltrating).

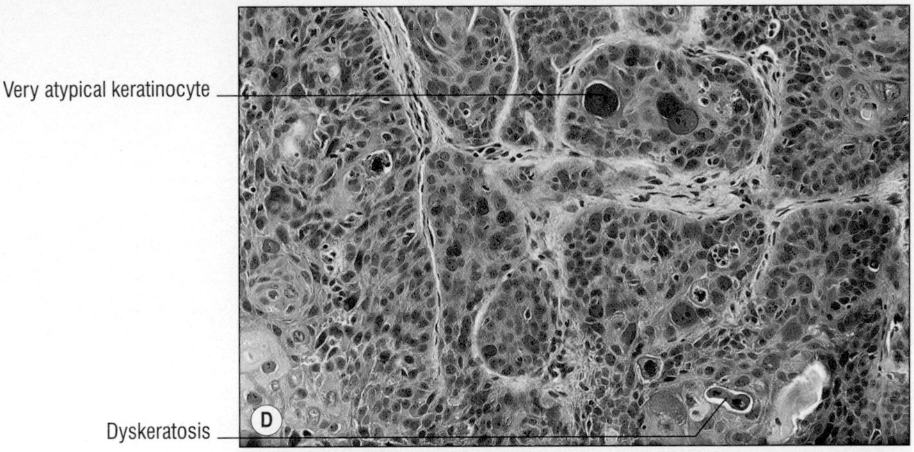

Very atypical keratinocyte

Dyskeratosis

Fig. 18.11 D Squamous cell carcinoma (poorly differentiated).

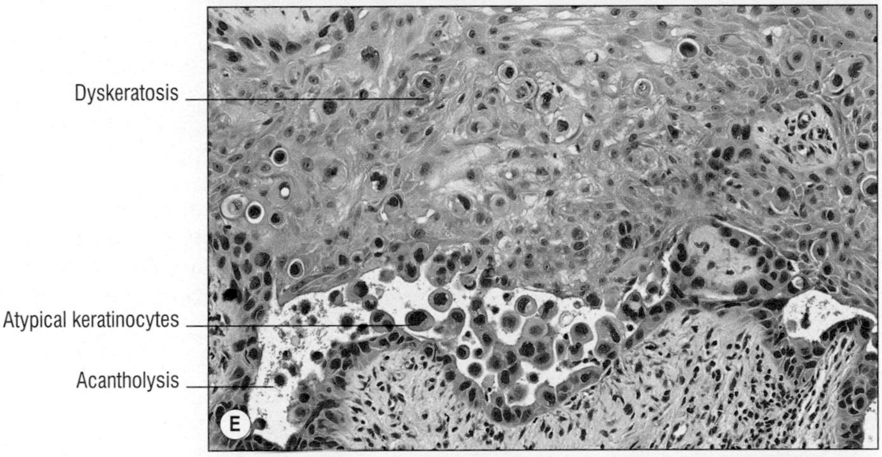

Dyskeratosis

Atypical keratinocytes

Acantholysis

Fig. 18.11 E Squamous cell carcinoma (acantholytic).

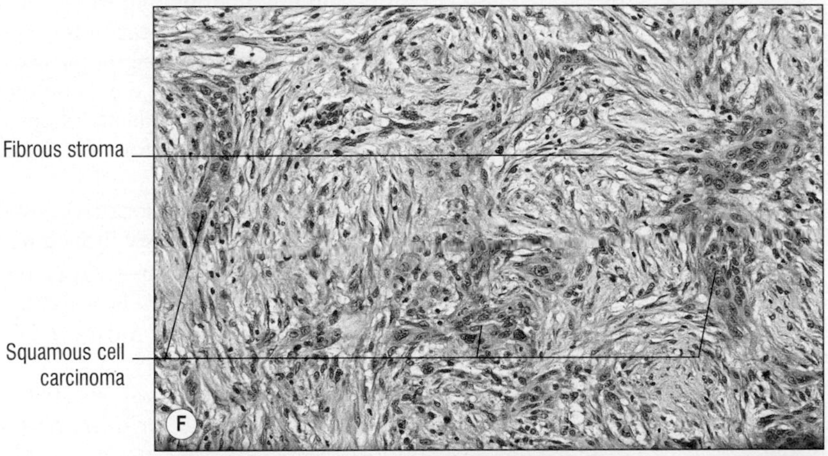

Fibrous stroma

Squamous cell carcinoma

Fig. 18.11 F Squamous cell carcinoma (spindle cell).

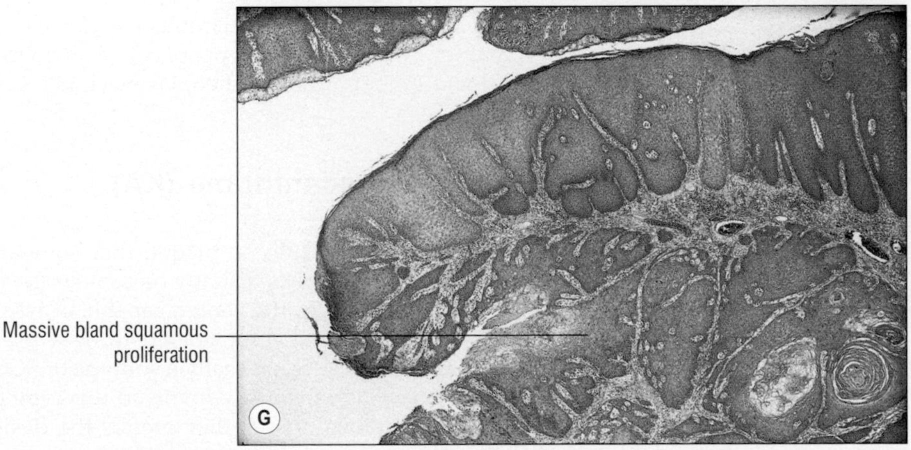

Massive bland squamous proliferation

Fig. 18.11 G Verrucous carcinoma.

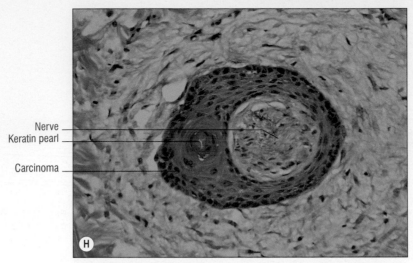

Nerve
Keratin pearl

Carcinoma

Fig. 18.11 H Perineural invasion of squamous cell carcinoma.

Variations

1. Well-differentiated SCC: epithelial proliferation is *pale and glassy*, more squamous eddies or pearls (1.134), *less atypicality*.
2. Poorly-differentiated SCC: more aggressive and infiltrating, less pale and glassy, fewer keratin pearls, *more severe atypicality*.
3. Adenoid SCC (acantholytic SCC, pseudoglandular SCC): considered an aggressive subtype. Gland-like changes, often due to *acantholysis* (1.2), may resemble an adenocarcinoma or sweat gland carcinoma but does not contain mucin and is CEAneg. About 70% of sweat gland carcinomas are S-100+, unlike adenoid SCC.
4. Adenosquamous cell carcinoma (mucoepidermoid carcinoma): very rare aggressive subtype of SCC as primary tumor in skin, more common in salivary glands, respiratory tract, and nasal mucosa. Goblet cells contain bluish mucin (positive for Alcian blue, PAS-D, and CEA), similar to sweat gland carcinomas (23.13), but unlike adenoid SCC.
5. Spindle cell SCC: aggressive subtype, prominent spindle cells, less keratinization; may be confused with other spindle cell tumors (1.131). Spindle cells may be positive for both vimentin and cytokeratin, whereas most tumor cells of ordinary SCC are negative for vimentin.
6. Verrucous carcinoma: *massive well-differentiated verrucous* proliferations usually related to human papillomavirus (14.1), including oral florid papillomatosis of the mouth, giant condyloma of Buschke–Lowenstein of the genitals, epithelioma cuniculatum of the soles, and subungual keratoacanthomas. Clinically slowly growing, locally invasive, typically does not metastasize unless irradiated. Histology has verrucous, well-differentiated SCC; pushing invasive border, but *very little atypia*. Differentiation from just a huge verruca may be an artificial distinction, and depends upon the threshold of the clinician and pathologist (viewing a deep enough biopsy) deciding that it is just too thick to be a verruca.
7. Lymphoepithelioma-like carcinoma of the skin: very rare, resembles nasopharyngeal carcinoma, *islands of squamous cells obscured by dense lymphocytic inflammatory nodules*, sometimes forming germinal centers. Sometimes keratin stains are needed to identify the squamous areas. Do not confuse with lymphadenoma (18.14).

Differential diagnosis

1. Pseudoepitheliomatous hyperplasia (PEH, 1.116): less atypia, look for another reason for its presence (wound site, acid fast bacilli or fungus infection, etc.). It is often present immediately above dermal fibrosis with more jagged edges than SCC. Elastic fibers jabbing into the epithelium can be a clue for PEH, but also can be seen with KA.
2. Pilar tumor (22.4): cystic localized subcutaneous nodule of scalp; some of these may indeed be SCC.
3. Irritated seborrheic keratosis (18.2): more stuck-on horizontal growth pattern, less atypia.
4. Keratoacanthoma (18.12): most probably really are a variant of SCC.
5. Hyperkeratotic actinic keratosis (18.8): no invasion of the dermis (the criteria for true invasion vary by the author).
6. Other irritated benign squamous neoplasms in this chapter, irritated adnexal neoplasms (Chapters 21 and 23) and other epithelioid neoplasms (1.38).

18.12 Keratoacanthoma (KA)

(see Fig. 18.12A,B)

Common volcano nodule or plaque that sometimes *erupts rapidly* over several weeks, usually on *sun-damaged skin*, with a keratin-filled *crater* in the center, capable of *resolving spontaneously*, so traditionally considered to be a pseudomalignancy (1.118). Most KAs are really a subtype of SCC, and rare reports of metastasis probably involved this type of KA. For most solitary lesions, this author prefers the designation of "SCC (KA type)". KAs may have some association with human papillomavirus.

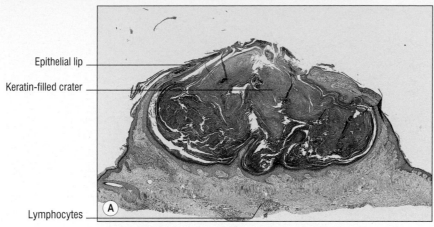

Epithelial lip

Keratin-filled crater

Lymphocytes

Fig. 18.12 A Keratoacanthoma (low mag.).

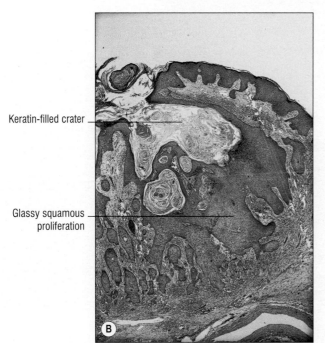

Keratin-filled crater

Glassy squamous proliferation

Fig. 18.12 B Keratoacanthoma (high mag.).

P
- Keratin-filled crater
- Pale, eosinophilic, glassy, well-differentiated epithelial proliferation, often with lips extending over both sides of crater, often with squamous eddies or keratin pearls (1.134)
- Sometimes microabscesses of neutrophils within the epithelium (1.117)
- Cytologic atypia of keratinocytes no more than mild
- Elastic fibers sometimes found within epithelium of base of lesion
- Perivascular or lichenoid infiltrate of lymphocytes, sometimes with eosinophils or plasma cells

Variations

1. Multiple KAs of Ferguson Smith: onset in childhood or adolescence, no more than a dozen lesions that may become large like solitary KAs.
2. Multiple eruptive KAs of Grzybowski: onset in adulthood, hundreds of 2–3-mm KAs, sometimes a mask facies.
3. Subungual KA: can invade bone under the nail. Most likely is a verrucous carcinoma (18.11).
4. Muir–Torre syndrome (21.3): sebaceous neoplasms plus KA.

Differential diagnosis

1. Well-differentiated SCC (18.11). While it is traditional for some texts to outline extensive criteria for distinguishing KAs from SCCs, most KAs are SCC variants, and the only reliable distinguishing feature of the benign type of KA from SCC is KAs capability to resolve spontaneously. When in doubt, consider a KA to be SCC, rather than waiting for spontaneous resolution that may never occur! Rapid growth and the keratin-filled crater can also occur in SCC. Diagnosis of KA is more certain in examples of the multiple KA syndrome variants. If atypia is more than mild, it is unwise to call a lesion a KA.
2. Other diseases with pseudoepitheliomatous hyperplasia (1.116).

18.13 Paget's disease

(see Fig. 18.13A–F)

Uncommon, *red scaly plaque* of *nipple* (1.90), breast, or axilla (1.10). Clinically resembles eczema, contact dermatitis, or Bowen's disease. Mammary Paget's disease has a nearly 100% association with intraductal breast cancer. *Extramammary Paget's disease* occurs on the groin (1.55), perianal (1.108), scrotum (1.126), or vulva (1.149), only 50% chance of an underlying carcinoma, unlike Paget's disease of the breast.

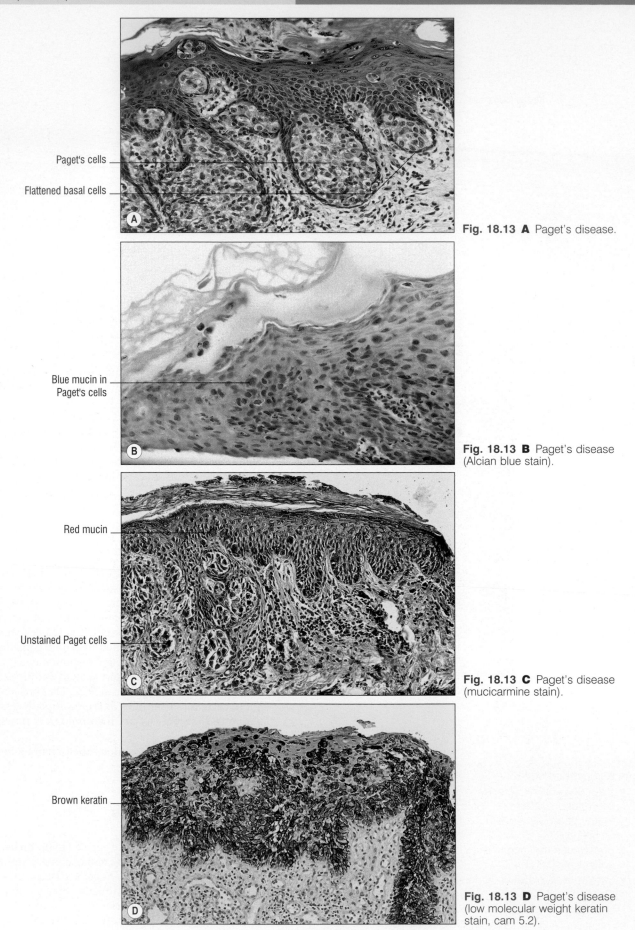

Paget's cells

Flattened basal cells

Fig. 18.13 A Paget's disease.

Blue mucin in Paget's cells

Fig. 18.13 B Paget's disease (Alcian blue stain).

Red mucin

Unstained Paget cells

Fig. 18.13 C Paget's disease (mucicarmine stain).

Brown keratin

Fig. 18.13 D Paget's disease (low molecular weight keratin stain, cam 5.2).

Parakeratosis

Keratinocyte

Pagetoid cell

Lymphocytes

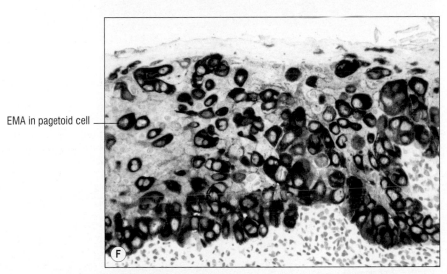

Fig. 18.13 E Paget disease of the breast.

EMA in pagetoid cell

Fig. 18.13 F Paget disease of the breast (EMA stain).

- *Pale staining Paget's cells* (often with atypical nuclei) scattered throughout the epidermis. Groups of them may compress and flatten the basal cells. May appear multifocal with skip areas
- Usually no dyskeratosis (1.27), unlike Bowen's disease
- Paget's cells usually positive for CEA, EMA, low molecular weight keratin such as keratin-8-18 (such as cam 5.2) or keratin-7, PAS with and without diastase, Alcian blue, and mucicarmine
- Gross cystic disease fluid protein is often positive, except in those cases where there is internal malignancy
- Underlying adenocarcinoma sometimes seen within the dermis

Differential diagnosis

1. Other diseases with epidermotropism or pagetoid cells (1.37) or clear cell lesions (1.22), especially Bowen's disease (18.10), and melanoma (20.11). As a practical point, Paget's disease and extramammary Paget's disease is not a consideration unless located on breast, axilla, groin, or genitals. S-100 more often positive in melanoma but sometimes positive in Paget's disease. Melanoma is negative for EMA and keratin staining, and often positive for HMB-45 or MART-1. Bowen's disease is negative for CK7, EMA, CEA, yet positive for high molecular weight keratins.

2. Toker cells are benign clear cells of the nipple which can be mistaken for Paget's disease. They are CK7+ but CEAneg and mucin stain negative.

18.14 Basal cell carcinoma (BCC)

(see Fig. 18.14A–I)

The most common type of skin cancer, usually slowly growing, occurs in 1 in 6 Americans. *Pearly* red macule, papule, nodule, or plaque, most common on *sun-exposed skin*, especially the nose (1.95), face (1.44), and ears (1.28). Telangiectasia over the neoplasm is often emphasized, but is not so helpful because these sun-damaged patients often have many telangiectasias from the sun in normal skin and over other lesions such as nevi. Rarely BCC arises in unusual sun-covered areas, such as the vulva. *Often annular* (1.5) with a *rolled up edge*. Sometimes ulcerated (1.142). BCC almost never metastasizes, but sometimes can be locally destructive. The

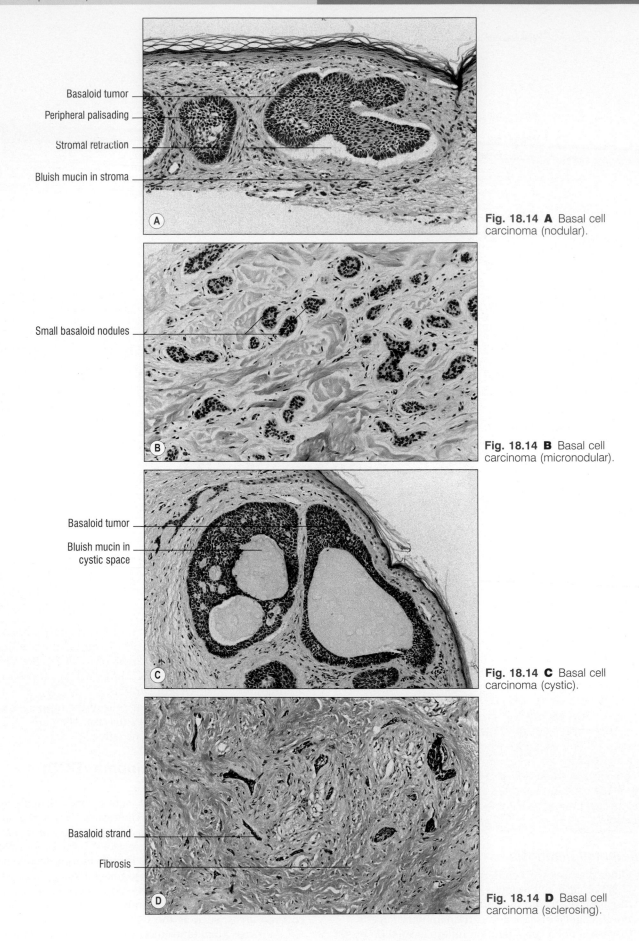

Basaloid tumor

Peripheral palisading

Stromal retraction

Bluish mucin in stroma

Fig. 18.14 A Basal cell carcinoma (nodular).

Small basaloid nodules

Fig. 18.14 B Basal cell carcinoma (micronodular).

Basaloid tumor

Bluish mucin in cystic space

Fig. 18.14 C Basal cell carcinoma (cystic).

Basaloid strand

Fibrosis

Fig. 18.14 D Basal cell carcinoma (sclerosing).

Stromal retraction

Basaloid proliferation

Squamoid proliferation

Keratin

Solar elastosis

Fig. 18.14 E Basosquamous cell carcinoma.

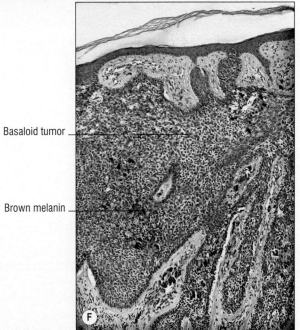

Basaloid tumor

Brown melanin

Fig. 18.14 F Basal cell carcinoma (pigmented).

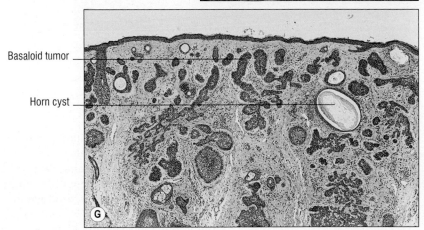

Basaloid tumor

Horn cyst

Fig. 18.14 G Basal cell carcinoma (keratotic).

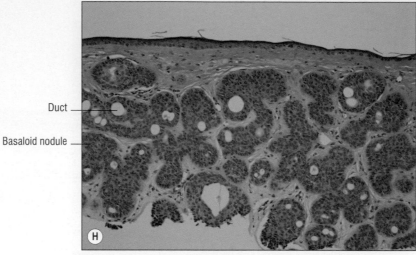

Fig. 18.14 H Basal cell carcinoma with eccrine differentiation (eccrine epithelioma) (courtesy Kenneth Tsai MD PhD).

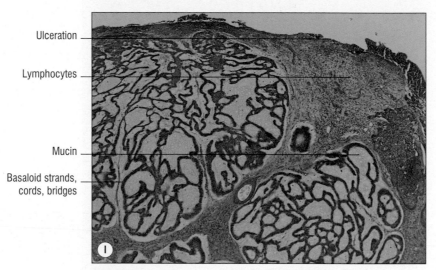

Fig. 18.14 I Basal cell carcinoma with adamantinoid pattern.

old name *basal cell epithelioma* uses the word epithelioma to mean a low-grade carcinoma.

- Ulceration of epidermis sometimes (1.142)
- *Basaloid tumor cells* budding from epidermis or follicles, or within the dermis, with variable atypia
- *Retraction artifact* (1.23, stroma separates from tumor lobules) often
- *Peripheral palisading* of nuclei often
- *Mucin* (1.83) in the stroma or within basaloid aggregates often
- *Solar elastosis* in the dermis (9.1)
- Perineural invasion in some aggressive forms (less often than in SCC)
- Variable infiltrate of lymphocytes, plasma cells, rarely lymphoid follicles around the tumor

Variations

1. Superficial BCC: small buds of basaloid tumor cells extending from epidermis.
2. Nodular BCC: solid basaloid tumor islands.
3. Cystic BCC: cystic space within tumor nodules, usually due to necrosis or mucin production.
4. Adenoid BCC: net-like or pseudoglandular pattern, often much mucin within basaloid aggregates. Do not confuse the name with adenocystic carcinoma (23.13) or adenoid cystic carcinoma (23.13).
5. Sclerosing (morpheaform, infiltrating) BCC: may resemble a scar clinically, more likely to be infiltrating or aggressive, thin strands of invasive basaloid cells in a fibrotic stroma.
6. Metatypical BCC (basosquamous carcinoma): combined features of basal and squamous cell carcinoma.
7. Pigmented BCC: more in darkly pigmented races, melanin and melanocytes within tumor.

8. BCC with sweat gland differentiation (eccrine epithelioma): areas of sweat gland differentiation.

9. BCC with sebaceous differentiation (sebaceous epithelioma): areas of sebaceous gland differentiation (21.4).

10. BCC with follicular differentiation (infundibulocystic BCC, keratotic BCC): horn cysts (1.59) or other follicular features present, suggesting follicular differentiation, may resemble a trichoepithelioma, SCC, or basosquamous carcinoma.

11. Fibroepithelioma of Pinkus: red plaque on the trunk, *net-like pattern* of thin anastomosing basaloid cells in a loose stroma, multiple connections to epidermis.

12. Nevoid BCC syndrome (basal cell nevus syndrome, Gorlin syndrome): *autosomal dominant* disease related to the patched (PTC) gene on chromosome 9, numerous BCCs may start in childhood, BCCs may resemble skin tags or brown nevi, palmoplantar pits (1.100), calcifications of the falx cerebri, bifid ribs (1.16), frontal bossing, hypertelorism, sometimes mental retardation, odontogenic keratocysts of the jaw, systemic malignancy.

13. Basaloid hyperplasia associated with dermatofibromas (27.1) or nevus sebaceus (21.2): whether these are true BCCs is debated.

14. Linear basal cell nevus: epidermal nevus variant (18.1) that is congenital and linear, but looks identical to BCC.

15. Linear BCC: clinically linear (1.73), no differences histologically.

16. Pleomorphic BCC[127] (giant cell BCC, BCC with monster cells): huge, impressive atypical cells, sometimes multinucleated, with no difference in clinical behavior.

17. Granular cell BCC:[142] granular cytoplasm, no different clinical significance.

18. Clear cell BCC (signet-ring BCC): clear cells (1.22) due to glycogen, no different clinical significance.

19. Follicular BCC: BCC arises from a follicle, and may clinically resemble a harmless comedo.

20. Adamantinoid BCC: rare, resembles adamantinoma of long bones or ameloblastoma (see below), thin connecting strands of stellate basaloid cells with amphophilic intercellular material and a fibromyxoid stroma.

21. Lymphadenoma: basaloid lobules in the dermis (pankeratin stain positive), with T and B lymphocytes within the lobules (stain with CD45). It might be considered to be a *calzone stuffed with lymphocytes*, with a shell of basaloid cells. Do not confuse with lymphoepithelioma-like carcinoma of the skin (18.11), which is an SCC variant in which the lymphocytic aggregates are mainly all around small squamous islands.

22. Bazex syndrome: rare, autosomal dominant, follicular atrophoderma (10.5), hypotrichosis, hypohidrosis, and facial BCCs. Don't confuse with the completely different paraneoplastic Bazex syndrome (acrokeratosis paraneoplastica, 2.15).

23. Rombo syndrome: rare, atrophoderma vermiculata (10.5), hypotrichosis, blepharitis, acneiform lesions, trichoepithelioma, BCCs, peripheral vasodilatation.

Differential diagnosis

1. Squamous cell carcinoma: epithelioid cells with more eosinophilic keratinizing cytoplasm (1.38), keratin pearls, occasionally more spindle cells (1.131). Ber-EP4 and bcl-2 are positive in BCC and negative in SCC.

2. Ameloblastoma: BCC-like benign but invasive neoplasm of odontogenic epithelium in the mouth (1.82).

3. Cloacogenic carcinoma: BCC-like malignancy of the anus that can metastasize.

4. Trichoepithelioma and trichoblastoma (22.2).

5. Other adnexal neoplasms (Chapters 21 and 23): sweat gland neoplasms more likely to be positive for CEA, EMA, or CD117.

6. Folliculocentric basaloid proliferation[85] (FBP, funny looking follicles): usually more vertically oriented, pinwheel-like extensions, not highly invasive.

7. BCC-like changes may occur in nevus sebaceus (21.2) and dermatofibroma (27.1). Some of these may be real BCCs, and others are not.

8. Other tumors with basaloid cells (1.11) or small cell tumors (1.130).

CHAPTER **19**

Cysts

A cyst is a walled-off cavity filled with keratin, mucin, or fluid, and a list of cystic lesions other than those in this chapter appears in Section 1.25. Most true cysts have an epithelial lining, but some, such as the digital mucous cyst or oral mucocele, do not. Cutaneous and subcutaneous cysts are classified on the basis of their location, contents, type of epithelial lining, and whether adnexa are attached to the wall. Although many physicians refer to all cysts as "sebaceous cysts", because they erroneously think the white cheesy material inside them is sebaceous rather than keratinous, only the steatocystoma (19.5) is a true sebaceous cyst. Surgeons have more important things to do than classify cysts; dermatopathologists rename them all so that we have at least 13 types, many of which have additional synonyms. Many of the cysts in this chapter may rupture and produce a mixed granulomatous infiltrate (1.51) with neutrophils, lymphocytes, histiocytes, plasma cells, or multinucleated giant cells. This does not necessarily mean infection, but secondary infection, particularly with *Staphylococcus*, can also occur.

19.1 Epidermoid cyst (epidermal inclusion cyst, follicular infundibular cyst)

(see Fig. 19.1)
Very common cyst found almost anywhere on the skin, especially head, neck, and trunk.

P
- Cyst contains lamellated keratin
- Cyst lined by squamous epithelium, sometimes flattened, with a granular layer

Variations

1. Milium (plural is milia): very small epidermoid cyst, less than 3 mm. Do not confuse with miliaria (10.6).
2. Hybrid cyst: part of the wall has a granular layer like an epidermoid cyst, while part of it lacks a granular cyst like a pilar cyst (19.2).
3. Gardner's syndrome: autosomal dominant paraneoplastic syndrome (1.105) of epidermoid cysts, lipomas (29.2), osteomas (29.8), pilomatricomas (22.3), desmoids (27.15), intestinal polyposis, and colorectal adenocarcinoma (1.49).

Differential diagnosis

1. Other cystic lesions (1.25).

©2012 Elsevier Ltd, Inc, BV
DOI: 10.1016/B978-0-323-06658-7.00019-1

19.2 Pilar cyst (trichilemmal cyst, isthmus-catagen cyst, wen)

(see Fig. 19.2A,B)
Common cyst, usually on the *scalp* (1.124).

P
- Cyst contains amorphous, dense and compact, *homogenized keratin*
- Cyst lined by squamous epithelium. The keratinocytes are often pale, and there is no *granular layer*
- *Calcification common* within the cyst (1.19)

Differential diagnosis

1. Proliferating pilar cyst (22.4), pilomatricoma (22.3).
2. Epidermoid cyst (19.1).

19.3 Dermoid cyst

(see Fig. 19.3)
Uncommon *congenital* cyst, especially on the *lateral eyebrow* (1.42), may extend into bone.

P
- Cyst contains lamellated keratin and *often hair shafts*
- Cyst lined by squamous epithelium with a *granular layer*
- Multiple *hair follicles open into the cyst*, sometimes with sebaceous glands or sweat glands

19.4 Vellus hair cyst

(see Fig. 19.4)
Uncommon small solitary cyst, or *multiple on the chest of children* (eruptive vellus hair cysts), *may spontaneously resolve.*

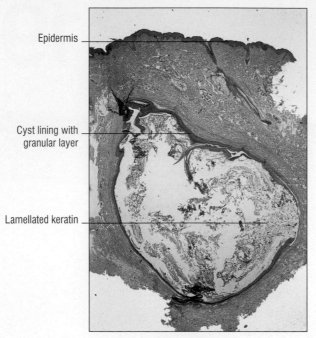

Epidermis

Cyst lining with
granular layer

Lamellated keratin

Fig. 19.1 Epidermoid cyst.

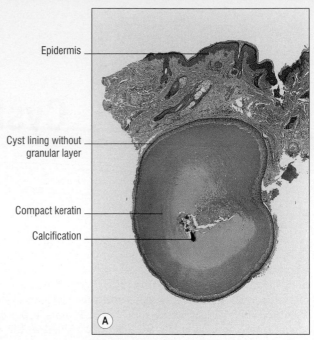

Epidermis

Cyst lining without
granular layer

Compact keratin

Calcification

Ⓐ

Fig. 19.2 A Pilar cyst (low mag.).

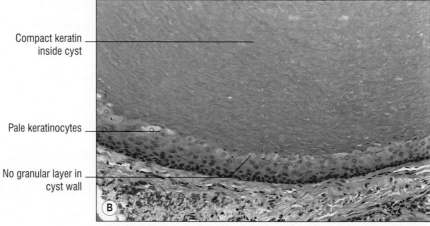

Compact keratin
inside cyst

Pale keratinocytes

No granular layer in
cyst wall

Ⓑ

Fig. 19.2 B Pilar cyst (high mag.).

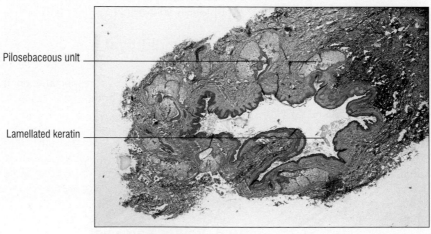

Pilosebaceous unit

Lamellated keratin

Fig. 19.3 Dermoid cyst.

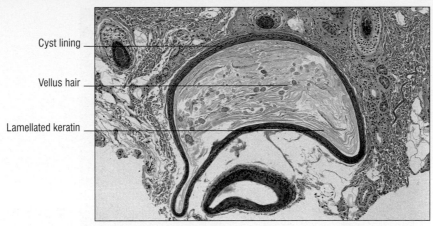

Cyst lining ⎯

Vellus hair ⎯

Lamellated keratin ⎯

Fig. 19.4 Vellus hair cyst.

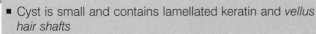
- Cyst is small and contains lamellated keratin and *vellus hair shafts*
- Cyst lined by squamous epithelium with a granular layer
- Hair follicles sometimes attached to cyst

Differential diagnosis

1. Trichofolliculoma (22.1): usually solitary multiple vellus follicles open into larger mother follicle.
2. Trichostasis spinulosa (22.7): clinically inapparent as an incidental finding, such as within nevi, or presenting as open comedones (blackheads). Histologically looks like a plugged follicle opening to the surface with numerous vellus hairs, rather than a cyst.
3. Steatocystoma (19.5): sometimes small like vellus hair cyst, has sebaceous glands in wall, eosinophilic cuticle.
4. Milium: small, like vellus hair cyst, but usually has no vellus hairs.

19.5 **Steatocystoma**

(see Fig. 19.5A,B)
Uncommon, usually on the trunk (1.141), head, neck (1.86), or earlobes (1.28), *contains yellowish oily lipid material* and keratin, *the only "true" sebaceous cyst.*

- Cyst may contain sparse keratin or hair shafts, but frequently *appears empty* because the oily sebaceous fluid dissolves during processing
- Cyst wall consists of ruggated squamous epithelium with a *wrinkled crenulated eosinophilic refractile cuticle* of keratin instead of a granular layer
- *Sebaceous glands* within or adjacent to the cyst wall, opening into the cyst

Variations

1. Steatocystoma simplex: solitary lesion.
2. Steatocystoma multiplex: multiple lesions, mutation in keratin 17 gene, the same gene defect found in some forms of pachyonychia congenita.

19.6 **Cervical thymic cyst**

Rare cyst of the neck (1.86) or anterior mediastinum.

- Cyst is often *multilocular and appears empty* because fluid washes out during processing
- Cyst wall varies from cuboidal, ciliated, and non-ciliated columnar to squamous epithelium
- Thymic tissue (aggregates of immature and mature lymphocytes) with *Hassall's corpuscles* (concentrically hyalinized collection of degenerating cells of 20–50 microns, sometimes calcified)
- Cholesterol clefts and granulomatous inflammation common

Differential diagnosis

1. The lymphoid proliferation in thymic cysts can resemble a lymph node. Hassall's corpuscles may rarely resemble squamous eddies of a metastatic squamous cell carcinoma (18.11).

19.7 **Cutaneous ciliated cyst**

Rare cyst, often on the sole (1.100), lower extremity, or buttock of women.

- Cyst usually appears empty because fluid runs out after biopsy
- Cyst lining consists of cuboidal or columnar *ciliated epithelium*, without goblet (mucin-secreting) cells

Differential diagnosis

1. Cilia may also be seen in bronchogenic, branchial cleft, thymic, and thyroglossal duct cysts.

19.8 **Thyroglossal duct cyst**

(see Fig. 19.8A–C)
Uncommon cyst, usually on the *midline of neck* (1.86), moves during swallowing.

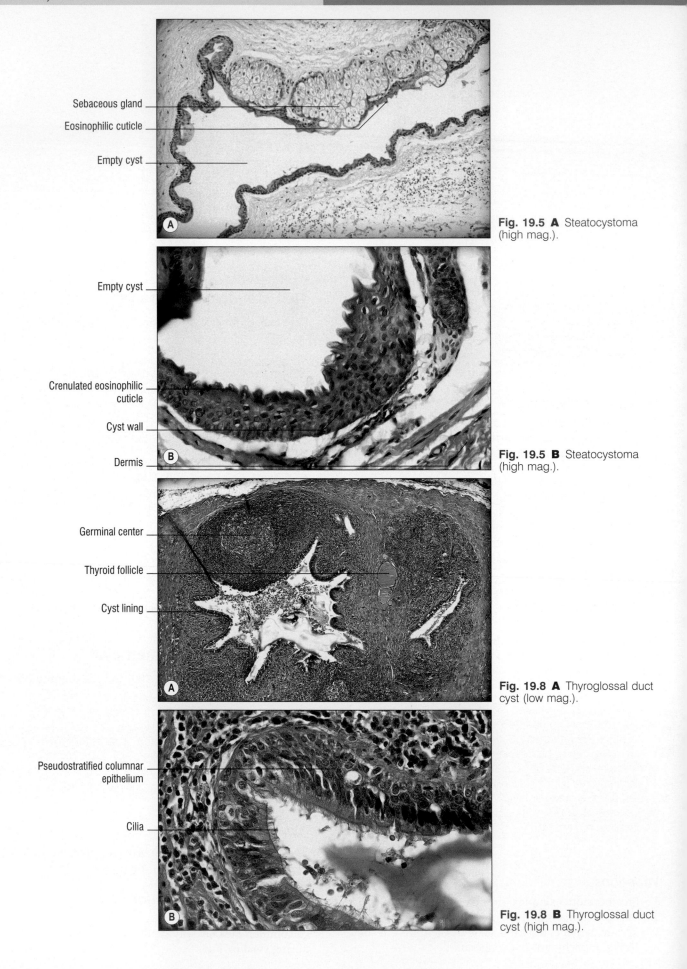

Sebaceous gland

Eosinophilic cuticle

Empty cyst

Fig. 19.5 A Steatocystoma (high mag.).

Empty cyst

Crenulated eosinophilic cuticle

Cyst wall

Dermis

Fig. 19.5 B Steatocystoma (high mag.).

Germinal center

Thyroid follicle

Cyst lining

Fig. 19.8 A Thyroglossal duct cyst (low mag.).

Pseudostratified columnar epithelium

Cilia

Fig. 19.8 B Thyroglossal duct cyst (high mag.).

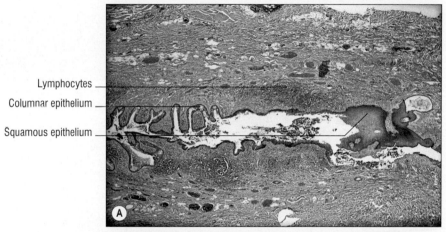

Thyroid follicle

Fig. 19.8 C Thyroglossal duct cyst (high mag.).

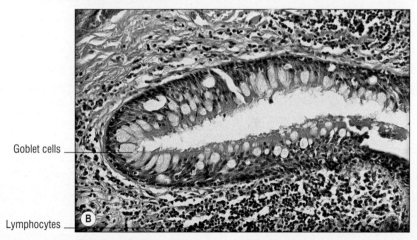

Lymphocytes

Columnar epithelium

Squamous epithelium

Fig. 19.9 A Branchial cleft cyst (low mag.).

Goblet cells

Lymphocytes

Fig. 19.9 B Branchial cleft cyst (high mag.).

P
- Cyst contains keratin or mucin
- Cyst lining varies from pseudostratified columnar (with or without goblet cells or cilia) to squamous epithelium. No smooth muscle, mucous glands, or cartilage adjacent to lining
- *Thyroid follicles or lymphoid follicles* may be present

P
- Cyst contains laminated keratin
- Sinus tract or cyst lined by squamous epithelium with a granular layer, or by columnar epithelium with or without cilia or goblet (mucus-secreting) cells
- Cyst often surrounded by *lymphoid follicles*

19.9 Branchial cleft cyst

(see Fig. 19.9A,B)
Uncommon cysts of the preauricular area, jaw, or lateral neck (1.86).

Differential diagnosis

1. Lymphoid follicles are often seen in lymph nodes, lymphocytoma cutis (24.14), thyroglossal duct cyst, thymic cyst, and bronchogenic cyst.

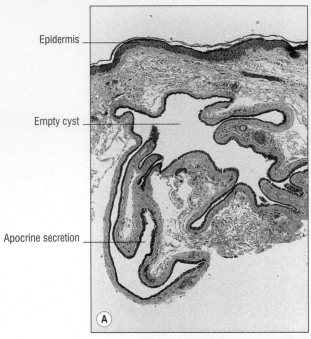

Fig. 19.11 A Apocrine hidrocystoma (low mag.).

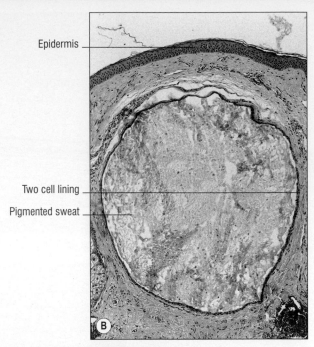

Fig. 19.11 B Apocrine hidrocystoma (pigmented).

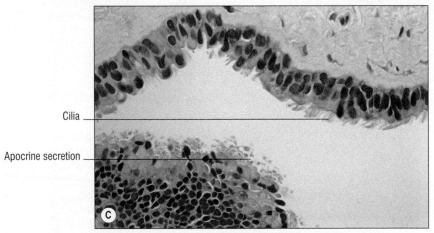

Fig. 19.11 C Apocrine hidrocystoma (high mag.).

19.10 Bronchogenic cyst

Uncommon cyst most common on the neck (1.86), especially the *suprasternal notch*.

P
- Cyst contains keratin or mucin
- Cyst lining varies from pseudostratified columnar (with or without goblet cells or cilia) to squamous epithelium
- Lining may be surrounded by mucous glands, *smooth muscle*, *lymphoid follicles*, or *cartilage*

19.11 Hidrocystoma (cystadenoma)

(see Fig. 19.11A–C)
Common translucent to bluish cyst, most common on eyelids (1.43), occasionally elsewhere, usually solitary, sometimes multiple.

P
- *Cyst appears empty* because fluid leaks out
- Cyst lined by thin cuboidal or columnar epithelium (often *two layers of cells*)

Variations

1. Apocrine hidrocystoma: apocrine decapitation secretion may be present; cyst more likely to be a neoplasm and is often *multiloculated*. Much more common than eccrine. The difference between apocrine and eccrine may not be so important.
2. Eccrine hidrocystoma: more likely to be a unilocular retention of sweat in a dilated duct or gland rather than a cystic neoplasm, no decapitation secretion. Sometimes found in areas of scar, such as cicatricial alopecia.

19.12 Median raphe cyst of the penis

Rare small cyst on the *midline ventral aspect of the penis* shaft (1.107).

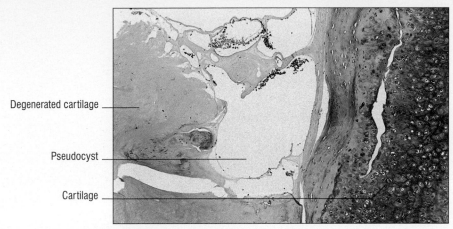

Degenerated cartilage

Pseudocyst

Cartilage

Fig. 19.13 Auricular pseudocyst.

 P
- Cyst appears empty because fluid leaks out after biopsy
- Cyst lined by pseudostratified columnar epithelium

- Intracartilaginous cystic space with degenerated cartilage and amorphous eosinophilic material
- Fibrosis, granulation tissue, or granulomatous inflammation may be present
P

19.13 Auricular pseudocyst
(see Fig. 19.13)
Tender cystic swelling of cartilaginous portion of the ear, usually in young males with trauma.

Differential diagnosis
1. Chondrodermatitis nodularis helicis (17.9).
2. Relapsing polychondritis (17.8).

CHAPTER 20

Melanocytic Neoplasms

20.1 Freckle (ephelis, plural is ephelides)

Very common multiple *red–brown macules* (1.18) on face (1.44) and shoulders, often genetically inherited in *fair-skinned patients*, especially those with red hair. Lesions darken easily with sun exposure.

P
- Increased melanin in basal layer
- Normal or decreased number of more active melanocytes
- No elongation of rete ridges or nesting of melanocytes

Differential diagnosis

1. Café-au-lait spot (20.2), lentigo simplex (20.3) and solar lentigo (20.4).

20.2 Café-au-lait spot (café-au-lait macule, CALM)

(see Fig. 20.2)
Common in normal individuals (10% of the population), *light brown macule* (1.18), larger than the average lentigo or freckle, French for "coffee with milk", sometimes associated with neurofibromatosis (26.1).

P
- Increased melanin in the basal layer
- Normal number of melanocytes (number of cells said to be normal but just more active at synthesizing increased melanin). This is the usual statement, but an increased number of melanocytes has been reported in NF-1 CALMs, so this dogma may not be so clear
- No elongation of rete ridges or nesting of melanocytes
- Macromelanosomes seen with electron microscopy have often been emphasized, but these are also seen in benign lentigo, melanocytic nevi, and other melanocytic proliferations

Variation

1. McCune–Albright syndrome (Albright syndrome, not to be confused with Albright's hereditary osteodystrophy, 29.8): *unilateral brown macule* with more *irregular jagged border* like the coast of Maine instead of the coast of California seen with the ordinarily lighter CALM, *polyostotic fibrous dysplasia* (1.16) often on same side of the body, *precocious puberty* in females, brown macules identical to café-au-lait spot histologically. Associated with embryonic post-zygotic somatic activating mutations in the GNAS1 gene.

Differential diagnosis

1. Freckles (20.1) are usually smaller, different clinically, but similar histologically.
2. Lentigo simplex (20.3) and solar lentigo (20.4) are different clinically, and usually have an increased number of melanocytes in elongated rete ridges.
3. Melasma and some other pigmented conditions may be nearly identical and impossible to distinguish without clinical information (17.10).

20.3 Lentigo simplex

(see Fig. 20.3A–C)
Common *brown macule* (1.18), especially on dorsum of forearms, usually less than 5 mm, and onset in children or young adults *unrelated to sun*. Lentigines is the plural of lentigo.

P
- Hyperpigmented, often elongated rete ridges, usually with increased melanocytes
- No nests of melanocytes
- No solar elastosis

Variations

1. Multiple lentigines (LEOPARD syndrome): *A*utosomal dominant, *L*entigines beginning in infancy, *E*lectrocardiographic conduction defects (1.57), *O*cular hypertelorism, *P*ulmonary stenosis, *A*bnormal genitalia, *R*etardation of growth, and neural *D*eafness. Not all of these features are present in any given case. Mutation in PTPN11 or RAF1 genes.
2. Peutz–Jeghers syndrome: autosomal dominant, brown macules on the *lips* (1.74) oral mucosa, or dorsal fingers, associated with *small bowel polyposis* (1.49) that is sometimes premalignant (1.105). Mutation related to serine/threonine kinase STK11 gene.
3. Becker's nevus (pigmented hairy epidermal nevus): *unilateral large pigmented hairy patch or plaque*, usually on

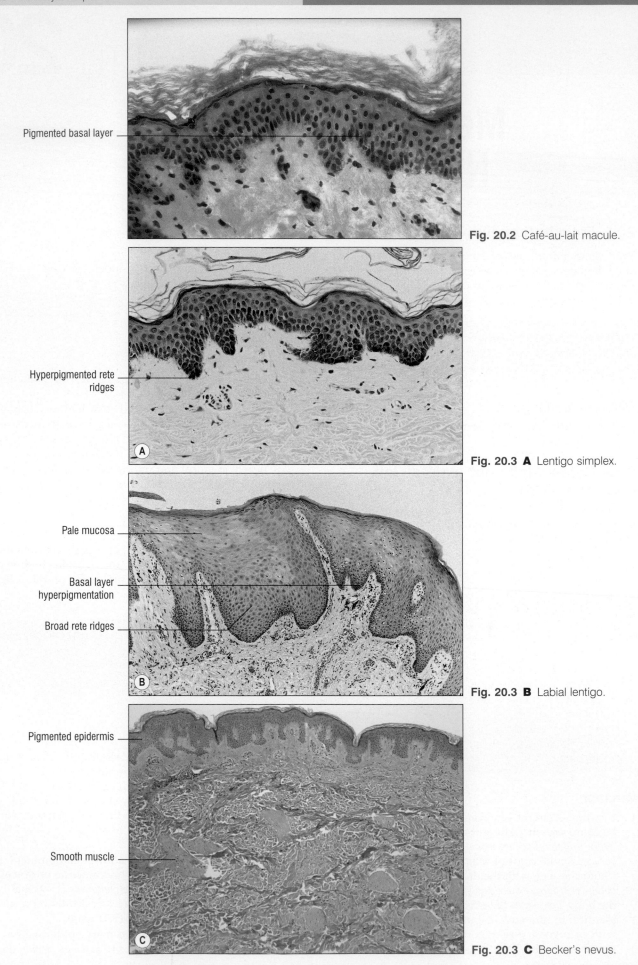

Pigmented basal layer

Fig. 20.2 Café-au-lait macule.

Hyperpigmented rete ridges

Fig. 20.3 A Lentigo simplex.

Pale mucosa

Basal layer hyperpigmentation

Broad rete ridges

Fig. 20.3 B Labial lentigo.

Pigmented epidermis

Smooth muscle

Fig. 20.3 C Becker's nevus.

the *shoulder* (1.141), *onset in adolescence*, may have epidermal papillomatosis-like epidermal nevus (18.1), *increased hair follicles or smooth muscle* (29.6) may be present.

4. Labial lentigo (labial melanotic macule): brown *lip* (1.74) macule, *rete ridges are broader*, and melanin usually stays limited to basal layer.
5. NAME and LAMB syndrome, Carney complex (27.17).
6. Melanonychia striata: brown longitudinal lentigo beneath the *nail* (1.85).
7. Laugier–Hunziker syndrome: melanonychia striata (1.85), lentigines of lips (1.74) or buccal mucosa, somewhat like Peutz–Jeghers syndrome.
8. Lentiginosis: *many clustered lesions of lentigo simplex*, especially common on the genital regions (1.107) or other areas.
9. Ink-spot lentigo: clinical term for black macule less than 5 mm in diameter, appearing like ink on skin with irregular borders, causes clinical concern regarding melanoma.

Differential diagnosis

1. Junctional nevus (20.5) may show features of lentigo simplex, but nests of melanocytes occur. Transitional lesions between the two occur, and have been called nevus incipiens or lentigo.
2. Solar lentigo (20.4) usually has more elongation of rete ridges and solar elastosis.
3. Ephelis (20.1): more orange–brown, more readily become darker with sun exposure.

20.4 Solar lentigo

(see Fig. 20.4)
Very common *brown macule* (1.18) *due to sun damage*, especially on the face (1.44) and dorsum of hands (1.56), often multiple, more in older adults. PUVA (psoralen plus ultraviolet A light) lentigines are often large and numerous, and are due to PUVA therapy.

- *Hyperpigmented basal layer*, often with elongated, clubbed rete ridges ("dirty feet"), usually with increased melanocytes
- No nests of melanocytes
- *Solar elastosis*

Differential diagnosis

1. Pigmented actinic keratosis (18.8): keratinocyte atypia, parakeratosis, hyperkeratosis, dyskeratosis.
2. Lentigo maligna (20.11): darker brown–black, asymmetrical variegated pigment pattern, notched or irregular border, epidermal atrophy or loss of rete ridges, atypical melanocytes, pagetoid cells, and lymphocytic infiltrate.
3. Lentigo simplex (20.3): smaller lesions, onset earlier in life, no solar elastosis, usually somewhat less rete ridge elongation.

20.5 Melanocytic nevus (poor synonyms: common mole, nevocellular nevus)

(see Fig. 20.5A–K)
Very common lesions with clinical presentation depending upon the specific type, found almost anywhere at any age. When the word "nevus" is used without an adjective, usually "melanocytic" is assumed, but really "melanocytic nevus" is more precise since there are many other non-melanocytic nevi (nevus sebaceus, epidermal nevus, eccrine nevus, etc). Some non-dermatologists assume any pigmented lesion is "nevus". The word "nevus" has actually been used for a variety of (a) hamartomas, and (b) congenital lesions, even though only less than 1% of melanocytic nevi are congenital.

- Epidermal changes vary greatly: atrophy (1.9), hyperplasia 1 (1.61), papillomatosis (1.102), or horn cysts (1.59) may be present
- *Nests (theques)* or cords of melanocytes ("nevus cells") at the dermal–epidermal junction or in the dermis. Nevus cells vary greatly in size and shape, and melanin may or may not be present (melanin most likely to be present in junctional nests or upper dermal nests). *Type A nevus cells* are usually present in the junctional zone or superficial dermis, and appear epithelioid (more cytoplasm, larger, pale nucleus). *Type B nevus cells* are usually present in the mid-dermis and resemble lymphocytes (less cytoplasm, small dark nucleus). *Type C nevus cells* are usually present in the deeper dermis; they are more spindled and have considerable pink cytoplasm, and may form neuroid structures. A fourth type of nevus cell is the nevus multinucleated giant cell (1.84). These are usually more prevalent in the superficial dermis and have clumped nuclei, but sometime they exhibit a rosette of nuclei
- Usually *no inflammation*, unless the lesion is irritated

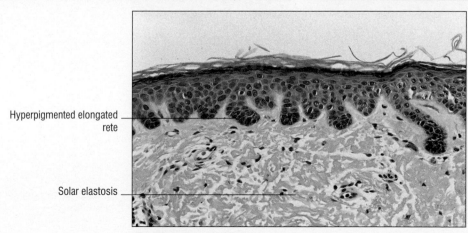
Hyperpigmented elongated rete

Solar elastosis

Fig. 20.4 Solar lentigo.

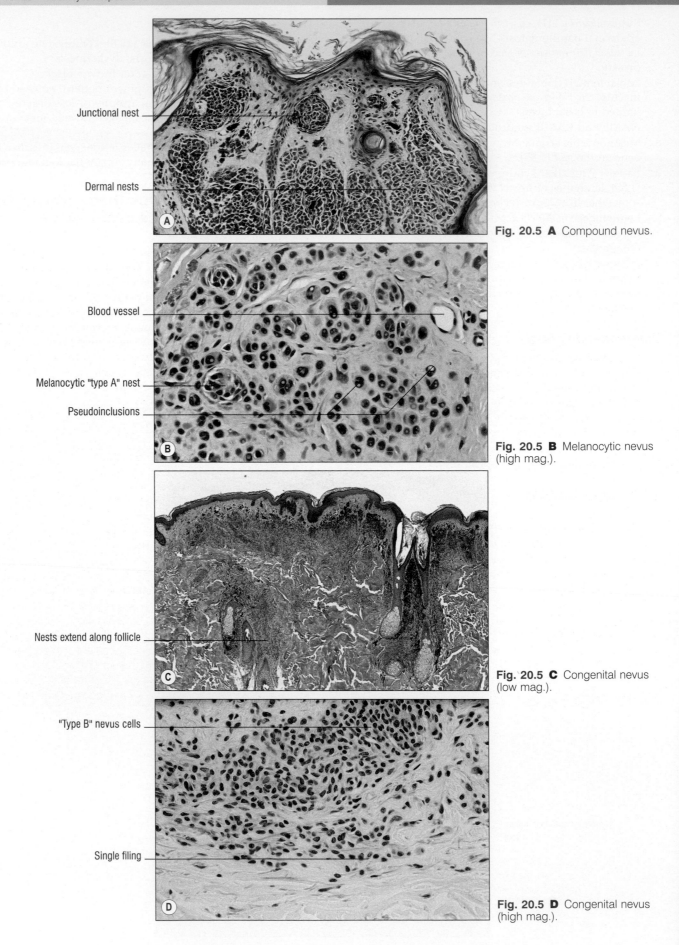

Junctional nest

Dermal nests

Fig. 20.5 A Compound nevus.

Blood vessel

Melanocytic "type A" nest

Pseudoinclusions

Fig. 20.5 B Melanocytic nevus (high mag.).

Nests extend along follicle

Fig. 20.5 C Congenital nevus (low mag.).

"Type B" nevus cells

Single filing

Fig. 20.5 D Congenital nevus (high mag.).

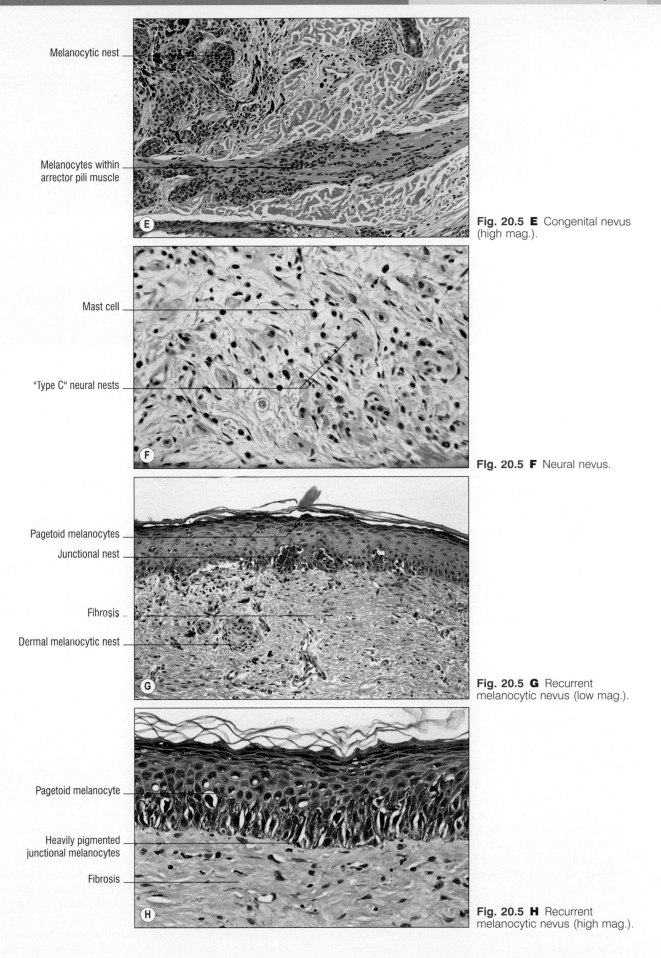

Melanocytic nest

Melanocytes within arrector pili muscle

Fig. 20.5 E Congenital nevus (high mag.).

Mast cell

"Type C" neural nests

Fig. 20.5 F Neural nevus.

Pagetoid melanocytes
Junctional nest

Fibrosis

Dermal melanocytic nest

Fig. 20.5 G Recurrent melanocytic nevus (low mag.).

Pagetoid melanocyte

Heavily pigmented junctional melanocytes

Fibrosis

Fig. 20.5 H Recurrent melanocytic nevus (high mag.).

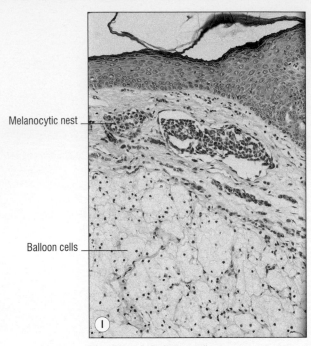

Melanocytic nest

Balloon cells

Fig. 20.5 I Balloon cell nevus.

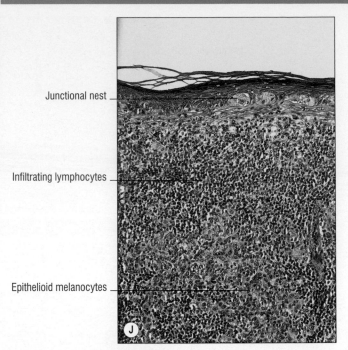

Junctional nest

Infiltrating lymphocytes

Epithelioid melanocytes

Fig. 20.5 J Halo nevus.

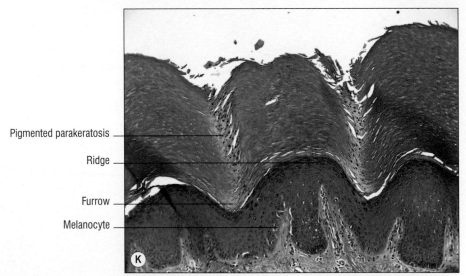

Pigmented parakeratosis

Ridge

Furrow

Melanocyte

Fig. 20.5 K Benign acral junctional nevus with pigmented parakeratosis over the dermatoglyphic furrows. "Furrows are fine, ridges are risky", meaning that pigmented parakeratosis in the peaks of the ridges is more often seen with melanoma.

Variations

1. Junctional nevus (JN): *brown macule* (1.18) usually, similar to lentigo simplex (20.3), nests limited to dermal–epidermal junction.
2. Intradermal nevus (IDN, BIN, benign dermal nevus): *skin-colored papule* (1.129), nests limited to dermis.
3. Compound nevus (CN): *brown papule* (1.18), nests present both at dermal–epidermal junction and in the dermis.
4. Congenital melanocytic nevus: present at birth, usually *more than 1 cm in* diameter. Superficial ones have been called *Zitelli nevus.*[52] Giant ones more than 20 cm in diameter have been called *Mark nevus,*[52] and those

definitely have an increased risk of development of melanoma. Congenital melanocytic nests are more likely to extend deeper (sometimes even into fascia), *invade into arrector pili muscles or extend around adnexal structures*, and *single-file* (1.128) or splay through the collagen. None of these features proves a nevus is congenital.

5. Neural (neurotized) nevus: nevus (usually intradermal) in which *type C nevus cells* are predominant; neuroid bundles may be present, may resemble a neurofibroma (26.1).
6. Recurrent melanocytic nevus (persistent nevus after shave excision): *fibrosis* in the dermis, *prominent*

junctional melanocytes, nested or not, basal layer usually *heavily pigmented*, often pagetoid, may resemble a melanoma (has been called *"pseudomelanoma"*), but pagetoid melanocytes (1.37) limited to central portion and do not proliferate into the shoulder beyond the scar.

7. Nevus spilus (speckled lentiginous nevus): common speckled nevus with childhood onset, features of lentigo simplex (20.3) in light brown areas, junctional or compound nevus in the darker speckles. The concept can be expanded to include any lesion with a light tan background with a "garden" of other melanocytic papules or nodules within it, such as agminated Spitz nevi, blue nevi, or dysplastic nevi within a lentiginous patch. Nevus sebaceus can be associated (21.2).

8. Balloon cell nevus: no distinct clinical appearance, large *ballooned melanocytes* with central nucleus and pale granular cytoplasm (often negative for lipid, glycogen, or mucin), with or without ordinary nevus cells. May be confused with other pale cell tumors (1.42).

9. Halo nevus: usually in older children or young adults, usually on the *trunk* (1.141), solitary, or sometimes multiple, white halo (1.150) around nevus, immunologic reaction to "aberrant" nevus, often a Clark's nevus (20.7), dense lichenoid *lymphocytes obscure melanocytic cells*, few melanocytes left in older lesions and lesion may become a completely white macule or papule. May be mistaken for other lichenoid diseases (1.72) or melanoma (20.5). S-100 protein stain may help identify hidden melanocytes. A white halo rarely occurs around a melanoma.

10. Acral melanocytic nevus[117] (melanocytic acral nevus with intraepidermal ascent of cells, MANIAC nevus[145]): nevi on acral skin (1.100), of which up to *one-third will have pagetoid melanocytes* over the central portion (1.37), possibly related to the direction of sectioning through dermatoglyphic lines,[160] but not pagetoid at the shoulders, and without atypia, simulating a melanoma. Clinically the pigment is more likely to be seen accentuated in the dermatoglyphic furrows in benign acral nevi, and at the peaks of the ridges in acral melanoma ("furrows fine, ridges risky"). This corresponds to pigmented parakeratosis more often seen in the furrows with benign acral nevus as opposed to the ridges in melanoma.

11. Clonal nevus[113] (nevus with focal epithelioid cell clusters): focal areas of superficial dermal pigmented epithelioid melanocytes that may resemble melanoma.

12. Ancient melanocytic nevus:[136] controversial term for a nodule in which there are melanocytic nests embedded in a degenerated hyalinized stroma, often with thrombi, sometimes with atypia, may resemble a melanoma.

13. Nevus of Nanta: melanocytic nevus with osteoma (29.8).

14. Nevus with cyst:[157] rather common phenomenon of melanocytic nevus associated with a ruptured cyst or prominent folliculitis with suppurative granulomatous reaction, which sometimes causes it to suddenly grow and cause concern regarding melanoma.

15. Unna nevus:[109] *papillated* (1.102) intradermal nevus.

16. Miescher nevus:[109] *smooth* compound or intradermal nevus.

17. Meyerson nevus:[30] red, scaling, pruritic, benign nevus with *spongiosis* (1.132).

Differential diagnosis

1. Malignant melanoma (20.11): less symmetry, more pagetoid, more cytologic atypia, less maturation of melanocytes (cells do not get smaller deeper into the dermis), more inflammation. Almost all melanomas originate at the dermal–epidermal junction, with rare exceptions being metastatic melanoma, malignant blue nevus (20.8), and some melanomas arising in congenital nevi.

20.6 Spitz nevus (antiquated synonyms: spindle and epithelioid cell nevus, S&E nevus, benign juvenile melanoma)

(see Fig. 20.6A–I)

Uncommon *pigmented papule or nodule* (75% of cases[158]) or *red* non-pigmented papule or nodule (25% of lesions) can resemble vascular neoplasms (Chapter 25) or other childhood nodules, famous for resembling melanoma histologically. Sophie Spitz originally thought she was studying melanomas of childhood (benign juvenile melanoma) that had an unexpected good prognosis. Most common on head or neck (most red lesions found there), and legs or trunk, but can occur anywhere. Usually in *children or young adults*, and the diagnosis made in older adults should be viewed suspiciously. May grow rapidly for a year or so, causing considerable concern, then usually remains stable.

- Symmetrical, sharply demarcated lesion **P**
- Epidermal hyperplasia (1.61), with rete ridges often clutching melanocytic nests
- Melanocytic nests (junctional, dermal, or compound), spindle-shaped or epithelioid, or both
- Clefts (1.23) often around melanocytic nests, sometimes pagetoid (1.37)
- Bizarre multinucleated or atypical melanocytes often in superficial portion of lesion, sometimes with mitoses limited to superficial portion, often with angulated or vertically oriented shape
- "Maturation" of melanocytes deeper in lesion (cells become smaller with less atypia). HMB-45 staining often shows zonal staining (stratification), more likely to be positive in superficial portion, unlike more prevalent staining found both superficial and deep in those melanomas that are positive[151]
- Melanin absent, sparse or prevalent
- Hyaline (Kamino) bodies sometimes at dermal–epidermal junction, thought to mostly contain basement membrane material more than degenerated keratinocytes (1.27)
- Vascular dilation often stressed, but not very helpful
- Lymphocytic infiltrate more likely patchy than lichenoid

Variations

1. Desmoplastic nevus (amelanotic blue nevus,[115] 20.8): skin-colored or light brown papule, prominent fibrosis and spindled melanocytes in the dermis, which may resemble a fibrohistiocytic lesion (Chapter 27). Melanin stain or S-100 protein stain is positive, unlike most fibrohistiocytic lesions. Desmoplastic melanoma is less likely to stain for Melan-A than desmoplastic nevus.

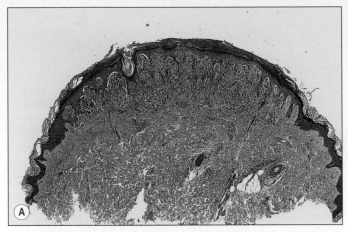

Fig. 20.6 A Spitz nevus (low mag.).

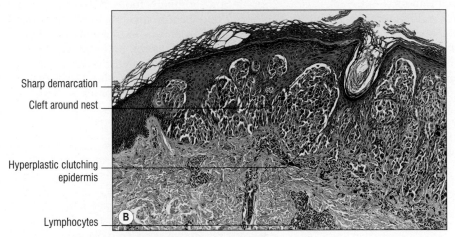

Sharp demarcation

Cleft around nest

Hyperplastic clutching epidermis

Lymphocytes

Fig. 20.6 B Spitz nevus (medium mag.).

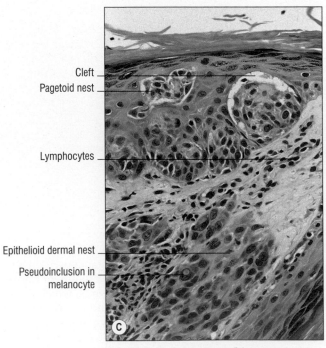

Cleft

Pagetoid nest

Lymphocytes

Epithelioid dermal nest

Pseudoinclusion in melanocyte

Fig. 20.6 C Spitz nevus (high mag.).

2. Pigmented spindle cell nevus (of Reed): black macule or papule, heavily pigmented spindled melanocytes, mainly junctional; lesion usually less than 6 mm in diameter, sometimes pagetoid (1.37), atypia usually mild.

3. Dermal Spitz nevus: red or skin-colored papule or nodule, lacks junctional nesting, usually melanocytes are plumper spindle cells than the desmoplastic nevus, sometimes epithelioid, with little or no melanin.

4. SPARK nevus: this has features of *Sp*itz nevus combined with C*lark* nevus (20.7).[137]

5. Agminated Spitz nevi: rare, localized grouping of multiple Spitz nevi.

6. Malignant Spitz nevus: controversial term for Spitz nevus in children that metastasizes to local lymph nodes, but apparently does not metastasize further, behaving in an otherwise benign manner, with long-term survival of the patients. Nodules are usually larger, deeper, with more atypia and necrosis.

Differential diagnosis

1. Ordinary melanocytic nevus (20.5).
2. Other nodules of childhood (1.93).

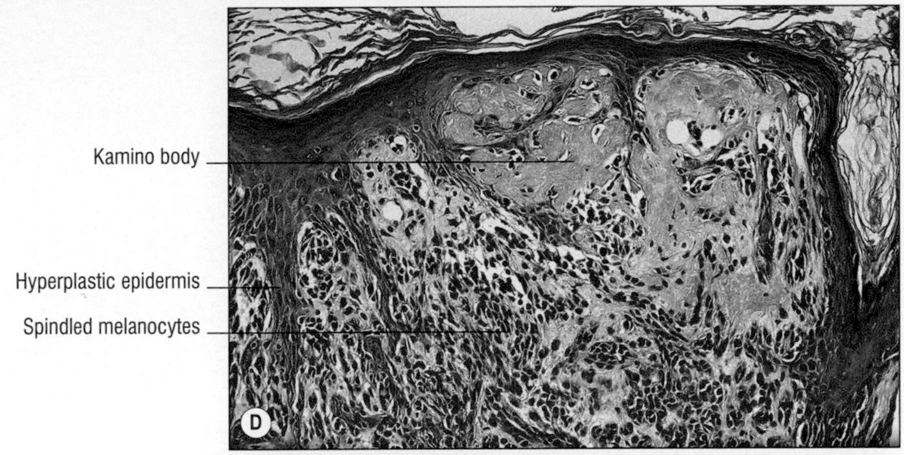

Kamino body

Hyperplastic epidermis

Spindled melanocytes

Fig. 20.6 D Spitz nevus (high mag.).

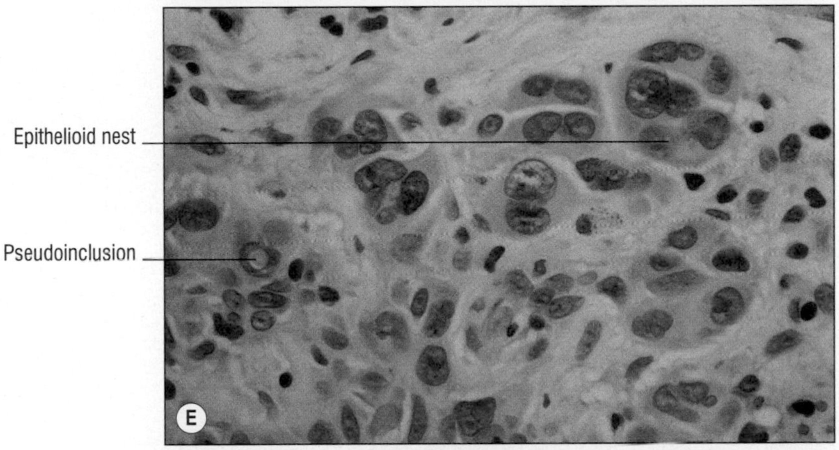

Epithelioid nest

Pseudoinclusion

Fig. 20.6 E Spitz nevus (epithelioid cell).

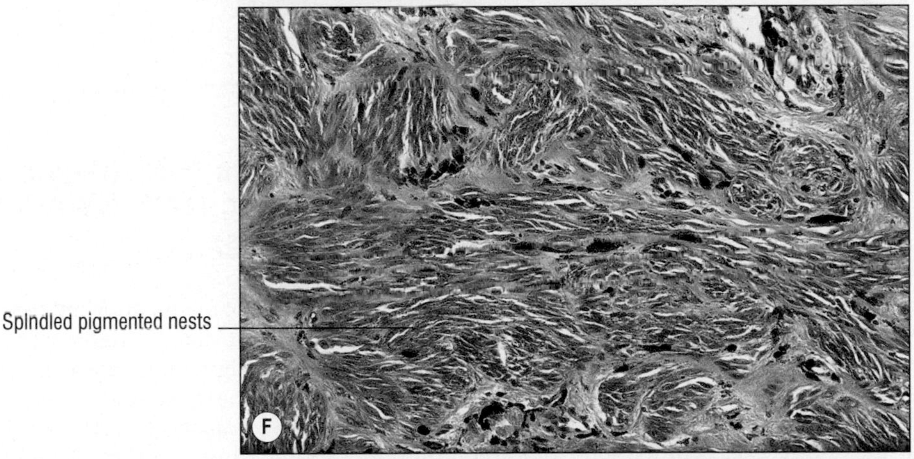

Splndled pigmented nests

Fig. 20.6 F Spitz nevus (spindle cell).

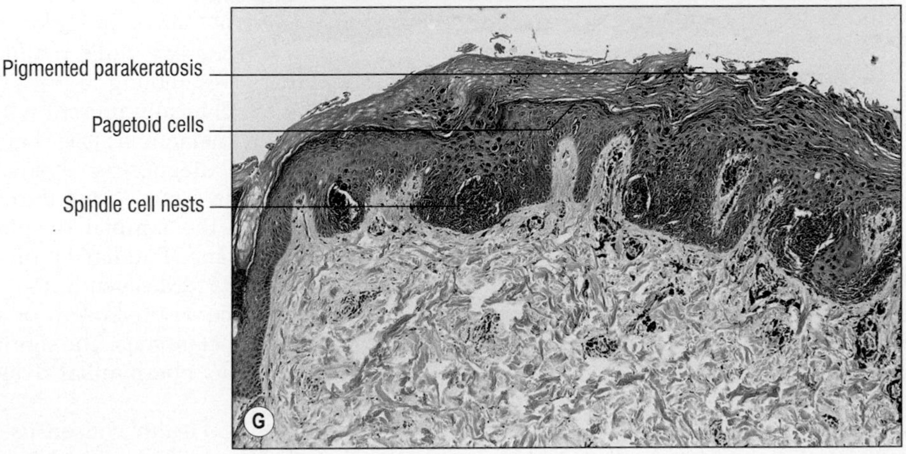

Pigmented parakeratosis

Pagetoid cells

Spindle cell nests

Fig. 20.6 G Pigmented spindle cell nevus (low mag.).

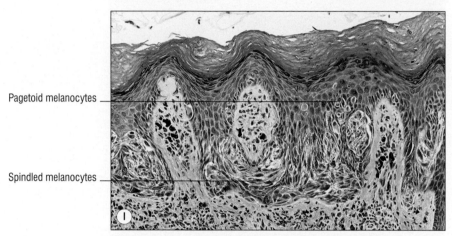

Pigmented parakeratosis

Pagetoid melanocytes

Spindle cell nests

Fig. 20.6 H Pigmented spindle cell nevus (high mag.).

Pagetoid melanocytes

Spindled melanocytes

Fig. 20.6 I Pigmented spindle cell nevus (high mag.).

3. Melanoma (20.11): can be difficult to distinguish, so complete excision of Spitz nevus is often recommended when there is significant uncertainty about the diagnosis. Usually not in children, more pagetoid melanocytes (1.37) at the shoulder instead of mainly over the central portion, more single pagetoid cells instead of groups of pagetoid cells in the epidermis, more cytologic atypia, more likely to have mitoses at the base, more likely to have regression, less symmetry, less maturation, more nest size variability, less sharp demarcation (except nodular melanoma), less epidermal hyperplasia, less clefting around nests, no Kamino bodies, lymphocytes more lichenoid than patchy, no stratified HMB-45 staining. S100A6, p16, and CD99 tend to be diffusely positive in Spitz nevus, while only patchy in melanoma. MIB-1 (Ki-67) is minimally positive in the dermis in Spitz nevus, and more positive in melanoma, especially in deeper component. In some cases, it may be impossible to differentiate between Spitz nevus and melanoma, and hedging terms such as atypical Spitz tumor and STUMP (spitzoid tumor of uncertain malignant potential) have been used for this legally treacherous situation.

4. Blue nevus (20.8): more melanin, cells more dendritic, limited to the dermis.

5. When amelanotic, Spitz nevus may resemble other neoplasms with spindle cells (1.131) or epithelioid cells (1.38).

20.7 Dysplastic nevus (DN) (nevus with architectural disorder, NAD, NWAD, Clark nevus, atypical nevus)

(see Fig. 20.7)

Common controversial type of nevus (most references say 5% of population has these, but since criteria vary, incidence reported as high as 50%). Pigmented macules, papules, or plaques, most common on the scalp and *trunk* (1.141), with clinical features *resembling melanoma* (20.11). Onset usually in older children and young adults. Common clinical features include *asymmetry, red–brown–black color, faded indistinct or notched borders, fried egg appearance* with papule within a macule, concentric circles resembling a target (cockade nevus). Essentially DNs can clinically present with the same ABCDE criteria used for melanoma (see below). Some dermatopathologists dislike diagnosing dysplastic nevus when the diameter is less than 6 mm, using terms like lentiginous junctional nevus. In the familial dysplastic nevus syndrome (B-K mole syndrome, familial atypical multiple mole–melanoma syndrome, FAMMM syndrome), these DNs have considerable significance as precursors or markers of patients prone to hereditary melanomas. The significance and histologic criteria for sporadic, non-familial dysplastic nevi are currently controversial.

The National Institutes of Health consensus conference published in the *Journal of the American Medical Association* in 1992 recommended that clinicians use the term "atypical

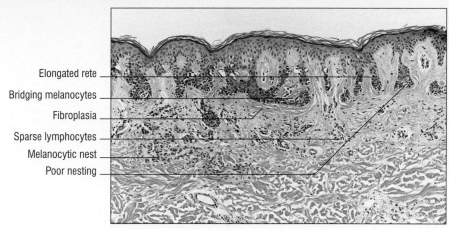

Elongated rete —
Bridging melanocytes —
Fibroplasia —
Sparse lymphocytes —
Melanocytic nest —
Poor nesting —

Fig. 20.7 Dysplastic nevus.

mole" and that pathologists abandon the term dysplastic nevus in favor of the term nevus with architectural disorder, because these lesions usually have more architectural atypia (bridging, single melanocytes, shouldering, fibroplasia, lymphocytes, described below) than cytologic atypia. The consensus conference recommended grading the cytologic atypia (see below) as mild, moderate, or severe. Because the architectural disorder is often more significant, some authorities grade both the architecture and the cytology. Other pathologists refuse to grade these at all, citing papers showing irreproducibility. Some pathologists use the term dysplastic nevus when the cytologic atypia is mainly within the epidermal melanocytes, using the term atypical nevus when it is in the dermis. Others use the two terms as synonyms. Unlike in gynecologic pathology, there is no uniform agreed-upon terminology for melanocytic neoplasms, and this is a big problem. Since melanocytic terminology is more like the Wild West, the clinician must know how a particular pathologist uses these terms. Some authorities have complained that dysplastic nevus is overdiagnosed when there are only minimal architectural changes; Ackerman sarcastically called it "the most common nevus in man". The term Clark nevus arose out of the aversion for calling these lesions truly "dysplastic".

Differential diagnosis

1. Melanoma (20.11): pagetoid cells, more severe atypia, more inflammation, less maturation. A lesion designated as severe dysplastic nevus may be melanoma, or at least difficult to distinguish from melanoma. Be very wary of diagnosing dysplastic nevus on skin with solar elastosis (especially face, forearms): some of these are melanoma (especially lentigo maligna)!
2. Ordinary melanocytic nevus (20.5): different clinical appearance, less horizontally oriented, more circumscribed, more nested, no cytologic atypia, less fibroplasia, less inflammation unless irritated.

20.8 Blue nevus

(see Fig. 20.8A–F)
Common *blue–black* (1.14) *papule or nodule,* usually beginning in early childhood. The prototypic heavily pigmented spindled form of common blue nevus has been called a *Tieche's*

- *Elongated, clubbed rete ridges* often similar to a lentigo (20.3)
- *Poorly circumscribed* melanocytic nests at the dermal–epidermal junction, often *bridging* between rete ridges. *Single melanocytes predominant* over nests (so-called lentiginous hyperplasia)
- Junctional melanocytes often extend beyond the dermal melanocytes at the periphery of the lesion (*shoulder phenomenon*) if it has a dermal component
- *Cytologic atypia of melanocytes* (absent in most cases per some authors, including this author, while others say it is the most important feature!). Nuclear size has been used as part of the grading: mild = melanocytic nuclear size less than 1.5× the size of basal keratinocytes, moderate = 1.5–2×, and severe 2×
- *Maturation* of melanocytes in the dermis if dermal nests are present (cells are smaller and less atypical in deepest portion)
- *Fibroplasia* in the papillary dermis around the junctional melanocytes, as if the body is walling off these melanocytes with collagen. Some think this is just compression of collagen by elongated rete ridges
- Mild to moderate perivascular *lymphocytes* in the dermis. An ordinary nevus should not have lymphocytes within it unless it is an irritated, halo, or Spitz nevus

nevus.[52] The term *dermal melanocytosis* has often been used collectively for those disorders in which there are dermal dendritic, spindled melanocytes, with or without melanophages: blue nevus, nevus of Ota (20.9), nevus of Ito (20.9), and Mongolian spot (20.10).

- Epidermis is normal
- *Spindle-shaped* (1.131) *dendritic melanocytes* in the dermis associated with abundant fine granules of melanin
- *Melanophages* (1.79, macrophages that have phagocytized clumps of melanin) often present
- *Sclerosis* of collagen common (1.125)

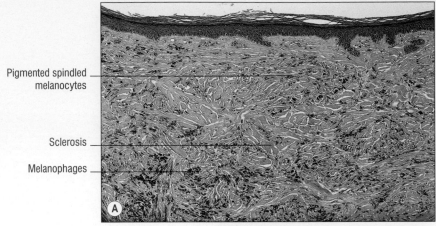

Pigmented spindled
melanocytes

Sclerosis

Melanophages

Fig. 20.8 A Blue nevus
(common type).

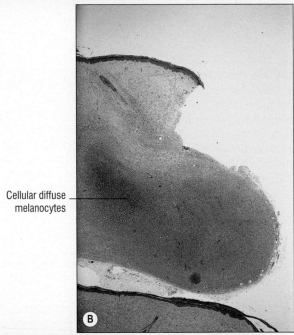

Cellular diffuse
melanocytes

Fig. 20.8 B Blue nevus (cellular
type, low mag.).

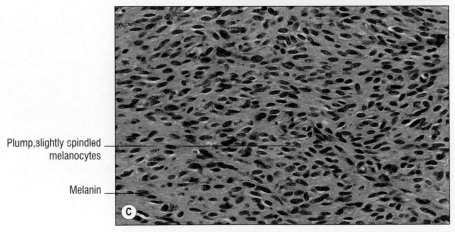

Plump, slightly spindled
melanocytes

Melanin

Fig. 20.8 C Blue nevus (cellular
type, high mag.).

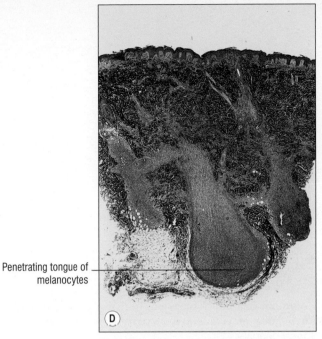

Penetrating tongue of melanocytes

Fig. 20.8 D Deep penetrating nevus (low mag.).

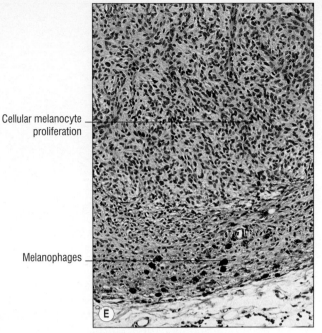

Cellular melanocyte proliferation

Melanophages

Fig. 20.8 E Deep penetrating nevus (high mag.).

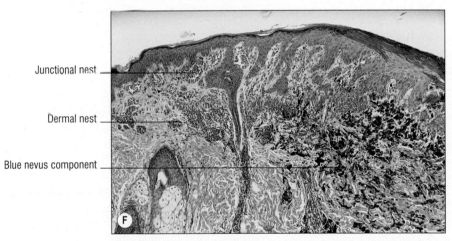

Junctional nest

Dermal nest

Blue nevus component

Fig. 20.8 F Combined nevus.

Variations

1. Cellular blue nevus (Jadassohn nevus[52]): densely packed plump melanocytes, some of which may not be so spindled, may be associated with very little melanin, may have a "biphasic" appearance (spindle cells and larger cells).

2. Deep penetrating nevus (Seab nevus[52]): vertically oriented diffuse infiltration of the dermis by melanocytes in a sharply demarcated nodule that extends into the fat, sometimes with nuclear pleomorphism.

3. Blue neuronevus (Masson nevus[52]): fascicles of plump neuroid melanocytes along with heavily pigmented spindled melanocytes.

4. Combined nevus: histology typical of an ordinary melanocytic nevus or Spitz nevus combined with focal changes of a blue nevus.

5. Amelanotic (hypomelanotic) blue nevus (desmoplastic nevus, 20.6): less melanin, resembles a dermatofibroma (27.1), desmoplastic melanoma (20.11), or other spindle cell neoplasms (1.131).

6. Compound blue nevus (Kamino nevus):[128] junctional melanocytes with prominent intraepidermal dendritic prolongations plus the usual dermal component.

7. Epithelioid blue nevus: predominance of epithelioid cells rather than spindle cells, but still may have considerable melanin and melanophages causing difficulty distinguishing from melanoma of the animal type. Pigmented epithelioid melanocytoma has been used collectively for epithelioid blue nevus and melanoma of the animal type, indicating this difficulty.

8. Pilar neurocristic hamartoma: controversial term for pigmented papule or plaque usually on head or neck, pigmented spindle cells arranged in perifollicular fascicles, may be melanoma in some cases.

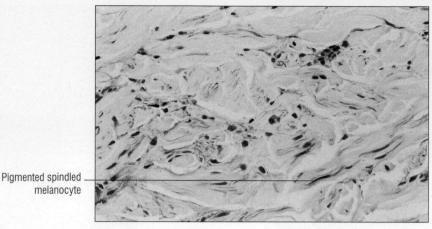

Pigmented spindled melanocyte

Fig. 20.9 Nevus of Ota.

Differential diagnosis

1. Malignant blue nevus: very rare, more densely cellular, atypical melanocytes, necrosis, and more inflammation.
2. Malignant melanoma (20.11): junctional melanocytes usually present except in metastatic lesions; often pagetoid, melanocytic atypia, more inflammation.
3. Other examples of "dermal melanocytosis": nevus of Ota, nevus of Ito, Mongolian spot (20.9, 20.10).

20.9 Nevus of Ota (nevus fuscocaeruleus ophthalmomaxillaris), nevus of Ito (nevus fuscocaeruleus acromiodeltoideus)

(see Fig. 20.9)
Uncommon unilateral *bluish–gray* (1.14) *patch on the face* (1.44, nevus of Ota), sometimes with blue sclera (1.14), or on the *shoulder* (1.141, nevus of Ito), onset at birth or early childhood, more common in females and Asians, very rare malignant degeneration.

- Epidermis is normal
- Spindle-shaped *dendritic melanocytes in the dermis* associated with abundant fine granules of melanin
- Melanophages usually not present

Variations

1. Dermal melanocytic hamartoma: pigmented blue–gray patch or plaque present at birth or early childhood, sometimes extensive, in another location other than face or shoulder.
2. Acquired unilateral nevus of Ota (Sun nevus): onset in adulthood.
3. Acquired bilateral nevus of Ota-like macules (Hori nevus): onset in adulthood, bilateral, often more speckled, no conjunctival involvement.

Differential diagnosis

1. Blue nevus (20.8): smaller papule or nodule, more cellular, more melanin, more melanophages.
2. Mongolian spot (20.10): onset in *sacral area* of *pigmented races at birth*, *regresses* spontaneously, less cellular, deeper in the dermis.

20.10 Mongolian spot

Common, but rarely biopsied, bluish–gray (1.14) macule of sacral area of pigmented races present at birth, regresses spontaneously.

- Epidermis is normal
- Spindle-shaped *dendritic melanocytes in the deep dermis* associated with abundant fine granules of melanin
- Melanophages usually not present

Differential diagnosis

1. Nevus of Ota (20.9), nevus of Ito (20.9), dermal melanocytic hamartoma (20.9), blue nevus (20.8).

20.11 Melanoma

(see Fig. 20.11 A–S)
The third most common type of skin cancer, sometimes called malignant melanoma (a redundant term that emphasizes its danger, but all melanomas are malignant by definition). Most commonly (not always) presents with the so-called ABCDE criteria: *Asymmetric* macule, papule, plaque, or nodule, with notched or *irregular Borders, Colors variegated* with red (inflammation), dark brown–black (1.13, melanin), blue (1.14, deep melanin) white (scarring), *Diameter more than 6 mm* in most cases. Since diameter more than 6 mm is relatively lame, since certainly many lesions more than 6 mm are not melanoma, and this criterion could result in missing really early small melanomas, it might be better to let the D stand for *Darkness*. Lesion is often *Evolving* (growing or changing).

Melanoma occurs in any location, but is most common in sun-covered areas (especially *shoulders, thighs*), despite all the hoopla over the fact that other more common skin cancers (basal cell and squamous cell carcinomas (BCC and SCC)) are most common in sun-exposed areas. BCC and SCC are often related to chronic long-term sun exposure in outdoor workers, while melanoma often occurs stereotypically in fair-skinned indoor workers who become acutely intermittently fried in the sun during childhood, weekends, or vacations. Sun exposure plays a role in melanoma, since the incidence is increased in latitudes closer to the equator, but genetic factors are also important. A minority of patients have genetic mutations,

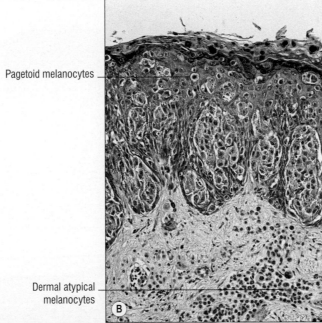

Pagetoid melanocytes

Atypical small melanocytes

Hemorrhage

Fig. 20.11 A Superficial spreading melanoma (low mag.).

Pagetoid melanocytes

Dermal atypical melanocytes

Fig. 20.11 B Melanoma (pagetoid cells).

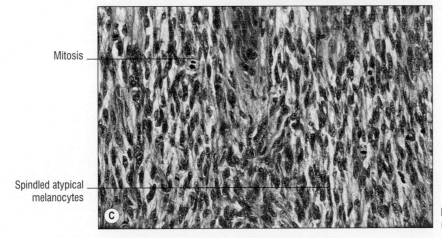

Mitosis

Spindled atypical melanocytes

Fig. 20.11 C Melanoma (spindle cells).

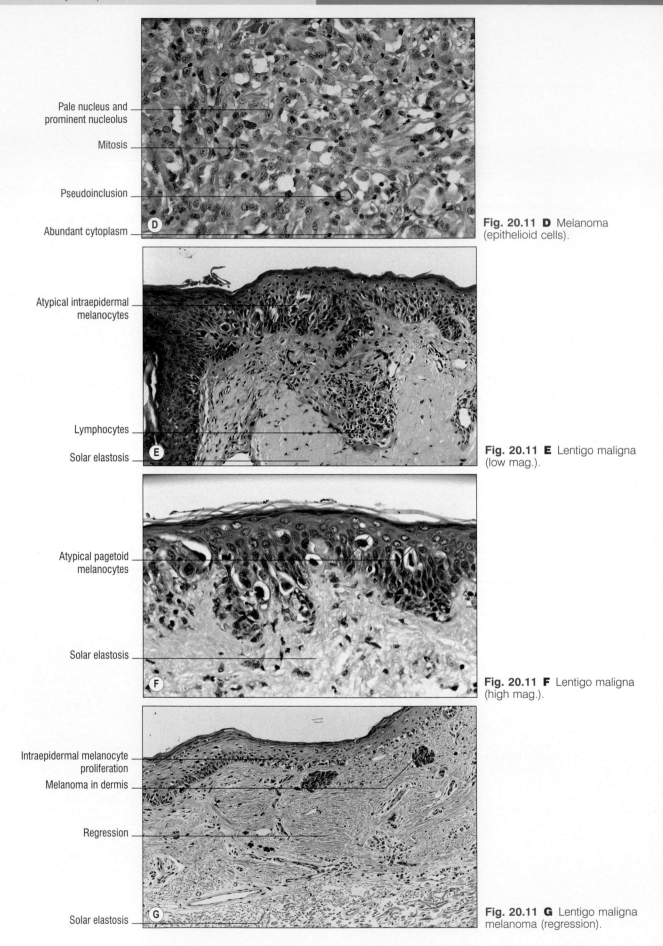

Pale nucleus and prominent nucleolus

Mitosis

Pseudoinclusion

Abundant cytoplasm

Fig. 20.11 D Melanoma (epithelioid cells).

Atypical intraepidermal melanocytes

Lymphocytes

Solar elastosis

Fig. 20.11 E Lentigo maligna (low mag.).

Atypical pagetoid melanocytes

Solar elastosis

Fig. 20.11 F Lentigo maligna (high mag.).

Intraepidermal melanocyte proliferation

Melanoma in dermis

Regression

Solar elastosis

Fig. 20.11 G Lentigo maligna melanoma (regression).

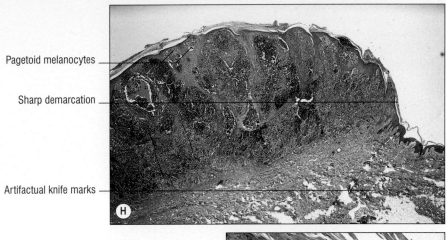

Pagetoid melanocytes

Sharp demarcation

Artifactual knife marks

Fig. 20.11 H Nodular melanoma (low mag.).

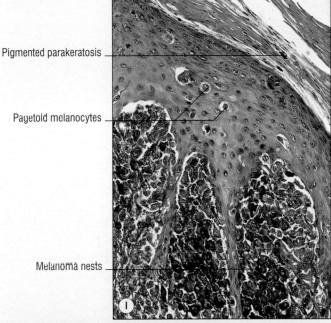

Pigmented parakeratosis

Pagetoid melanocytes

Melanoma nests

Fig. 20.11 I Nodular melanoma (high mag.).

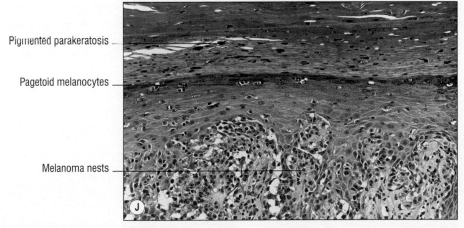

Pigmented parakeratosis

Pagetoid melanocytes

Melanoma nests

Fig. 20.11 J Acral lentiginous melanoma.

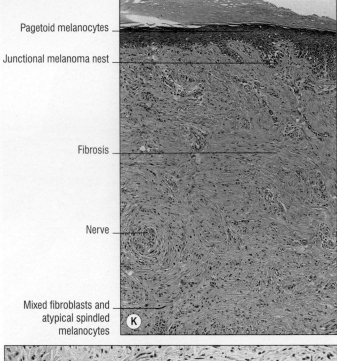

Pagetoid melanocytes

Junctional melanoma nest

Fibrosis

Nerve

Mixed fibroblasts and atypical spindled melanocytes

Fig. 20.11 K Desmoplastic melanoma.

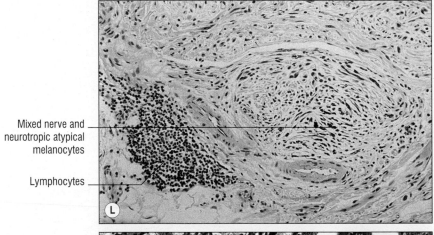

Mixed nerve and neurotropic atypical melanocytes

Lymphocytes

Fig. 20.11 L Neurotropic melanoma.

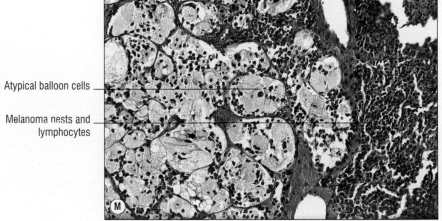

Atypical balloon cells

Melanoma nests and lymphocytes

Fig. 20.11 M Balloon cell melanoma.

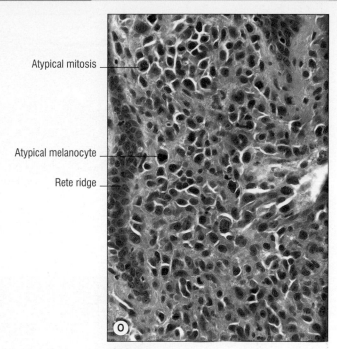

Atypical mitosis

Atypical melanocyte

Rete ridge

Atypical melanocytes

Pseudoinclusion

Fig. 20.11 N Metastatic melanoma (low mag.).

Fig. 20.11 O Metastatic melanoma (high mag.).

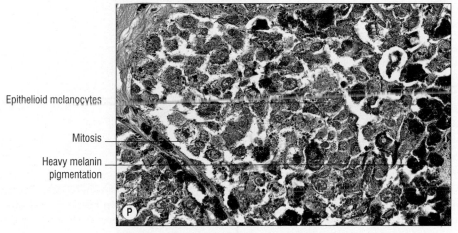

Epithelioid melanocytes

Mitosis

Heavy melanin pigmentation

Fig. 20.11 P Melanoma of animal type.

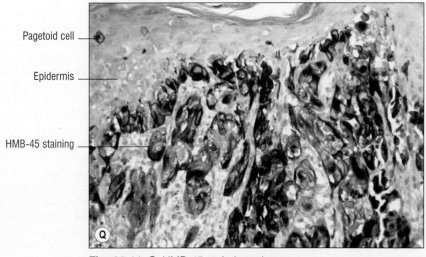

Pagetoid cell

Epidermis

HMB-45 staining

Fig. 20.11 Q HMB-45 stain in melanoma.

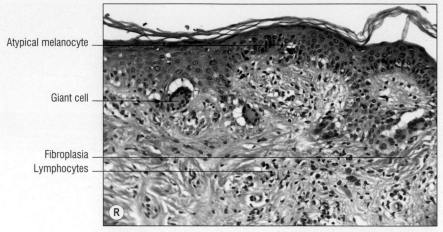

Atypical melanocyte

Giant cell

Fibroplasia
Lymphocytes

R

Fig. 20.11 R Starburst giant cells in lentigo maligna.

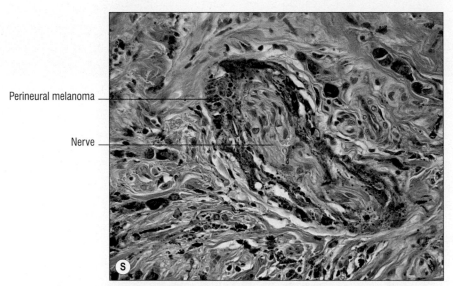

Perineural melanoma

Nerve

S

Fig. 20.11 S Perineural invasion by melanoma.

especially CDKN2A (p16, a cyclin-dependent kinase inhibitor). Only one-third of melanomas arise in *pre-existing melanocytic nevi* (20.5, 20.7), while two-thirds arise de novo. Melanoma lifetime incidence is increasing more rapidly than any other cancer, doubling every 10–20 years, and is estimated to be 1 in 50 Americans in 2010. In Australia, lifetime risk is 1 in 25 males. Various devices for dermoscopy (dermatoscopy) have been used to use light sources with magnification in the clinic to aid in distinguishing benign pigmented lesions from melanoma prior to biopsy. Five-year survival is 85%, which is that high only because of earlier diagnosis today as compared to the past.

Variations

1. Superficial spreading melanoma (SSM): most common type, found on non-sun-exposed skin. More likely to have pagetoid cells and epithelioid melanocytes, and no solar elastosis.
2. Lentigo maligna (LM): melanoma in situ (limited to epidermis) of *sun-exposed skin* with solar elastosis. If a melanoma in situ does not have solar elastosis, then it is simply called melanoma in situ, and is not called LM. LM is a pigmented macule usually on the face or sun-exposed skin. Prolonged in situ stage may last for

years (probably longer than melanoma in situ of non-sun-exposed areas), and only 5% become invasive. More likely to have epidermal atrophy, spindled melanocytes, and extension of malignant melanocytes along adnexal structures, and less likely to have pagetoid cells. LM can be very subtle, and is easily confused clinically and histologically with benign solar lentigo (20.4), macular seborrheic keratosis (SK, 18.2), and pigmented actinic keratosis (AK, 18.8). Some lesions called dysplastic nevus on sun-damaged skin are actually LM or invasive LM melanoma. All sorts of euphemisms are used for lesions that fall short of definitive LM diagnosis: such as atypical intraepidermal melanocytic proliferation or solar intraepidermal melanocytic proliferation (SIMP). Margins of LM are difficult to evaluate because sun-damaged skin often has solar melanocytic hyperplasia (SMH). Pigmented AKs and solar lentigo can lurk around the vicinity of LM in a mottled pattern, making small biopsies hazardous if they are not representative. Using immunostaining such as HMB-45 or S-100 to determine margins is highly overrated in this author's opinion. MART-1 can cause overdiagnosis of melanoma in the margin, partly because keratinocytes and other cells in the dermis can stain positively.

P

- Epidermis normal, atrophic, or hyperplastic (*ulceration*, 1.142, means worse prognosis)
- *Asymmetrical* proliferation melanocytes, often with poorly demarcated border (except in nodular melanoma)
- *Atypical melanocytes*, small, spindled, or epithelioid, often finely dusted with melanin, *arise at the dermal–epidermal junction* and invade the dermis. Melanoma almost never begins in the dermis (except in malignant blue nevus, congenital nevus, and other rare cases). Sometimes cytologic atypia is slight. Pleomorphism, hyperchromatism, increased mitoses, and prominent nucleoli are not always present
- *Mitoses* are often not present, but when they are present in dermal melanocytes, this is usually a sign of malignancy. Junctional mitoses are less important, usually (but sometimes also can indicate melanoma!). Counting mitoses per mm squared in the dermis is now part of the newest American Joint Committee on Cancer staging system. Even one mitosis per mm squared has been argued by some to be an indication for sentinel lymph node biopsy
- *Poor maturation* of the melanocytes (deeper cells are just as large and atypical as the superficial ones)
- *Pagetoid* melanocytes often
- Lymphatic or vascular invasion may be present (usually deeply invasive cases)
- Often *lichenoid* (1.72) lymphocytes in the dermis, less commonly perivascular (1.109) or sparse
- Precursor benign melanocytic nevus or dysplastic nevus present in only one-third of melanomas histologically (at least two-thirds arise de novo)
- *Regression* sometimes present (vascular fibrous tissue in the papillary dermis, sometimes with melanophages)
- *Special stains:* for difficult cases, stain for melanocytes may be helpful. The most sensitive stains are Sox10 and S-100 protein, both positive in more than 90% of cases. HMB-45 and MART-1 are more specific but less sensitive, and tend to be negative in spindle cell melanoma. Other more specific melanocytic stains include nuclear stain Mitf and tyrosinase. S-100neg desmoplastic melanomas can be stained with NGFR (nerve growth factor receptor)[155]
- *Depth of invasion* into the dermis is the most important *prognostic indicator*. Depth of invasion is often measured by antiquated *Clark levels*:
  - Level I: in situ within the epidermis
  - Level II: invades papillary dermis
  - Level III: fills papillary dermis and reaches reticular dermis
  - Level IV: invades reticular dermis
  - Level V: invades subcutaneous fat
- Clark levels are problematic because of the vague boundary between papillary and reticular dermis, and because the levels change in an abrupt stair-step manner. A more accurate way to gauge the depth of invasion is by

Breslow's thickness. Measure the thickness of invasion in millimeters with a micrometer from the top of the granular layer to the deepest point of invasion. Cure rate 99% if Breslow thickness is less than 0.76 mm. Extension of melanoma down the adnexal structures does not count for the measurement. Some authors prefer to define thin melanomas as those less than 0.85 mm or 1.0 mm. Those more than 4 mm are usually considered deep, and have a high chance of metastasis

- *Staging*. Do not confuse Clark levels with stages. The American Joint Committee on Cancer staging system for cutaneous melanoma was updated in 2009, adding consideration of mitoses per square mm in the dermis, immunostaining of nodal metastases, and deleting Clark levels:[112]
  - Stage 0: melanoma in situ (no invasion)
  - Stage Ia: localized. Breslow less than or equal to 1 mm with no ulceration or dermal mitoses
  - Stage Ib: localized. Breslow less than or equal to 1 mm with ulceration or one mitosis or more per square mm, *or* tumor 1.01 to 2 mm without ulceration
  - Stage IIa: localized. Breslow 1.01 to 2 mm with ulceration, *or* 2.01 to 4 mm without ulceration
  - Stage IIb: localized. Breslow 2.01 to 4 mm with ulceration, *or* greater than 4 mm without ulceration
  - Stage III: regional metastasis. Satellite skin metastasis (defined as within 2 cm of main tumor, or "in transit metastasis" in skin (defined as beyond 2 cm of the main tumor but still within nodal basin), or any regional node metastasis (even any size micrometastasis detected with immunostaining by HMB-45 or MART-1/ Melan-A. Stage III is further subcategorized based upon the number of nodes and whether a node has macrometastasis (clinically detected), or whether metastasis was satellite or in transit without nodal involvement
  - Stage IV: distant metastasis. Any distant skin, distant subcutaneous, distant node, or visceral metastasis. Stage IV can be further subcategorized depending upon the site of metastasis (distant skin, lung versus other visceral) and elevation of the serum lactate dehydrogenase
- *Features for the pathology report* that may be worth identifying include: subtype (SSM, LMM, NM, ALM, or others below), Clark level and Breslow thickness, presence of radial growth phase (spread of tumor through epidermis), or vertical growth phase (defined as invasion into dermis whereby largest dermal nest is larger than largest epidermal nest, or any mitosis in the dermis), mitotic figures per square millimeter, ulceration, regression, vascular invasion, perineural invasion, microscopic satellitosis, briskness of tumor infiltrating lymphocytes (TILs), associated nevus, cytologic type (epithelioid, spindle, or small cell), and surgical margins.

3. Lentigo maligna melanoma (LMM): same as lentigo maligna, but dermal invasion has occurred.

4. Nodular melanoma (NM): intraepidermal spread (*radial growth phase*) *absent* or limited to area above nodule plus no more than three rete ridges beyond nodular invasion of dermis.

5. Acral lentiginous melanoma (ALM): location on hands (1.56) or feet (1.48), more common in Asians and blacks, more likely to have benign-appearing melanocytes, spindled melanocytes, and lentiginous elongation of rete ridges.

6. Desmoplastic melanoma: spindled melanocytes in a fibrotic stroma, often amelanotic, usually arises from lentigo maligna. Often resembles other spindle cell proliferations (1.43), especially scars (1.125), and desmoplastic nevus but atypical melanocytes usually found, lymphocytic aggregates are present, lentigo maligna changes often found in the epidermis. S-100 stain usually positive, but HMB-45 usually negative (unlike most other melanomas). MART-1 also usually negative, but positive in desmoplastic nevi. If S-100neg, sometimes p75 (NGFR) positivity will help.

7. Neurotropic melanoma: variant of desmoplastic melanoma; fascicles of tumor invade nerves; often amelanotic.

8. Amelanotic melanoma: melanin not apparent clinically, or minimally present with H&E stain. Special stains for melanin, S-100 protein, HMB-45, MART-1, or electron microscopy (more historical, looking for melanosomes) may help differentiate it from other tumors.

9. Balloon cell melanoma: ballooned melanocytes with other malignant melanocytes; similar to balloon cell nevus (20.5), but other features of melanoma are present (consider other clear cell tumors 1.22).

10. Pedunculated melanoma: polypoid (1.106) tumor on a pedicle; measurement of depth of invasion is inaccurate in predicting prognosis.

11. Nevoid melanoma (minimal deviation melanoma): controversial term for a nodule of expansile melanocytes in the dermis that may resemble a nevus with scanning microscopy.

12. Metastatic melanoma: very rarely exhibits junctional melanocytes except in the very rare epidermotropic metastatic melanoma; inflammation uncommon.

13. Clear cell sarcoma (melanoma of soft parts): large, deep, soft tissue multilobulated neoplasm with clear cells (1.22) and multinucleated cells, sometimes with melanin, most common on the foot (20.11), resembles sarcomas (28.6).

14. Spitzoid melanoma: resembles Spitz nevus (20.6).

15. Myxoid melanoma: prominent mucinous stroma (1.83), resembles mucinous carcinoma (23.13) or malignant nerve sheath tumor (26.9).

16. Pigmented epithelioid melanocytoma[124] (melanoma of the animal type, equine melanoma, melanophagic melanoma[8]): dermal epithelioid or spindled melanocytes obscured by impressive amounts of melanin, histologically resembling melanoma of animals. In animals, particularly gray horses, melanoma can be slow growing and have a benign course, but in humans this type of melanoma is more likely to have a long indolent course than ordinary melanoma, though it may metastasize. Difficult to distinguish from epithelioid blue nevus (20.8).

17. Small cell melanoma: uniform small cells, may appear benign, may resemble other small cell neoplasms (1.130).

18. Other unusual cell types can make melanoma a great mimick, such as rhabdoid, myxoid, clear cell, chondroid, osteoid.

Differential diagnosis

1. Other melanocytic neoplasms (this chapter).

2. Melanocytic nevus (20.5): less likely to have cytologic atypia, mitoses, inflammation, and pagetoid cells. More likely to have symmetry, well-circumscribed nests of melanocytes in the junction region, nest size uniformity, maturation of melanocytes deeper in the dermis, and sharp lateral circumscription. Lymphocytes can be a valuable clue for melanoma because they can be considered smart bombs that can see melanoma antigens that we cannot see with H&E. Lymphocytes are uncommon in benign nevus, with noteworthy exceptions being irritated nevus, halo nevus, dysplastic nevus and Spitz nevus. Lymphocytes are more common in a band deep to a melanoma in the dermis, whereas in halo nevus the lymphocytes mingle more freely with the melanocytes. To help distinguish melanoma from nevus, some authorities have relied upon immunostaining, while others feel this is not so helpful. HMB-45 stain in benign nevus tends to stain the superficial portion, but not the deeper dermal component, whereas in melanoma it stains patchy or diffuse in the dermis ("stratification" of staining, analogous to the "maturation" described above with H&E stain). Ki-67 (MIB-1) staining of less than 5% of the dermal melanocytes suggests nevus, whereas staining more than 10% of the cells favors melanoma. S-100 and Melan-A usually stain both nevus and melanoma, except that desmoplastic melanoma tends to be negative for Melan-A as opposed to desmoplastic nevus. In some cases, it may not be possible to distinguish melanoma from benign nevus, and disclaimers, euphemisms, or hedging terms are used, such as borderline melanocytic tumor, AMP (atypical melanocytic proliferation), MELTUMP (melanocytic tumor of uncertain malignant potential), or SAMPUS (superficial atypical melanocytic proliferation of uncertain significance).

3. Spitz nevus (20.6).

4. Dysplastic nevus (20.7).

5. Other neoplasms with pagetoid cells (1.37), or pagetoid melanocytes (1.37).

6. Especially if melanin is lacking, consider other epithelioid neoplasms (1.38) or spindle cell malignancies (1.131). Melanoma is usually S-100+, Sox10+, HMB45+, MART-1+, pankeratin negative, desmin negative. CD68 sometimes can be positive, causing confusion with fibrohistiocytic proliferations.

Sebaceous Neoplasms

21.1 Sebaceous hyperplasia

(see Fig. 21.1)
Common whitish (1.150) to yellowish (1.151) papules, often with a rolled edge or central umbilication, most common on the face (1.145).

P
- Enlarged, otherwise normal sebaceous gland, often with a large central orifice
- Solar elastosis frequent

Variations

1. Fordyce spots: enlarged sebaceous glands of the lips (1.74) and rarely on other mucosal surfaces such as the vulva.
2. Montgomery's tubercles: enlarged sebaceous glands of the nipples (1.90).
3. Folliculosebaceous cystic hamartoma (22.1).
4. Sebocrine adenoma (23.10).
5. Rhinophyma: enlarged nose related to sebaceous gland hyperplasia or acne rosacea (10.1).

Differential diagnosis

1. Basal cell carcinoma (18.14), milium (19.1), syringoma (23.7), intradermal nevus (20.5), and fibrous papule (27.3), often resemble sebaceous hyperplasia clinically.
2. Nevus sebaceus (21.2): onset at birth or at childhood, growth at puberty, linear larger plaque, more papillomatosis, and apocrine glands.
3. Sebaceous adenoma (21.3).

21.2 Nevus sebaceus (organoid nevus)

(see Fig. 21.2)
Somewhat common *congenital, yellowish, verrucous, linear plaque,* usually on the head or neck, especially *on or near the scalp* (1.124), usually with alopecia (1.4) in the area. Often is more macular at birth, but the papillomatosis increases and sebaceous glands *enlarge at puberty,* bringing the patient into the office with a changing birthmark. Nevus sebaceus syndrome (Schimmelpenning–Feuerstein–Mims syndrome), analogous to epidermal nevus syndrome, is the sporadic

association of nevus sebaceus with ocular, CNS, and skeletal abnormalities. Phacomatosis pigmentokeratotica is a variant of nevus sebaceus syndrome, in which a nevus sebaceus is combined with a speckled lentiginous nevus (20.5) in a checkerboard pattern, sometimes with segmental hyperhidrosis.

P
- Epidermal hyperplasia (1.61) and *papillomatosis*
- Many normal or *enlarged sebaceous glands,* usually unassociated with mature hair shafts. Early in childhood, the entire pilosebaceous unit is poorly developed and appears as small buds
- Many *apocrine glands*
- *Basaloid hyperplasia,* true basal cell carcinoma (BCC, less than 5% incidence, some authors call them trichoblastoma instead, 22.7), syringocystadenoma papilliferum (23.3), trichilemmoma, or other adnexal tumors commonly develop within a nevus sebaceus after puberty

Differential diagnosis

1. Other linear (1.73), yellowish (1.151), papillomatous (1.102), or verrucous lesions (1.146).
2. Epidermal nevus (18.1): usually on extremities or trunk instead of head near scalp, no proliferation of sebaceous and apocrine glands. Nevus sebaceus may be considered to be an epidermal nevus variant by the "lumpers".
3. Other sebaceous gland neoplasms in this chapter. Nevus sebaceus is the only one that is congenital, linear, and spelled without the "o" because of Latin derivation. The patient may mislead by erroneously stating that it primarily started at puberty when nevus sebaceus enlarges.

21.3 Sebaceous adenoma

(see Fig. 21.3A,B)
Uncommon papule, usually solitary, usually on the face (1.44). Usually not diagnosed clinically. Considered to be benign by nearly all authorities, but has been considered to be malignant by Ackerman and coworkers[107] (some large sebaceous adenomas with Muir–Torre syndrome certainly can be aggressive).

©2012 Elsevier Ltd, Inc, BV
DOI: 10.1016/B978-0-323-06658-7.00021-X

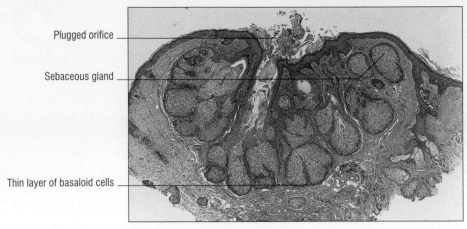

Plugged orifice

Sebaceous gland

Thin layer of basaloid cells

Fig. 21.1 Sebaceous hyperplasia.

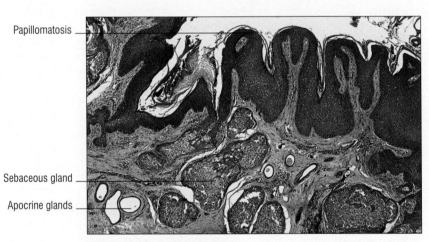

Papillomatosis

Sebaceous gland

Apocrine glands

Fig. 21.2 Nevus sebaceus.

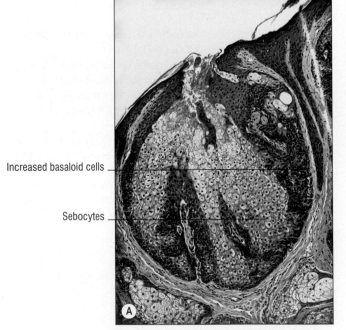

Increased basaloid cells

Sebocytes

Fig. 21.3 A Sebaceous adenoma (low mag.).

- Distinctly circumscribed lobular tumor of mature sebaceous cells (sebocytes) and basaloid (germinative) cells, with about *50% or more of the cells being mature sebaceous cells*
- *Minimal cytologic atypia*, although mitoses may be prevalent in some lesions

Variation

1. Muir–Torre syndrome (a subset of Lynch syndrome, hereditary non-polyposis colorectal cancer, HNPCC): paraneoplastic syndrome (1.105) of sebaceous neoplasms (usually multiple), especially sebaceous adenoma or sebaceous carcinoma, keratoacanthomas (18.12), associated with gastrointestinal malignancy (1.49), and less commonly genitourinary malignancy. Tumors may have mutations and lack of immunostaining for DNA mismatch repair proteins MSH2 (most common), MLH1, MLH3, PMS2, MSH1 or MSH6. Immunostains for these are commercially available, although some patients still have the syndrome despite retaining positive staining for all of these proteins. Genetic testing is available.

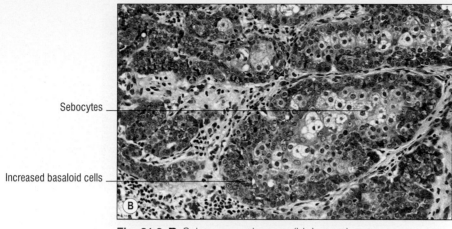

Fig. 21.3 B Sebaceous adenoma (high mag.).

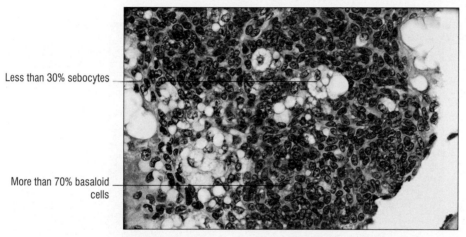

Fig. 21.4 Basal cell carcinoma with sebaceous differentiation.

Differential diagnosis

1. Other pale cell tumors (1.22) or lesions with foam cells (1.46).
2. BCC with sebaceous differentiation (21.4): most cells are basaloid, more atypia, more stromal retraction, with less than 30% (often only focal) sebaceous cells.
3. Sebaceous hyperplasia (21.1): more than 90% of the cells are mature sebocytes, with basaloid cells limited to the edges of the lobules (usually about one or two layers of cells).
4. Sebaceous epithelioma and sebaceoma are poorly defined. It is unclear whether they represent BCC with sebaceous differentiation, sebaceous adenoma, or some other sebaceous neoplasm variant. In this author's opinion, those terms should be avoided. The antiquated word epithelioma usually means a low-grade carcinoma, but some authorities have labeled sebaceous epithelioma as benign.

21.4 Basal cell carcinoma with sebaceous differentiation

(see Fig. 21.4)
Uncommon papule, nodule, or plaque most common on sun-exposed skin.

- Features of BCC (18.14) with less than 30% mature sebocytes (often only focal areas).

Differential diagnosis

1. Other neoplasms with basaloid cells (1.11).
2. Sebaceous carcinoma (21.5): more cytologic atypia (hyperchromatic, pleomorphic cells with many mitoses), poorly defined lobules, sometimes pagetoid cells.
3. Sebaceous adenoma (21.3): more sebaceous cells, less atypia, no stromal retraction.
4. Sebaceous epithelioma and sebaceoma have been unclear in the literature as to whether they represent BCC with sebaceous differentiation, sebaceous adenoma, or some other sebaceous neoplasm variant. In this author's opinion, those terms should be avoided.

21.5 Sebaceous carcinoma

(see Fig. 21.5A–C)
Rare papule, nodule, or plaque, most common on the *eyelid* (1.43), where it is thought to usually arise from Meibomian glands. Often mistaken for chalazion (10.1), blepharitis, or BCC. Metastasis is common. May be associated with Muir–Torre syndrome (21.3).

- *Pagetoid cells* sometimes in the epidermis or conjunctiva
- Disordered invasion of dermis by poorly defined lobules of *basaloid or squamoid cells and poorly developed sebaceous cells*
- *Moderate to severe atypia*

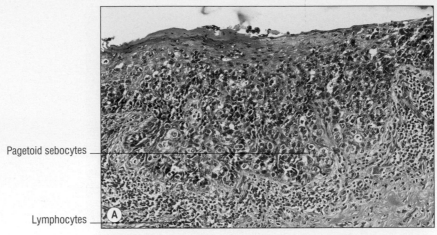

Pagetoid sebocytes

Lymphocytes

Fig. 21.5 A Sebaceous carcinoma (pagetoid, low mag.).

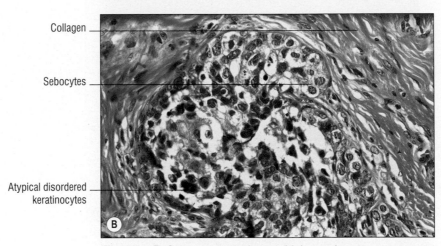

Collagen

Sebocytes

Atypical disordered keratinocytes

Fig. 21.5 B Sebaceous carcinoma (high mag.).

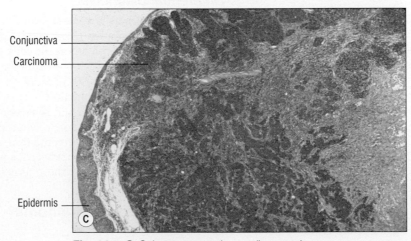

Conjunctiva

Carcinoma

Epidermis

Fig. 21.5 C Sebaceous carcinoma (low mag).

P
- *Oil-red-O* or Sudan black stain for lipid must be done with frozen section, but is important because the sebaceous areas may be subtle, focal, and easily missed
- Positive staining for EMA; is more weakly positive or negative in both BCC and squamous cell carcinoma (SCC) compared with sebaceous carcinoma. Sebaceous carcinoma tends to have nuclei scalloped by lipid vacuoles.

Differential diagnosis

1. BCC with sebaceous differentiation (21.4).
2. SCC (18.11): no sebocytes, but may have clear cells that are PAS-positive, but oil-red-O and cam 5.2 (low molecular weight keratin) negative. EMA is positive in both SCC and sebaceous carcinoma.
3. Other neoplasms with clear cells (1.22), foam cells (1.46), or pagetoid cells (1.37).

Follicular Neoplasms

22.1 Trichofolliculoma

(see Fig. 22.1A–E)
Uncommon solitary papule on the face (1.44), sometimes with a plugged orifice in which vellus hairs are seen.

P
- Large open or closed *comedo-like lesion* (sometimes resembling a cyst if there is no orifice) into which numerous *small hair follicles with trichohyaline granules and vellus hairs open*
- Fibrotic stroma

Variations

1. Dilated pore of Winer: solitary 1–3 mm orifice on face, buds of epithelium with no associated hair shafts connect into open comedo (1.24).
2. Pilar sheath acanthoma: usually on *upper lip*, buds of epithelium from open comedo *more massive*, without hair shafts in the buds.
3. Trichostasis spinulosa (10.4): common finding of *multiple vellus hairs within a comedonal plug*, either as an acneiform clinical condition of open comedones (1.24) or as an incidental histologic finding, not apparent clinically, in many different lesions, particularly melanocytic nevi.
4. Folliculosebaceous cystic hamartoma (sebaceous trichofolliculoma): sebaceous glands associated with the comedo-like lesion, in adults.

Differential diagnosis

1. Dermoid cyst (19.3): larger, congenital cyst, with larger hairs and hair shafts.

22.2 Trichoepithelioma

(see Fig. 22.2A–F)
Somewhat common *skin-colored papule or nodule* (1.129), most common on the *central face* (1.44). Lesions more commonly are *solitary*, but *multiple* trichoepitheliomas with childhood onset may be associated with cylindromas (23.4) and spiradenomas (23.11), inherited as the autosomal dominant Brooke–Spiegler syndrome, related to the CYLD gene mutation. Trichoepithelioma is a benign neoplasm, even though the word epithelioma usually means low-grade carcinoma. It can sometimes be very difficult to distinguish trichoepithelioma from a basal cell carcinoma (basal cell epithelioma).

P
- Circumscribed *basaloid tumor islands*, *often in a reticulated pattern* or cribriform pattern (interconnecting cords), sometimes resembling poorly developed hair follicles
- *Horn cysts* common
- Peripheral palisading of nuclei, but *no artifactual retraction* between tumor and stroma
- Loose *stroma with many fibroblasts* surrounds basaloid islands
- *Papillary mesenchymal bodies* (clusters of fibroblasts adjacent to epithelial buds as in the germinative portion of the normal hair papilla)

Variations

1. Trichoadenoma of Nikolowski: tumor cells are not basaloid and are *more squamous* like normal epithelium, having more pink cytoplasm and a pale nucleus, *horn cysts numerous*.
2. Desmoplastic trichoepithelioma: *thinner strands of basaloid cells, horn cysts* usually present, resembling a sclerosing basal cell carcinoma.
3. Basaloid follicular hamartoma:[166] *small papules*, often multiple, usually on the face, *vertically-oriented* basaloid cells *centered upon a comedo-like follicle*.

Differential diagnosis

1. Multiple facial papules may cause clinical confusion, but are much different histologically: Cowden's disease (22.5), Birt–Hogg–Dube syndrome (22.6), and tuberous sclerosis (27.3).
2. Keratotic basal cell carcinoma (BCC, 20.14) or BCC with follicular differentiation is more likely to have a pearly translucent clinical appearance rather than a fleshy papule or nodule with minimal history of growth, solar elastosis, stromal retraction, ulceration, necrosis, fewer fibroblasts in the stroma, less hair papilla formation with papillary mesenchymal bodies, and bcl-2 expression more than just in the basal layer. CD34 is more likely to stain stroma immediately against the basaloid aggregates in trichoepithelioma, with a rim of sparing around basaloid aggregates of BCC, but this is highly overrated as helpful. Desmoplastic trichoepithelioma is usually negative for CK7, whereas a minority of BCCs are positive (another stain of limited help). Some studies show BCC is more likely to express

©2012 Elsevier Ltd, Inc, BV
DOI: 10.1016/B978-0-323-06658-7.00022-1

Ber-EP4 than desmoplastic trichoepithelioma or trichoadenoma, but this varies by the study. Because it may be difficult to be sure of the distinction, a solitary trichoepithelioma in sun-damaged skin is usually best treated as if it were a BCC (when in doubt, cut it out).

3. Trichoblastoma (22.7): Ackerman considered trichoepithelioma to be a superficial type of trichoblastoma with a cribriform or germinative pattern, while Santa Cruz says that trichoepitheliomas mainly differ by being closer to the epidermis.
4. Microcystic adnexal carcinoma (23.13).
5. Other basaloid neoplasms (1.11).

22.3 Pilomatrixoma (pilomatricoma, calcifying epithelioma of Malherbe)

(see Fig. 22.3A–C)
Somewhat common dermal or subcutaneous nodule (1.135), clinically *mistaken for a cyst* (1.25, Chapter 19), often on the head or neck of children (1.93), sometimes occurs in adults of any age. Often becomes inflamed and red. Often exhibits *"tent sign"* of elevating the surface of the skin like a tent. When incised, it contains shards of keratinous material like a cyst, but it is often *chalky* due to calcification. Some pilomatrixomas are caused by mutation in the beta-catenin gene (CTNNB1).

- *Circumscribed nodule resembling a cyst* in the dermis, sometimes with a squamous epithelial lining of the periphery
- *Basaloid cells* in younger lesions, especially around periphery of nodule
- *Shadow (ghost) cells*, which have a pale, empty space where the nucleus used to be, with abundant pink cytoplasm. *Transitional cells* may be present, not to be confused with transitional epithelium, with pyknotic nuclei in the process of becoming shadow cells
- *Shards of keratinous debris*, shadow cells, *calcification*, or *ossification* may be predominant in older lesions (basaloid cells gradually decrease in number)
- *Foreign body multinucleated giant cells* (1.84) and *granulomatous inflammation* (1.51) often present as a reaction to abundant keratin

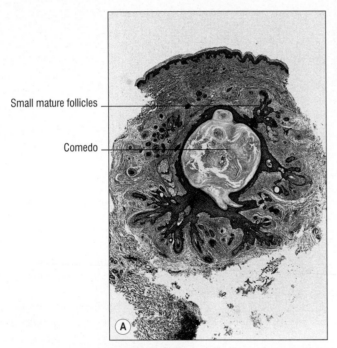

Small mature follicles

Comedo

Fig. 22.1 A Trichofolliculoma (low mag.).

Differential diagnosis

1. Shadow cells are rarely present in small numbers in epidermal inclusion cysts (19.1), pilar cysts (19.2), or other adnexal neoplasms.
2. Completely calcified or ossified lesions may resemble other diseases with calcification (1.19) or osteoma cutis (29.8).
3. Pilomatrix carcinoma: rare malignant counterpart of pilomatrixoma, larger, more infiltrating, more atypia, might just be a squamous cell carcinoma (SCC) with shadow cells.
4. Other basaloid neoplasms (1.11) rarely cause difficulty once shadow cells are identified.

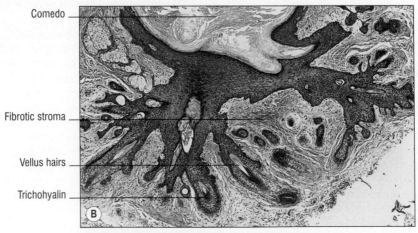

Comedo

Fibrotic stroma

Vellus hairs

Trichohyalin

Fig. 22.1 B Trichofolliculoma (high mag.).

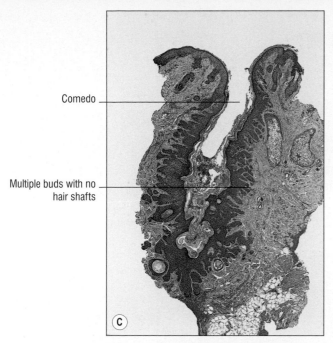

Fig. 22.1 C Dilated pore of Winer.

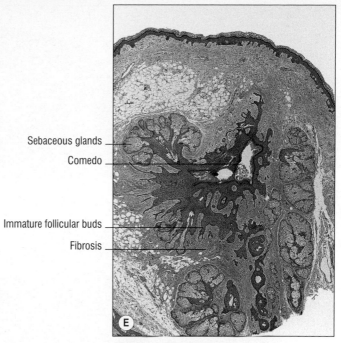

Fig. 22.1 E Folliculosebaceous cystic hamartoma.

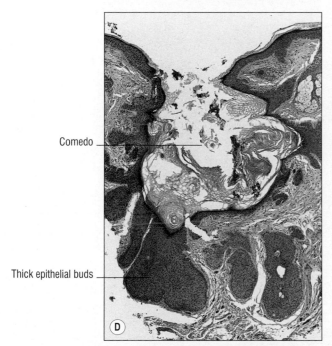

Fig 22.1 D Pilar sheath acanthoma.

22.4 Proliferating trichilemmal cyst (proliferating pilar cyst, pilar tumor, proliferating follicular cystic neoplasm, giant hair matrix tumor)

(see Fig. 22.4A,B)

Uncommon enlarging nodule, usually on the *scalp* (1.124), appearing to be largely *circumscribed and subcutaneous*. Traditionally considered in nearly all cases to be a benign pseudomalignancy (1.118), but examples of so-called malignant proliferating trichilemmal cyst with metastasis have been reported. Ackerman and coworkers[149] have taken the

minority view that all proliferating trichilemmal cysts are malignant!

- This tumor apparently *arises in a trichilemmal cyst* (19.2) in which the wall has proliferated, often with squamous eddies and pearls (1.134), and abrupt *trichilemmal keratinization without a granular layer*. Sometimes evidence of the previous cyst is apparent, while in other cases the tumor is more solid
- Clear cells sometimes present (1.22)

Differential diagnosis

1. Squamous cell carcinoma (18.11): more cytologic atypia, less well circumscribed, does not "shell out", clinically more obvious broad connection to surface epidermis in setting of solar elastosis. Most examples of metastasizing malignant proliferating pilar cyst have been large, recurrent, or very atypical cytologically.
2. Pseudoepitheliomatous hyperplasia (1.116): broad connection to surface epidermis, not a subcutaneous nodule.

22.5 Trichilemmoma (tricholemmoma)

(see Fig. 22.5A–D)

Uncommon *warty or smooth papule of the face* (1.44), often not diagnosed clinically unless multiple lesions are present. It has been considered to be a viral wart, but molecular genetic studies generally have not shown papillomavirus.

- Hyperkeratosis with *downward lobular growth* of epidermis
- *Keratinocytes are clear cells* because of glycogen within the cells (PAS positive, diastase labile)
- Thin rim of basal cells palisade at edge of lobule of clear cells
- Thickened basement membrane sometimes

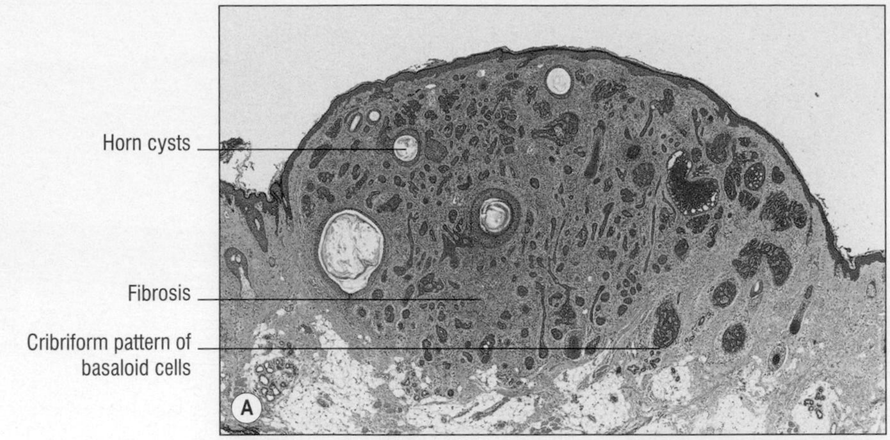

Horn cysts

Fibrosis

Cribriform pattern of
basaloid cells

Fig. 22.2 A Trichoepithelioma
(low mag.).

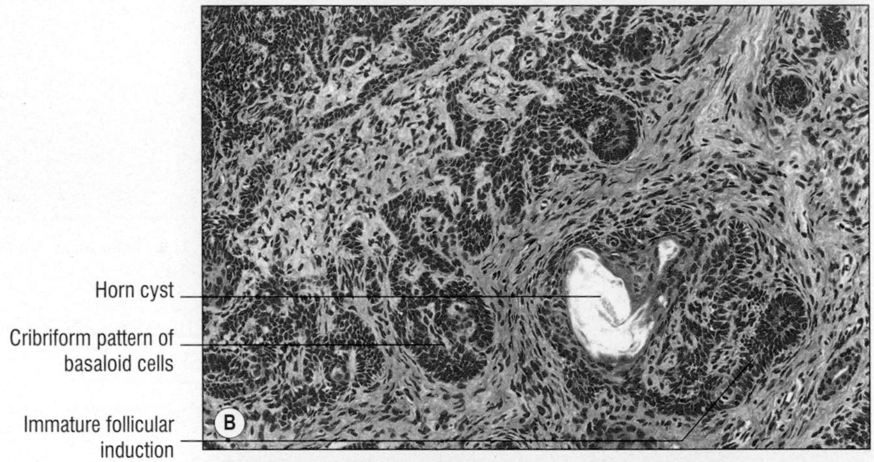

Horn cyst

Cribriform pattern of
basaloid cells

Immature follicular
induction

Fig. 22.2 B Trichoepithelioma
(medium mag.).

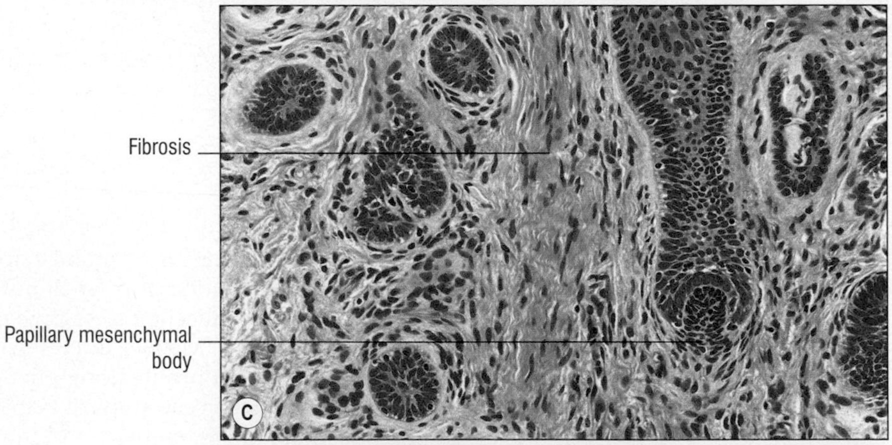

Fibrosis

Papillary mesenchymal
body

Fig. 22.2 C Trichoepithelioma
(high mag.).

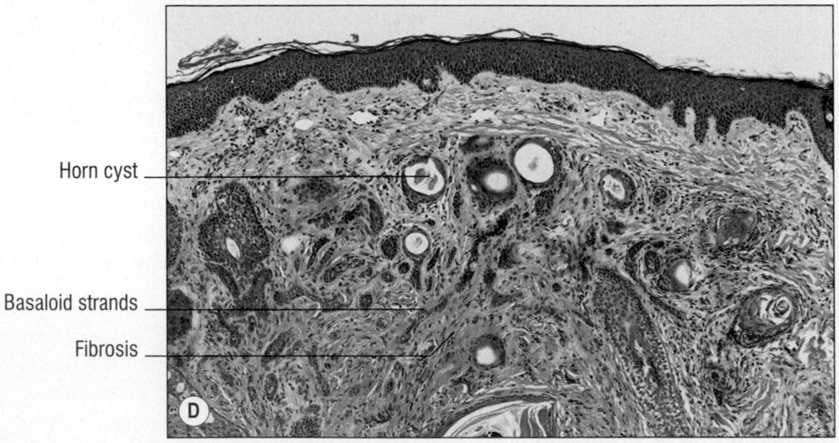

Horn cyst

Basaloid strands

Fibrosis

Fig. 22.2 D Desmoplastic
trichoepithelioma.

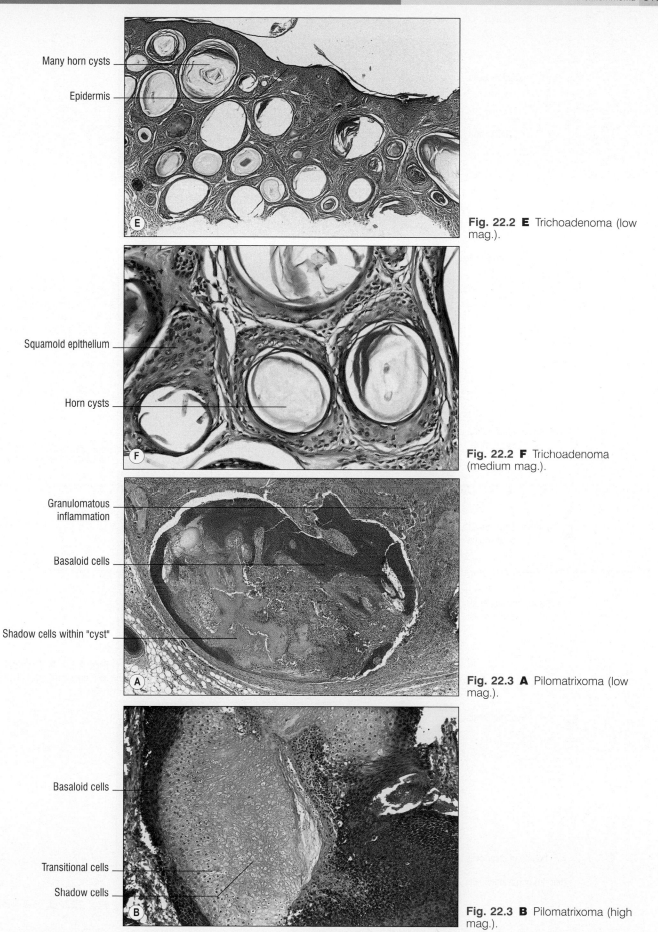

Many horn cysts
Epidermis

Fig. 22.2 E Trichoadenoma (low mag.).

Squamoid epithelium

Horn cysts

Fig. 22.2 F Trichoadenoma (medium mag.).

Granulomatous inflammation

Basaloid cells

Shadow cells within "cyst"

Fig. 22.3 A Pilomatrixoma (low mag.).

Basaloid cells

Transitional cells

Shadow cells

Fig. 22.3 B Pilomatrixoma (high mag.).

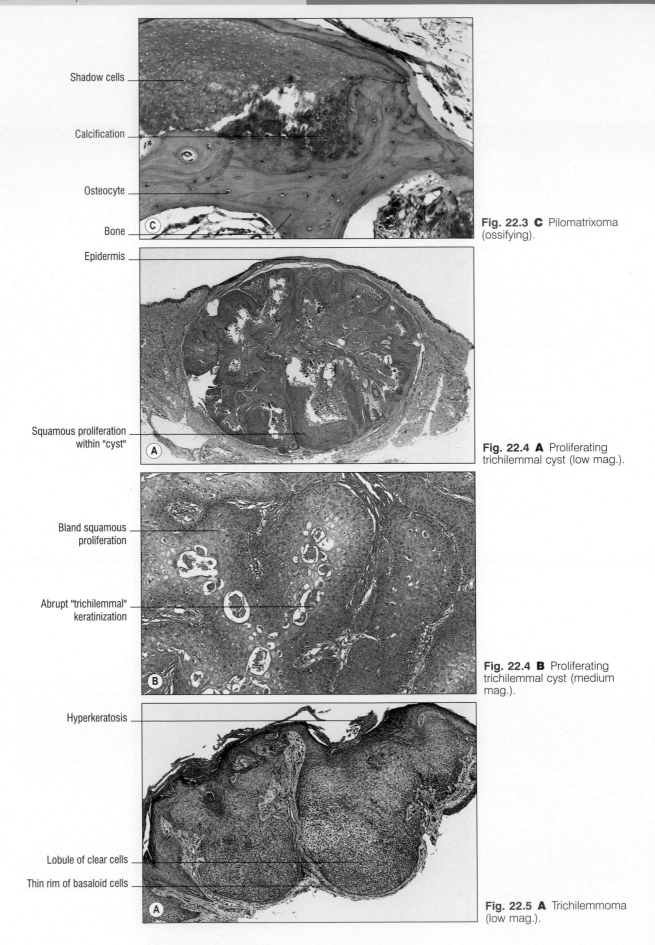

Shadow cells

Calcification

Osteocyte

Bone

Fig. 22.3 C Pilomatrixoma (ossifying).

Epidermis

Squamous proliferation within "cyst"

Fig. 22.4 A Proliferating trichilemmal cyst (low mag.).

Bland squamous proliferation

Abrupt "trichilemmal" keratinization

Fig. 22.4 B Proliferating trichilemmal cyst (medium mag.).

Hyperkeratosis

Lobule of clear cells

Thin rim of basaloid cells

Fig. 22.5 A Trichilemmoma (low mag.).

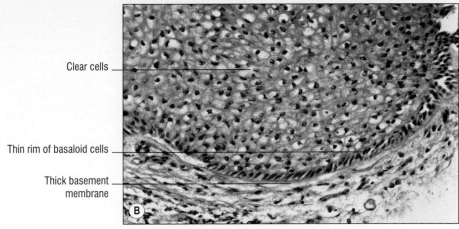

Clear cells

Thin rim of basaloid cells

Thick basement membrane

Fig. 22.5 B Trichilemmoma (high mag.).

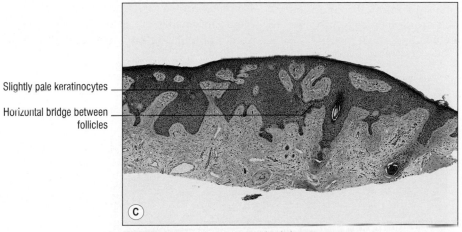

Slightly pale keratinocytes

Horizontal bridge between follicles

Fig. 22.5 C Tumor of follicular infundibulum.

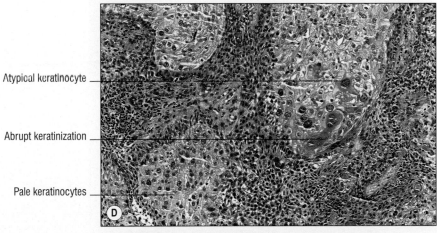

Atypical keratinocyte

Abrupt keratinization

Pale keratinocytes

Fig. 22.5 D Trichilemmocarcinoma.

Variations

1. Cowden's disease (multiple harmartoma syndrome): autosomal dominant paraneoplastic syndrome (1.105), 80% of patients have PTEN mutation, which also occurs in Bannayan–Riley–Ruvulcaba syndrome and Proteus syndrome. Multiple facial trichilemmomas, acral keratoses, palmoplantar keratoses, mucosal papillomas or fibromas, sclerotic fibromas (27.1), and breast or thyroid malignancy.
2. Tumor of the follicular infundibulum: thin anastomosing strands of clear cells, extending parallel to the epidermis, bridging between the infundibular portions of adjacent follicles, also considered a variant of seborrheic keratosis (18.2).

Differential diagnosis

1. Verruca vulgaris (14.1): fewer clear cells, more hypergranulosis, koilocytosis, papillomavirus may be demonstrated.
2. Inverted follicular keratosis (18.2): downward-growing seborrheic keratosis, cells not as clear, more squamous eddies sometimes.

3. Trichilemmal carcinoma (tricholemmocarcinoma): rare malignant counterpart of trichilemmoma, probably is just a squamous cell carcinoma with clear cells resembling trichilemmoma.
4. Clear cell acanthoma (18.6): most common on the leg, more of a horizontal plaque resembling psoriasis with clear cells instead of a downward-growing lobule.
5. Clear cell Bowen's disease (18.10): more severe atypia.
6. Other clear cell tumors (1.22).

22.6 Fibrofolliculoma and trichodiscoma

(see Fig. 22.6A,B)
Rare skin-colored papules of the face, usually multiple, rarely solitary. Usually associated with *Birt–Hogg–Dube syndrome*, autosomal dominant, due to mutation in the folliculin (FLCN) gene, multiple fibrofolliculomas, trichodiscomas, acrochordons, a paraneoplastic syndrome associated with renal cell carcinoma (1.105). Trichodiscoma and fibrofolliculoma are probably two expressions of the same neoplasm, just like cylindroma and eccrine spiradenoma.

■ Hair follicle with thin extensions of epithelium into surrounding mucinous stroma (fibrofolliculoma)
■ Loose fibrosis with thin collagen bundles and blood vessels localized to a subepidermal area adjacent to a hair follicle (the so-called hair disk or Haarscheibe, which probably has nothing to do with this), without the follicular extensions in older lesions (trichodiscoma)

Differential diagnosis

1. Angiofibroma, fibrous papule, perifollicular fibroma (27.3): collagen encircles follicles or is oriented perpendicular to epidermis, sometimes with plump fibroblasts and vascular dilation.
2. Dermatofibroma (27.1).
3. Neurofibroma (26.1).
4. Tumor of follicular infundibulum (22.5).

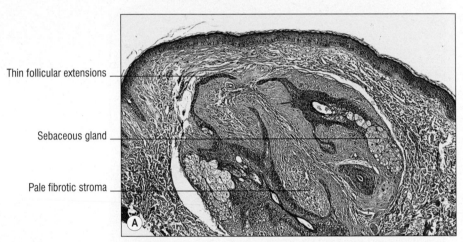

Thin follicular extensions
Sebaceous gland
Pale fibrotic stroma

Fig. 22.6 A Fibrofolliculoma.

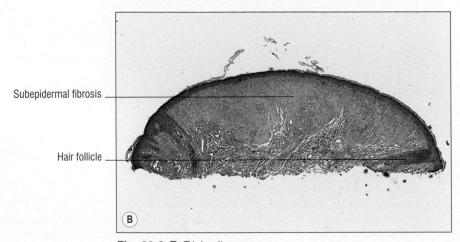

Subepidermal fibrosis
Hair follicle

Fig. 22.6 B Trichodiscoma.

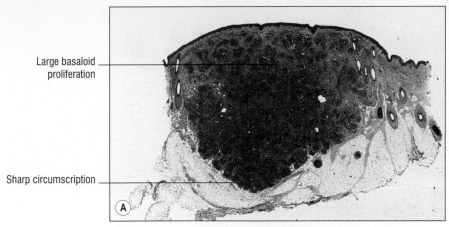

Large basaloid proliferation

Sharp circumscription

Fig. 22.7 A Trichoblastoma (low mag.).

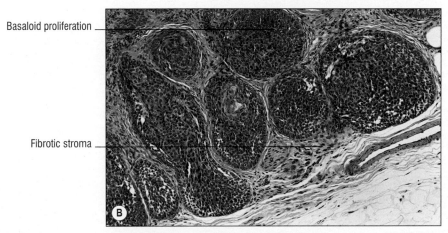

Basaloid proliferation

Fibrotic stroma

Fig. 22.7 B Trichoblastoma (medium mag.)

22.7 Trichoblastoma

(see Fig. 22.7A,B)

Uncommon basaloid neoplasm that used to be very rare, but now is diagnosed more commonly, ever since Ackerman and coworkers published their book on follicular neoplasms[92] and expanded the scope of this lesion to include many lesions formerly called trichoepithelioma. The diagnosis is now so much in vogue that many basal cell carcinomas associated with nevus sebaceus (21.2) are now being called trichoblastoma. Different dermatopathologists and textbooks use divergent criteria and terminology. Headington[131] originally described variants such as trichoblastic fibroma, trichogenic trichoblastoma, and trichogenic myxoma. Ackerman describes five main types: large nodular, small nodular, cribriform,

racemiform, and retiform. Trichogerminoma also belongs in this group. Classifying snowflakes is easier.

- Circumscribed large basaloid neoplasm usually greater than 1 cm
- Location deep dermis or subcutaneous tissue
- No solar elastosis, no connection to surface epithelium
- No significant numbers of mitoses or cytologic atypia

Differential diagnosis

1. Trichoepithelioma (22.2).
2. Basal cell carcinoma (18.14).
3. Other basaloid neoplasms (1.11).

CHAPTER 23

Sweat Gland Neoplasms

23.1 Eccrine nevus and apocrine nevus

Very rare plaque or patch of hyperhidrosis, onset at birth or early childhood, sometimes with one or many sweat pores.

P
- Basaloid hyperplasia of the epidermis sometimes
- *Increased size or number of apocrine or eccrine glands*

Variation

1. Angiomatous eccrine nevus (eccrine angiomatous hamartoma): blood vessels proliferate along with eccrine glands.

Differential diagnosis

1. Increased numbers of sweat glands are normal for certain anatomic areas.
2. Nevus sebaceus (21.2): also has increased apocrine glands, but usually is on the head near the scalp, is linear and yellowish, and sebaceous glands are proliferating.

23.2 Hidradenoma papilliferum

(see Fig. 23.2)
Uncommon papule or nodule *almost always on the vulva* (1.149) or perianal area (1.108) of women.

P
- Circumscribed tumor in the dermis with many *maze-like glandular spaces*, *apocrine* differentiation, and *papillary folds*
- Usually *no connection of the tumor to the epidermis*
- Usually minimal inflammation around the tumor

Differential diagnosis

1. Syringocystadenoma papilliferum (SCAP) (23.3): connects to epidermis, plasma cells, head or neck
2. Papillary eccrine adenoma (23.8).
3. Nipple adenoma (23.5): location on the nipple.
4. Tubular apocrine adenoma (23.6).

23.3 Syringocystadenoma papilliferum

(see Fig. 23.3A,B)
Uncommon red papillomatous plaque usually on the *scalp* (1.124).

P
- Papillomatous epidermis (1.102) connecting to underlying tumor
- Cystic space within *tumor opens to surface of skin*. Tumor lined by squamous epithelium in the upper portion; lower portion lined by sweat glandular epithelium
- *Apocrine* decapitation secretion usually present (sometimes is eccrine)
- *Papillary projections into cystic space*
- *Plasma cell infiltrate* (1.111) around tumor
- *Nevus sebaceus* (21.2) is often present as a precursor lesion

Differential diagnosis

1. Same differential as hidradenoma papilliferum (23.2).
2. Malignant syringocystadenocarcinoma: very rare, more atypia, more necrosis, more invasive.

23.4 Cylindroma of skin

(see Fig. 23.4A,B)
Uncommon smooth red nodules, usually of the *scalp* (1.124), invoking the name "turban tumor". Multiple lesions can be autosomal dominant, associated with the CYLD gene. Sometimes associated with multiple trichoepitheliomas in Brooke–Spiegler syndrome (22.2). Cylindroma and eccrine spiradenoma (23.11) may coexist within the same neoplasm (spiradenocylindroma), and may be two expressions of the same neoplasm, just like fibrofolliculoma and trichodiscoma.

P
- Tumor of *basaloid cells* in the dermis arranged in islands that often fit together like a *jigsaw puzzle*. Basaloid cells are of two types: one type is larger and has a paler nucleus than the other
- *Hyalinized cylinders* (partly due to a thickened basement membrane, PAS positive, containing type IV collagen) around each tumor island
- *Hyalinized droplets* often within the tumor
- *Sweat duct lumina* often present within tumor islands

©2012 Elsevier Ltd, Inc, BV
DOI: 10.1016/B978-0-323-06658-7.00023-3

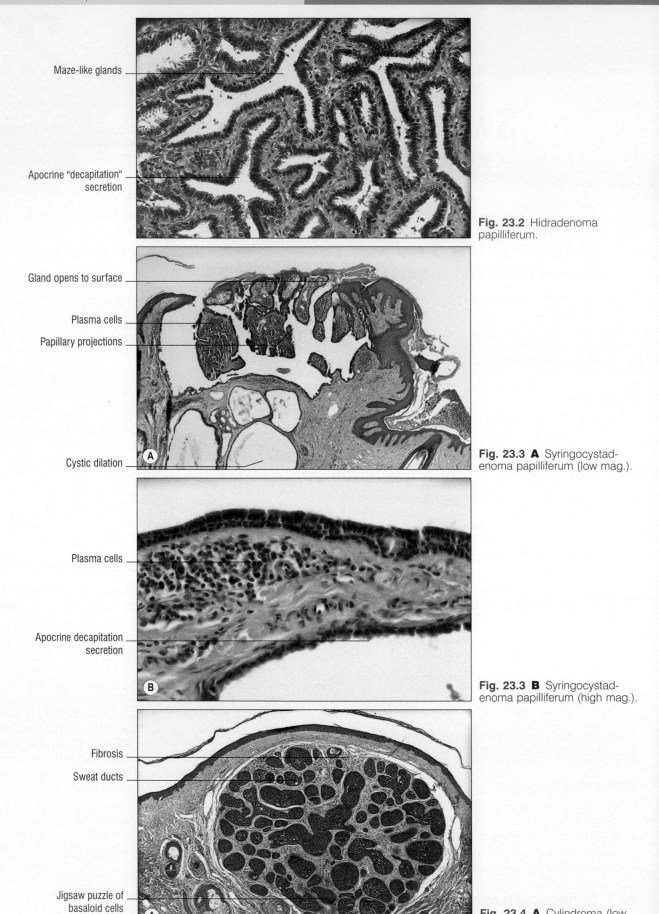

Maze-like glands

Apocrine "decapitation" secretion

Fig. 23.2 Hidradenoma papilliferum.

Gland opens to surface

Plasma cells

Papillary projections

Cystic dilation

Fig. 23.3 A Syringocystadenoma papilliferum (low mag.).

Plasma cells

Apocrine decapitation secretion

Fig. 23.3 B Syringocystadenoma papilliferum (high mag.).

Fibrosis

Sweat ducts

Jigsaw puzzle of basaloid cells

Fig. 23.4 A Cylindroma (low mag.).

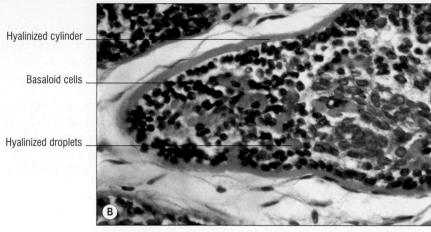

Hyalinized cylinder

Basaloid cells

Hyalinized droplets

B

Fig. 23.4 B Cylindroma (high mag.).

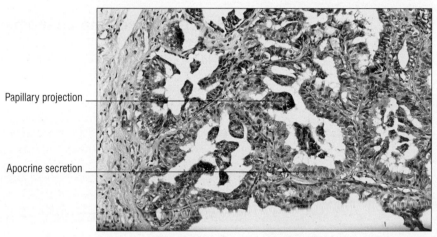

Papillary projection

Apocrine secretion

Fig. 23.5 Nipple adenoma.

Differential diagnosis

1. Malignant cylindroma: very rare.
2. Cylindromas (pleomorphic adenomas) may also originate from salivary glands instead of skin, and can be mistaken for malignancy.
3. Other basaloid neoplasms (1.11), especially resembles basal cell carcinoma (BCC, 18.14) clinically (and histologically at first glance).

23.5 Nipple adenoma (erosive adenomatosis of the nipple, papillary adenoma of the nipple)

(see Fig. 23.5)
Uncommon crusted papule or plaque on the *nipple* (1.90), usually in females.

P
- Circumscribed tumor, many glandular spaces with *apocrine* decapitation secretion and *papillary* projections into the lumina, sometimes filling the lumina
- Tumor often connects to surface of epidermis
- Infiltrate of lymphocytes or plasma cells around the tumor sometimes

Differential diagnosis

1. Paget's disease and carcinoma of the breast: cytologic atypia.
2. Other papillary sweat gland neoplasms in this chapter.

23.6 Tubular apocrine adenoma

Rare, slowly growing, solitary, large nodule, no characteristic location.

- Epidermis sometimes hyperplastic (1.61)
- Circumscribed tumor in dermis or subcutaneous tissue consisting of many glandular spaces
- *Apocrine* decapitation secretion usually present
- *Papillary projections without stroma* extend into the lumina of the tubules
- No connection to the surface epithelium

Differential diagnosis

1. Papillary eccrine adenoma (23.8): eccrine differentiation, otherwise may be the same neoplasm.
2. Hidradenoma papilliferum (23.2): almost always on the vulva, maze-like pattern.

3. Syringocystadenoma papilliferum (23.3): more superficial, always connects to surface epithelium, more plasma cells.
4. Sweat gland carcinoma (23.13).
5. Metastatic adenocarcinoma (28.2).

23.7 Syringoma

(see Fig. 23.7A,B)
Somewhat common *small* (less than 3 mm) papules, *often multiple on the eyelids* (1.43), and more rarely disseminated over the trunk, mostly in females, or on the penis or on the labia.

- *Proliferation of eccrine ducted structures* in the dermis. When sectioned at an angle, they appear to *resemble tadpoles*
- No aggressive infiltration of the deeper dermis
- Horn cysts may be present, and *milia may coexist* (19.1)
- *Stroma is often fibrotic* or sclerotic

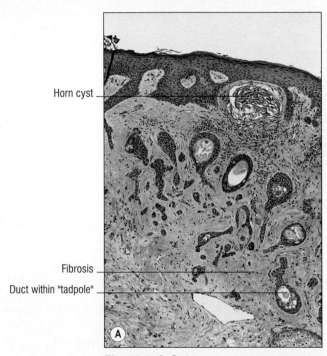

Horn cyst

Fibrosis

Duct within "tadpole"

Fig. 23.7 A Syringoma.

Variation

1. Clear cell syringoma: clinically identical, clear cells (1.22) containing glycogen (PAS positive, diastase labile) are present.

Differential diagnosis

1. Sclerosing basal cell carcinoma (18.14): pearly appearance clinically instead of skin-colored papules, ductal spaces uncommon, more solar elastosis, stromal retraction, atypia.
2. Desmoplastic trichoepithelioma (22.2): more horn cysts, no sweat ducts.
3. Sweat gland carcinoma (23.13): much larger infiltrating neoplasm, particularly easy to miss when only small inadequate biopsy is performed, more cytologic atypia and more invasive.
4. Metastatic adenocarcinoma (28.2): larger, cytologic atypia.

23.8 Papillary eccrine adenoma

(see Fig. 23.8)
Rare, slowly growing nodule on *extremities* of *black women*.

- Circumscribed dermal tumor consisting of *many glandular spaces* with eccrine (sometimes apocrine) differentiation
- *Papillary* projections into the lumina only in some portions of the neoplasm
- Focal or no connection to the surface epithelium
- Fibrous stroma
- Positive staining for CEA and S-100

Differential diagnosis

1. Tubular apocrine adenoma (23.6): apocrine differentiation, otherwise similar entity.
2. Sweat gland carcinoma, especially aggressive digital papillary adenocarcinoma (23.13): larger ductal structures, more cytologic atypia, and more aggressive infiltration.
3. Metastatic adenocarcinoma (28.2): cytologic atypia.

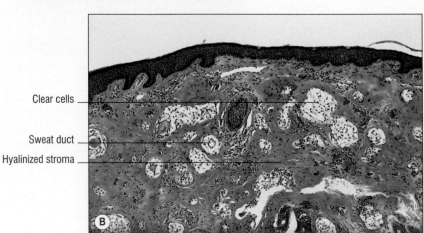

Clear cells

Sweat duct

Hyalinized stroma

Fig. 23.7 B Syringoma (clear cell).

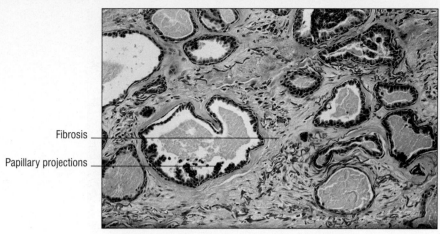

Fig. 23.8 Papillary "eccrine" adenoma (low mag.).

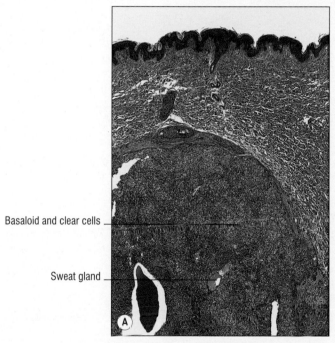

Basaloid and clear cells

Sweat gland

Fig. 23.9 A Nodular hidradenoma.

23.9 Nodular hidradenoma (eccrine acrospiroma)

(see Fig. 23.9A,B)
Uncommon nodule without a characteristic location or clinical appearance.

Variations
1. Clear cell hidradenoma: clear cells (1.22) containing glycogen (PAS positive, diastase labile).
2. Solid-cystic hidradenoma: prominent cystic spaces plus solid areas.
3. Dermal duct tumor: no connection to surface epithelium, otherwise is a synonym.

Differential diagnosis
1. Malignant eccrine acrospiroma: rare, more atypia, more invasive.
2. Eccrine poroma (23.10): in the same family with nodular hidradenoma, broad-based connection to epidermis, resembles a seborrheic keratosis on low power, most common on the sole or scalp.
3. Eccrine spiradenoma (23.11): confusing name, sounds similar to acrospiroma, rosettes of two sizes of basaloid cells.
4. Other basaloid neoplasms (1.11) or clear cell neoplasms (1.22) mostly do not have sweat ducts.

23.10 Eccrine poroma
(see Fig. 23.10A–C)
Some authorities prefer to call it simply "poroma" because they protest that they believe it is really apocrine. This seems to be a lot to do about nothing, and dermatopathologists have debated eccrine versus apocrine on many of the sweat gland tumors for decades. It is an uncommon *eroded friable papule or plaque* most common on the *sole* (1.100) or *scalp* (1.124), sometimes with an indented moat around it. Clinically resembles pyogenic granuloma (25.3).

P
- Nodular tumor in the dermis or subcutaneous tissue made up of mainly *one cell type of basaloid cells*, sometimes with focal connection to epidermis
- Sweat duct lumina usually present within the tumor, varying from small ducts to large cystic spaces
- Usually eccrine differentiation, rarely apocrine decapitation secretion is present
- Hyalinized collagen in the stroma sometimes
- Keratinous cysts sometimes

- Tumor of cuboidal or *basaloid "poroid"* cells within the lower portion of an acanthotic epidermis, extending into the dermis
- Often *sharp demarcation* or moat between normal epidermis and tumor
- Tumor cells may be clear (1.22) due to glycogen accumulation (PAS positive, diastase labile)
- Small sweat ducts usually present within tumor

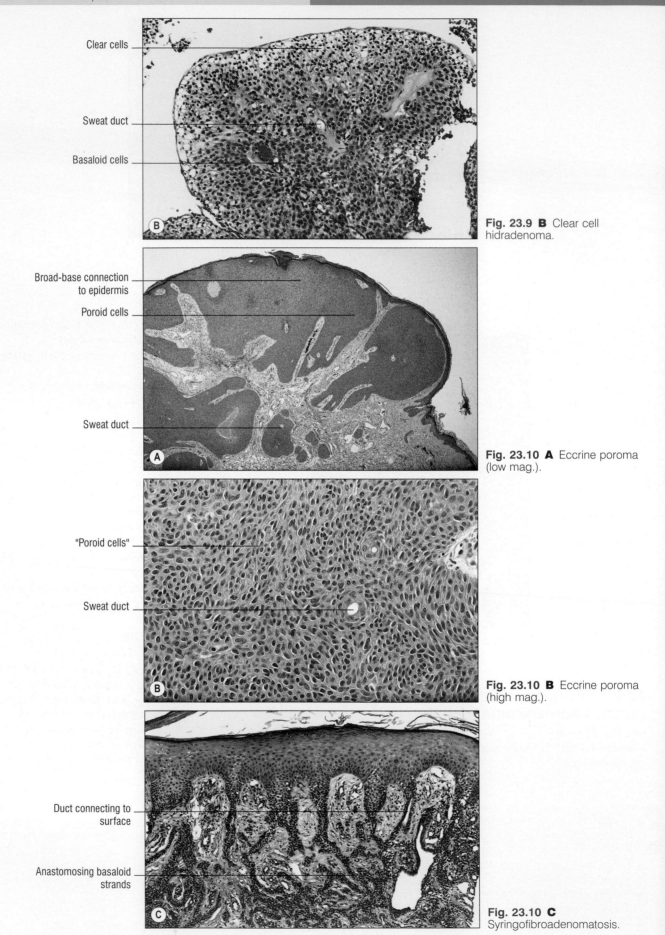

Clear cells

Sweat duct

Basaloid cells

Fig. 23.9 B Clear cell hidradenoma.

Broad-base connection to epidermis

Poroid cells

Sweat duct

Fig. 23.10 A Eccrine poroma (low mag.).

"Poroid cells"

Sweat duct

Fig. 23.10 B Eccrine poroma (high mag.).

Duct connecting to surface

Anastomosing basaloid strands

Fig. 23.10 C Syringofibroadenomatosis.

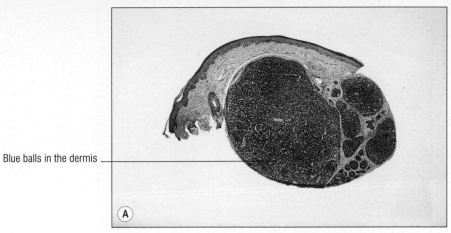

Blue balls in the dermis

Fig. 23.11 A Eccrine spiradenoma (low mag.).

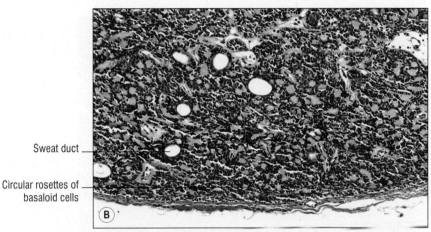

Sweat duct

Circular rosettes of basaloid cells

Fig. 23.11 B Eccrine spiradenoma (high mag.).

Variations

1. Hidroacanthoma simplex: proliferation of clones of basaloid or clear cells and ductal lumina *completely within epidermis*, similar to Borst–Jadassohn intraepidermal epithelioma (1.37).
2. Syringofibroadenomatosis: rare *anastomosing net-like ductal proliferation* in the dermis with a broad connection to the surface, similar to a fibroepithelioma (18.14) with sweat ducts. May be found in *Schopf–Schulz–Passarge syndrome* (23.10, associated with mutation in the WNT10A gene).
3. Sebocrine adenoma: *sebaceous and apocrine* differentiation in a poroma-like lesion.

Differential diagnosis

1. Malignant eccrine poroma (porocarcinoma): rare, larger, more cytologic atypia, more necrosis, more invasive, resembles squamous cell carcinoma but has sweat ducts.
2. Nodular hidradenoma (23.9): eccrine poroma may be considered to be a variant of hidradenoma. The major difference is that eccrine poroma has a *broad-based connection to the surface epidermis*, while hidradenoma is a dermal or subcutaneous nodule. The "poroid cells" are otherwise identical.

3. Seborrheic keratosis (18.2): basaloid cell can look poroid, but has no increased sweat ducts.
4. Other basaloid neoplasms (1.11).

23.11 Eccrine spiradenoma

(see Fig. 23.11A,B)

Uncommon, painful (1.96), usually solitary, dermal, or subcutaneous nodule (1.135). Like many subcutaneous nodules, it occasionally can have a bluish appearance (1.14). Rarely multiple, sometimes associated with trichoepithelioma (22.2) and cylindroma (23.4). Like eccrine poroma, some authorities have argued that this tumor is also apocrine.

- Sharply demarcated nodules of basaloid cells in dermis or subcutaneous tissue ("blue balls")
- Almost never any connection to the epidermis
- Basaloid cells are often said to be of two types, which might not be so apparent: one is more pale with more cytoplasm than the darker cells
- Basaloid cells tend to be arranged in rosettes, sometimes called trabeculae
- Sparse small sweat ductal lumina usually present
- Lymphocytes with Langerhans cells usually scattered in the stroma and in the epithelial aggregates
- Stroma often vascular

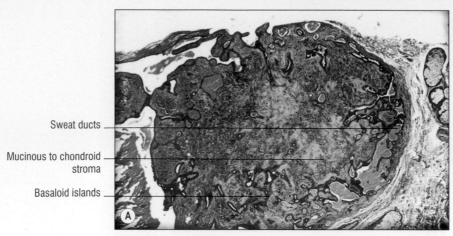

Sweat ducts

Mucinous to chondroid stroma

Basaloid islands

Fig. 23.12 A Chondroid syringoma (low mag.).

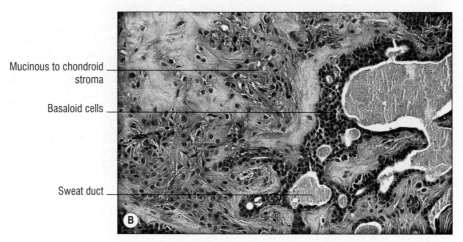

Mucinous to chondroid stroma

Basaloid cells

Sweat duct

Fig. 23.12 B Chondroid syringoma (medium mag.).

Differential diagnosis

1. Malignant eccrine spiradenoma: very rare, more atypia, more necrosis, more invasive.
2. Nodular hidradenoma (23.9).
3. Spiradenocylindroma: lesion with combined cylindroma (23.4) and spiradenoma components.
4. Other basaloid neoplasms (1.11).

23.12 Chondroid syringoma (mixed tumor of skin)

(see Fig. 23.12A,B)

Uncommon dermal or subcutaneous nodule or cyst, no specific location. It is called a mixed tumor because of the prominent mixture of epithelial and stromal components (a ludicrous concept, because nearly all epithelial neoplasms have a stromal component, but the point is that this one makes impressive cartilage-like stroma).

- Epithelial islands *small to medium sweat ductal structures*, eccrine or apocrine
- Prominent *mucinous stroma* (positive with acid mucopolysaccharide stains, eventually becoming *chondroid*)
- Hyalinized areas in the stroma sometimes

Variation

1. Combined adnexal tumor: term used for difficult to classify adnexal neoplasms with divergent differentiation toward sweat ductal, sebaceous, and pilar structures. Unusual divergent adnexal tumors are encountered frequently and many of these are difficult to categorize in our man-made classification. Adnexal tumors are not necessarily derived from the type of adnexal structure seen in the neoplasm. On the contrary they actually are differentiating in the direction of the type of structures that are seen. So a sweat gland tumor does not necessarily derive from sweat glands.

Differential diagnosis

1. Malignant chondroid syringoma: very rare, more atypia, more necrosis, more invasive.
2. Pleomorphic adenoma (mixed tumor of the salivary gland): similar histologically, may extend into the skin.
3. Chondroid lipoma (29.2).
4. Extraskeletal chondroma (cutaneous cartilaginous tumor): slowly growing benign mass, especially around small joints of hands and feet, localized mature cartilage (S-100 positive), sometimes with granulomatous reaction, fibrosis, calcification, or ossification. No epithelial or sweat gland component.

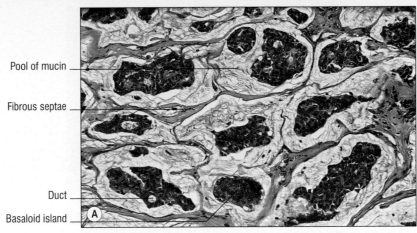

Pool of mucin

Fibrous septae

Duct

Basaloid island

Fig. 23.13 A Mucinous carcinoma.

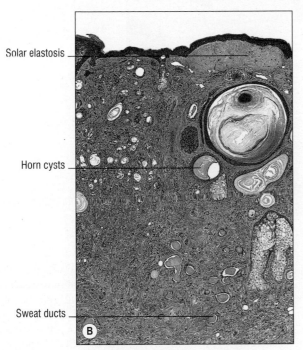

Solar elastosis

Horn cysts

Sweat ducts

Fig. 23.13 B Microcystic adnexal carcinoma (low mag.).

5. Chondrosarcoma and osteochondroma.
6. Accessory tragus (29.10) can contain cartilage.
7. Other lesions with mucin (1.83).

23.13 Sweat gland carcinoma

(see Fig. 23.13A–D)
There are several varieties of uncommon malignancies with sweat gland differentiation.

P ■ Tumor infiltrating the dermis and consisting of *ductal or glandular structures*
■ *Atypia* (hyperchromatism, pleomorphism, increased numbers of mitoses) or *necrosis* often present

---

Variations

1. Malignant counterparts of cylindroma, eccrine poroma, eccrine spiradenoma, and chondroid syringoma have been described, with characteristics in common with each of those benign entities.
2. Primary mucinous carcinoma (adenocystic carcinoma): small ductal structures embedded in *abundant pools of mucin*, separated by fibrous septae.
3. Adenoid cystic carcinoma: confusing name sounds similar to adenocystic carcinoma, glandular proliferations containing mucin, often *cribriform pattern* (net-like bridges between ductal spaces). More likely to be CD117+, whereas basal cell carcinoma is negative.
4. Microcystic adnexal carcinoma (MAC): indurated plaque (1.125) that may be clinically subtle but nevertheless large, most common on nose (1.95) and upper lip (1.74), resembles a large aggressive sclerosing basal cell carcinoma, *basaloid strands with small lumina, horn cysts* may be present, especially in superficial portion, sometimes thought to show dual differentiation toward sweat glands and follicular structures. Perineural invasion is common.
5. Sclerosing sweat duct carcinoma: infiltrating strands of *basaloid cells with small ductal lumina*, sometimes used as a synonym for MAC, except that "splitters" separate it out mainly because of the lack of horn cysts.
6. Epidermotropic adnexal carcinoma: similar to Paget's disease (18.13), but this term is used when an underlying sweat duct carcinoma (as opposed to an adenocarcinoma of internal organ origin) *infiltrates the epidermis*.
7. Aggressive digital papillary adenoma and adenocarcinoma: these two lesions are often lumped together because the benign form is so difficult to distinguish from the malignant form. Solitary nodule of *acral skin*, often *cystic*. Papillary projections extend into a cystic space, sometimes with atypia, increased mitoses, invasion into bone.
8. Mucoepidermoid carcinoma: basaloid or squamoid neoplasm with ductal differentiation and *mucin within individual cells*, "lumpers" might consider it to be synonym for adenosquamous carcinoma (18.11).

Hyalinized stroma —

Basaloid strands —

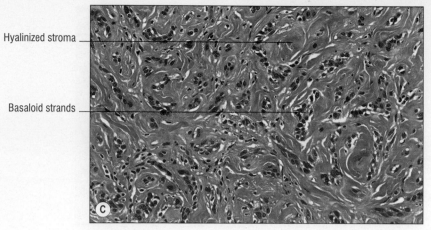

Fig. 23.13 C Microcystic adnexal carcinoma (medium mag.).

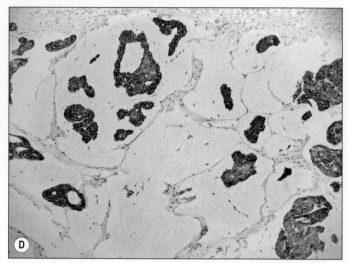

Fig. 23.13 D Primary mucinous carcinoma (CK-7 stain).

Differential diagnosis

1. Metastatic adenocarcinoma (28.2): sometimes impossible to distinguish, may require a search in other organs for possible primary sites of origin. Primary adnexal carcinomas will stain for D2-40 and p63 in 90% of cases, except for mucinous carcinoma, which typically is p63neg. Metastatic adenocarcinomas are almost always negative for p63 and negative for D2-40.[134,139]

2. Adenoid basal cell carcinoma (18.14): mucinous spaces in the basaloid aggregates are pale blue instead of the more eosinophic color found in sweat glands, and there is no eosinophilic cuticle as is found lining true sweat ducts. MAC and desmoplastic trichoepithelioma are usually positive for CK15, whereas BCC is negative. MAC is more likely to be CEA+ and EMA+. Basal cell carcinoma is more likely to stain for Ber-EP4 than desmoplastic trichoepithelioma.

CHAPTER 24

Myeloproliferative Disorders

A detailed classification of myeloproliferative disorders is complex and constantly in flux, with continued advances in immunophenotyping, gene rearrangement studies, fluorescence in situ hybridization, microarrays, comparative genomic hybridization, and laser-based microdissection. Indeed, this chapter was without a doubt the worst chapter in the first edition of this book, so a complete overhaul was needed. Many classification schemes have come and gone over the years.[91,93] The most recent one in common use is that of the World Health Organization (WHO).[163] In this book, some of the original headings have been preserved, even though they do not correspond exactly to the WHO schema. It has been joked that a more simplified classification of lymphomas should consist of good ones, bad ones, in-between ones, and the ones that are not what they seem.[132] This chapter will focus mainly on lymphomas that are primary in the skin. Systemic lymphomas (often called nodal lymphomas) may secondarily involve the skin, often with a worse prognosis. Although selected features of skin biopsies can help to distinguish primary from systemic lymphoma, typically a more detailed workup, including imaging, flow cytometry, bone marrow assessement, and other ancillary studies, are needed. The services of a hematopathologist or a dermatopathologist with a special interest in these disorders may be needed for an exact classification of a case.

Lymphomas are difficult to distinguish from benign reactive lymphoid proliferations (24.14). One problem is that reactive lymphoid cells may interact with or obscure the malignant clone, causing difficulty in its identification. For example, reactive CD20+ B cells can be found in some cases of T-cell lymphoma. Another problem is that monoclonality does not always indicate malignancy. For example, abnormal gene rearrangement results have been reported in apparently benign conditions, such as lichen planus (2.11), pityriasis lichenoides (2.14), purpura pigmentosa chronica (4.8), lichen sclerosus (9.5), and pseudolymphoma (24.14). It is important to realize that most benign "rashes" involve mostly T lymphocytes, so that looking for T-cell lymphoma is much more complicated than just looking for T cells! Immunomarkers have become more important, as oncologists develop more targeted therapies directed against specific antigens, such as zanolimumab (anti-CD4), rituximab (anti-CD20, expressed in most B-cell lymphomas), alemtuzumab (anti-CD52), and denileukin diftitox (anti-CD25). Refer to Chapter 30 for summaries of many of the immunostains used heavily for these disorders.

24.1 Mycosis fungoides (MF)

(see Fig. 24.1A–G)

MF has nothing to do with fungus, despite the unfortunate name. It is the most common prototypic form of cutaneous T-cell lymphoma (CTCL), hence it has its own section in this book. Most CTCL is MF, but MF is just one type of CTCL. The other T-cell lymphomas have been moved to Sections 24.2 through 24.7. The classical Alibert–Bazin type of MF has three stages. Initially, *eczematous* patches (1.29), especially of the *hip and buttock*, often persist for years and are difficult to distinguish from eczema. Second, *papulosquamous plaques* develop (1.103). Third, *tumor nodules* (1.92) appear. About 90% of patients never progress to tumor stage and do not develop systemic disease. Therefore routine staging investigations (imaging scans, bone marrow biopsies, etc.) are not recommended in patch stage patients. Lymph node, liver, spleen, lung, and bone marrow involvement are usually late findings. Dermatopathic lymphadenopathy (benign nodes reacting to the skin) is difficult to distinguish from lymph node involvement by malignant cells.

©2012 Elsevier Ltd, Inc, BV
DOI: 10.1016/B978-0-323-06658-7.00024-5

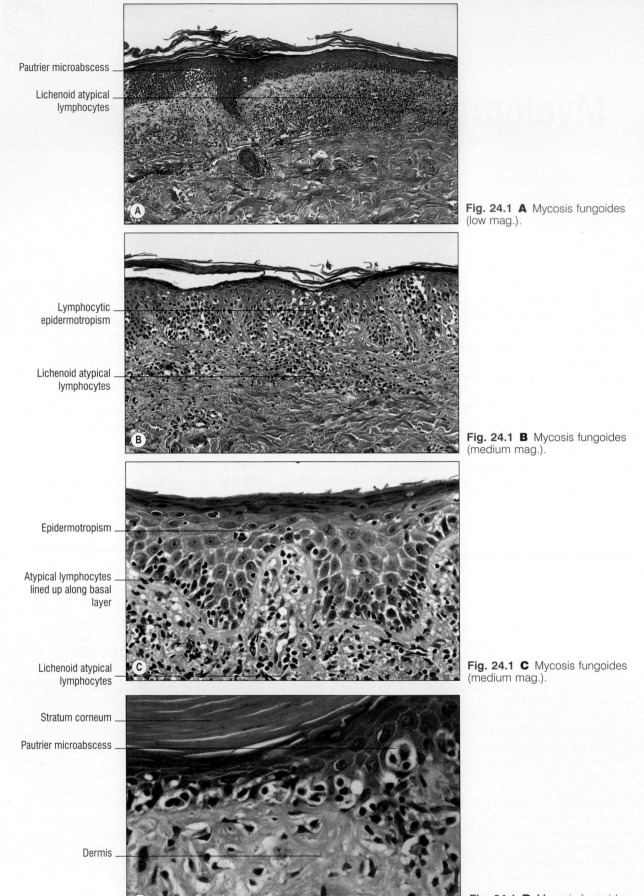

Pautrier microabscess

Lichenoid atypical lymphocytes

Fig. 24.1 A Mycosis fungoides (low mag.).

Lymphocytic epidermotropism

Lichenoid atypical lymphocytes

Fig. 24.1 B Mycosis fungoides (medium mag.).

Epidermotropism

Atypical lymphocytes lined up along basal layer

Lichenoid atypical lymphocytes

Fig. 24.1 C Mycosis fungoides (medium mag.).

Stratum corneum

Pautrier microabscess

Dermis

Fig. 24.1 D Mycosis fungoides (high mag.).

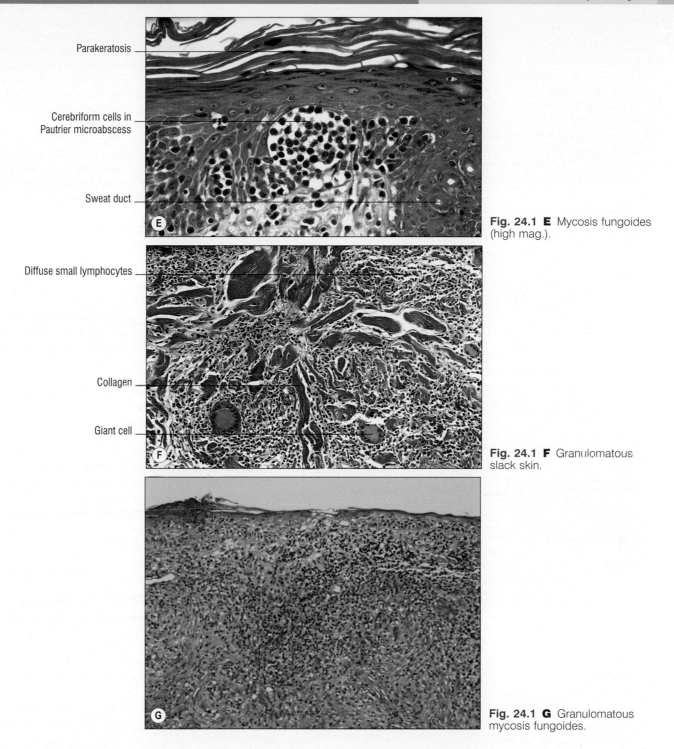

Parakeratosis

Cerebriform cells in
Pautrier microabscess

Sweat duct

Fig. 24.1 E Mycosis fungoides
(high mag.).

Diffuse small lymphocytes

Collagen

Giant cell

Fig. 24.1 F Granulomatous
slack skin.

Fig. 24.1 G Granulomatous
mycosis fungoides.

- Epidermis may be atrophic (1.9), hyperplastic (1.61), or ulcerated (1.142)
- *Lichenoid* or diffuse (1.91), less commonly just perivascular (1.109), atypical lymphocytes, sometimes with *cerebriform nuclei,*, but sometimes just small banal-appearing lymphocytes, with eosinophils (1.36), and plasma cells (1.111)
- *Epidermotropism of the atypical lymphocytes* often, sometimes producing single cell "punched-out" holes ("haloed nuclei") in the epidermis, or larger spaces filled with these lymphocytes (*Pautrier microabscesses*, also known as Darier's nests since he described it first), or prominently lining up at the dermal–epidermal junction. Epidermal lymphocytes tend to be larger and more atypical than those in the dermis. Epidermotropism often less prominent in older nodules
- Spongiosis usually not seen in most cases, unlike eczema. MF has too much epidermotropism for too little spongiosis ("too much for too little")
- *Follicular mucinosis* sometimes present (10.8)
- Most lymphocytes exhibit positive staining with *T-cell markers* (CD2, *CD3*, CD5), most often with increased T-helper cells (CD4) and fewer suppressor-cytotoxic T cells (CD8), ratio CD4:CD8 usually more than 3:1. *Loss of pan-T-cell markers such as CD7* and less commonly CD5, has been stressed as helpful, but this may not be as specific as advertised
- Identification of CD25 (IL-2 receptor) positive cells is useful prior to therapy with denileukin diftitox (Ontak). Positive staining for CD52 is useful for possible alemtuzumab (anti-CD52, Campath) treatment. Positive staining for cytotoxic proteins (granzyme, perforin, TIA-1) indicates more aggressive subtype (some would not classify this as true mycosis fungoides)
- Clonal *T-cell receptor* (TCR) *gene rearrangements* may be present, more commonly in later stages, less in patch stage, usually alpha–beta, but sometimes gamma–delta
- Papillary dermal collagen often said to be wiry, resembling fettuccine, but this is overrated as a diagnostic help

Variations

1. Woringer–Kolopp disease (pagetoid reticulosis): *solitary patch or plaque of MF* with *prominent epidermotropism*, most common on the distal limbs. The atypical cells are characteristically CD3+, CD4neg, CD8+, CD45RO+, CD20neg, CD30neg, CD79a neg. Sometimes CD4+ more than CD8+. Good prognosis.
2. Poikiloderma atrophicans vasculare (PAV): *poikilodermatous changes* are dominant (1.112), more common on trunk, more *epidermal atrophy* (1.9), interface (1.64), or lichenoid lymphocytes (1.72), *telangiectasia* (1.136), melanin incontinence (1.79), and extravasated erythrocytes (1.40).
3. Granulomatous T-cell lymphoma: very rare form of MF in which *granulomatous* infiltrates in the dermis may cause confusion with benign granulomas (1.51). Epidermotropism may be helpful when present.
4. Granulomatous slack skin: very rare, patches or plaque eventually result in *hanging folds of skin*, especially in the

axilla (1.10) and groin (1.55), due to *fragmented elastic fibers* (1.31) like in cutis laxa (9.10). Sometimes associated with Hodgkin lymphoma (24.15). Pathology similar to granulomatous T-cell lymphoma: *diffuse small lymphocytes*, immunostaining as in MF, epidermotropism sometimes slight, *multinucleated giant cells* (1.84) that contain lymphocytes or elastic fibers stain with macrophage stains such as lysozyme and CD68.

5. Hypopigmented MF: hypopigmented (1.150) macules, often in *young patients* with *black skin*, more likely to express CD8. It may be difficult to distinguish from atopic dermatitis (2.1) and the inflammatory stage of vitiligo (17.2). The term *white spot parapsoriasis* has been used when there is insufficient evidence to confirm the diagnosis as MF or eczema.
6. MF in young patients: MF is rarely found in children, more likely to be hypopigmented or resemble pityriasis lichenoides (2.14). In most cases, there are patches with an indolent and non-aggressive course.
7. MF palmaris et plantaris (dyshidrosiform MF): scaly plaques or vesicles of the *palms or soles* (1.100), which may resemble eczema (2.1), and may be an example of overdiagnosis based upon excessive reliance on lymphocyte marker studies.
8. MF d'emblee: aggressive subtype wherein tumor *nodules develop without the usual previous patch or plaque stages*. Most of these patients actually have CD30-positive anaplastic large cell lymphoma (24.5) or natural killer (NK)/T-cell cytotoxic lymphoma (24.6), and generally no longer considered to have a type of MF.
9. Follicular MF (folliculotropic, pilotropic MF): prominent clinical and pathological *follicular involvement* (1.47), often sparing epidermis, sometimes with infundibular cyst formation, not necessarily with follicular mucinosis (10.8), often head and neck.
10. Syringotropic MF: prominent involvement around the sweat glands.
11. MF with gamma-delta (γ–δ) gene rearrangement and MF with CD8+ predominance has the normal progression of chronic patches and plaques of ordinary MF, unlike the more aggressive primary cutaneous γ–δ T-cell lymphoma and the aggressive primary cutaneous epidermotropic CD8+ T-cell lymphoma (both 24.6).
12. Interstitial MF: resembles interstitial granuloma annulare (7.1). Epidermotropism may be a clue toward the diagnosis.
13. Papular MF: small papules are present instead of patches or plaques, does not have spontaneous regression as found in lymphomatoid papulosis type B (24.5).
14. Invisible MF: patients have no visible patches or other skin lesions, but biopsy shows MF.
15. Erythrodermic MF: generalized *exfoliative erythroderma* (1.39), but lacks the leukemic phase of Sezary syndrome (24.1).
16. MF with large cell transformation: large cells are usually but not always CD30+, usually appears with later stage of MF with worse prognosis, may overlap with other CD30+ lymphoproliferative diseases (24.5).

Differential diagnosis

1. Other lymphomas and leukemias in this chapter.
2. Eczema (2.1) and contact dermatitis (2.2): clinically more responsive to corticosteroids, more spongiosis, less epidermotropism, less lichenoid and more perivascular lymphocytes, no atypical lymphocytes, no abnormal T-cell gene rearrangements, less likely to have CD7 depletion. In paraffin sections, epidermal lymphocytes of contact dermatitis are more commonly CD45RBneg, CD45RO+, whereas epidermotropic lymphocytes in MF are CD45RB+, CD45ROneg. In frozen sections and flow cytometry, MF lymphocytes are strangely typically CD45RO+.
3. Parapsoriasis (2.9): often used as a controversial term for persistent eczematous lesions for which it is uncertain as to whether they represent MF or not.
4. Actinic reticuloid (2.2): a chronic photodermatitis (like chronic actinic dermatitis or persistent light reactor) with atypical lymphocytes resembling MF, usually benign but persistent course.
5. Other diseases with epidermotropism (1.37), not to be confused with spongiosis (1.132). Langerhans microgranulomas (24.18) have been rarely reported in the epidermis of MF.
6. Lichenoid (1.72), interface (1.64), nodular and diffuse (1.91), and spongiotic[118] (1.132) dermatitis. The following disorders are often mistaken for MF: lichenoid keratosis (18.8), lichen planus (2.11), pityriasis lichenoides (2.14), purpura pigmentosa chronica (4.8). T-cell receptor gene rearrangments have even been found in some of these disorders, compounding the problem.

24.2 Sezary syndrome

(see Fig. 24.2)
This can be considered to be the *leukemic phase of MF*, but now is considered a separate entity by WHO.[163] Patients usually have *exfoliative erythroderma* (1.39), palmar–plantar involvement, and lymphadenopathy from the start, instead of progressing more slowly with patches or plaques as in MF. If a patient lacks sufficient Sezary cells in the blood,

they are designated as having erythrodermic MF instead of Sezary syndrome.

> ■ By definition, more than 1000 Sezary cells per cubic millimeter in the peripheral blood (large cerebriform atypical CD4+ lymphocytes greater than 14 microns). The CD4+:CD8+ ratio is often more than 10:1 with flow cytometry with most cells CD7–. Sezary cells are negative for CD4.
> ■ Otherwise routine histology and immunopathology similar to MF (24.1). In some cases the skin biopsy is non-specific and the diagnosis is made from the blood.
> ■ Clonal T-cell gene rearrangments in skin or blood as in MF.

24.3 Adult T-cell leukemia–lymphoma (ATLL)

This is associated with infection by the *human T-cell lymphotropic virus type I* (HTLV-1). Serology for this virus is available, and it can be detected within the atypical lymphocytes (transmitted sexually or by blood transfusion), not to be confused with HTLV-III (which is now called HIV-1, 14.12). Often called *ATLL* since it primarily affects adults, and latent infection with this virus prior to apparent disease is prolonged. Other patients have acute aggressive disease. More common in Japan, Africa, Caribbean, and south-eastern US. Systemic involvement, *lymphadenopathy*, *hypercalcemia*, and *osteolytic bone lesions* (1.16) are common. Half of the patients have skin lesions: papules, nodules or plaques.

> ■ Histology similar to MF in many cases (24.1), with or without epidermotropism, but lymphocytes in skin and blood sometimes multilobed (called "flower cells" in peripheral blood)
> ■ Usually CD3+, CD4+. *CD25 routinely positive* (unlike many cases of MF). CD30neg even though some patient have large atypical lymphocytes like CD30+ lymphoma (24.5). CD7 usually remains positive and does not become depleted
> ■ Gene rearrangements like MF often present

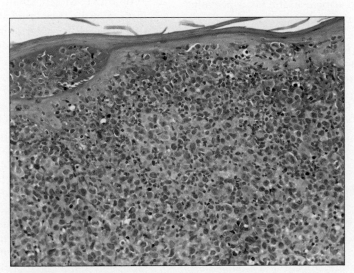

Fig. 24.2 Sezary syndrome.

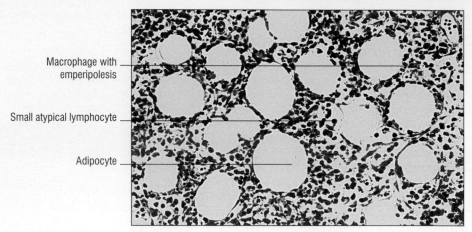

Fig. 24.4 Subcutaneous T-cell lymphoma.

24.4 Subcutaneous T-cell lymphoma

(see Fig 24.4)
Subcutaneous "panniculitis-like" T-cell lymphoma (SPTCL) presents as nodules (1.92) or plaques, most common on the legs (1.67). Many cases are non-aggressive and indolent; other cases rapidly fatal. *Hemophagocytic syndrome* may occur, consisting of macrophages in bone marrow, liver, spleen or lymph nodes with cytophagocytosis, hepatosplenomegaly (1.75), fever (1.45), pancytopenia, and aggressive course.

- Lobular panniculitis (often lace-like pattern of lymphocytes rimming adipocytes), without significant dermal or epidermal involvement
- The malignant small lymphocytes are usually CD3+, CD8+, granzyme+, TIA-1+, perforin+ (*cytotoxic phenotype*). Sometimes the lymphocytes may be larger with more cytologic atypia
- CD68+ macrophages often exhibit *cytophagocytosis* of erythrocytes or nuclear debris ("*bean bag cells*")
- Sometimes an alpha–beta (α–β) T-cell receptor gene rearrangement is present (BF-1 positive)

Differential diagnosis

1. Other lymphomas can also appear in the fat, especially γ–δ T-cell lymphoma (24.6).
2. Panniculitis (Chapter 16). *Cytophagic histiocytic panniculitis* is a term used for panniculitis with cytophagocytosis, some cases of which can be benign and reactive instead of lymphoma. May overlap with lupus panniculitis (17.6).
3. Similar emperipolesis can be seen also in Rosai–Dorfman disease (7.13). Phagocytosed erythrocytes and neutrophils are rarely seen in melanoma or squamous cell carcinoma.

24.5 CD30+ lymphoproliferative disorders

(see Fig. 24.5A–G)
This is an uncommon group of lymphomas in which large atypical lymphocytes express CD30. Lymphomatoid papulosis (LyP) is a rare disorder, in which *crops of papules or nodules*, which sometimes ulcerate, appear and *spontaneously regress*. Lymphomatoid means resembling lymphoma, since

the suffix -oid means resembling. The disease has a *benign course in 90% of cases*, but in 10% of cases, a bona fide lymphoma, usually *Hodgkin's disease* or *mycosis fungoides*, develops. There is debate whether the patients all actually have lymphoma from the start, which is low grade and may regress, or whether benign disease (pseudomalignancy) actually transforms into lymphoma. DNA flow cytometry or T-cell receptor gene rearrangement tests do not predict which patients develop lymphoma.

- Epidermal necrosis (1.87) often, or ulceration
- Nodular infiltrate of ordinary lymphocytes, very *atypical CD-30 positive activated T lymphocytes*, with *epidermotropism* (1.37) into the epidermis
- Neutrophils and eosinophils sometimes present
- Extravasated erythrocytes (1.40), often with red blood cells in the epidermis

Variations

1. Type A LyP: Most common subtype, large CD30-positive atypical lymphocytes resemble histiocytes, found within localized wedge-shaped dermal infiltrate of lymphocytes, neutrophils and eosinophils as above, often with epidermotropism resembling MF.
2. Type B LyP: Mostly smaller cerebriform lymphocytes instead of the very large atypical cells, usually CD30neg, with epidermotropism as in MF, but papules and nodules spontaneously remit.
3. Type C LyP: More impressive sheets of CD30+ large atypical lymphocytes, resembles ALCL below except lesions often come and go.
4. Primary cutaneous anaplastic large cell lymphoma (ALCL): If this is primary in the skin, it tends to regress, but if there is systemic (nodal) involvement, it can be rapidly progressive and fatal. Many examples of malignant histiocytosis (24.7) have been reclassified here. ALK-1 (expressed when chromosomal translocation t(2;5) occurs) and EMA are more likely to be expressed in systemic large cell CD30+ lymphoma than by primary cutaneous anaplastic CD30+ lymphoma, but staging systemic workup is needed to make definitive distinction.
5. Nodal (systemic) anaplastic large cell lymphoma: usually presents with larger nodules or sheets of cells

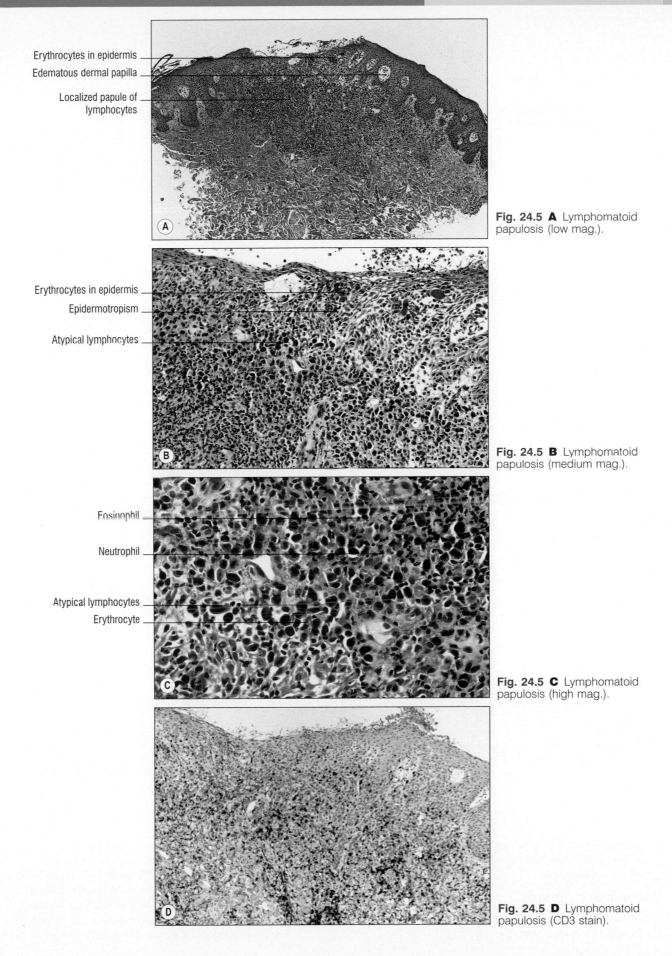

Erythrocytes in epidermis

Edematous dermal papilla

Localized papule of
lymphocytes

Fig. 24.5 A Lymphomatoid
papulosis (low mag.).

Erythrocytes in epidermis

Epidermotropism

Atypical lymphocytes

Fig. 24.5 B Lymphomatoid
papulosis (medium mag.).

Eosinophil

Neutrophil

Atypical lymphocytes

Erythrocyte

Fig. 24.5 C Lymphomatoid
papulosis (high mag.).

Fig. 24.5 D Lymphomatoid
papulosis (CD3 stain).

Epidermis

Brown staining of CD 30 positive lymphocytes

Fig. 24.5 E Lymphomatoid papulosis (CD30 stain).

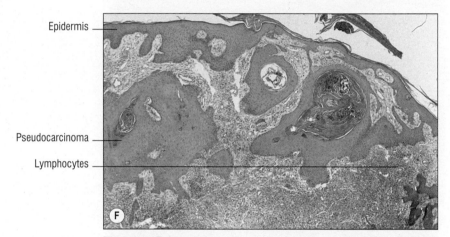

Epidermis

Pseudocarcinoma

Lymphocytes

Fig. 24.5 F Lymphomatoid papulosis with pseudocarcinomatous hyperplasia.

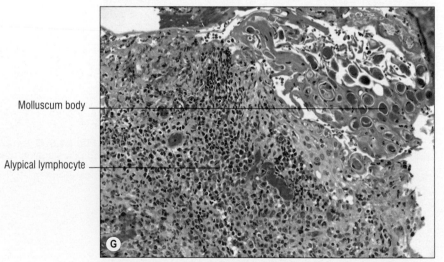

Molluscum body

Alypical lymphocyte

Fig. 24.5 G Atypical CD30+ pseudolymphomatous reaction in molluscum contagiosum.

instead of smaller papules or nodules that come and go, worse prognosis, distinguished from primary cutaneous ALCL as above.

Differential diagnosis

1. Mycosis fungoides (24.1).
2. Hodgkin's lymphoma (24.15).

3. Mucha–Habermann disease (2.14, pityriasis lichenoides et varioliformis acuta, PLEVA): clinically and histologically very similar, but little or no cellular atypia (lymphomatoid papulosis has been called "evil" PLEVA), fewer eosinophils, and CD30 is negative.

4. CD30+ cells have been reported in some apparently benign examples of atopic dermatitis, drug eruptions,

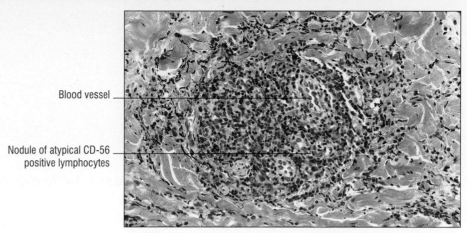

Blood vessel

Nodule of atypical CD-56 positive lymphocytes

Fig. 24.6 Nasal NK/T-cell lymphoma (CD56 positive).

orf, milker's nodule, papillomaviral warts, herpes virus infections, molluscum contagiosum, scabies, and arthropod bites. Scattered CD30+ cells are often seen in many other benign inflammatory conditions.

24.6 Natural killer (NK) cell and cytotoxic lymphomas

(see Fig. 24.6)

This is a rare group of aggressive peripheral T-cell lymphomas (see also 24.7), some formerly called angiocentric immunoproliferative lesions (AIL), some related to Epstein–Barr virus, with large *ulcerating, destructive violaceous plaques or nodules*. Do not confuse "angiocentric" with the equally antiquated term angiotropic lymphoma (24.13). Many of these cytotoxic lymphomas were previously called *malignant histiocytosis*.

Variations

1. Extranodal NK/T-cell lymphoma, nasal type (formerly called lethal midline granuloma): red plaques or nodules, either solitary or localized to a region, commonly around the *central face*, sometimes ulcerated. Aggressive course, nasal and palate destruction may occur. No history of chronic patches or plaques of MF.

P
- Epidermis often ulcerated, sometimes pseudocarcinomatous hyperplasia
- Diffuse or perivascular *polymorphous infiltrate* of atypical lymphocytes, histiocytes, plasma cells, and eosinophils
- Epidermotropism sometimes, invasion of adnexa and nerves common
- *Infiltration of blood vessel walls* by lymphocytes, sometimes with changes suggesting *vasculitis* (necrosis of vessel walls, with thrombi, 1.145)
- CD2+, *CD56+*, TIA-1+, but with frequent loss of T-cell markers CD3, CD4, CD5, or CD7 (therefore formerly called null cells). *Epstein–Barr positive* (by in situ hybridization, for example)
- Usually negative for gene rearrangements

2. Cutaneous aggressive epidermotropic CD8+ cytotoxic T-cell lymphoma: usually adults, plaques or nodules, often ulcerated and hemorrhagic, often involving mucous membranes and skin. Often rapidly progressive. No previous history of chronic patches or plaques of MF.

P
- Nodular or diffuse atypical lymphocytes with prominent epidermotropism
- Less involvement of the fat than the other two conditions in this section
- CD3+, CD7+, *CD8+*, CD45RA+, *TIA-1+*, *granzyme+, perforin+*. CD4neg, CD30neg, *CD56neg*
- Clonal T-cell receptor (TCR) gene rearrangement often present (usually BF-1+)

3. Primary cutaneous γ–δ T-cell lymphoma: red plaques and tumor nodules, often ulcerated. Usually adults, rarely children. Aggressive course. By definition, does not start out as MF-like chronic patches or plaques (24.1).

P
- Erosion, necrosis, or ulceration common
- Lichenoid or nodular pattern of atypical lymphocytes with prominent epidermotropism and frequent extension into the fat
- Papillary dermal edema, and lymphocytic angiotropism and vascular destruction are common
- Macrophages with phagocytosis of lymphocytes or erythrocytes (hemophagocytic syndrome) common
- Lymphocytes are CD3+, CD5+, CD56+, CD57neg, CD30neg, CD4neg. CD8 variable. *Cytotoxic phenotype*: TIA-1, granzyme, perforin positive. Epstein–Barr negative
- γ–δ T-cell gene rearrangement present by definition (not α–β)

Differential diagnosis

1. γ–δ T-cell lymphoma often resembles subcutaneous "panniculitis-like" T-cell lymphoma (24.4), but has worse prognosis, usually involves epidermis and dermis as well as fat, and is α–β T-cell receptor gene rearrangement negative (BF-1neg). Hemophagocytic syndrome may occur in both.
2. CD8+ cytotoxic T-cell lymphoma mainly differs from CD8+ mycosis fungoides (24.1) and pagetoid reticulosis

(24.1) by the clinical setting (more aggressive, no Alibert-like progression of patches to plaques, no solitary lesion presentation).

3. Wegener's granulomatosis (4.6): sometimes granulomatous, more vasculitis, not CD56+, no T-cell receptor gene rearrangments.

4. Blastic plasmacytoid dendritic cell neoplasm (24.7) has less vascular destruction and is CD123+.

5. Other lymphomas in this chapter, and polymorphous diffuse inflammatory conditions (1.91).

24.7 Other T-cell lymphomas

Some other forms of T-cell lymphoma are still not as clearly defined.

Variations

1. Primary cutaneous CD4+ small/medium-sized pleomorphic T-cell lymphoma: this is a provisional entity in the WHO classification. Nodules or plaques are usually localized. Prognosis is good.

P
- Diffuse small to medium-sized lymphocytes in dermis or subcutaneous fat, sometimes epidermis
- CD3+, CD4+, CD8neg, CD30neg, sometimes CD7 depleted. Clonal T-cell receptor gene rearrangements may be present

2. Angioimmunoblastic T-cell lymphoma. This was formerly called angioimmunoblastic lymphadenopathy. Elderly adults, rarely children, develop papules or nodules with more specific histologic findings, or other skin lesions with non-specific histology: morbilliform rashes (1.81), purpura (1.120), or exfoliative erythroderma (1.39).

P
- Usually diagnosed from lymph node rather than skin
- Diffuse lymphocytes, macrophages, eosinophils, plasma cells, and immunoblasts in the dermis
- Superficial venules have prominent endothelial cells ("high endothelial venules")
- CD3+, CD4+, CD5+, CXCL13+, CD21+ (non-malignant follicular dendritic cells around vessels), CD8neg. CD10 may be positive
- T-cell receptor gene rearrangements often present

3. Peripheral T-cell lymphoma. This is a term used for a heterogeneous group of "other" cutaneous T-cell lymphomas that are mainly in the dermis and subcutaneous fat ("peripheral" to nodes and internal organs), a provisional "diagnosis of exclusion" for those cases which don't fit into the other categories in this chapter, *without MF clinical features or epidermotropism*.

4. Blastic plasmacytoid dendritic cell neoplasm (hematodermic neoplasm, blastic NK-cell lymphoma). This is a malignancy of immature cells. Patients may present with solitary or multiple plaques or nodules. Prognosis is poor, with dissemination to lymph nodes, blood, and bone marrow.

P
- Diffuse lymphoid infiltrate in dermis and fat, sparing epidermis
- Not angiocentric (no vascular destruction), unlike other CD56+ lymphomas in 24.6
- CD4+, *CD56+, CD123+* (plasmacytoid dendritic cells), CD3neg, myeloperoxidase negative (unlike myeloid leukemia)
- No clonal T-cell receptor gene rearrangement; Epstein–Barr virus negative

24.8 Primary cutaneous follicular center lymphoma (PCFCL)

Adults present with red nodules or plaques, usually without ulceration, often localized to one site, more on head, neck, or trunk. Good prognosis unless nodal type of follicular center cell lymphoma with secondary skin involvement. Crosti's lymphoma (reticulohistiocytoma of the dorsum), a term no longer used, is an indolent low-grade plaque or nodule of the back with centrifugal expansion, without systemic involvement, now considered a variant of follicular center cell lymphoma.

P
- Diffuse or nodular lymphoid infiltrate in dermis and fat, sparing epidermis
- Germinal centers with reduced mantle zones and reduced tingible body macrophages are present except in the "diffuse type", and Ki-67 proliferation is decreased compared to normal germinal centers (see below)
- CD20+, CD79a+, Bcl-6+. CD10+ in the follicular type, but not diffuse type. Bcl-2neg, CD5neg, CD43neg, MUM-1neg, FOX-P1neg (worse prognosis if positive). CD21+ follicular dendritic cells show an irregular network
- Usually no t(14;18) translocation

Differential diagnosis

1. Mantle cell lymphoma (24.11) and marginal zone lymphoma (24.9) lack bcl-6 expression. Diffuse large B-cell lymphoma of leg type (24.10) is usually bcl-2+, MUM-1+, FOX-P1+.

2. Nodal (systemic) follicular center cell lymphoma is positive for bcl-2, unlike the purely cutaneous form, and unlike normal germinal centers or reactive lymphoid hyperplasia (pseudolymphoma, 24.14). Translocation t(14;18) is more likely to be present.

3. Pseudolymphoma (24.14). Ki-67 stains more than 90% of the cells in reactive germinal centers, but less than 50% of cells in the follicular centers of follicular center lymphoma of the non-diffuse type.

24.9 Primary cutaneous marginal zone lymphoma (PCMZL)

(see Fig. 24.9)

This B-cell lymphoma is often said to be related to mucosa-associated lymphoid tissue (MALT), though there really is no comparable skin-associated lymphoid tissue (SALT). Solitary or multiple nodules, low grade, good prognosis. Most common on trunk. Upper extremities more common

4. Mantle cell lymphoma (24.11) is rare in skin and is bcl-1+, CD43+, CD23neg.
5. Secondary cutaneous marginal zone lymphoma (SCMZL) is mainly distinguished by imaging showing systemic involvement with secondary skin involvement. It usually has larger numbers of the malignant B cells compared with reactive T cells, more head and neck involvement, less likely to have germinal centers, and patients are older.

24.10 Primary cutaneous diffuse large B-cell lymphoma, leg type (DLBCLLT)

(see Fig. 24.10A,B)
Solitary or just a few localized red to red–brown nodules, often ulcerated, usually legs of patients more than 70 years old. More common in women. If on the legs or in multiple sites, the prognosis is worse than most other cutaneous B-cell lymphomas. If localized to one site, it has a good prognosis.

P
- Diffuse infiltrate (1.91) of large atypical lymphocytes with prominent nucleoli in the dermis. As with many lymphomas and Merkel cell carcinoma, cells often fragile and may show crush artifacts
- Grenz zone common (1.53), but epidermotropism may be present in some cases (1.37). Adnexa often destroyed
- B cells positive for CD20, CD79, MUM-1, FOX-P1. Usually positive for both bcl-2 and bcl-6. Sometimes CD10+. Negative for CD30 despite the larger cells.
- Gene rearrangement for J heavy chain may be found

Differential diagnosis

1. Mantle cell lymphoma (24.11) and marginal zone lymphoma (24.9) lack bcl-6 expression.
2. Primary follicular center cell lymphoma of the diffuse type (24.8) is bcl-2neg, CD10neg and MUM-1-neg.

24.11 Other B-cell lymphomas

(see Fig. 24.11)
Uncommon, usually presenting as red nodules (1.92) in the skin. Prototypic pathologic findings below do not apply to all variations.

P
- Epidermis usually normal, without epidermotropism
- *Nodular or diffuse infiltrate of lymphoid cells* in the dermis
- Grenz zone common
- *Single filing* of cells (1.128) between collagen bundles often
- Cytologic atypia and mitoses often
- Cells often fragile and may show crush artifacts
- *Monoclonal staining* common. This means that the malignant cells may express only one immunoglobulin heavy chain and one light chain (κ or λ), although some inflammatory cells associated with the lymphoma may be polyclonal (some cells express κ, while others express λ)
- Positive staining for *B-cell markers such as CD20, CD79a, PAX-5*. Reactive T cells often are present. TIA-1 is negative.

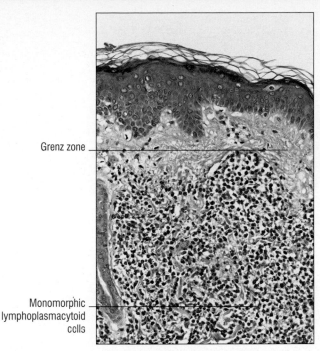

Grenz zone

Monomorphic lymphoplasmacytoid cells

Fig. 24.9 Immunocytoma.

than lower extremities. Primary cutaneous immunocytomas, associated with *Borrelia* are now included in this group.

P
- Nodular or diffuse (1.91) small lymphocytes with eosinophils (1.36) and plasma cells (1.111), in dermis and superficial fat, sparing epidermis. Sometimes a top-heavy infiltrate of mostly small lymphocytes (more superficial in dermis than most other B-cell lymphomas). Many of the cells are reactive to a malignant clone which may be represented by a minority of cells. May have a cutaneous *inverse pattern* (compared with normal lymph nodes): central small, dark reactive lymphocytes, with surrounding malignant clone of lymphocytes with increased pale cytoplasm (marginal zone cells, hence the name marginal zone lymphoma)
- Sometimes folliculocentric or syringotropic orientation (invades hair follicles and sweat glands)
- Reactive germinal centers present in 30% of cases
- In the immunocytoma variants, there may be plasmacytoid cells with intranuclear immunoglobulin deposits (Dutcher bodies)
- Malignant clone positive for CD20, CD79a, bcl-2. Sometimes positive for CD23. Negative for CD43, CD5, CD10, bcl-6. Often monoclonal kappa or lambda restriction. Reactive CD3+ T cells may equal the numbers of CD20+ B cells in many cases, with only 15% of cases really having a predominance of CD20+ cells even though this is a B-cell lymphoma
- Often heavy chain gene rearrangement
- Translocation t(14;18) in small number of cases

Differential diagnosis

1. Other diseases with plasma cells (1.111), including myeloma (24.12).
2. Other diseases with nodular or diffuse infiltrates (1.91).
3. Primary cutaneous follicular center lymphoma (24.8) is bcl-6+, bcl-2neg.

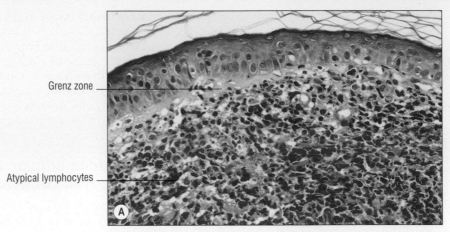

Grenz zone

Atypical lymphocytes

Fig. 24.10 A Large B-cell lymphoma of the leg.

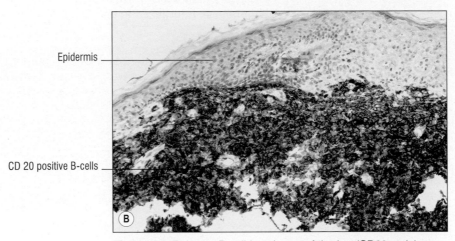

Epidermis

CD 20 positive B-cells

Fig. 24.10 B Large B-cell lymphoma of the leg (CD20 stain).

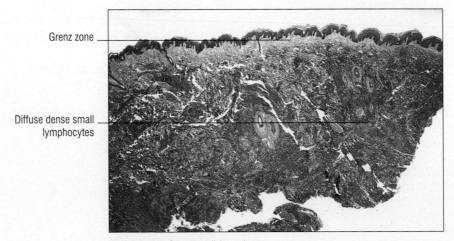

Grenz zone

Diffuse dense small
lymphocytes

Fig. 24.11 Small cell lymphoma.

Variations

1. Burkitt lymphoma: skin involvement is *secondary*, one form is endemic in *Africa*, most common in *children*, diffuse medium-sized lymphocytes often contain lipid-filled vacuoles, mixed with reactive macrophages that phagocytize debris producing a *"starry-sky" appearance*, CD10+, CD19+, CD20+, CD22+, CD79a+, Ki-67 (MIB-1)+ in nearly 100% of cells. Negative staining for CD5, CD23, bcl-2, TdT.

2. Mantle cell lymphoma: a systemic lymphoma generally not found in the skin, so-named because it resembles the mantle zone of the lymphoid follicle. It resembles marginal zone lymphoma, and is CD5+, CD10+, CD20+, CD43+, bcl-2+, and *bcl-1+ (Cyclin Dl)*. CD10, bcl-6, and CD23 are negative. Cyclin D1 translocation t(11;14) usually present.

3. Lymphomatoid granulomatosis: this Wegener's granulomatosis-like process (4.6) was thought to

resemble a lymphoma (hence lymphomatoid, since the suffix -oid means resembling), but now it is considered to be an angiocentric lymphoma (granulomatous vasculitis with vessel necrosis often present). Prominent pulmonary involvement is almost always present. CD20+ large atypical B cells, often EBER+, with background CD3+ reactive T cells (which may be in the majority).

Differential diagnosis

1. Pseudolymphoma (lymphocytoma, 24.9).
2. Other diseases with nodular or diffuse lymphocytes (1.91).
3. Myeloma, immunocytoma, and plasmacytoma (25.5).
4. The so-called "polymorphous" lymphomas (with reactive cells mixed with the malignant ones), such as Hodgkin's disease (24.2), mycosis fungoides (24.3), marginal zone lymphoma (24.9), also tend to show a mixed infiltrate of lymphocytes, histiocytes, plasma cells, and eosinophils. Immunostaining or gene rearrangement studies may be helpful.

24.12 Multiple myeloma (plasma cell myeloma)

(see Fig. 24.12)
Uncommon in skin, presenting as nodules similar to lymphoma (24.1), with involvement in the bone marrow. Paraproteinemia is usually present (1.80).

P
- *Diffuse plasma cells* in the dermis. These cells may be lymphoplasmacytoid and difficult to recognize as plasma cells because of their atypicality. Multinucleated plasma cells, Russell bodies, or Dutcher bodies are sometimes present. Mitoses often prevalent
- Plasma cells are CD38+ and CD138+. CD56+ and CD79a are often positive. CD20 and CD45 (leukocyte common antigen, LCA) are usually negative
- *Methyl green pyronin* (MGP) stains the cytoplasm of plasma cells red, but is not commonly done nowadays
- Immunostaining for κ or λ light chains, IgG, IgA, or IgD often reveals *monoclonality*

Variations

1. Extramedullary plasmacytoma (primary cutaneous plasmacytoma): multiple myeloma is called multiple because usually there are multiple sites in bone involved. When it appears solitary, it is called plasmacytoma. Extramedullary plasmacytoma is a solitary lesion outside of bone. Many of these have been reclassified as marginal zone lymphoma, whereas others are myeloma. Very rare, histology similar to multiple myeloma, except there tends to be less atypicality and the *bone marrow is uninvolved*, at least initially, but metastasis may occur later. CD20 is negative, but CD79a may be positive.
2. Primary cutaneous immunocytoma (lymphoplasmacytoid lymphoma): many of these have been reclassified as marginal zone lymphoma (24.9). More common in Europe, related to infection with *Borrelia* (12.14), *lymphoplasmacytoid cells*, macrophages, eosinophils, considered to be a low-grade B-cell lymphoma, but CD20 staining is often negative, as is CD5, CD10, and CD23.
3. Waldenstrom's macroglobulinemia: histology similar to multiple myeloma, except that direct immunofluorescence demonstrates *monoclonal IgM* within and around the cells and in the blood (1.80), and *PAS-positive hyalinized deposits* resembling amyloid (8.4) are prominent.
4. POEMS syndrome (Takatsuki syndrome, Crow–Fukase syndrome): *P*olyneuropathy *O*rganomegaly, *E*ndocrinopathies, *M* paraprotein produced by plasmacytoma or multiple myeloma, *S*kin diffuse hyperpigmentation, hirsuitism, *glomeruloid hemangiomas* (25.1) or microvenular hemangiomas.

Differential diagnosis

1. Other diseases with numerous plasma cells (1.111). Plasma cells are CD138 positive, but so are fibroblasts, endothelial cells, keratinocytes, and melanocytes (including some squamous cell carcinomas and melanomas). Sometimes cytokeratin, HMB45, or CD30 can be positive, causing misdiagnosis as carcinoma, melanoma, or anaplastic large cell lymphoma.
2. Other diseases with nodular or diffuse infiltrates (1.91).

Atypical plasma cells —

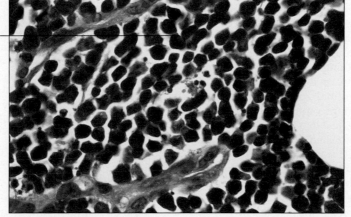

Fig. 24.12 Multiple myeloma.

24.13 Intravascular lymphoma

Very rare, high grade, often fatal, usually with CNS involvement (due to vascular occlusion), red, violaceous, purpuric, indurated woody, or reticulated livedoid plaques (1.123).

> P
> - *Intravascular large atypical lymphocytes*, often with occlusion or thrombi (1.137). Therefore formerly called angiotropic lymphoma (not to be confused with the other antiquated name angiocentric lymphoma, which is now called lymphomatoid granulomatosis (24.11) or NK lymphoma (24.6). Mainly intravascular, sometimes extravascular also
> - Most cases are B cells (CD20+, CD79a+). Sometimes CD5+, CD10+, CD11a+, bcl-2+, MUM-1+. CD10, EBER, and bcl-6 are positive in a minority of cases. Bcl-1 negative. Rare cases of intravascular NK/T-cell lymphoma (CD3+ and/or CD56+) have been described

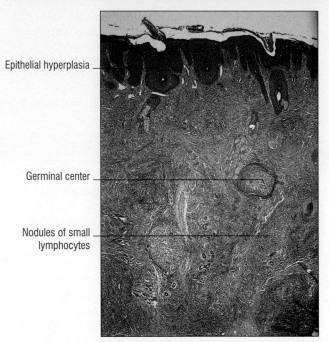

Epithelial hyperplasia

Germinal center

Nodules of small lymphocytes

Fig. 24.14 Lymphocytoma cutis.

Differential diagnosis

1. Reactive angioendotheliomatosis (25.1) can resemble intravascular lymphoma (formerly called malignant angioendotheliomatosis) because the malignant cells can appear like the proliferating endothelial cells (CD31+, CD34+) or histiocytes (CD68+) in the reactive condition. Other lymphomas can become intravascular.
2. Other diseases with vascular thrombi (1.137).

> P
> - Epidermis unremarkable or often *hyperplastic* (1.61)
> - *Nodular or diffuse dermal infiltrate* of mostly lymphocytes, also with *mixed* sparse or many eosinophils (1.36), macrophages (1.76), multinucleated giant cells (1.84), or plasma cells (1.111)
> - Grenz zone (1.53), with no lymphocytes in the epidermis
> - *Germinal centers* with tingible body macrophages (nuclear dust within macrophages) sometimes present
> - Endothelial hyperplasia common

24.14 Pseudolymphoma (cutaneous lymphoid hyperplasia, lymphocytoma cutis, lymphadenosis benigna cutis, Spiegler–Fendt sarcoid, Bäfverstedt syndrome)

(see Fig. 24.14)

The term pseudolymphoma has been criticized, but it is used here to represent a collection of disorders that resemble bona fide lymphoma. "Real" pathologists often prefer the term reactive lymphoid hyperplasia and have a real disdain for the term lymphocytoma preferred by many dermatologists. Lymphadenosis benigna cutis is a term from the literature of the ancients. Nowadays, many lesions previously considered to be pseudolymphoma have been reclassified as low-grade lymphoma by immunoprofiling and molecular techniques, even though bad things infrequently happen to those patients. Prominent examples of this include follicular center cell lymphoma and marginal zone lymphoma (24.1). Pseudolymphoma is usually an uncommon indolent *solitary, red, smooth, non-scaly papule or nodule* (1.92), most common on the face (l.44), sometimes biopsied with the clinical diagnosis of basal cell carcinoma. Pseudolymphoma less commonly presents as multiple or disseminated lesions. Some cases are due to drugs (3.5, such as phenytoin), reaction to red tattoos, contact dermatitis (2.2), or arthropod bites (15.7), especially ticks, which may spread spirochetes such as *Borrelia* (12.14).

Variations

1. Acral pseudolymphomatous angiokeratoma (APACHE): unilateral scaly, red–brown papules on *acral sites*, especially hands (1.56) and feet (1.48) of children, *collarette of epidermis* clutches a dome-shaped nodule of *mixed B and T lymphocytes* (both CD4+ and CD8+), histiocytes, multinucleated giant cells, plasma cells, and eosinophils, with thick-walled *proliferating blood vessels* and hyperplasia of endothelial cells.
2. Kikuchi syndrome: an *influenza-like illness* possibly due to Epstein–Barr virus, cytomegalovirus, parvovirus, or herpes type 6, mainly with *lymphadenopathy* (especially cervical), rash in 30% with *polymorphous morbilliform* (1.81), urticarial, or papular lesions. Lymph nodes often with CD8 predominance, and *histiocytic aggregates may resemble lymphoma* or lupus lymphadenitis. Skin lesions usually are non-specific but may have perivascular or interstitial lymphohistiocytic infiltrate with nuclear dust, but without neutrophils.
3. Actinic reticuloid (2.2).
4. Reactive CD30+ pseudolymphoma (24.5).

Differential diagnosis

1. Lymphoma and leukemia (24.16). The distinction can be really difficult, and hematopathology consultation, immunostaining, gene rearrangement studies, and

evaluation of lymph nodes, peripheral blood, and bone marrow may be needed. This is a common place for hedging on the diagnosis, often with the use of the term *atypical lymphoid proliferation* for difficult cases. The passing of time often makes the correct diagnosis more apparent, but low-grade lymphomas can go on for years. Pseudolymphoma is more likely to have the dermal infiltrate more superficial and less "bottom heavy" toward the deeper dermis, more vascular proliferation with endothelial swelling and epithelial hyperplasia, a more mixed infiltrate (plasma cells, eosinophils, giant cells), but real lymphomas can have a mixture of T and B cells, plasma cells, and eosinophils too. Reactive T cells can obscure a malignant B-cell proliferation. Lymphoma is more likely to be CD10+ and bcl-6+ outside follicles (24.8), and bcl-2+ within lymphoid follicles, if lymphoid follicles are present. Ki-67 stains more than 90% of the cells in reactive germinal centers, but less than 50% of cells in the follicular centers of follicular center lymphoma of the non-diffuse type. Tingible body macrophages are less common within follicles of lymphoma. κ and λ show a polyclonal pattern in pseudolymphoma, instead of a strong preponderance of κ or λ in some B-cell lymphomas.

2. Angiolymphoid hyperplasia with eosinophilia (25.4): more prominent vessels with larger endothelial cells.
3. Jessner's lymphocytic infiltrate (17.6).
4. Other diseases with nodular or diffuse dermatitis (1.91).
5. See mycosis fungoides differential diagnosis (24.1) for other inflammatory conditions that might be called pseudolymphoma because they resemble MF.

24.15 Hodgkin lymphoma

(see Fig. 24.15)

An uncommon, potentially curable lymphoma (5 year survival 65–90%, depending upon the stage). Bimodal age distribution (children and young adults, and those over 55 years). Specific malignant lesions of Hodgkin lymphoma uncommonly involve the skin in 0.5% of cases, and more commonly involve lymph nodes, liver, and spleen. There are different histologic subtypes in the lymph nodes (nodular lymphocyte predominant, nodular sclerosis, mixed cellularity, lymphocyte rich, lymphocyte depleted), but skin lesions cannot be classified this way. Skin lesions are usually red nodules or plaques, and indicate a poor prognosis. Pruritus without lesions (1.115) and several non-specific skin lesions may also occur. Most Hodgkin lymphomas are considered to be B-cell lymphomas, often associated with Epstein–Barr virus.

- Epidermis usually normal, often with a Grenz zone (1.53)
- *Polymorphous nodular or diffuse lymphocytes* (1.91) in the dermis of *atypical Hodgkin's cells* (often positive for CD15 and CD30, negative for CD45R and TIA-1), eosinophils (1.36), plasma cells (1.111), neutrophils, and multinucleated giant cells. CD45, CD20, CD79a, PAX5, and bcl-6 are variable, depending upon the subtype.
- Characteristic *Reed–Sternberg cells* are difficult to find in the rare skin lesions of Hodgkin's disease. They are large, binucleated cells with prominent nucleoli surrounded by a halo, resembling owl's eyes

Differential diagnosis

1. Other lymphomas, especially anaplastic large cell lymphoma (24.3), cutaneous T-cell lymphoma (24.3), lymphomatoid papulosis (24.8), and leukemia cutis (24.4).

24.16 Leukemia cutis

(see Fig. 24.16A–D)

Leukemia commonly produces a variety of non-specific skin lesions, but specific leukemic infiltration of the skin is less common, producing papules, nodules, plaques, or purpura (1.120), especially of the head, neck, and trunk. Special stains, mainly using peripheral blood and bone marrow, and evaluations for chromosomal translocations are necessary to diagnose and classify leukemia. A detailed discussion is beyond the scope of this book.

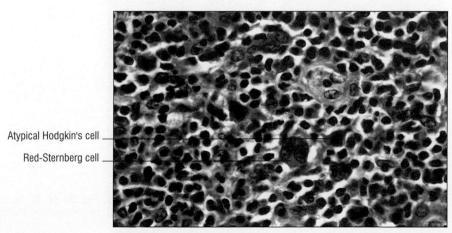

Atypical Hodgkin's cell

Red-Sternberg cell

Fig. 24.15 Hodgkin lymphoma.

Atypical myeloid cell

Erythrocyte

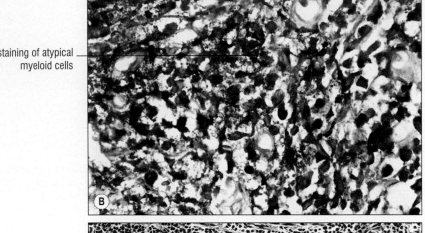

Fig. 24.16 A Myelocytic leukemia cutis.

Red staining of atypical myeloid cells

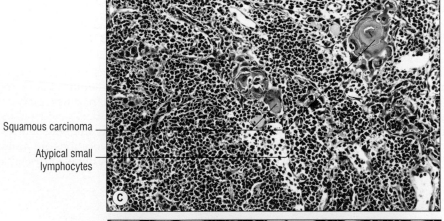

Fig. 24.16 B Myelocytic leukemia cutis (Leder stain).

Squamous carcinoma

Atypical small lymphocytes

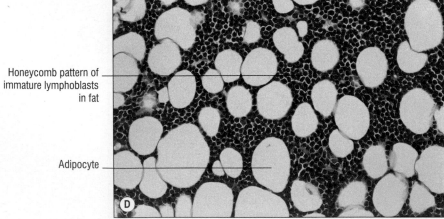

Fig. 24.16 C Chronic lymphocytic leukemia with squamous cell carcinoma of lip.

Honeycomb pattern of immature lymphoblasts in fat

Adipocyte

Fig. 24.16 D Acute lymphoblastic leukemia.

P
- Epidermis usually normal, without epidermotropism
- Nodular or *diffuse cells in the dermis*, often with a Grenz zone (1.53)
- Infiltrating cells may appear *monomorphic*, *atypical*, or *immature*, and often are fragile, showing crush artifacts
- Single filing of cells (1.128) between collagen bundles sometimes
- Most leukemias will stain in the skin with the less specific stains, CD43 and CD45 (leukocyte common antigen), and are negative with most T-cell stains such as CD3 and CD45RO. Mature B-cell stains such as CD20 are negative, except sometimes it is weakly positive in CLL

Variations

1. Myeloid leukemia (myelogenous, myelocytic, acute or chronic granulocytic leukemia, AML, CML, called "granulocytic sarcoma" when in tissue other than blood): dusky gray lesions (1.14) are called "chloromas". Myeloid leukemia is the type of leukemia most commonly encountered in the skin. Infiltrating myeloid cells (except myeloblasts, M1) stain with Leder stain (naphthol AS-D, chloroacetate esterase) and myeloperoxidase (MPO). They are usually CD4+, CD13+, CD14+, CD15+, CD33+, CD43+, CD45+, CD3neg, CD20neg. Myeloblasts stain positive for CD117 and lysozyme, sometimes CD68, but not MPO.
2. Acute monocytic leukemia (M5, AMoL), acute myelomonocytic leukemia (M4, AMMoL), and chronic myelomonocytic leukemia (CMMoL): granulocytic cells stain as in granulocytic leukemia. Monocytes stain blue with alphanaphthol acetate esterase (non-specific esterase), HAM56, MAC387, and CD68.
3. Chronic lymphocytic leukemia (CLL): the most common leukemia in adults after age 50 years, especially men, usually low grade, often blurs with small lymphocytic lymphoma when tissue other than blood is involved (24.1). B-cell CLL (B-CLL) is more common than T-cell CLL: diffuse dermal *small lymphocytes* usually CD 5+, CD19+, CD23+, CD43+. CD20 is variably positive, and it is CD3neg, CD10neg, bcl-1neg, and lysozyme negative. Monoclonal κ or λ expression commonly found.
4. T-lymphoblastic leukemia–lymphoma and B-lymphoblastic leukemia–lymphoma (formerly acute lymphoblastic leukemia–lymphoma, ALL): patients may present with skin nodules as well as blood, lymph node, and bone involvement. Accounts for 80% of *childhood* leukemias, typically CD10+, CD19+, CD22+, CD79a+, CD99+, TdT+. CD34+ in 75%. CD20 variable.
5. Hairy cell leukemia (HCL): hairy cell cytoplasmic projections cannot be visualized in fixed sections. Hairy cells usually CD20+, CD22+.
6. Adult T-cell leukemia/lymphoma (ATLL, 24.3).
7. Chronic eosinophilic leukemia: idiopathic hypereosinophilic syndrome is defined as unexplained eosinophilia (1.34) for more than 6 months. A subset of those patients are reclassified as chronic eosinophilic leukemia if there is an increase in blasts or there is a clonal chromosomal abnormality.
8. Aleukemic leukemia cutis: dermal infiltrate as in other cases of leukemia cutis, but no leukemic cells found in the blood.

Differential diagnosis

1. Extramedullary hematopoiesis (24.12): clinical correlation is very important.
2. Other diseases with nodular or diffuse infiltrates (1.91), or small cell infiltrates (1.130), especially lymphomas in this chapter.

24.17 Mastocytosis

(see Fig. 24.17A–D)
Somewhat common *infiltration of the skin by mast cells*, mostly in *children*, with a benign course, usually without systemic disease, and usually resolving by adulthood. In adults, there is a higher incidence of systemic disease, such as involvement of the gastrointestinal tract (with pain, vomiting, or diarrhea), bone marrow (with osteolysis), with very rare mast cell leukemia. Scratching of the pruritic lesions (1.114) causes mast cell degranulation, producing urtication (*Darier's sign*), and rarely severe flushing or syncope. Lesions may blister (*bullous mastocytoma*). Some drugs can cause flares due to mast cell degranulation.

P
- Perivascular or diffuse *dermal mast cells*, often with a few eosinophils (1.36)
- Dermal edema (1.30) or subepidermal blister formation sometimes
- Mast cells (1.78) usually can be recognized with H&E stain, but are better demonstrated with *Giemsa*, *Leder*, toluidine blue, tryptase, or CD117 (c-kit)

Variations

1. Urticaria pigmentosa: *multiple brown–red macules* (1.18) mostly in children on the trunk (1.141), basal layer hyperpigmentation.

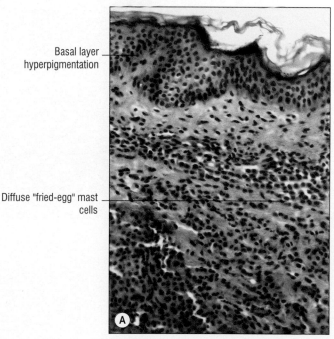

Basal layer hyperpigmentation

Diffuse "fried-egg" mast cells

Fig. 24.17 A Urticaria pigmentosa.

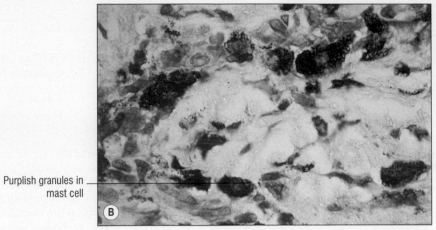

Purplish granules in mast cell

Fig. 24.17 B Urticaria pigmentosa (Giemsa stain).

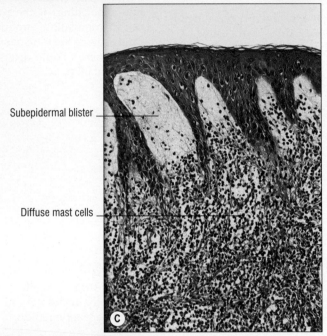

Subepidermal blister

Diffuse mast cells

Fig. 24.17 C Bullous mastocytoma.

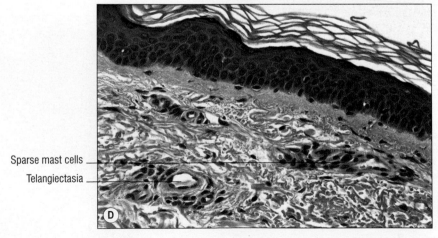

Sparse mast cells

Telangiectasia

Fig. 24.17 D Telangiectasia macularis eruptiva perstans.

2. Solitary mastocytoma: *red nodule* (1.93), usually in children.

3. Telangiectasia macularis eruptiva perstans (TMEP): rare, *poikilodermatous* (1.112) or reticulated (1.123) *macules* on the *trunk of adults*, usually without systemic disease, usually without Darier's sign, with *telangiectasia* (1.136) and only *sparse perivascular mast cells*.

Differential diagnosis

1. As long as the majority of cells in the dermis are mast cells, the biopsy is diagnostic. Other disorders with mast cells seldom cause difficulty (1.78). If mast cells are not recognized, mastocytosis can be confused with other causes of perivascular (1.109) or diffuse dermatitis (1.91), particularly other nodules in childhood (1.93).

2. If blisters are present, it may be confused with a blistering disorder (1.147).

3. Myeloblasts in myelocytic leukemia, clear cell sarcoma, some melanocytic tumors, and some carcinomas will stain for CD117.

24.18 Langerhans cell histiocytosis (LCH, histiocytosis X)

(see Fig. 24.18A–E)

Rare proliferation of Langerhans cells (not true histiocytes, see 1.76) mainly found in *children*. The most common presentation is *red–brown purpuric* (1.120) *seborrheic dermatitis-like*

(2.1) lesions, especially of the scalp (1.124), trunk, and intertriginous areas (1.10, 1.55). Solitary or multiple papules or nodules (1.93) may ulcerate. Internal organ involvement in the *bone marrow, liver, spleen, or lungs indicates a worse prognosis*, and the disease may be fatal. *Osteolytic lesions* (1.16) with *diabetes insipidus* may occur. Some patients have exophthalmos. In other cases, it behaves in a benign manner, and may spontaneously resolve.

> **P**
> - Epidermis may be ulcerated (1.142)
> - *Epidermotropism* of Langerhans cells into the epidermis is common
> - *Lichenoid or diffuse* dermal infiltrate of Langerhans cells (often have an atypical kidney-shaped *reniform nucleus*), may be foamy or resemble Touton histiocytes (1.84)
> - Polymorphous infiltrate of accompanying lymphocytes, eosinophils (1.36), neutrophils (1.89), or plasma cells (1.111) often present
> - Extravasated erythrocytes often (1.40)
> - Positive staining of Langerhans cells for *S-100 protein* and *CDla* (more specific, commonly used). Peanut agglutinin stains them but is not as widely used. CD207 (langerin) stains Langerhans cell specifically but is a newer stain not yet as commonly used
> - *Birbeck granules* appear like tennis rackets with electron microscopy of Langerhans cells

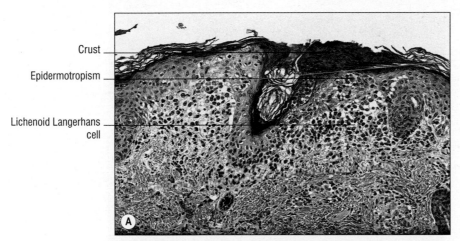

Fig. 24.18 **A** Langerhans cell histiocytosis (low mag.).

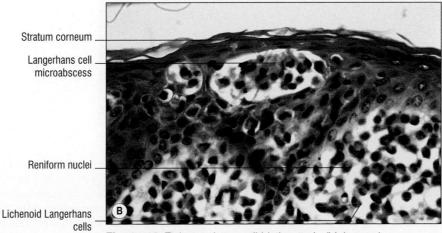

Fig. 24.18 **B** Langerhans cell histiocytosis (high mag.).

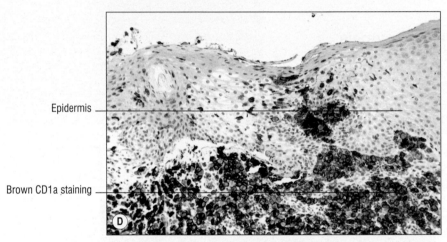

Fig. 24.18 C Eosinophilic granuloma.

Eosinophils

Langerhans cells

Epidermis

Brown CD1a staining

Fig. 24.18 D Eosinophilic granuloma (CD1a stain).

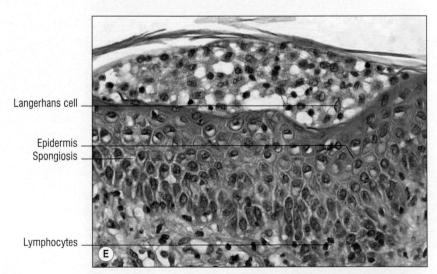

Langerhans cell

Epidermis
Spongiosis

Lymphocytes

Fig. 24.18 E Langerhans microgranuloma in a case of eczema.

Variations

1. Letterer–Siwe disease: *young infants, more fulminant, more epidermotropism,* and fewer foamy cells.
2. Hand–Schuller–Christian disease: children beyond infancy, less epidermotropism, *more foamy cells* and *more giant cells.*
3. Eosinophilic granuloma: *older children* and young adults, more benign course, *mostly in the bone* (presenting as fracture or otitis media), with uncommon skin lesions, less epidermotropism, fewer foamy cells, more diffuse infiltrate with *more eosinophils,* histiocytes, and giant cells.

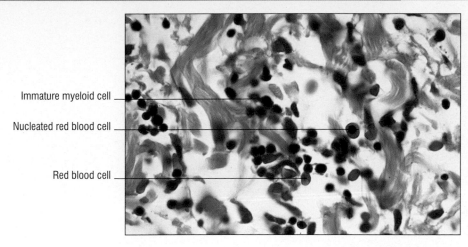

Immature myeloid cell

Nucleated red blood cell

Red blood cell

Fig. 24.19 Cutaneous extramedullary hematopoiesis.

4. Congenital self-healing reticulohistiocytosis (Hashimoto–Pritzker disease): usually no systemic disease, *spontaneous resolution* takes place in several months.

5. Indeterminate cell histiocytosis: proliferating cells are positive for S-100 and CD1a, but *Birbeck granules are absent* with electron microscopy.

Differential diagnosis

1. Other diseases with epidermotropism (1.37). In particular, CD1a+ Langerhans cell microabscesses[118,154] (epidermal "microgranulomas") can sometimes be seen in the epidermis in spongiotic conditions (1.132) such as eczema (2.1) or contact dermatitis (2.2). Usually these conditions do not have CD1a+ Langerhans cells proliferating in the dermis.

2. Other diseases with epithelioid cells (1.38) or foam cells (1.46).

3. Other diseases with lichenoid (1.72) or nodular and diffuse (1.91) infiltrate.

4. Juvenile xanthogranuloma (7.10): also more common in children, not clinically seborrheic dermatitis-like, has proliferating cells that are true histiocytes instead of Langerhans cells, so is usually negative for S-100 and CD1a (the latter is more specific), no epidermotropism.

5. Other rare "non-X" histiocytic disorders (7.13) are generally CD1a negative.

24.19 Cutaneous extramedullary hematopoiesis

(see Fig. 24.19)
Rare, most commonly occurring with *congenital infections* (especially cytomegalovirus, rubella, Coxsackie virus, and toxoplasmosis) and neonatal hemolytic conditions, producing purpuric macules or nodules (1.120) called the *blueberry muffin baby*. In adults it is usually associated with *myelofibrosis*.

- Bone marrow precursors of one or all three lineages may present (myeloid, erythroid, and megakaryocytes), usually sparse in dermis or subcutaneous tissue (not nodular or densely diffuse).
- Immature myeloid cells are CD14+, CD34+, CD68+, CD117+, and CD163+. They also stain with Leder, lysozyme, and myeloperoxidase stains.
- Nucleated red blood cells (nucleated erythrocytes, normoblasts, erythroblasts) are positive for hemoglobin or glycophorin stains.
- Megakaryocytes are CD41+, CD42b+, and CD61+.
- Vascular or myxoid stroma (1.83).

Differential diagnosis

1. Leukemia cutis (24.16), especially myeloid leukemia, can stain in a similar manner, so clinical correlation may be needed. Both leukemias and lymphomas usually have a much denser infiltrate.

2. Extramedullary hematopoiesis has been found within exceptional examples of ossifying pilomatricomas, pyogenic granulomas, chronic leg ulcers, and involuting infantile hemangiomas.

Vascular Proliferations and Neoplasms

25.1 Hemangioma and vascular malformation

(see Fig. 25.1A–E)

Pediatric dermatologists split most vascular neoplasms into two groups, true hemangiomas and vascular malformations, based upon the tendency of true hemangiomas in childhood to proliferate and then involute spontaneously, while vascular malformations persist.[147] This is a somewhat artificial classification, because many mixed lesions may be found. Other dermatologists tend to use the term hemangioma more loosely for most benign vascular neoplasms. They also tend to drop the prefix "heme" and call very small lesions "angiomas"! Even smaller vascular dilations are called telangiectasias (1.136). Most hemangiomas are *red macules, plaques or nodules* (1.121), but some may be bluish (1.14).

- Epidermis usually normal or atrophic
- *Proliferation of blood vessels* and endothelial cells
- GLUT-1 positive in proliferating and involuting infantile hemangiomas (and placentas), negative in other vascular neoplasms, vascular malformations, non-involuting congenital hemangioma (NICH), and rapidly involuting congenital hemangioma (RICH).

Variations

1. Infantile hemangioma (IH, historically called strawberry hemangioma): origin at birth or soon after, classically with proliferative phase, and involution phase, usually largely scarred by age 7 years. Nodules or plaques may become very large, histologically with more endothelial proliferation. Younger proliferative lesions may resemble angiosarcoma, *whitish fibrosis in involuting lesions*.

2. NICH and RICH appear to be distinct from IH. RICH proliferates in utero, and rapidly resolves within 2 years. NICH proliferates rapidly but does not involute and is more likely to need surgical excision.

3. Cherry hemangioma: very common, *adults* after age 30 years, *small papule* usually less than 5 mm, often multiple, most common on the *trunk* (1.141), small vessels proliferate.

4. Verrucous hemangioma: onset in childhood, most common on legs, verrucous epidermis, with dermal vascular proliferation more likely to be a malformation.

5. Nevus flammeus: red or purple *macule*, includes the congenital salmon patch ("stork bite") of the posterior scalp, which may involute, and the port-wine stain on the face (1.44) which usually persists.

6. Cavernous hemangioma: onset soon after birth, *extensive, deep dilated vessels* in the dermis and subcutaneous tissue.

7. Arteriovenous hemangioma (cirsoid aneurysm): *face* (1.44) or acral skin of adults, solitary *small papule, thick-walled vessels*, localized to the dermis.

8. Glomeruloid hemangioma: multiple red to purple papules on the trunk or extremities of adults, especially Japanese, associated with *POEMS syndrome* (24.12), or Castleman's syndrome (giant lymph node hyperplasia), small capillaries protrude into a dilated vascular space *resembling a glomerulus*, with plump endothelial cells having *PAS-positive hyaline globules* containing immunoglobulins or cryoproteins. It may be reactive rather than neoplastic and is similar to reactive angioendotheliomatosis (see below).

9. Tufted hemangioma (angioblastoma of Nakagawa): childhood red macule or plaque, most common on the neck or upper trunk, associated with Kasabach–Merritt syndrome (see below), *"cannonball" clusters* of glomeruloid capillary proliferations separated by normal dermis.

10. Kaposiform hemangioendothelioma: *childhood aggressive violaceous, purpuric plaque* (1.148), high mortality if not treated, associated with Kasabach–Merritt syndrome like the tufted hemangioma, thrombosed capillaries (1.137), and *slit-like vascular spaces*.

©2012 Elsevier Ltd, Inc, BV
DOI: 10.1016/B978-0-323-06658-7.00025-7

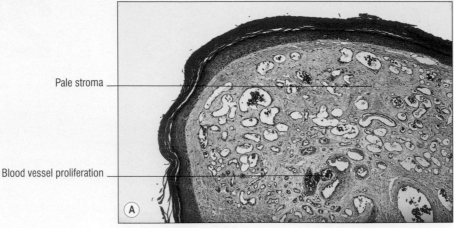

Pale stroma

Blood vessel proliferation

Fig. 25.1 A Cherry hemangioma.

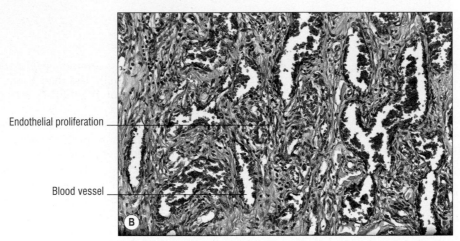

Endothelial proliferation

Blood vessel

Fig. 25.1 B Hemangioma of infancy.

11. Microvenular hemangioma: adults, solitary plaque mostly on extremities, *small slit-like spaces* dissect through the dermis, and may not be readily recognized as vascular spaces (CD31+, CD34+), may resemble Kaposi sarcoma (25.9). Pericytes around the endothelial cells often SMA+. May occur in healthy adults, pregnancy, or POEMS syndrome (24.5).

12. Neonatal hemangiomatosis:[147] *multiple congenital hemangiomas involving three separate organ systems*.

13. Sturge–Weber syndrome: port-wine stain associated with ipsilateral brain lesions.

14. PHACES syndrome: *P*osterior fossa malformations (Arnold–Chiari and Dandy–Walker), *H*emangiomas (large cervicofacial or laryngeal), *A*rterial anomalies (carotid, cerebral, vertebral *C*ardiac defects), *E*ye abnormalities, *S*ternal or abdominal clefting.

15. PELVIS syndrome: perineal hemangioma with external genital abnormalities, lipomyelomeningocele, renal or bladder abnormalities, imperforate anus, or acrochordon.

16. Kasabach–Merritt syndrome: bleeding diathesis associated with platelet trapping in children having tufted hemangioma or kaposiform hemangioendothelioma.

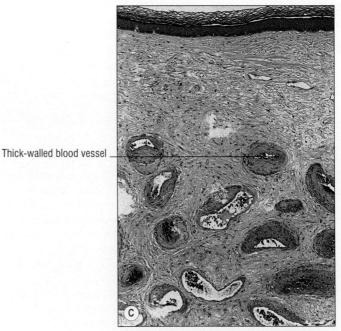

Thick-walled blood vessel

Fig. 25.1 C Arteriovenous hemangioma.

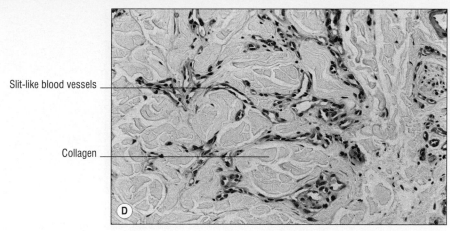

Fig. 25.1 D Microvenular hemangioma.

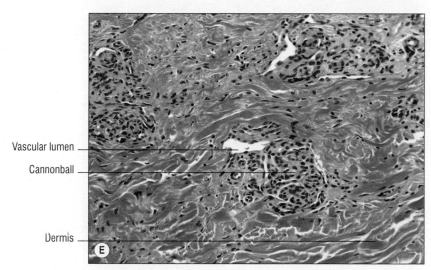

Fig. 25.1 E Tufted hemangioma.

17. Klippel–Trenaunay Weber syndrome: *hypertrophy of a limb* associated with a hemangioma or vascular malformation.
18. Maffucci syndrome: multiple enchondromas and osteochondromas associated with hemangioma or vascular malformation.
19. Blue rubber bleb nevus syndrome: soft bluish papules or nodules associated with GI hemangiomas (1.49).
20. Reactive angioendotheliomatosis: purpuric red macules (1.120), papules or plaques, or reticulated erythema, reacting to infection or cryoglobulinemia (4.9), but usually idiopathic, with lobular proliferations of capillaries in the dermis, thrombi (1.137), and *endothelial cells that occlude the lumina*. It is not to be confused with malignant angioendotheliomatosis, which is now called intravascular lymphomatosis (24.10). Intravascular histiocytosis has been considered a form of reactive angioendotheliomatosis.
21. Diffuse dermal angiomatosis: variant of reactive angioendotheliomatosis, mostly on trunk or extremities, especially pendulous breasts with skin ulcerations, associated with peripheral vascular disease, chronic renal disease, diabetes mellitus, and

antiphospholipid antibody syndrome. There is endothelial proliferation which may resemble microvenular hemangioma or lymphangiosarcoma.

Differential diagnosis

1. Angiokeratoma (25.2): epidermal hyperplasia, vessels more dilated without endothelial proliferation.
2. Pyogenic granuloma (25.3): often related to trauma, more inflammation, pale stroma, and often ulcerated.

25.2 Angiokeratoma

(see Fig. 25.2A–D)

Uncommon solitary or multiple red, *purple* (1.148), or *black* (1.13) *papules* or plaques.

- Hyperkeratosis, epidermal rete ridges often encircle dilated vessels
- Dilated vessels in superficial dermis, without much endothelial proliferation
- Thrombi common (1.137)

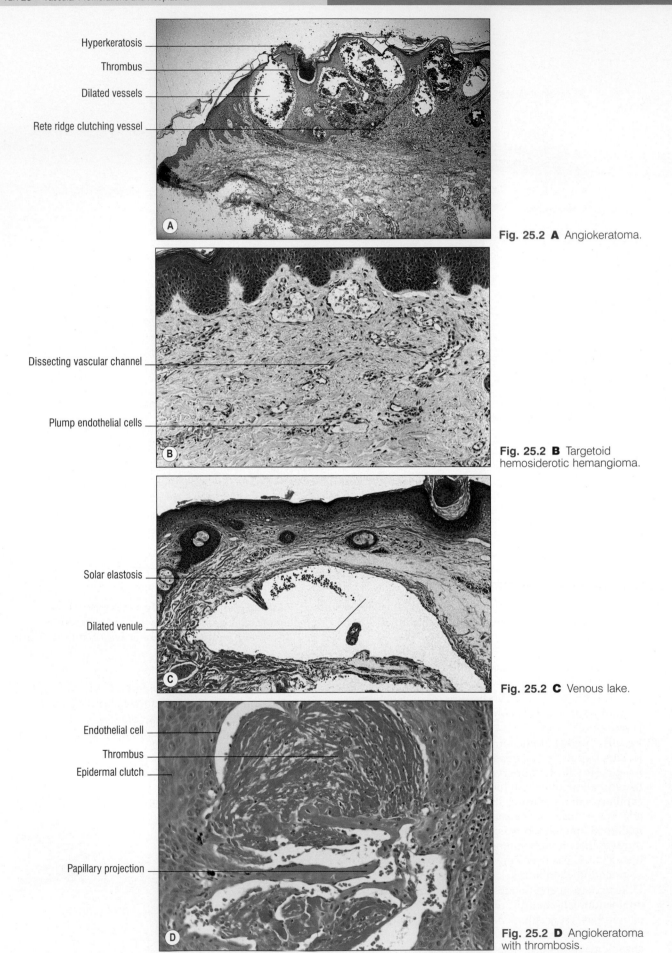

Hyperkeratosis

Thrombus

Dilated vessels

Rete ridge clutching vessel

Fig. 25.2 A Angiokeratoma.

Dissecting vascular channel

Plump endothelial cells

Fig. 25.2 B Targetoid hemosiderotic hemangioma.

Solar elastosis

Dilated venule

Fig. 25.2 C Venous lake.

Endothelial cell

Thrombus

Epidermal clutch

Papillary projection

Fig. 25.2 D Angiokeratoma with thrombosis.

Variations

1. Angiokeratoma of Mibelli: *dorsal fingers and toes* (1.56); arises in *childhood*.
2. Angiokeratoma scroti of Fordyce: *scrotum* (1.126, and rarely of vulva) of adults.
3. Papular angiokeratoma: solitary or multiple small papules in adults, especially on the *legs* (1.67).
4. Angiokeratoma circumscriptum: *larger* lesion, usually extremities, deeper vessels; arises *at birth* or early in childhood.
5. Angiokeratoma corporis diffusum (Fabry's disease): X-linked recessive, alpha-galactosidase deficiency (commercially available test) related to mutation in the GLA gene, resulting in trihexosylceramide accumulation in several organs, *bathing trunk distribution* of many small angiokeratomas, *painful peripheral neuritis*, no hyperkeratosis, small *lipid deposits in endothelial cells* (PAS positive, frozen sections positive with Sudan black B, birefringent under polarized light; visible with electron microscopy).
6. Beta-galactosidase deficiency: very rare, similar to Fabry's disease.
7. Fucosidosis: very rare autosomal recessive disorder, alpha-fucosidase deficiency, related to mutation in the FUCA1 gene, similar to Fabry's disease.
8. Targetoid hemosiderotic hemangioma: usually solitary red–brown macule or barely elevated plaque in an adult, sometimes with *annular target appearance* (1.5), no hyperkeratosis, superficial dilated vessels, with deeper dissecting slit-like vascular channels. Plump "hobnail" endothelial cells protrude into lumen of the dilated vessels, *hemosiderin* (1.58) and erythrocyte extravasation (1.40) common, may mimic Kaposi sarcoma (25.9). The term *hobnail hemangioma* has been proposed as a synonym for targetoid hemosiderotic hemangioma, but unfortunately hobnail endothelial cells have also been used to describe angiolymphoid hyperplasia (25.4), retiform hemangioendothelioma (25.7), Dabska's tumor (25.7), and acquired progressive lymphangioma (25.10).
9. Venous lake: *blue–black* (1.14) macule, no epidermal change, large *dilated venule in sun-damaged skin*, especially of the *ear* (1.28), *lip* (1.74), cheek, or neck, which is often biopsied to rule out melanoma, especially if it becomes thrombosed.

25.3 Pyogenic granuloma (PG, lobular capillary hemangioma)

(see Fig. 25.3A–C)
Common, *friable, often bleeding* (patients come in to the office with the so-called Band-Aid sign), often *pedunculated* (1.106), solitary papule or nodule, often with rapid growth following *trauma* or during *pregnancy* (1.113), especially in the mouth (1.82), or *on the fingers* (1.56), especially in children (1.93) or young adults.

- *Epidermis atrophic or ulcerated*, often with crust with neutrophils (pyo-) on surface (1.89)
- *Collarette of epidermis* often demarcates the lesion
- Pyogenic granuloma is a misnomer, as it is characterized by excessive *granulation tissue* ("proud flesh"), *often arranged in vascular lobules*, rather than a granuloma. Granulation tissue is vascular proliferation in a *pale stroma* with an inflammatory sparse or prominent infiltrate of *neutrophils or lymphocytes*

Differential diagnosis

1. Other hemangiomas (25.1).
2. Bacillary angiomatosis (12.15).
3. Kaposi sarcoma (25.9).

25.4 Angiolymphoid hyperplasia with eosinophilia (antiquated name: histiocytoid hemangioma)

(see Fig. 25.4A–C)
Uncommon red nodules around the scalp (1.124).

- Epidermis normal
- Vascular proliferation with prominent "*hobnail*" endothelial cells (25.2) protruding into the lumina, often associated with vacuoles
- Nodular or *diffuse infiltrate of lymphocytes and eosinophils*

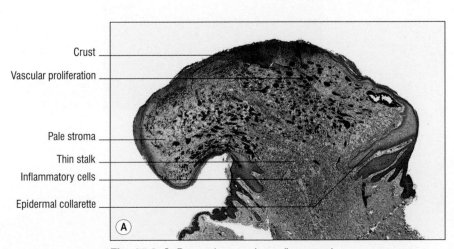

Fig. 25.3 A Pyogenic granuloma (low mag.).

Crust
Vascular proliferation
Pale stroma
Thin stalk
Inflammatory cells
Epidermal collarette
(A)

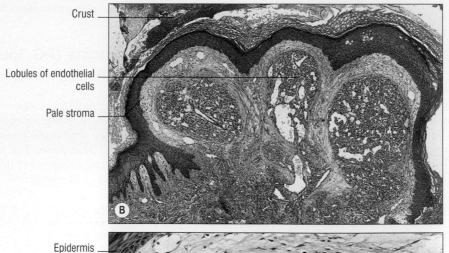

Crust

Lobules of endothelial cells

Pale stroma

Fig. 25.3 B Pyogenic granuloma (medium mag.).

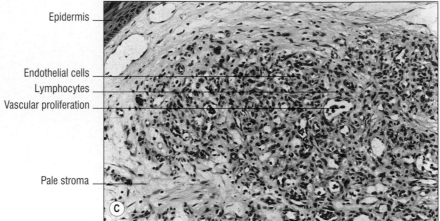

Epidermis

Endothelial cells

Lymphocytes

Vascular proliferation

Pale stroma

Fig. 25.3 C Pyogenic granuloma (high mag.).

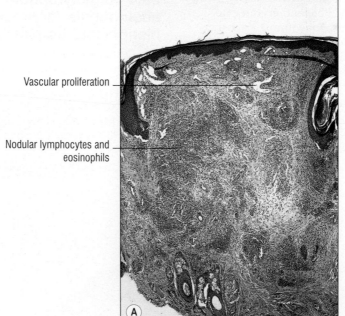

Vascular proliferation

Nodular lymphocytes and eosinophils

Fig. 25.4 A Angiolymphoid hyperplasia with eosinophilia (low mag.).

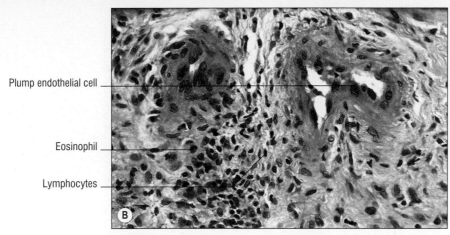

Plump endothelial cell

Eosinophil

Lymphocytes

Fig. 25.4 B Angiolymphoid hyperplasia with eosinophilia (high mag.).

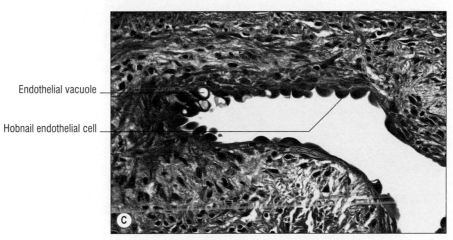

Endothelial vacuole

Hobnail endothelial cell

Fig. 25.4 C Angiolymphoid hyperplasia with eosinophilia (high mag.).

Variations

1. Kimura's disease: some authors use this as a synonym for angiolymphoid hyperplasia, while others use it for the deeper lesions with *prominent lymphoid follicles with germinal centers*, usually on the *posterior neck* (1.86), more common in Japan.
2. Papular angioplasia: very rare, *multiple papules on the face or scalp* of *elderly* patients with *bizarre atypical endothelial cells.*

Differential diagnosis

1. Prominent endothelial cells can be seen with angiosarcoma (25.7) and hobnail hemangioma (25.2).
2. Lymphocytoma cutis (24.14): more prominent lymphoid infiltrate with less impressive vessels.
3. Angiosarcoma (25.7): more of a hemorrhagic plaque, less nodular, more atypical, more necrosis, no eosinophils.
4. Arthropod bite reaction (15.7): acute onset clinically, often more epidermal changes, less prominent endothelial cells.
5. Other diseases with eosinophils (1.36).

25.5 Glomus tumor

(see Fig. 25.5)

Uncommon *painful* (1.96), solitary, *blue* (1.14) subungual macule (1.85) or nodule elsewhere, or multiple less likely painful nodules. Glomus cells are modified smooth muscle cells that normally line the Sucquet–Hoyer canal, an arteriovenous fistula that is involved in temperature regulation in the digits.

- Proliferation of blood vessels surrounded by *glomus cells* (monotonous cells with a dense, *round nucleus* and abundant pink cytoplasm), often *single-filing* (1.128) through the stroma
- Stroma often pale (1.30)
- Positive staining for smooth muscle actin in glomus cells. Desmin is positive in a minority of cases

P

Variations

1. Glomangioma: this term is usually used for the solitary or multiple glomus tumors that are less painful, *unencapsulated*, that have *predominant vessels and fewer*

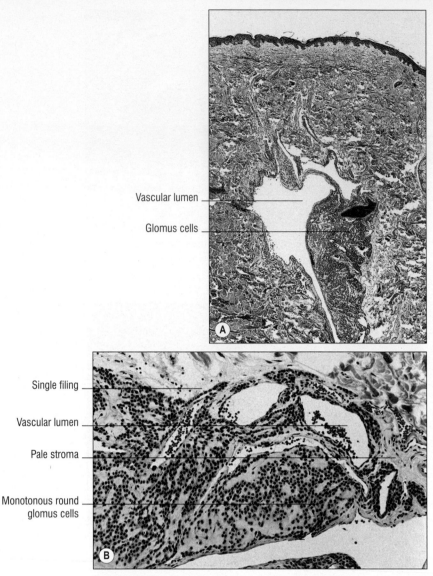

Vascular lumen

Glomus cells

Single filing

Vascular lumen

Pale stroma

Monotonous round glomus cells

Fig. 25.5 Glomus tumor.

glomus cells. Some cases related to glomulin gene mutation.

2. Solitary glomus tumor: tends to be more common in the *nail bed*, more painful, encapsulated, *smaller vessels*, more glomus cells, more nerve fibers seen with Bodian stain.

Differential diagnosis

1. Eccrine spiradenoma (23.11): basaloid cells can resemble glomus cells, but has sweat ducts instead of vascular proliferation.
2. Hemangioma (25.1): no monotonous rounded glomus cells.
3. Glomangiosarcoma: very rare, malignant, more atypical cells.

25.6 **Hemangiopericytoma**

Uncommon *subcutaneous nodule or mass* (1.135), rarely dermal (rarely encountered by dermatologists), most common on upper and lower extremities or retroperitoneal, in adults. Most are benign, but some are malignant.

- Epidermis normal
- Circumscribed nodule of *spindle-shaped or polygonal-shaped pericytes* with variable cytologic atypia
- Increased number of blood vessels, sometimes with *antler-like branching* ("stag horn")
- Reticulum stain shows that the pericytes are outside the reticulum fibers that surround the endothelium
- Malignant lesions more likely to show more extravasated erythrocytes (1.40), necrosis, more cellularity and more than four mitoses per ten high-power fields
- Positive staining for vimentin, CD34, and p75. Negative for keratin, S-100, CD31, factor VIII-related antigen, *Ulex europaeus*, smooth muscle actin, and desmin

Differential diagnosis

1. Kaposi sarcoma (25.8): slit-like vascular spaces.
2. Angiosarcoma (25.7): less circumscribed, more atypia, endothelial cells are inside the vascular reticulum fibers.

3. Glomus tumor (25.5): usually smaller, cells more rounded.
4. Other spindle cell tumors (1.43): some consider hemangiopericytoma a poorly defined diagnosis that is made only after other soft tissue neoplasms have been excluded, since most stains are negative.

25.7 Angiosarcoma

(see Fig. 25.7A–D)
Uncommon purpuric (1.120) or black (1.13) plaque on the *face* (1.44), especially near the *scalp* (1.124) of *elderly* individuals, or as a complication of chronic lymphedema.

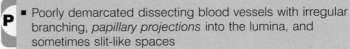

- Poorly demarcated dissecting blood vessels with irregular branching, *papillary projections* into the lumina, and sometimes slit-like spaces
- Proliferating infiltrating *spindled or epithelioid atypical endothelial cells*. If well-differentiated, proliferating vessels may be readily identified and atypia is mild to moderate, but poorly differentiated angiosarcomas have very pleomorphic, atypical hyperchromatic endothelial cells with many mitoses, and poorly recognizable vessels
- Prominent *extravasated erythrocytes* (1.40), sometimes hemosiderin (1.58)
- Reticulum stain shows endothelial cells to be surrounded by reticulum fibers
- *Positive staining with endothelial cell markers* such as CD31, CD34, factor VIII-related antigen, and *Ulex europaeus*

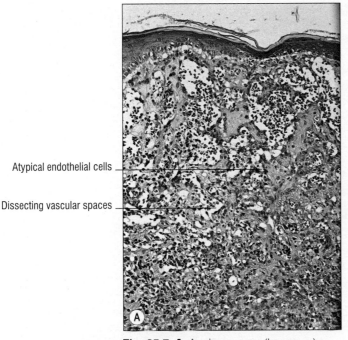

Atypical endothelial cells

Dissecting vascular spaces

Fig. 25.7 A Angiosarcoma (low mag.).

Variations

1. Epithelioid angiosarcoma: rare in skin, predominance of monotonous *atypical epithelioid cells*, with *more solid areas than vascular spaces*, more closely resembles carcinoma or melanoma.
2. Lymphangiosarcoma and Stewart–Treves syndrome: usually occurs in *lymphedematous extremity*, especially *after radical breast surgery* and axillary dissection, fewer red blood cells in vascular spaces.
3. Spindle cell hemangioendothelioma: rare, considered benign, but radiation treatment may induce sarcoma with metastasis, is like a cavernous hemangioma (25.1) with solid proliferative areas, thrombosis, papillary projections, and often thick-walled muscular vessels.
4. Epithelioid hemangioendothelioma: a low-grade or borderline malignancy, poorly defined (some feel that the term hemangioendothelioma should be avoided), more in soft tissue and internal organs, rare in skin, deep nodule with 30% incidence of metastasis, atypical epithelioid and spindle cells in a *myxoid or hyalinized stroma*.
5. Retiform hemangioendothelioma: rare, *young adults*, more on *lower leg*, deep tumor with rare metastasis, similar to Dabska tumor in children, infiltrating *branching vascular spaces with hobnail endothelial cells,*

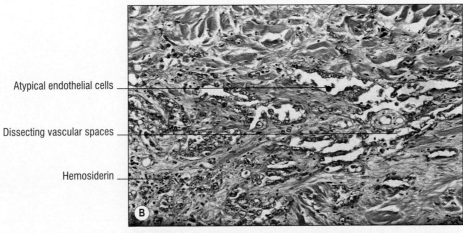

Atypical endothelial cells

Dissecting vascular spaces

Hemosiderin

Fig. 25.7 B Angiosarcoma (medium mag.).

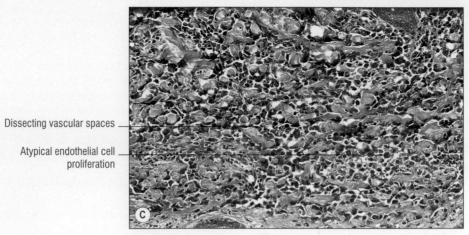

Dissecting vascular spaces

Atypical endothelial cell proliferation

Fig. 25.7 C Angiosarcoma (medium mag.).

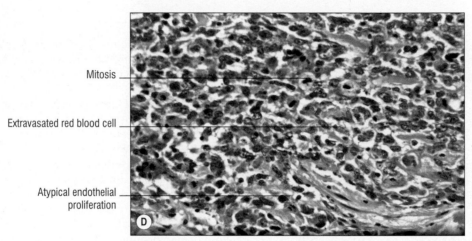

Mitosis

Extravasated red blood cell

Atypical endothelial proliferation

Fig. 25.7 D Angiosarcoma (high mag.).

often with *many lymphocytes*. The name "retiform" refers to the resemblance to rete testis.

6. Dabska tumor (malignant endovascular papillary angioendothelioma): rare, *childhood*, deep, *locally destructive* neoplasm which rarely metastasizes to regional nodes, *cavernous vascular spaces lined by hobnail endothelial cells with projecting papillary tufts with hyalinized cores, many lymphocytes.*

Differential diagnosis

1. Kaposi sarcoma (25.9).
2. Hemangiopericytoma (25.6).
3. Intravascular papillary endothelial hyperplasia (25.8).
4. Poorly differentiated angiosarcoma may resemble spindle cell (1.131) or epithelioid cell (1.38) neoplasms, especially squamous cell carcinoma (18.11), melanoma (20.11), or metastatic neoplasms (Chapter 28).

25.8 Intravascular papillary endothelial hyperplasia (IPEH, Masson's pseudoangiosarcoma)

(see Fig. 25.8A,B)
Uncommon benign nodule in young adults, most common on the head, neck, or extremities, thought to be an unusually *proliferative organizing thrombus* (1.137).

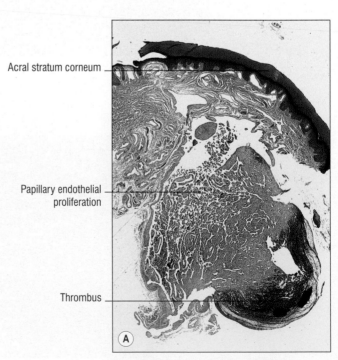

Acral stratum corneum

Papillary endothelial proliferation

Thrombus

Fig. 25.8 A Intravascular papillary endothelial hyperplasia (low mag.).

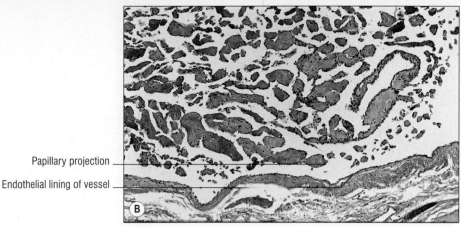

Papillary projection
Endothelial lining of vessel

Fig. 25.8 B Intravascular papillary endothelial hyperplasia (high mag.).

Differential diagnosis

1. Angiosarcoma (25.7): not intravascular, more atypical cells and mitoses.

25.9 Kaposi sarcoma (KS)

(see Fig. 25.9A–D)

Rare except in association with AIDS (14.12) or other immunodeficiency, KS is thought to be a vascular reaction related to co-infection with herpes virus type 8 (14.7). *Multiple red, purplish (1.148) to brownish (1.18) macules (patch stage), plaques, or nodules* occur. The *classic type* of KS occurs mostly in persons of Eastern European heritage, after age 50 years, and usually on the *legs* (1.67). The *African endemic form* and the *epidemic AIDS-related type* may occur with HIV infection of other immunosuppression, lesions occur anywhere, but particularly on the face, nose, mouth, palate, neck, trunk, lower extremities, and soles. Internal involvement may occur in any type, but is more common in the epidemic type, especially lungs, bowel, liver, and spleen, and it may result in death. KS may be a vascular proliferative response to a virus rather than a true sarcoma, because it begins in multiple foci at once (instead of cancer starting from one site and then metastasizing), the cells are not very atypical, the AIDS patients with KS have a survival slightly better than those without it, and KS may resolve spontaneously with an improved immune status.

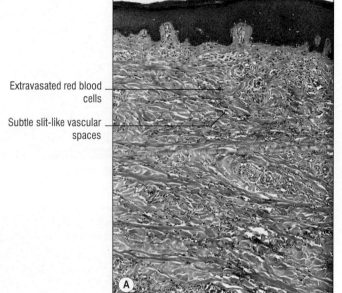

Extravasated red blood cells

Subtle slit-like vascular spaces

Fig. 25.9 A Kaposi sarcoma (patch stage, low mag.).

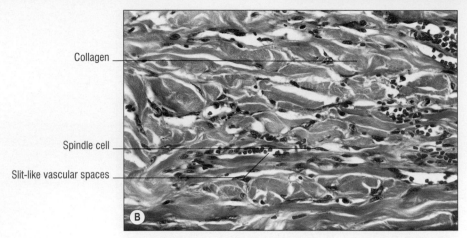

Fig. 25.9 B Kaposi sarcoma (patch stage, medium mag.).

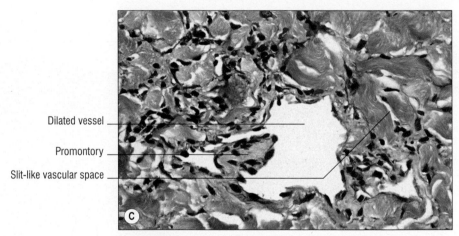

Fig. 25.9 C Kaposi sarcoma (medium mag.).

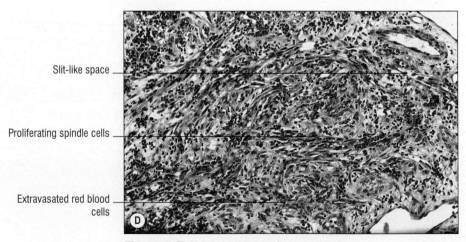

Fig. 25.9 D Kaposi sarcoma (tumor stage).

Differential diagnosis

1. Acroangiodermatitis (pseudo-KS) (2.1): related to stasis, clinically more diffuse and less papulonodular, not associated with HIV, may have spongiosis, mature small vessels and less slit-like.
2. Multinucleate cell angiohistiocytoma (7.13): atypical multinucleated cells.
3. Bacillary angiomatosis (12.15): smudgy amphophilic areas containing bacteria.
4. Kaposiform hemangioendothelioma (25.1): large plaque in childhood.
5. Microvenular hemangioma (25.1): solitary plaque on extremity, HIV negative.
6. Hobnail hemangioma (25.2): targetoid appearance, more epithelioid.
7. Pyogenic granuloma (25.3): rapid onset, more inflammation, and fewer slit-like spaces.
8. Hemangiopericytoma: (25.6): deep mass.

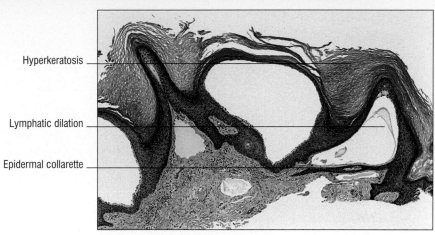

Fig. 25.10 Lymphangioma.

9. Angiosarcoma (25.7): more cytologic atypia, different clinical setting.
10. Sclerosing hemangioma type of dermatofibroma (27.1): epidermal hyperplasia, whorling pattern.
11. Young scar with hemorrhage (27.2): fibroblasts run parallel to epidermis.
12. Other spindle cell tumors (1.131).

25.10 Lymphangioma

(see Fig. 25.10)
Uncommon grouped papulovesicles (resembling *frog spawn*), sometimes purplish if bleeding occurs, usually multiple, usually *congenital*, sometimes arising later in childhood, rare in adulthood. A deep cavernous component may exist, even when lesions appear superficial.

P
- Epidermal hyperplasia sometimes (1.61)
- Proliferation and dilation of lymph vessels in dermis (especially papillary dermis) or deep soft tissue, lined by endothelial cells

Variations

1. Cavernous lymphangioma and cystic hygroma: common on *neck* (1.86), or *axilla* (1.10), larger lymphatic vessels (like cavernous hemangioma without the blood, 25.1), *deeper* in the dermis or subcutaneous tissue.
2. Lymphangioma circumscriptum: hyperkeratosis, *collarette of acantholic epidermis* extends around dilated lymph vessels in the upper dermis. Sometimes a few dilated lymph vessels present in the deeper or subcutaneous tissue.
3. Acquired progressive lymphangioma: rare, benign red patch that *gradually enlarges over years*, mostly in adults, *dissecting horizontally-oriented pattern of lymphatic spaces* (possibly are blood vessels), resembles targetoid hemosiderotic hemangioma (25.2), well-differentiated angiosarcoma (25.7), or Kaposi sarcoma (25.9). KS is often multiple, has more erythrocytes, hemosiderin, and plasma cells.

Differential diagnosis

1. Angiokeratoma (25.2): more red cells in the vessels.
2. Hemangioma (25.1): more red cells in the vessels.

CHAPTER 26

Neural Neoplasms

26.1 Neurofibroma (NF)

(see Fig. 26.1A–D)

Common *soft, skin-colored or violaceous papules or nodules* (1.129), *pedunculated* (1.106) or subcutaneous (1.135), may exhibit "buttonhole sign" whereby they can be invaginated with finger compression.

P

- Somewhat demarcated nodule in the dermis or subcutaneous tissue of spindle cells with wavy nuclei, sometimes in strands said to resemble shredded carrots
- Pale "bubblegum" pink stroma, mucinous or myxoid
- Mucinous stroma (1.83) stains positive for acid mucopolysaccharides (Chapter 30)
- Mast cells common (1.78)
- Positive staining for S-100, CD34, PGP9.5, factor XIIIa, myelin basic protein, and neurofilaments. Bodian stain rarely performed, but should reveal axons since the neurofibroma is a neoplasm of the entire peripheral nerve

Variations

1. Subcutaneous NF: subcutaneous mass, often has a true capsule.
2. Diffuse NF: diffuse infiltration of dermis or subcutaneous tissue.
3. Pigmented NF: melanin pigmentation (understandable since melanocytes, like Schwann cells, are from neural crest).
4. Blue–red macule NF: red or blue tint due to increased thickened blood vessels, usually with NF-1 (see below).
5. Pseudoatrophic macule NF (neurofibromatous dermal hypoplasia): slightly depressed NFs due to decreased reticular dermis: NF tissue more whorled around vessels and nerves.
6. Plexiform NF: large *"bag of worms" mass*, nearly pathognomonic for NF-1.
7. Neurofibromatosis type I (NF-1, von Recklinghausen's disease, peripheral neurofibromatosis, the most common type of NF): autosomal dominant, mutation in neurofibromin (NF1) gene, two or more neurofibromas or a plexiform neurofibroma, six or more *café-au-lait macules* (20.2) that are greater than 1.5 cm in adults or 0.5 cm in children, axillary or inguinal freckling (Crowe sign, onset in childhood, present in 90% of adults), optic gliomas (15% of patients), *Lisch nodules* (iris hamartomas, 15% of children by age 6 years old, 95% of adults), osseous lesions such as sphenoid dysplasia,

hypertension due to renal artery stenosis or pheochromocytomas, dysplasia of long bones such as the tibia (10% of patients), kyphoscoliosis (less than 10% of patients), sometimes seizures or below average intelligence.

8. Neurofibromatosis type II (NF-2, acoustic neurofibromatosis, central neurofibromatosis): mutation in gene encoding neurofibromin-2 (merlin). Hereditary bilateral eighth nerve masses, neurofibromas, meningiomas, gliomas or Schwannomas, fewer café-au-lait macules.
9. NF-3, NF-4, NF-8: these terms are no longer in vogue (atypical NF variants).
10. Segmental neurofibromatosis (NF-5, now called segmental NF-1): NFs or café-au-lait macules restricted to one sector of the body, without crossing the midline, usually without a family history.
11. NF-6: familial café-au-lait macules (autosomal dominant, without neurofibromas and without other NF-1 manifestations, rare).
12. NF-7: schwannomatosis (26.2).

Differential diagnosis

1. Dermatofibroma (27.1): indurated, more likely to be brown, more fibrotic stroma, less demarcated, epidermal hyperplasia, tabled rete ridges.
2. Leiomyoma (29.6): blunt-ended cigar nuclei.
3. Schwannoma (26.2): Verocay bodies, no axons with Bodian stain.
4. Neuroma (26.3): more delineated nerves.
5. Neurotized melanocytic nevus (20.5): melanocytic nests, melanin, myelin basic protein negative.
6. Other spindle cell tumors (1.131).

26.2 Schwannoma (neurilemmoma)

(see Fig. 26.2A,B)

Uncommon neoplasm of the nerve sheath (not the entire peripheral nerve as in neurofibroma and neuroma), presenting as a *dermal or subcutaneous nodule* (1.135), sometimes *painful* (1.96), especially on the extremities. Usually solitary tumor, may be associated with NF-1.

DOI: 10.1016/B978-0-323-06658-7.00026-9

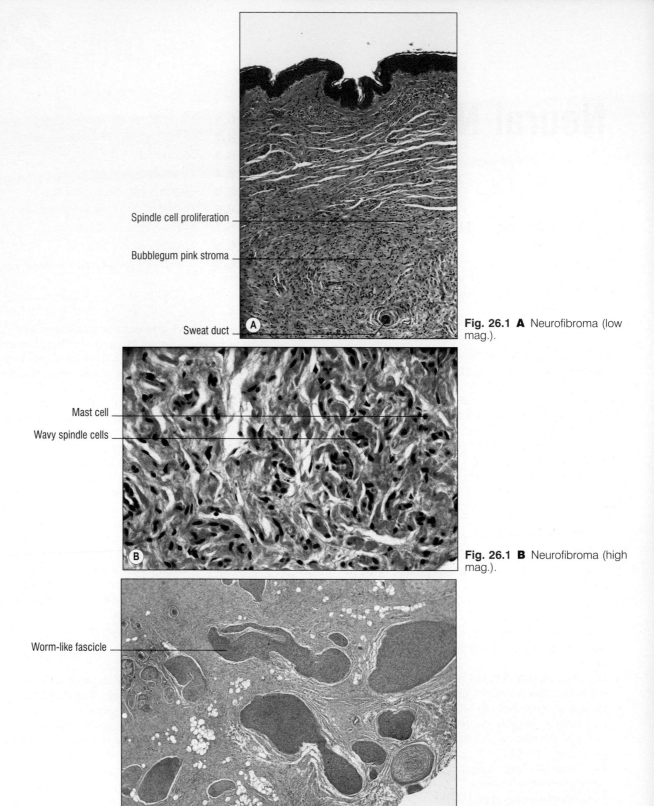

Spindle cell proliferation

Bubblegum pink stroma

Sweat duct

Fig. 26.1 A Neurofibroma (low mag.).

Mast cell

Wavy spindle cells

Fig. 26.1 B Neurofibroma (high mag.).

Worm-like fascicle

Fig. 26.1 C Plexiform neurofibroma.

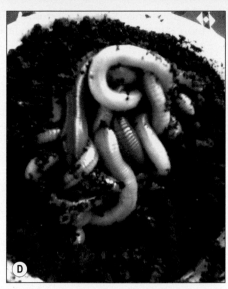

- Encapsulated subcutaneous tumor with cellular areas (Antoni A tissue) and/or edematous myxoid areas (Antoni B tissue)
- Spindle cells in Antoni A tissue line up in two parallel rows separated by areas without nuclei (Verocay bodies)
- Mucinous stroma stains positive for acid mucopolysaccharides (Chapter 30)
- Mast cells common (1.78)
- Positive staining for S-100 and myelin basic protein (MBP) in the Antoni A areas, negative for neurofilaments. Bodian stain usually demonstrates no axons
- Tumor may be attached to large nerve

Fig. 26.1 D Bag of worms appearance of plexiform neurofibroma (for non-fishermen).

Variations

1. Ancient schwannoma: degenerative changes such as hyalinization, calcification or thrombi, sometimes pleomorphic cytology, but no mitoses, mostly Antoni B tissue.
2. Plexiform schwannoma: interconnecting fascicles of Antoni A tissue.
3. Cellular schwannoma: usually deeper masses, rare in skin, hypercellular nodules with atypia, might be a low-grade malignancy.

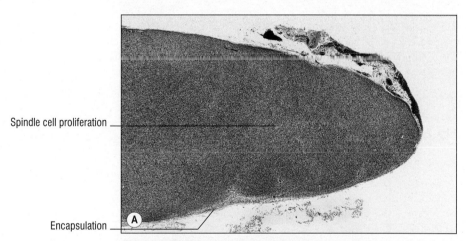

Spindle cell proliferation

Encapsulation

Fig. 26.2 A Schwannoma (low mag.).

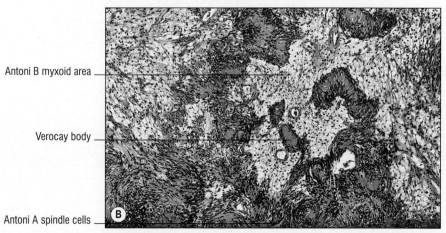

Antoni B myxoid area

Verocay body

Antoni A spindle cells

Fig. 26.2 B Schwannoma (high mag.).

4. Schwannomatosis (NF-7, neurilemmomatosis): rare multiple form.
5. Psammomatous melanotic schwannoma: rare component of Carney's complex (27.17), usually found in the bone, deep soft tissue, spinal nerve roots, or GI tract, and rarely in skin. Pigmented melanocytes (S-100 and HMB-45 positive) are present along with melanin and psammoma bodies (1.35).

Differential diagnosis

1. Rare examples of dermatofibroma have been reported to have Verocay-like bodies (27.1).
2. Other neoplasms with mucin (1.83).
3. Other spindle cell neoplasms (1.131).
4. Neurofibroma (26.2): consists of both the axons (demonstrated with Bodian stain) and the sheath portion of the nerve, no Verocay bodies.

5. Palisaded encapsulated neuroma (26.3): smaller lesion, more superficial, usually on face, fascicles with clefts, axons present.

26.3 Neuroma
(see Fig. 26.3A–C)
Somewhat common, often painful (1.96), papules or nodules consisting of all of the usual components of a peripheral nerve, including axons and Schwann cells.

- Bundles of somewhat well-delineated fascicles of peripheral nerves
- Stroma often fibrotic
- Positive staining for S-100, myelin basic protein, and neurofilaments

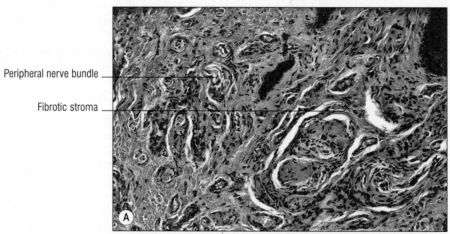

Fig. 26.3 **A** Traumatic neuroma.

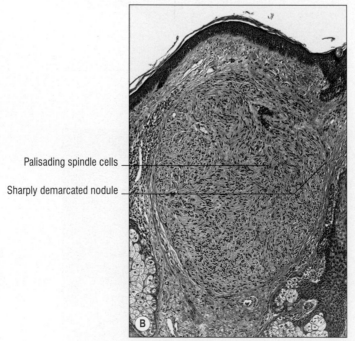

Fig. 26.3 **B** Palisaded encapsulated neuroma (low mag.).

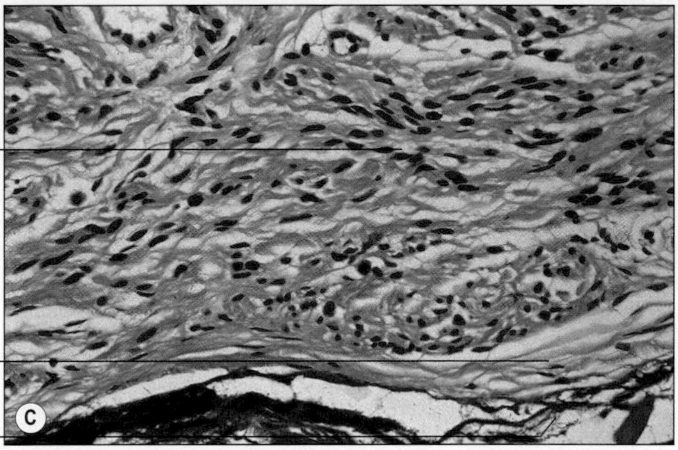

Fig. 26.3 C Palisaded encapsulated neuroma (high mag.).

Variations

1. Traumatic neuroma: follows *trauma*, such as an amputation, after which nerve fibers attempt to regenerate in an irregular tangled growth pattern.
2. Palisaded encapsulated neuroma (PEN, solitary circumscribed neuroma): asymptomatic, skin-colored or pink, smooth, non-descript, usually solitary, *papule of the face* (1.44) of adults, usually *smaller than 6 mm*, without other associations. Well-circumscribed but poorly encapsulated (somewhat of a misnomer), fascicles separated by clefts.
3. Multiple mucosal neuroma syndrome, also called multiple endocrine neoplasia (MEN) type 2b, or multiple endocrine adenomatosis (MEA) type 2b or MEN type 3: rare autosomal dominant paraneoplastic (1.105) disorder, possibly due to RET gene mutation, with multiple soft papular *mucosal neuromas of the lips* (1.74) and tongue (1.139), thick lips (1.74), marfenoid habitus, *pheochromocytoma, medullary carcinoma of the thyroid* (1.138).
4. Morton's neuroma: painful, usually between 3rd and 4th toes (1.48), distorted nerves, perineural fibrosis, sometimes thrombi.
5. Supernumerary digit (27.5): somewhat like a traumatic neuroma that forms in utero, and is not a true neuroma.
6. Perineurioma: benign subcutaneous circumscribed nodule of extremities or trunk of middle-aged adult, made of perineurial cells, may be intraneural. Interweaving fascicles of spindle cells may have a storiform pattern, sometimes with perivascular whorls. Tumor is vimentin+, EMA+, CD34+, Glut-1+, collagen IV+. SMA is variable. S100, GFAP, and neurofilaments are negative. May resemble dermatofibrosarcoma protuberans (27.10) or myoepithelioma (29.6).

Differential diagnosis

1. Neurofibroma: softer nodule clinically, pale stroma, less discrete neural bundles.
2. Schwannoma: larger, deeper nodule, more palisading and Verocay bodies, and no axons.
3. Other spindle cell neoplasms (1.131).

26.4 Granular cell tumor

(see Fig. 26.4A,B)

Uncommon, firm nodule, solitary or multiple, found on the *tongue* (1.139) in 40% of cases, but anywhere on the skin in 60%.

> - *Epidermal hyperplasia*, sometimes pseudoepitheliomatous hyperplasia
> - Infiltration of the dermis or subcutaneous tissue by large cells with a *granular cytoplasm* and small, centrally located nuclei
> - Larger eosinophilic intracytoplasmic granules are called *pustulo-ovoid bodies of Milian*
> - Granules are *positive with PAS stain* (diastase resistant) or PTAH, and usually negative with lipid stains
> - Tumor stains positive for myelin basic protein, NSE, S-100 protein (nuclear and cytoplasmic), and CD68

Differential diagnosis

1. The pseudoepitheliomatous hyperplasia (1.116) may be mistaken for a squamous cell carcinoma (18.11), especially in superficial biopsies. Unfortunate aggressive tongue excisions have occurred.
2. Xanthoma (7.9) and other lesions with foam cells (1.46) usually have more distinct cell boundaries, less granularity, no pustulo-ovoid bodies, positive for lipid stains, negative staining with PAS, PTAH, S-100, myelin basic protein.
3. Malignant granular cell tumor: very rare; larger, deeper tumor, sometimes cytologic atypia, but nearly impossible to distinguish with certainty until after metastasis occurs.
4. Granular cell changes have been reported in dermatofibroma, ameloblastoma, leiomyoma, leiomyosarcoma, angiosarcoma, malignant fibrous histiocytoma, melanoma, and renal cell carcinoma.

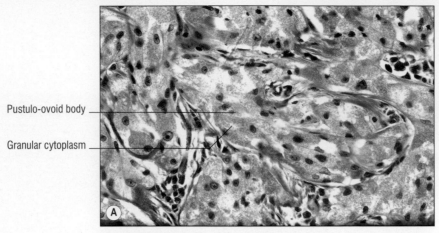

Fig. 26.4 A Granular cell tumor.

Pustulo-ovoid body

Granular cytoplasm

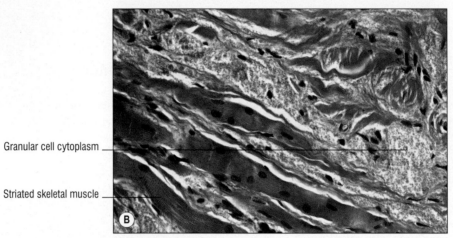

Fig. 26.4 B Granular cell tumor.

Granular cell cytoplasm

Striated skeletal muscle

26.5 Heterotopic neuroglial tissue

(see Fig. 26.5)

These uncommon lesions include meningomyeloceles, meningoencephaloceles, and heterotopic brain tissue, which are usually present in the *midline cranial area*. Imaging studies are recommended before biopsy, because there may be a connection to the central nervous system. Biopsy may result in encephalitis, so neurosurgical consultation should be sought if these lesions are considered. Heterotopic or herniated brain tissue is often called *nasal glioma*, because it is most common as a *congenital*, skin-colored, pink, smooth, very large nodule resembling a hemangioma on the *nasal bridge* or intranasally (1.95).

P
- Epidermis atrophic (1.9)
- *Astrocytes* (glial cells with small round nuclei, distinct nuclear membrane, and prominent nucleolus) and *neurons* (cells with eccentric nuclei and Nissl's granules in the cytoplasm) in a pale *neurofibrillary stroma* (neuropil matrix, resembles tangled phone lines)
- Multinucleated giant cells common (1.84)
- Calcification sometimes (1.19)

P
- Fibrotic stroma, vascular ectasia common
- *Glial fibrillary acid protein* stains glial cells, *neuron-specific enolase* stains the neurons
- Bodian silver stain or neurofilament stain demonstrates neurites (axons) extending from neurons

Differential diagnosis

1. Ganglioneuroma: very rare nodule at any site, sometimes paravertebral, many rounded *ganglion cells* (large oval or stellate cells with eccentric nuclei and prominent nucleoli, and toluidine-positive Nissl's granules in the cytoplasm) in a myxoid stroma, positive staining for neurofilament and glial fibrillary acidic protein. Wavy fibers with spindle cells or nerve fibers also sometimes present.
2. Other neural neoplasms in this chapter.

26.6 Heterotopic meningeal tissue

(see Fig. 26.6)

Heterotopic (rudimentary) meningoceles are uncommon congenital malformations or herniations. A *meningioma* belongs in this group, but is defined as an independent proliferation

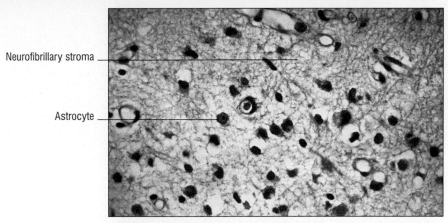

Neurofibrillary stroma

Astrocyte

Fig. 26.5 Nasal glioma.

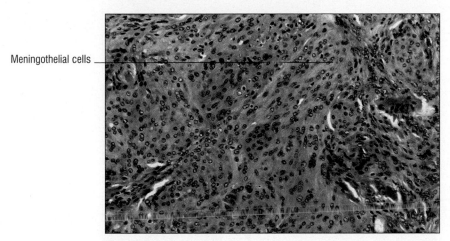

Meningothelial cells

Fig. 26.6 Meningioma.

of displaced meningothelial cells. All of these present as hemorrhagic cysts, nodules, or plaques, sometimes pedunculated (1.106), usually on the scalp (1.124), forehead, temple, or along cranial nerves, sometimes associated with bony defects that may be seen with imaging studies. Sometimes a collarette of increased hair surrounds the lesion (*hair collar sign*), which can also be seen with aplasia cutis congenita (17.4).

P
- Sharply demarcated connection *through skull* to central nervous system
- *Meningothelial cells* are epithelioid or spindled, with vesicular nuclei, abundant pink cytoplasm with indistinct borders, often in a hyalinized stroma
- Pseudovascular spaces sometimes, dense fibrous stroma often
- *Psammoma bodies* (1.35, laminated, hyalinized, or calcified structures) sometimes present (also may be seen in metastatic papillary thyroid carcinoma and ovarian carcinoma)
- Positive staining for vimentin (rather non-specific) and *epithelial membrane antigen* in meningothelial cells, with variable staining for S-100, neuron-specific enolase, and cytokeratin

Differential diagnosis

1. Aplasia cutis congenita (17.4) and intradermal melanocytic nevus (20.5) have a similar clinical resemblance.
2. Heterotopic neuroglial tissue (26.5).
3. Chordoma: deep dermal or subcutaneous nodule, often paraspinal by direct extension from a sacral tumor or rarely by metastasis, sometimes appearing in extremities near tendons or joints, vacuolated epithelioid cells called physalipherous cells, myxoid stroma, positive for S-100, EMA, and pankeratin, resembles extraskeletal chondroma (23.12).
4. Squamous cell carcinoma (18.11): keratin pearls, pankeratin positive.
5. Pseudovascular spaces can resemble hemangioma, but CD31 and CD34 staining is negative in the lining cells.
6. Giant cell fibroblastoma is CD34 positive and EMA negative.

26.7 Myxoid neurothekeoma (nerve sheath myxoma)

(see Fig. 26.7A–F)
Rare *soft papule or nodule* in young adults, especially head, neck, or upper extremities.

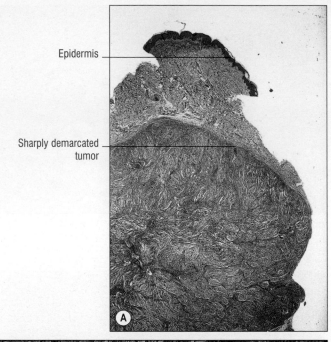

Epidermis

Sharply demarcated tumor

Fig. 26.7 A Neurothekeoma (low mag.).

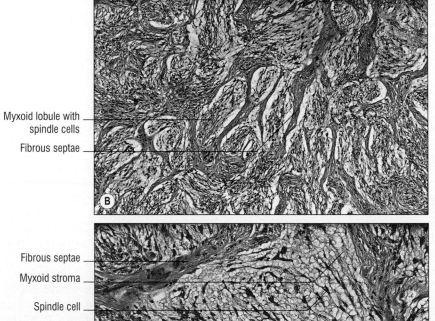

Myxoid lobule with spindle cells

Fibrous septae

Fig. 26.7 B Neurothekeoma (medium mag.).

Fibrous septae

Myxoid stroma

Spindle cell

Atypical cell

Fig. 26.7 C Neurothekeoma (high mag.).

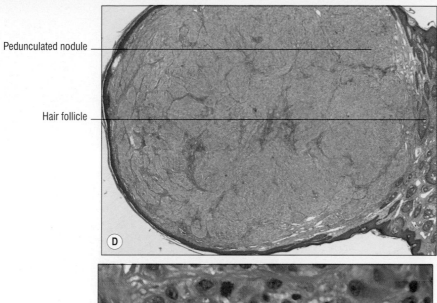

Pedunculated nodule

Hair follicle

Fig. 26.7 D Cellular neurotheke-oma (low mag.).

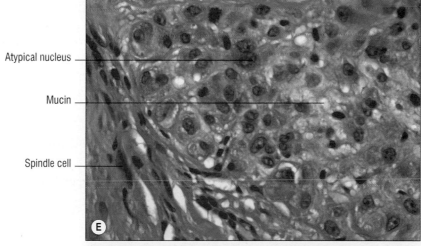

Atypical nucleus

Mucin

Spindle cell

Fig. 26.7 E Cellular neurotheke-oma (high mag.).

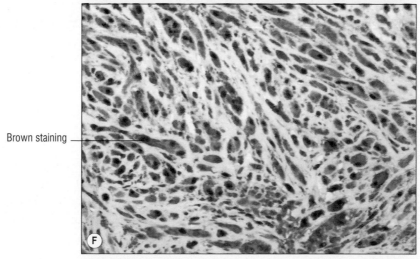

Brown staining

Fig. 26.7 F Cellular neurotheke-oma (S-100A6 stain).

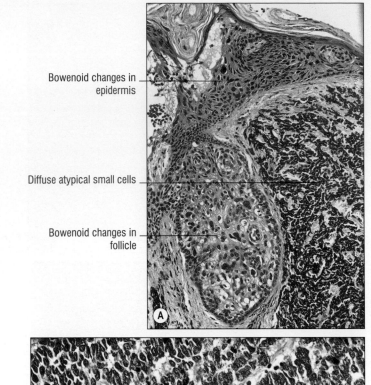

Bowenoid changes in epidermis

Diffuse atypical small cells

Bowenoid changes in follicle

Fig. 26.8 A Merkel cell carcinoma (with bowenoid changes, low mag.).

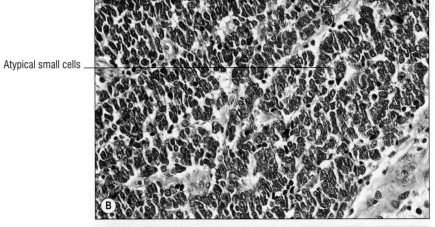

Atypical small cells

Fig. 26.8 B Merkel cell carcinoma (medium mag.).

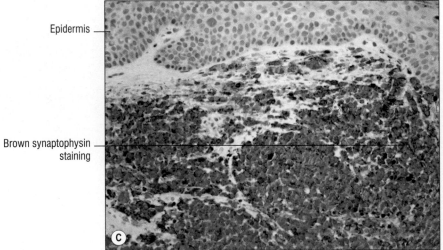

Epidermis

Brown synaptophysin staining

Fig. 26.8 C Merkel cell carcinoma (synaptophysin stain).

- *Pale myxoid sharply demarcated* or encapsulated dermal or subcutaneous nodule *divided into lobules* or fascicles by fibrous septae
- *Spindle cell nuclei may be pleomorphic*, sometimes epithelioid (1.38)
- Mucinous stroma stains positive for acid mucopolysaccharides (Chapter 30)
- Positive staining for S-100, weak for NSE, negative for axons (neurofilament immunostain or Bodian stain)

Variation

1. Cellular neurothekeoma is really a completely different neoplasm. Nodule in any location of young adults, poorly circumscribed, *hypercellular*, benign nodule with epithelioid cells (1.38) and spindle cells, more mitoses, more cytoplasm, more infiltrating, and less mucin than ordinary neurothekeoma. Resembles Spitz nevus, but is negative for S-100 and HMB45. Usually positive staining with NSE, S-100A6, PGP9.5, microphthalmia transcription factor (Mitf), NKI-C3, and the non-specific stain vimentin. Desmin is negative. Since SMA is positive in half of cellular neurothekeomas, it has been speculated that this tumor might be a muscle tumor without any relationship to ordinary neurothekeoma (especially since cellular neurothekeoma is S-100neg, unlike most other neural neoplasms).

Differential diagnosis

1. Focal mucinosis of the skin (8.11), myxomas (27.17), and mucous cysts (8.9) are negative for S-100 and are not divided into lobules or fascicles.
2. Schwannoma (26.2) is more cellular, at least in some areas.
3. Neurofibroma contains evidence of axons, staining positively for neurofilaments.
4. Other diseases with considerable mucin (1.83) or spindle cells (1.131).

26.8 Merkel cell carcinoma (MCC, neuroendocrine carcinoma of the skin, trabecular carcinoma)

(see Fig. 26.8A–C)
Rare, *quickly growing red nodule or plaque*, often ulcerated (1.142), thought to be related to Merkel cells in the epidermis, but this is uncertain and it has been called a "murky cell carcinoma". Recent evidence points to an association with polyoma virus in 80% of cases, but this virus has also been found in two-thirds of basal cell carcinomas. Usually found on the *head* (1.44), neck, or legs of older adults, especially in sun-damaged areas. *Rapid metastasis* and death are common, making this tumor worse than the average melanoma.

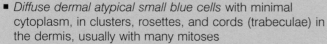

- *Diffuse dermal atypical small blue cells* with minimal cytoplasm, in clusters, rosettes, and cords (trabeculae) in the dermis, usually with many mitoses
- Epidermotropism of the small cells, or coexisting bowenoid change (18.10) may be present

- Positive staining often with *neuron-specific enolase* (NSE), epithelial membrane antigen (EMA), *CD56*, neurofilament, *synaptophysin, chromogranin*, or argyrophil stains. There is often a *classic paranuclear dot staining pattern* with low molecular weight keratin, such as *CK20*, cam 5.2, AE-1. Negative staining for S-100, TTF-1, CK5-6, CEA, and LCA. Some rare CK20neg cases will stain with CK7, but CK7 is usually negative. Bombesin may be positive in Merkel cell carcinoma, but some studies found it to be negative and more likely positive in metastatic neuroendocrine carcinoma in the skin, so it is mainly used as an exam question and not in clinical use. CM2B4 stains the large T-antigen of the polyoma virus, and is highly specific for MCC but not sensitive (only 60% of MCCs are positive)
- Neuroendocrine dense-core granules seen with electron microscopy

Differential diagnosis

1. Metastatic small cell (oat cell) carcinoma of the lung: more likely to stain with high molecular weight keratins (such as CK7) instead of low molecular weight (such as CK20), positive for TTF-1. CEA positive in 50% of cases, less likely to stain for neurofilament.
2. Other small cell tumors (1.130, 28.5).
3. Tumors with basaloid cells (1.11).

26.9 Malignant peripheral nerve sheath tumor (MPNST, malignant schwannoma, antiquated name neurofibrosarcoma)

Uncommon *nodule or mass*, usually in the *subcutaneous* or deep tissue (1.135), often associated with malignant transformation of neurofibroma in *von Recklinghausen's disease* (26.1).

- Poor circumscription of mass
- Proliferation of spindle cells with wavy nuclei in a pale mucinous stroma (1.83)
- Positive for p75. Usually S-100+ and Sox10+,[152] but some are negative and then may be very difficult to distinguish from other spindle cell tumors
- Cytologic atypia (pleomorphism, hyperchromatism, increased numbers of mitoses) often present, but not always prominent
- Necrosis sometimes present

Differential diagnosis

1. Neurofibroma: usually less cellular, no atypical cells or mitoses, less likely to be p53+.
2. Fibrosarcoma (27.13).
3. Other spindle cell neoplasms (1.131).

CHAPTER 27

Fibrohistiocytic Proliferations and Neoplasms

27.1 Dermatofibroma (DF, benign fibrous histiocytoma, subepidermal nodular fibrosis)

(see Fig. 27.1A–I)

Brownish (1.18) nodules most common on the *legs* (1.67), also seen on upper extremities and trunk, rarely on the head or neck, probably originating from folliculitis, arthropod bites, or some other initial inflammatory condition. Some authors prefer to think of a dermatofibroma as fibrosing dermatitis rather than a neoplasm. Often mistaken for "nevi" (20.5) by the non-dermatologist, but they are more indurated than nevi. DFs often have the *dimple sign* when inwardly compressed.

P
- *Epidermal hyperplasia* (1.61) often, sometimes with *flattened "tabled" rete ridges* or basaloid proliferation simulating a basal cell carcinoma
- *Hyperpigmented basal layer* often
- Poorly circumscribed proliferation of boomerang-shaped *spindled fibroblasts* or histiocytes in the dermis, often *whorling* about, blending into the surrounding dermis like a bomb was dropped in the dermis, sometimes extending into the subcutaneous fat
- Multinucleated giant cells (1.84), Touton giant cells, or foamy histiocytes (1.46) sometimes
- *Hemosiderin* often (1.58)
- Large bundles of collagen ("*keloidal collagen*") often present at *periphery* of lesion, with fibroblasts around the bundles ("collagen trapping")

Variations

1. Hemosiderotic DF (aneurysmal DF, sclerosing hemangioma): hemosiderin (1.58), prominent pseudovascularity, erythrocyte extravasation (1.40), may resemble Kaposi sarcoma (25.9).
2. Xanthomatous DF: foamy histiocytes, sometimes Touton giant cells (1.46).
3. Atrophic DF: atrophic epidermis (1.9) instead of hyperplastic.
4. DF with monster cells: occasional bizarre atypical giant cells are present, but still has benign behavior.
5. Palisading DF: Verocay-like bodies may resemble a schwannoma (26.2).
6. Cellular DF: larger, more numerous fibroblasts, may infiltrate fat, may closely resemble dermatofibrosarcoma protuberans (DFSP, 27.10).
7. Epithelioid cell histiocytoma: majority of cells are epithelioid (1.38), often with angulated shapes that may resemble Spitz nevus (20.6) or reticulohistiocytoma (7.8).
8. Sclerotic fibroma (circumscribed storiform collagenoma, plywood fibroma): sharply circumscribed, hyalinized *plywood pattern* of dense collagen, clefts between thick collagen bundles (1.23), mucin sometimes in the clefts (1.83), very few CD34+ and factor XIIIa+ fibroblasts (hypocellular), some cases associated with Cowden's disease (22.5). The presence of ongoing type I collagen synthesis and positive staining for PCNA and Ki-67 suggest that it is a growing neoplasm rather than just a DF variant. Similar sclerotic changes may occur within an ordinary DF, however. EMA is negative.
9. Dermatomyofibroma (myoid fibroma): red or white plaque of upper trunk or neck of young adults, slowly growing to several centimeters, usually does not recur. *Myofibroblasts are oriented parallel to the epidermis,* resemble leiomyoma or DFSP, and are actin positive and negative for CD34, factor XIIIa, and desmin.
10. Oral fibroma (bite fibroma): very common mouth (1.82) nodule (especially buccal mucosa, lower lip, lateral tongue) related to trauma in the mouth.
11. Solitary fibrous tumor:[123] firm mass on head and neck of middle-aged adults, without atypia, with a "*patternless*

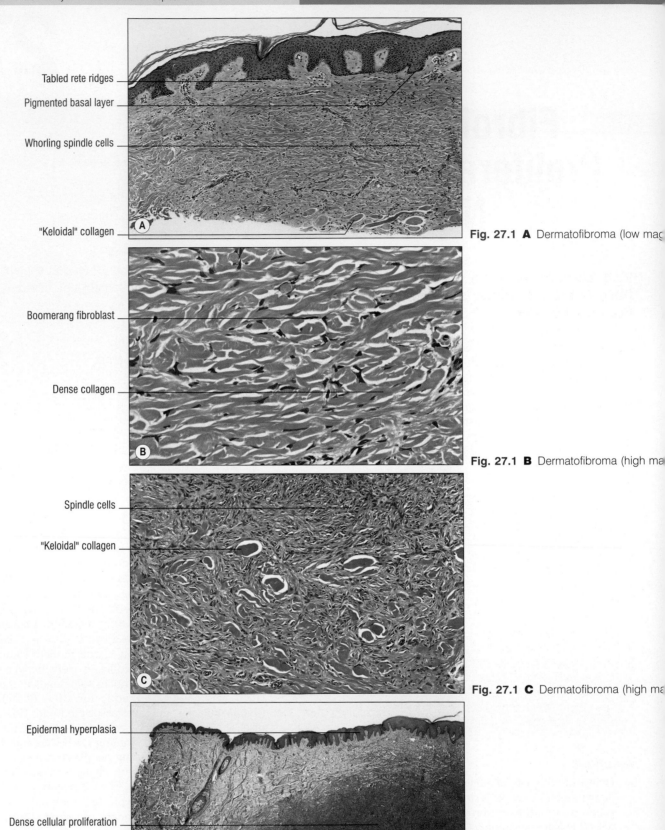

Tabled rete ridges

Pigmented basal layer

Whorling spindle cells

"Keloidal" collagen

Fig. 27.1 A Dermatofibroma (low mag

Boomerang fibroblast

Dense collagen

Fig. 27.1 B Dermatofibroma (high ma

Spindle cells

"Keloidal" collagen

Fig. 27.1 C Dermatofibroma (high ma

Epidermal hyperplasia

Dense cellular proliferation

Fig. 27.1 D Dermatofibroma (cellular

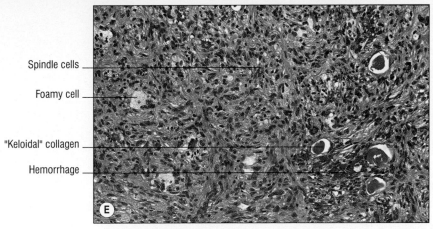

Spindle cells

Foamy cell

"Keloidal" collagen

Hemorrhage

E

Fig. 27.1 E Xanthomatous dermatofibroma.

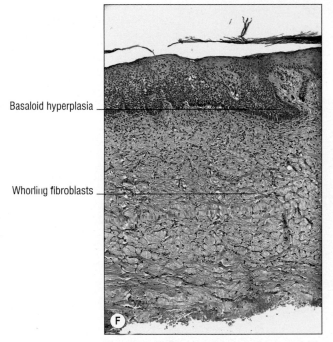

Basaloid hyperplasia

Whorling fibroblasts

F

Fig. 27.1 F Dermatofibroma with basaloid hyperplasia.

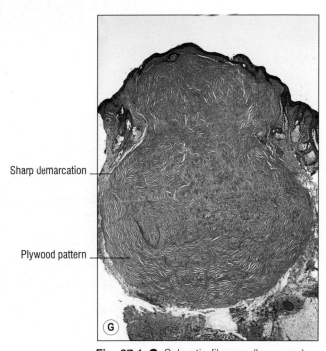

Sharp demarcation

Plywood pattern

G

Fig. 27.1 G Sclerotic fibroma (low mag.).

pattern" of any combination of spindle cells in a nodule, slit-like staghorn vascular channels, has a benign course despite being CD34 positive as in DFSP (27.10).

Differential diagnosis

1. Scar (27.2): epidermal atrophy, fibroblasts tend to be oriented more parallel to the epidermis instead of whorling, with blood vessels more perpendicular.
2. Dermatofibrosarcoma protuberans (27.10): large size, location usually on the trunk, infiltrating bands of spindle cells extend into adipose, more prominent storiform pattern, mild cytologic atypia, no epidermal hyperplasia, usually no multinucleated giant cells or foam cells. DFSP is typically CD34+, factor XIIIaneg, stromelysin-3neg, D2-40neg (all four stains are the opposite in DF). Intermediate lesions with worrisome

histology and equivocal immunostaining are not rare and might be called fibrous neoplasm of uncertain malignant potential (FRUMP).
3. Leiomyoma (29.6).
4. Neurofibroma (26.1).
5. Desmoplastic nevus (20.5).
6. Other spindle cell neoplasms (1.131), epithelioid cell neoplasms (1.38), or granulomas (1.51).

27.2 Scar (cicatrix)

(see Fig. 27.2A,B)

Although not a neoplasm, a scar is included here for comparison with other fibrohistiocytic proliferations. Scars are red initially, and then may become white (1.150) and sometimes indurated papules or plaques.

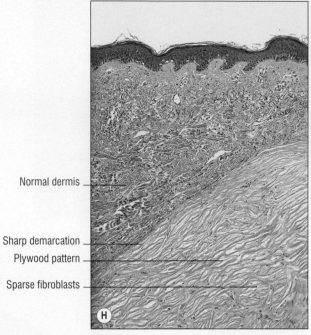

Normal dermis

Sharp demarcation
Plywood pattern
Sparse fibroblasts

Fig. 27.1 H Sclerotic fibroma (medium mag.).

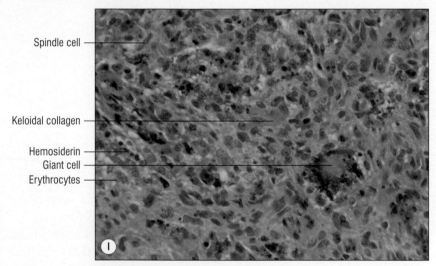

Spindle cell

Keloidal collagen

Hemosiderin
Giant cell
Erythrocytes

Fig. 27.1 I Hemosiderotic dermatofibroma.

P
- *Epidermis atrophic* or normal, often with loss of rete ridges
- Subepidermal blister artifact is common (1.147)
- Bands of fibroblasts and dense collagen, often *oriented parallel to the epidermis*
- Young scars may have a pale or mucinous stroma and more fibroblasts, sometimes extravasated erythrocytes, while older ones have more collagen, less paleness, and fewer fibroblasts (more sclerotic)
- *Blood vessels tend to be more perpendicularly oriented* with respect to the epidermis

Variations

1. Hypertrophic scar: thick scar that is significantly elevated above the skin surface to a greater degree than average.
2. Keloid: large nodule or plaque that *grows like a neoplasm beyond the original site of injury*, more in black skin, *thicker hyalinized bands of collagen* ("keloidal collagen").

3. Striae distensae: linear tears in the skin, violaceous lesions later become white, usually in areas of tension, loss of elastic fibers in these areas.
4. Anetoderma (9.11): perhaps an unusual variant of scar.

Differential diagnosis

1. Dermatofibroma (27.1), and other fibrous neoplasms (Chapter 27).
2. Other spindle cell neoplasms (1.131).
3. Other alterations of connective tissue (1.125, Chapter 9).

27.3 Angiofibroma (fibrous papule)

(see Fig. 27.3A–E)

Common small (1.5 mm), *red to skin-colored papule*, usually on the *nose* (1.95) or central face (1.44).

- Collagen oriented concentrically around follicles or oriented more perpendicular to the epidermis
- Sometimes increased numbers of stellate, plump fibroblasts
- Few dilated blood vessels

Variations

1. Tuberous sclerosis (epiloia, Bourneville's disease): autosomal dominant, type 1 due to mutation in TSC1 gene which codes for hamartin, type 2 is more common, more severe, and due to mutation in TSC2 gene which codes for tuberin. Multiple angiofibromas (misnamed adenoma sebaceum) on the central face that begin at puberty and are mistaken for acne (10.1), forehead angiofibrotic plaques, periungual fibromas (1.85), ash leaf white macules (1.150) since early childhood, café-au-lait macules (20.2), connective tissue nevi (Shagreen patch of the sacral area, 27.6), enamel teeth pits, epilepsy, and low intelligence (epiloia stands for this plus adenoma sebaceum), basal ganglia calcification, and a variety of internal neoplasms such as cerebral tubers and gliomas, retinal phakomata, cardiac

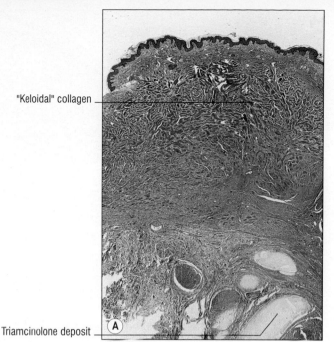

"Keloidal" collagen

Triamcinolone deposit

Fig. 27.2 A Keloid (low mag.).

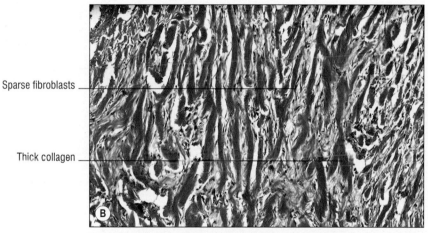

Sparse fibroblasts

Thick collagen

Fig. 27.2 B Keloid (high mag.).

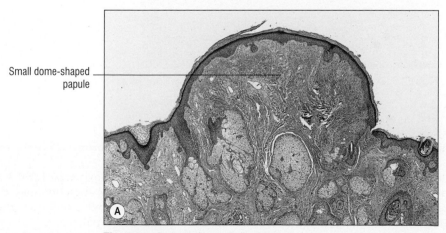

Small dome-shaped papule

Fig. 27.3 A Angiofibroma (low mag.).

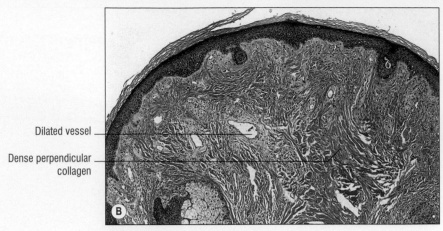

Dilated vessel

Dense perpendicular collagen

Fig. 27.3 B Angiofibroma (medium mag.).

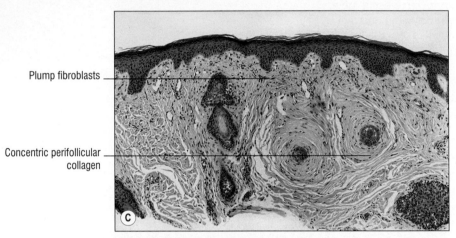

Plump fibroblasts

Concentric perifollicular collagen

Fig. 27.3 C Perifollicular fibroma.

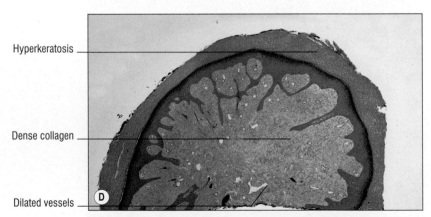

Hyperkeratosis

Dense collagen

Dilated vessels

Fig. 27.3 D Periungual fibroma of tuberous sclerosis (low mag.).

rhabdomyomas, renal angiomyolipomas, and many other systemic lesions.

2. Pearly penile papules: multiple tiny 1-mm or smaller papules around the coronal sulcus of the penis (1.107) sometimes mistaken for warts (14.1).

3. Perifollicular fibroma: perifollicular accentuation of the fibrous tissue.

4. Familial myxovascular fibromas:[153] rare papules on the hands (1.56).

5. Multiple endocrine neoplasia type 1 (MEA type 1, Wermer syndrome): facial angiofibromas, collagenomas (27.6), lipomas, parathyroid, pancreatic (glucagonoma, 3.2), pituitary tumors (1.105).

6. Multinucleate cell angiohistiocytoma (7.13).

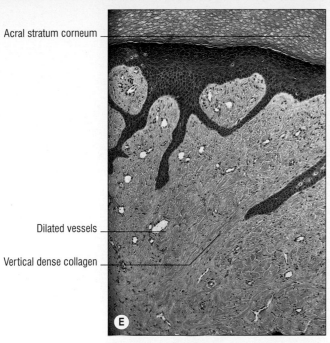

Acral stratum corneum

Dilated vessels

Vertical dense collagen

E

Fig. 27.3 E Periungual fibroma of tuberous sclerosis (medium mag.).

Differential diagnosis

1. Fibrofolliculoma and trichodiscoma (22.6), trichilemmomas (22.5), and trichoepitheliomas (22.2) can also be multiple on the face.
2. Fibrosing melanocytic nevus (20.5).
3. At first glance, these subtle papules may resemble normal skin (1.94).
4. Folliculitis (10.2) or acne (10.1) with fibrosis.

27.4 Acrochordon (skin tag, soft fibroma, fibroepithelial polyp, FEP)

(see Fig. 27.4)
Very common, often *pedunculated* (1.106), skin-colored (1.129) to brown, *papules* of *eyelids* (1.43), *neck* (1.86), *axilla* (1.10), or *groin* (1.55). Increased incidence with aging and obesity, controversial association with intestinal polyps.

P
- *Pedunculated papule* (1.106), epidermis often extends almost completely around the specimen when it is sectioned
- Papillomatosis and acanthosis common, sometimes epidermal atrophy (1.9)
- Dermis consists of loose connective tissue that is often pale
- Dilated blood vessels often

Variations

1. Dermatosis papulosa nigra (18.2).
2. Birt–Hogg–Dube syndrome (22.6).
3. Lipofibroma ("fibroma molle"): larger tag with *adipose in the stroma*, not to be confused with nevus lipomatosus (29.1).

4. Pleomorphic fibroma (pseudosarcomatous polyp): large *atypical fibroblasts* and histiocytes in the stroma, sometimes multinucleated, a pseudomalignancy (1.118).

Differential diagnosis

1. Other papillomas (1.102).
2. Improper orientation of a thin, folded shave biopsy can resemble a tag.

27.5 Acquired digital fibrokeratoma

(see Fig. 27.5A,B)
Uncommon finger-like projection from a digit or acral skin (1.56, 1.48).

P
- *Massive orthokeratosis*, usually no parakeratosis, with acanthosis
- *Thickened collagen* in the dermis, often *oriented parallel to the long axis* of the lesion

Differential diagnosis

1. Supernumerary digit: congenital, mostly related to the fifth digit where a sixth digit would be expected, increased peripheral nerves present (26.3).
2. Acrochordon (27.4): different location, softer and less hyperkeratotic, less dense connective tissue.
3. Viral wart (14.1): more papillomatosis, hypergranulosis, koilocytosis, columns of parakeratosis, less dense connective tissue.
4. Periungual fibroma (27.3): association with tuberous sclerosis, more blood vessels, plump fibroblasts.
5. Other lesions with hyperplasia of epidermis (1.61) or scars, sclerosis, or fibrosis (1.125).

27.6 Connective tissue nevus

(see Fig. 27.6A,B)
Uncommon *skin-colored* (1.129) *papules, nodules or plaques, present at birth*, or arising in childhood. Clinically and histologically, may be subtle and may resemble normal skin (1.94).

P
- *Poorly demarcated nodule with increased collagen* and normal, decreased, or increased elastic fibers. Sometimes the changes are easily missed unless *surrounding normal skin is biopsied for comparison*

Variations

1. Shagreen patch of tuberous sclerosis (27.3): pigskin cobble-stoned plaque most common in the *sacral area*, no increased elastic tissue.
2. Nevus elasticus: increased elastic fibers (1.31).
3. Buschke–Ollendorff syndrome (BOS): rare, autosomal dominant, mutation resulting in loss of function of LEMD3, affecting BMP signaling, resulting in upregulation of SMAD and transforming growth factor (TGF)-β. Multiple scattered papules are mostly

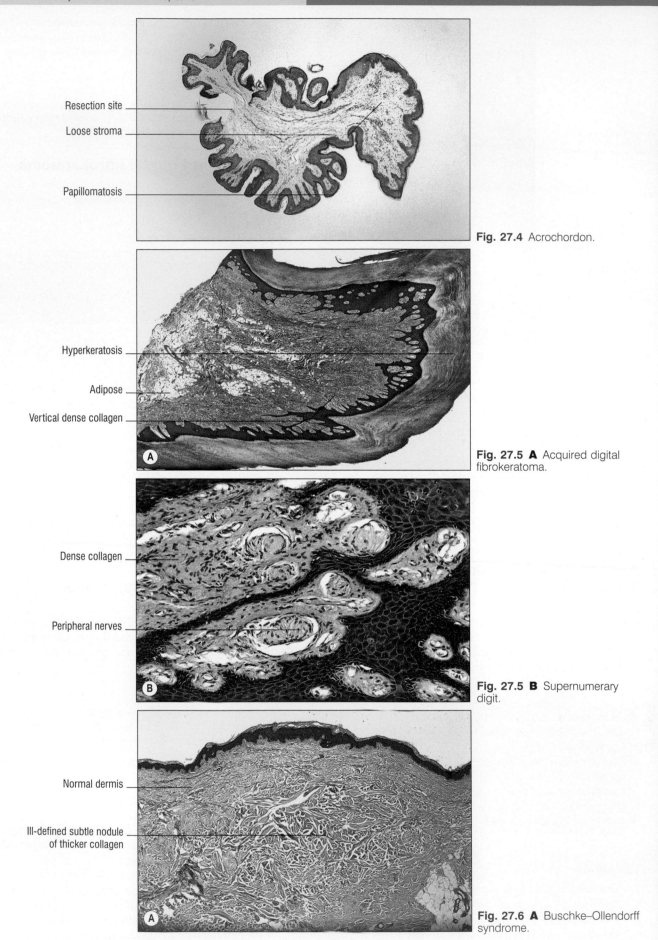

Resection site

Loose stroma

Papillomatosis

Fig. 27.4 Acrochordon.

Hyperkeratosis

Adipose

Vertical dense collagen

A

Fig. 27.5 A Acquired digital fibrokeratoma.

Dense collagen

Peripheral nerves

B

Fig. 27.5 B Supernumerary digit.

Normal dermis

Ill-defined subtle nodule of thicker collagen

A

Fig. 27.6 A Buschke–Ollendorff syndrome.

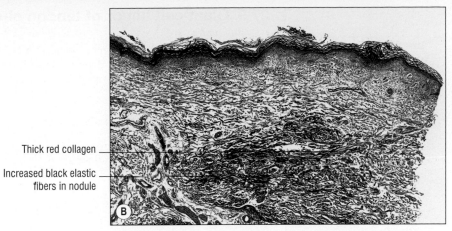

Thick red collagen

Increased black elastic fibers in nodule

Fig. 27.6 B Buschke–Ollendorff syndrome (WG stain).

connective tissue nevi with increased elastic fibers (nevus elasticus), but some have mostly increased collagen (dermatofibrosis lenticularis disseminata), osteopoikilosis (spotted bones, 1.16).

Differential diagnosis

1. Other diseases with altered connective tissue (Chapter 9), and scars, sclerosis, and fibrosis (1.125).
2. Elastofibroma: actually no resemblance to nevus elasticus except its name, large subcutaneous mass on shoulder with increased clumped elastic fibers.

27.7 Infantile digital fibromatosis (inclusion body fibromatosis)

(see Fig. 27.7A–C)
Rare indurated, solitary or multiple *recurrent nodules or plaques* on acral skin, especially *fingers* (1.56), of *children* in the first year of life. They usually regress in a few years, but may cause deforming contractures.

- Dense bands of collagen and many plump spindled myofibroblasts
- *Eosinophilic cytoplasmic inclusion bodies* (3–10 microns) in the myofibroblasts, often adjacent to the nuclei. They can be seen with H&E stain but are easier to identify with PTAH, actin, or trichrome stains. Negative with PAS.

Differential diagnosis

1. Other hand and finger lesions (1.56).
2. Other spindle cell neoplasms (1.131), and scars, sclerosis and fibrosis (1.125) generally have a different clinical presentation and do not have the inclusion bodies.

27.8 Nodular fasciitis (pseudosarcomatous fasciitis)

(see Fig. 27.8A,B)
Uncommon *subcutaneous rapidly growing nodule* in a *young adult*, most common on upper extremity, or in *children* on the head or neck, sometimes related to trauma. These lesions may resemble a sarcoma histologically (1.118), but clinically they

regress and are not neoplastic. If the lesion recurs following excision, the diagnosis should be reconsidered (distinction from a bona fide sarcoma can be difficult).

- Subcutaneous somewhat circumscribed nodular proliferation of myofibroblasts in a loose, mucinous stroma, resembling "tissue-culture fibroblasts"
- Muscle-specific actin or smooth muscle actin often positive, but desmin is usually negative
- Sometimes infiltration through muscle or along fibrous septae of fat
- Fibroblasts may be moderately pleomorphic, hyperchromatic, or may show increased mitoses that are not atypical
- Multinucleated osteoclast-like giant cells may be present (27.9)
- Often prominent vascularity, sometimes slit-like spaces
- Lymphocytes often present within the nodule to a greater extent than usual in a sarcoma, especially at the margin

Variation

1. Proliferative fasciitis: large polygonal cells with amphophilic cytoplasm resembling ganglion cells are present.

Differential diagnosis

1. Fibrosarcoma (27.13): more herringbone pattern, more densely cellular, less inflammation, less mucinous stroma.
2. Malignant fibrous histiocytoma (27.11): usually more prominent atypia and more atypical mitoses, less inflammation.
3. Benign fibrous histiocytoma (27.1): slower growing, usually more dermal, less myxoid, usually more collagen trapping.
4. Fibromatosis (27.15): more dense collagen, fewer fibroblasts, less myxoid.
5. Dermatofibrosarcoma protuberans (27.10): more on the trunk, more storiform, CD34 positive.
6. Other spindle cell proliferations (1.131).

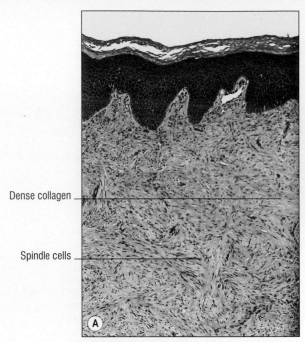

Dense collagen

Spindle cells

Fig. 27.7 A Infantile digital fibromatosis (low mag.).

27.9 Giant cell tumor of tendon sheath
(*see Fig. 27.9A,B*)
Uncommon nodule of the *finger or acral skin* (1.56) of adults, which might be considered a deep variant of benign fibrous histiocytoma or dermatofibroma (27.1) that *is fixed to tendon sheath or fascia.*

- Sharply demarcated localized lobule
- Proliferation of fibroblasts and histiocytes, sometimes foamy (1.46)
- Large osteoclast-like giant cells (1.84) with many haphazard nuclei usually present
- Hemosiderin often present (1.58)

Differential diagnosis

1. The lesion is rather histologically distinct, but might be mistaken for other diseases with multinucleated giant cells (1.84), or other spindle cell neoplasms (1.131).

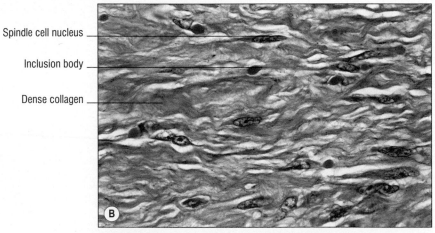

Spindle cell nucleus

Inclusion body

Dense collagen

Fig. 27.7 B Infantile digital fibromatosis (high mag.).

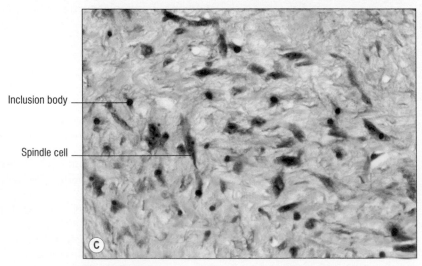

Inclusion body

Spindle cell

Fig. 27.7 C Inclusion body fibromatosis (trichrome stain).

27.10 Dermatofibrosarcoma protuberans (DFSP)

(see Fig. 27.10A–D)

Rare large nodule or plaque, indolently growing, often with *multiple protuberances*, most common on the *trunk* (1.141) of young to middle-aged adults, *unrelated to sun damage*. Locally infiltrating, often recurs after excision, but almost never metastasizes unless fibrosarcomatous change occurs. Most DFSPs, including all variants below, including giant cell fibroblastoma, are caused by a specific fusion of COL1A1 gene with the PDGFB gene. Cytogenetic analysis most often reveals ring chromosomes r(17;22) or linear t(17;22)(q22;q13). Usually treated with wide excision or Mohs surgery. The tyrosine kinase inhibitor drug, imatinib, can result in shrinkage of the tumor.

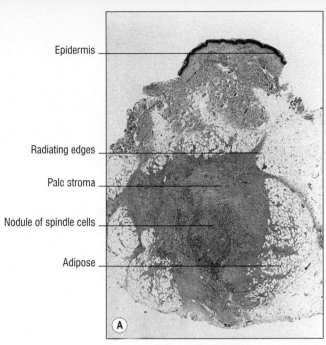

Epidermis

Radiating edges

Pale stroma

Nodule of spindle cells

Adipose

Fig. 27.8 A Nodular fasciitis (low mag.).

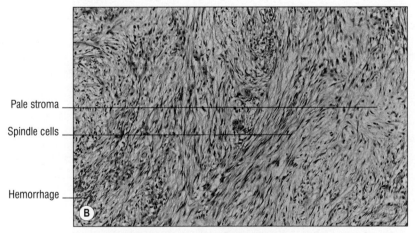

Pale stroma

Spindle cells

Hemorrhage

Fig. 27.8 B Nodular fasciitis (high mag.).

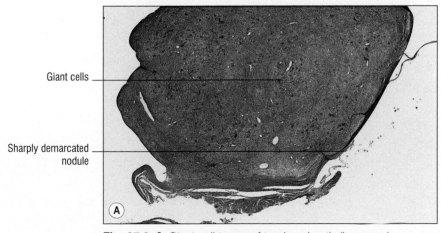

Giant cells

Sharply demarcated nodule

Fig. 27.9 A Giant cell tumor of tendon sheath (low mag.).

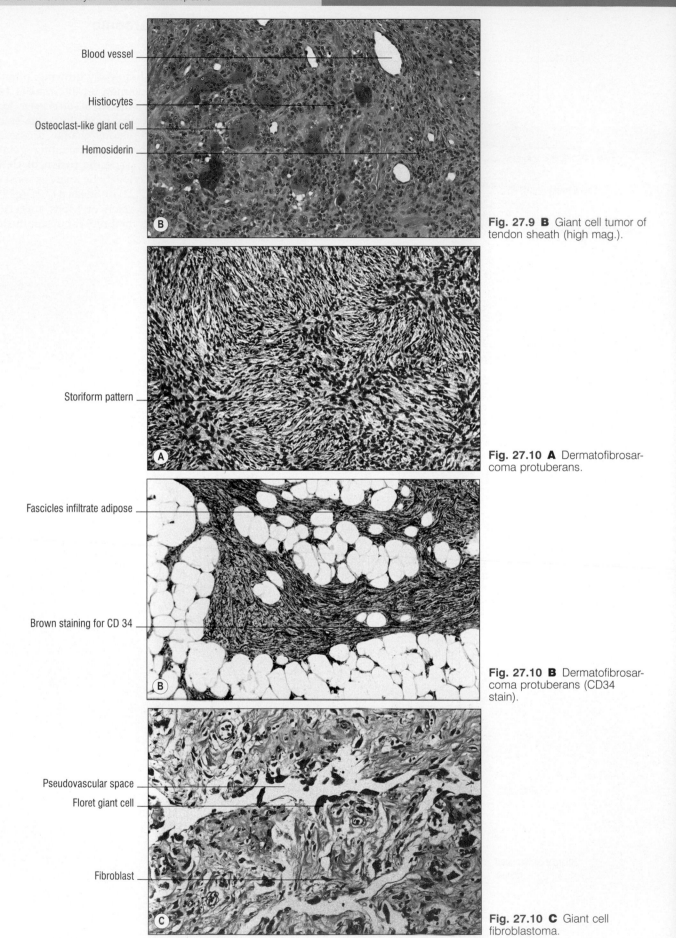

Blood vessel

Histiocytes

Osteoclast-like giant cell

Hemosiderin

Fig. 27.9 B Giant cell tumor of tendon sheath (high mag.).

Storiform pattern

Fig. 27.10 A Dermatofibrosarcoma protuberans.

Fascicles infiltrate adipose

Brown staining for CD 34

Fig. 27.10 B Dermatofibrosarcoma protuberans (CD34 stain).

Pseudovascular space

Floret giant cell

Fibroblast

Fig. 27.10 C Giant cell fibroblastoma.

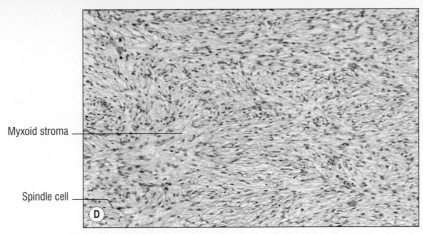

Myxoid stroma —

Spindle cell —

(D)

Fig. 27.10 D Myxoid dermatofibrosarcoma protuberans.

P
- Epidermis normal, atrophic, or ulcerated (rarely hyperplastic)
- Very cellular proliferation of thin spindled fibroblasts and collagen in the dermis, extending into the subcutaneous fat
- *Cartwheel pattern* (fibroblasts whorl around like spokes of a wheel) or *storiform* (whirligig or mat-like) pattern
- Usually no foamy cells or multinucleated giant cells, unlike dermatofibroma
- *Infiltration of fat in a fascicular or honeycomb pattern*
- Cytologic *atypia mild to moderate*, very few mitoses
- CD34+, stromelysin-3neg, factor XIIIaneg, D2-40neg (all four opposite of dermatofibroma). S-100 is negative

Variations

1. Atrophic DFSP: flat indurated macule or slightly elevated plaque instead of the more common protuberant nodules. Not very cellular, so it is easy to misdiagnose on a punch biopsy.
2. Myxoid DFSP: myxoid (1.83) stroma, may resemble myxoid neoplasms such as myxoid liposarcoma (29.5), but usually extends more superficially than liposarcoma, and lacks chicken wire vasculature and lipoblasts.
3. Bednar tumor (pigmented DFSP): more common with black skin, melanin and some melanocytes present, may be S-100+.
4. Fibrosarcomatous degeneration in DFSP (dedifferentiation): foci with more atypia and mitoses, transformation to fibrosarcoma (27.13) or malignant fibrous histiocytoma (27.11) with risk of metastasis.
5. Giant cell fibroblastoma (GCF): DFSP-like tumor of childhood, especially boys, trunk and lower extremities, jagged *pseudovascular spaces* lined by floret-like *multinucleated giant cells* (1.84), and spindle cells, sometimes storiform, in a hyalinized (1.35) or myxoid (1.83) stroma. Since CD34+ staining is found in this tumor as well as vascular neoplasms (Chapter 25), negative staining of the pseudovascular spaces with endothelial cell markers is important.
6. Subcutaneous DFSP: deep mass with normal surface changes on the skin.

Differential diagnosis

1. Dermatofibroma (27.1), especially cellular type.
2. Fibrosarcoma (27.13).
3. Atypical fibroxanthoma (27.12): very atypical, sun exposed in older patients.
4. Other spindle cell tumors (1.131).
5. Whorling or storiform pattern may be seen in sclerotic fibroma (27.1), cellular dermatofibroma (27.1), myoepithelioma (29.6), and perineurioma (26.3).

27.11 Pleomorphic sarcoma (malignant fibrous histiocytoma, MFH)

(see Fig. 27.11)

Uncommon *mass of the deep subcutaneous tissue*, usually not encountered by dermatologists, high risk of metastasis. Since this appears to be a wastebasket for a heterogeneous group of poorly differentiated tumors with striking atypia, some newer classifications prefer the term pleomorphic sarcoma over MFH.

- Subcutaneous cellular proliferation of fibroblasts, histiocyte-like cells, and bizarre giant cells **P**
- Severe pleomorphism, hyperchromatism, *many bizarre cells or highly atypical mitoses* often
- Vimentin+: variable positivity with fibrohistiocytic markers CD68, alpha-1 antitrypsin, and alpha-1-antichymotrypsin. Variable positivity with muscle markers desmin and actin. CD34 is negative.

Variations

1. Myxoid MFH (myxofibrosarcoma): myxomatous stroma (1.83), curvilinear vessels, pseudolipoblasts (29.5).
2. Inflammatory MFH (fibroxanthosarcoma): neutrophils, foamy histiocytes, and giant cells.
3. Angiomatoid MFH: vascular proliferation and hemorrhage.
4. Giant cell variant: osteoclast-like giant cells.

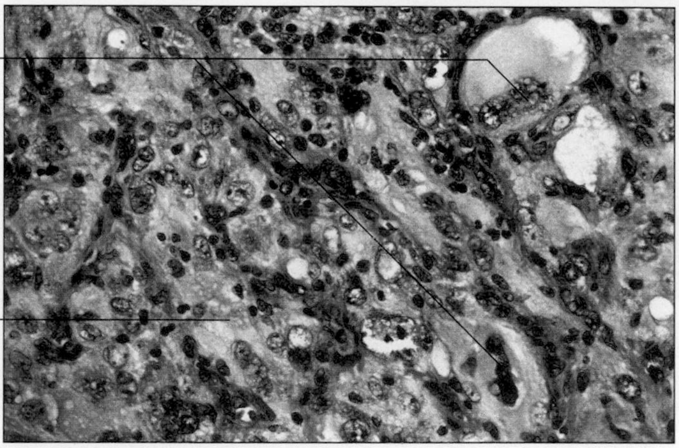

Fig. 27.11 Malignant fibrous histiocytoma.

Differential diagnosis

1. Atypical fibroxanthoma (27.12): sun-damaged skin of ears or face, smaller, more superficial, solar elastosis, less chance of metastasis.
2. Melanoma (20.11).
3. Nodular fasciitis (27.8).
4. Myxoid liposarcoma (29.5).
5. Other spindle cell (1.131) or epithelioid (1.38) neoplasms.

27.12 Atypical fibroxanthoma (AFX, superficial malignant fibrous histiocytoma)

(see Fig. 27.12)

Uncommon, red plaque or nodule of *sun-damaged skin*, often ulcerated (1.142), especially on the *ear* (1.28), small risk of metastasis (behaves like sun-induced squamous cell carcinoma). It is not as aggressive as the severe atypia would suggest.

P
- Dermal cellular proliferation of *bizarre spindle cells*, epithelioid cells, or multinucleated giant cells (1.84), and *sometimes foamy* cells, *often extending up against the epidermis*
- *Severe pleomorphism*, hyperchromatism, *many very atypical mitoses*
- *Solar elastosis*
- Positive staining for vimentin, CD68 and other histiocytic stains, CD99, calponin, procollagen-1, and strongly positive for CD10. Negative for S-100, desmin, and pankeratin. SMA and EMA may be focally positive

Variation

1. Myxoid, granular cell, osteoclast-like, clear cell, and pseudoangiomatous variants have been described.

Differential diagnosis

1. Malignant fibrous histiocytoma (MFH, 27.11): deep mass, not sun exposed, more likely to stain for CD74 (rarely done).

2. The other two most commonly encountered malignancies of sun-damaged skin that resemble AFX are spindle cell squamous cell carcinoma (18.11, pankeratin positive, sometimes weakly positive for CD10) and melanoma (20.11, S-100+).
3. Other spindle cell neoplasms (1.131), epithelioid cell neoplasms (1.38), or foamy neoplasms (1.46).

27.13 Fibrosarcoma

(see Fig. 27.13)

Rare tumor presenting as a *deep mass*, rarely encountered by dermatologists. It used to be a wastebasket category for many tumors which has been reclassified elsewhere.

P
- Subcutaneous densely cellular proliferation of uniform spindle cells, sometimes with a *herringbone pattern* (nuclei radiate off on either side of a central "vertebral" column)
- Cytologic *atypia mild to moderate*, depending upon how well differentiated it is. Necrosis and mitoses common
- Vimentin+. Negative staining for pankeratin, S100, CD34, desmin, SMA

Differential diagnosis

1. Dermatofibrosarcoma protuberans (27.10): more superficial, prominent storiform pattern.
2. Malignant fibrous histiocytoma (27.11): more common, far more atypia, and no herringbone pattern.
3. Nodular pseudosarcomatous fasciitis (27.8).
4. Other spindle cell tumors (1.130).

27.14 Epithelioid sarcoma

(see Fig. 27.14)

Rare nodule on distal forearms or *acral skin*, especially hand or finger (1.56) of *young adults*. Often recurs, metastasizes in 50% of patients.

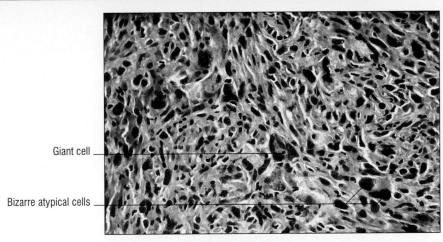

Giant cell

Bizarre atypical cells

Fig. 27.12 Atypical fibroxanthoma.

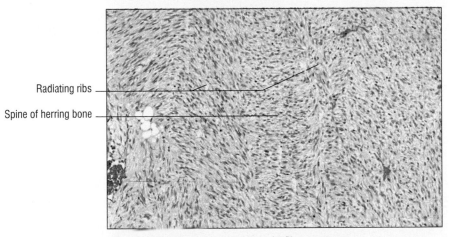

Radiating ribs

Spine of herring bone

Fig. 27.13 Herringbone pattern in fibrosarcoma.

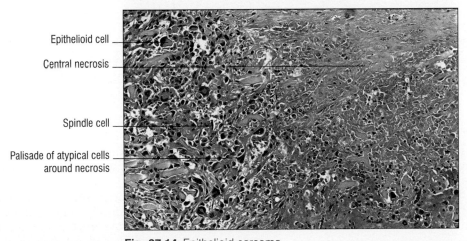

Epithelioid cell

Central necrosis

Spindle cell

Palisade of atypical cells around necrosis

Fig. 27.14 Epithelioid sarcoma.

P

- Poorly circumscribed proliferation of polygonal atypical epithelioid cells and spindled cells often palisade around central necrosis, resembling a palisading granuloma
- Pleomorphism, hyperchromatism, numerous mitoses
- Lymphocytes common, especially at tumor periphery
- Positive staining with both pankeratin and vimentin (hence the tumor's name, which refers to epithelial-like staining with keratin, as well as sarcomatous staining with vimentin). Epithelial membrane antigen is also positive. CD34 is positive in 50% of cases

Differential diagnosis

1. Malignant fibrous histiocytoma: bizarre atypical cells, foamy cells (27.11).
2. Palisading granulomas (1.51), especially granuloma annulare (7.1), which is common in the same location: no atypia, keratin negative.

27.15 Fibromatosis

(see Fig. 27.15A,B)

This is a group of fibrous proliferations with plenty of collagen, but with low cellularity. They are considered benign, but

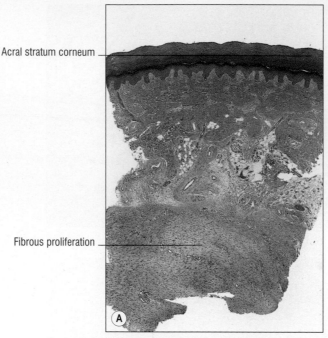

Fig. 27.15 A Plantar fibromatosis (low mag.).

Acral stratum corneum

Fibrous proliferation

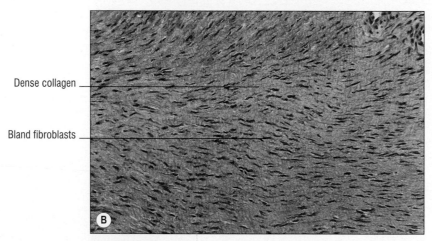

Fig. 27.15 B Plantar fibromatosis (medium mag.).

Dense collagen

Bland fibroblasts

some forms can be locally infiltrative, and may recur after excision. Fibromatosis may occur in childhood or be acquired in adulthood. Some patients may have more than one of these forms of fibromatosis at the same time.

■ Dense hyalinized collagenous neoplasm with poorly defined borders
■ Scattered fibroblasts, sometimes with corkscrew nuclei (may be more cellular in early lesions) without atypia or mitoses

Variations

1. Palmar fibromatosis (Dupuytren's contracture): older males, increased incidence of alcoholism, often develops clinically chord-like bands on the palms (1.100) with flexion contractures.

2. Plantar fibromatosis (Ledderhose's disease): young to middle-aged adults, thick soles (1.100) may interfere with walking.

3. Penile fibromatosis (Peyronie's disease): middle-aged to older adult males slowly develop fibrous thickening of the penis, often with dorsal curvature of the penis with pain, more commonly inflamed, calcified, or ossified than other forms of fibromatosis.

4. Knuckle pads: thick plaques on dorsum of finger joints in adults, usually without significant symptoms or contracture, usually with acanthosis and hyperkeratosis in addition to the fibrous proliferation.

5. Desmoid tumor: some cases are due to mutation in APC gene. Solitary, rarely multiple, deep, indurated, non-tender, slowly growing mass of the fascia or muscle, which sometimes extends up into the fat. *Abdominal desmoids* tend to occur during or after pregnancy. *Extra-abdominal desmoids* occur in children and young adults, most common on the trunk, neck, or thigh. *Fibromatosis coli* is a desmoid of the neck that causes

torticollis. *Intra-abdominal desmoids* occur in the mesentery and retroperitoneum in Gardner's syndrome (19.1). Desmoids are difficult to excise, frequently recur, but do not metastasize.

6. Infantile digital fibromatosis (27.7).

Differential diagnosis

1. Well-differentiated fibrosarcoma (27.13): used as a synonym for some of the larger fibromatosis lesions by some authorities, more than one mitosis per high-power field, more cellular.
2. Dermatofibrosarcoma protuberans (27.10).
3. Solitary fibrous tumor (27.1).
4. Fibrous hamartoma of infancy (27.19).
5. Other conditions with scarring, fibrosis, or sclerosis (1.125).

27.16 Calcifying aponeurotic fibroma

Rare nodule or plaque on the *hands* (1.56), and less commonly on the *feet* of *children*, and less commonly in adults, usually attached to tendons or fascia, with a tendency to recur, without pain or contractures.

- Spindle or epithelioid fibroblasts tend to palisade around areas of dense collagen and calcification (1.19)
- Cartilage may form in the calcified areas in older lesions

Differential diagnosis

1. Fibromatosis (27.15): less cellular, less epithelioid, less calcification, less palisading, no metaplastic cartilage.
2. Gout (8.5) and pseudogout.
3. Epithelioid sarcoma (27.14): positive staining for keratin, CD34+ in 50% of cases, more necrosis, no calcification.
4. Palisading granulomas (1.51).

27.17 Myxoma (cutaneous myxoma, superficial angiomyxoma)

Rare, slowly growing dermal or subcutaneous nodule, most common on head or neck of adults, may recur after excision.

- Poorly demarcated, paucicellular nodule of vimentin+ stellate spindle cells in *vascular myxoid stroma*. Occasionally multinucleated cells may be present
- Variable staining for S100, CD34, factor XIIIa, SMA, MSA. Desmin is negative
- Often contains epithelial strands, cysts, or trichoblastic changes
- Minimal cytologic atypia, but mitoses may be present

Variations

1. Aggressive angiomyxoma: deeper, more infiltrating and less circumscribed, in anogenital region, may grow larger than 5 cm, local recurrence common but does not metastasize. Positive for vimentin, focal positive smooth muscle actin, desmin-neg, S-100neg, negative XIIIaneg, CD34neg.

2. Superficial acral angiomyxoma: hand nodule (1.56), especially around nail (1.85). Similar myxoid stroma, but mild nuclear atypia, CD34+. EMAneg, actin-neg, desmin-neg, S-100neg. CD99 is sometimes positive. If multiple papules present on hands, consider familial myxovascular fibromas (27.3).

3. Carney complex: autosomal dominant disorder (CNC1 or PRKAR1A gene, or CNC2 gene), myxomatous lesions (cutaneous myxomas, psammomatous melanotic schwannoma, 26.2, cardiac myxomas, or myxoid fibroadenomas of the breast), pigmented skin lesions (ephelides, lentigines, or blue nevi), and endocrine disorders. Related entities include NAME syndrome (nevi, atrial or cutaneous myxomas, ephelides) or LAMB syndrome (lentigines, atrial or cutaneous myxomas, blue nevus).

Differential diagnosis

1. Other mucinous or myxoid lesions (1.33).
2. Focal mucinosis of the skin (8.11) and mucous cysts (8.9): does not grow like a neoplasm, less vascular, more superficial, no association with Carney complex, less cellular, more sharply demarcated.
3. Nerve sheath myxoma (26.7): more cellular, more lobules or fascicles, S-100+.
4. Myxoid MFH (27.11): larger tumor, more nuclear atypia, and curvilinear vascular pattern.
5. Myxoid liposarcoma (29.5): lipoblasts, chicken-wire vascular pattern.

27.18 Plexiform fibrohistiocytic tumor

Nodule or mass in *children or young adults*, most common on the *upper extremity*. *Behavior* varies from spontaneous regression, recurrence after excision, to occasional local metastasis.

- Fascicles of spindle or epithelioid cells in complex plexiform pattern
- Nodular aggregates CD68+, SMA+ histiocytes, multinucleated giant cells (1.84), and lymphocytes, suggesting granulomas seen in an infectious process
- Mild to absent pleomorphism, mitoses rare
- Extravasated erythrocytes (1.40) and hemosiderin (1.58) often
- Atypia mild, mitoses uncommon
- May contain myofibroblasts positive for actin

Differential diagnosis

1. Granulomas (1.51).
2. Fibrous hamartoma of infancy (27.19): similar location, usually more myxoid.
3. Fibromatosis (27.15).
4. Other neoplasms with spindle cells (1.131) or epithelioid cells (1.38).

27.19 Fibrous hamartoma of infancy

(see Fig. 27.19A,B)

Slowly growing, *solitary subcutaneous mass*, onset in *first 3 years of life*, more in boys, especially of the *axilla* (1.10) or

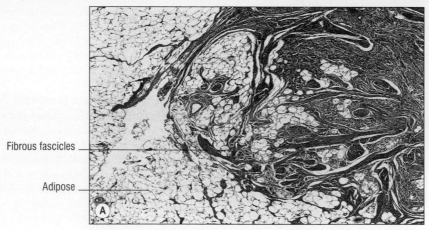

Fig. 27.19 A Fibrous hamartoma of infancy (low mag.).

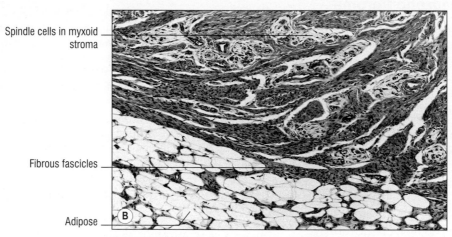

Fig. 27.19 B Fibrous hamartoma of infancy (high mag.).

shoulder. It usually does not recur after excision, but does not regress spontaneously.

 ■ Ill-defined subcutaneous nodule with *three components:* whorled cellular islands of round or spindle cells in a myxoid stroma (1.83), hypocellular fibrous fascicles, and islands of adipose tissue

Differential diagnosis

1. Infantile myofibromatosis (multiple lesions) and solitary myofibroma: young male children, head, neck, or trunk, may recur after excision but eventually often spontaneously regresses. In adults it is more common on the extremities. It contains myofibroblasts like fibrous hamartoma of infancy, but has more vascular hemangiopericytoma-like areas (25.6), and usually has a biphasic pattern of bundles of spindle cells resembling smooth muscle (vimentin+, SMA+, desmin-neg), with fascicles of more rounded cells around the vessels (SMAneg, desmin-neg).
2. Fibromatosis (27.15).

27.20 Solitary fibrous tumor (SFT)

Rare soft tissue mass most common in pleura and rarely in skin. It is a borderline neoplasm that is not considered malignant, but uncommonly recurs locally.

■ Spindle cell proliferation (1.131) said to have a "*patternless pattern*".
■ Immunoprofile is vimentin+. CD34+ in 80%, SMA+ in 30% of cases. Staining is negative for factor XIIIa, EMA, and S100.

27.21 Cutaneous PEComa

The PEComa (perivascular epithelioid cell tumor) has been rarely reported in the skin. The tumor has an uncertain nosologic standing, but appears to be benign.

■ Clear cells (1.22) within a dermal nodule, accentuated in perivascular distribution
■ Immunoprofile may suggest a melanocytic tumor, except that S100 is negative. HMB-45, Mitf, NKI-C3, and PAS (glycogen) are positive. MART-1, desmin and CD68 are variable. SMA, pankeratin, and EMA are negative.

CHAPTER 28

Metastatic Neoplasms to Skin

Chapter Contents

It is beyond the scope of this book to discuss all of the neoplasms that may metastasize to the skin.[159] The more common or characteristic tumors are mentioned below. Breast cancer most commonly metastasizes to skin, hence it is covered in its own section, 28.3. Colon and lung cancer are also common. Breast, colon, and lung happen to be three of the most common internal malignancies in man. Prostate cancer is a common cancer, but tends not to metastasize to skin. Renal cell carcinoma, the other exception, is uncommon, but seems to have an exceptional affinity for skin, hence a separate section (28.4). Metastatic melanoma is also common in skin, and is considered in Chapter 20.

28.1 Metastatic squamous cell carcinoma

(see Fig. 28.1A–D)
Dermal or subcutaneous nodule, most common on the trunk or scalp, most commonly originating from a lung, head, or neck malignancy.

- Tumor in the dermis showing features of squamous cell carcinoma (18.11), usually with *keratin pearls or squamous eddies* if well differentiated, with no connection to the epidermis
- Pleomorphism and hyperchromatic nuclei, increased numbers of mitoses, more prominent if poorly differentiated
- Usually not possible to determine the site of origin of the tumor based upon histologic features
- Pseudoglandular spaces without mucin may be due to acantholysis (1.2)
- Positive staining for pankeratin useful in difficult cases

Differential diagnosis
1. Other epithelioid neoplasms (1.38) or spindle cell neoplasms (1.131).

28.2 Metastatic adenocarcinoma

(see Fig. 28.2A–C)
Dermal or subcutaneous nodule, most common on the trunk or scalp, most commonly originating from *breast* (28.3) or *gastrointestinal tract*, or lung.

©2012 Elsevier Ltd, Inc, BV
DOI: 10.1016/B978-0-323-06658-7.00028-2

- Tumor in the dermis with variable small *glandular formations or signet-ring cells* (if tumor is differentiated)
- Pleomorphism, hyperchromatism, and increased numbers of mitoses
- Usually not possible to determine the site of origin of the tumor based upon histologic features, with some exceptions
- Mucin stains, such as mucicarmine, often stain *mucin* within the tumor cells
- Positive staining for pankeratin useful to prove the tumor is carcinoma (epithelial origin rather than mesenchymal or hematopoietic) when needed. A battery of more specific cytokeratin stains, such as CK5/6, CK7, and CK20 can be used to predict the origin of the primary tumor, using a table of probabilities of expression of these keratins found in general pathology books, but this is not completely reliable and usually clinical work-up of the patient is needed. Colon cancer, for example, is usually CK20+ and CK7neg. Lung cancer is usually CK7+, CK20neg. Breast and ovarian cancer are usually CK7+. Prostate cancer is usually CK7neg
- Other immunostains might help identify primary site. CA-125 is positive in ovarian carcinoma and tumors of the fallopian tube, endometrium, endocervix, and mesothelioma, but negative in breast and colon carcinoma. PSA staining is very sensitive for prostate carcinoma, though that cancer rarely metastasizes to skin. Thyroglobulin immunostain identifies papillary and follicular thyroid carcinoma and is negative in non-thyroid adenocarcinomas

Differential diagnosis
1. Primary sweat gland carcinoma (23.13).
2. Pseudoglandular primary or metastatic squamous cell carcinoma (SCC, 18.11, 28.1): keratin pearls, acantholysis in pseudoglandular areas. SCCs are usually CK18neg whereas adenocarcinomas are mostly CK18+.
3. Endometriosis (29.9) and omphalomesenteric duct polyp (29.11).

28.3 Metastatic breast carcinoma

(see Fig. 28.3A–E)
This carcinoma is considered in a separate section because it is the *most common* malignancy to metastasize to skin,

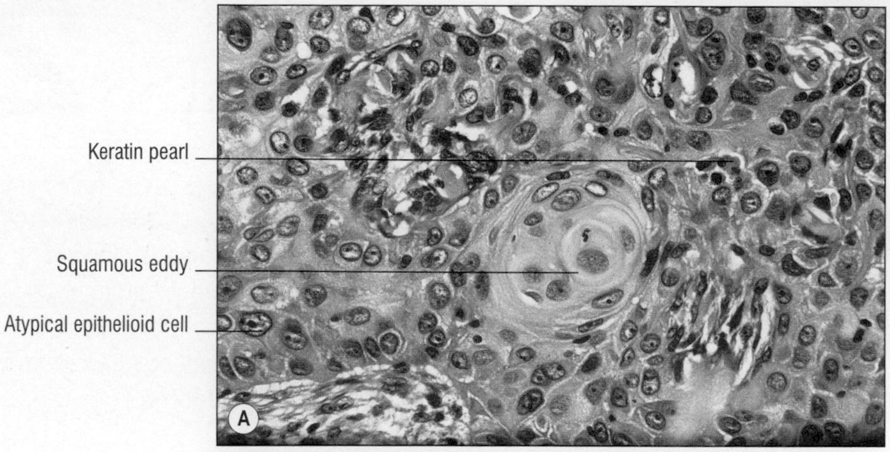

Keratin pearl

Squamous eddy

Atypical epithelioid cell

Fig. 28.1 A Metastatic squamous cell carcinoma.

Tumor in lymphatic

Atypical epithelioid cell

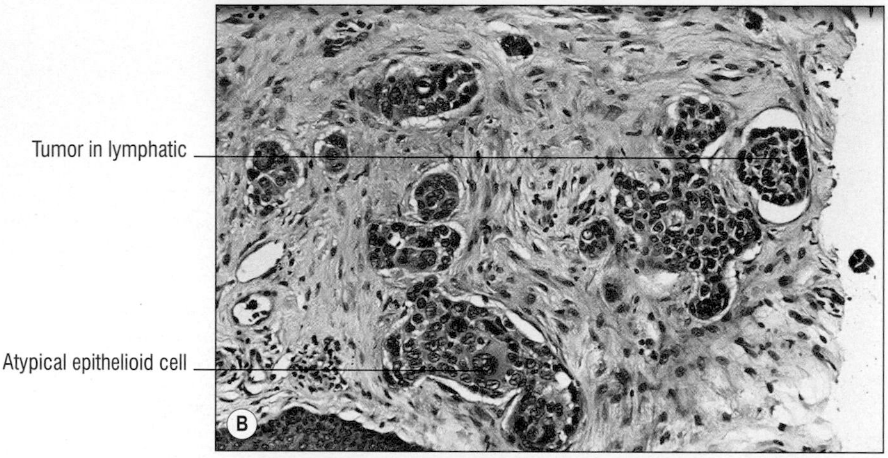

Fig. 28.1 B Metastatic squamous cell carcinoma (in lymphatics).

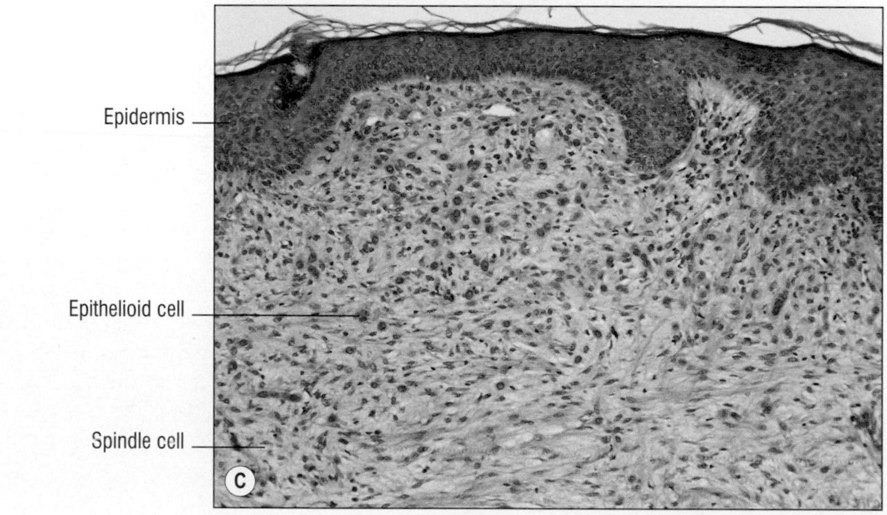

Epidermis

Epithelioid cell

Spindle cell

Fig. 28.1 C Poorly differentiated metastatic carcinoma in dermis.

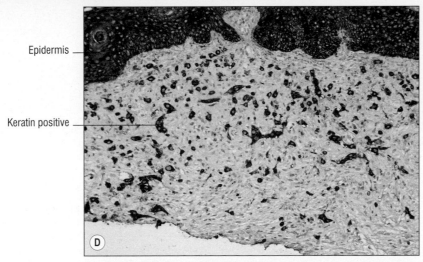

Epidermis ⎯

Keratin positive ⎯

Fig. 28.1 D Same carcinoma seen in 28.1C, stained with pankeratin.

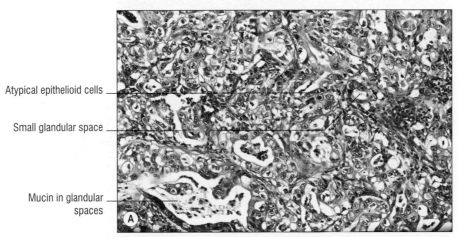

Atypical epithelioid cells ⎯

Small glandular space ⎯

Mucin in glandular spaces ⎯

Fig. 28.2 A Metastatic adenocarcinoma from colon.

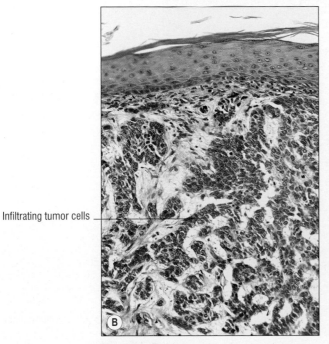

Infiltrating tumor cells ⎯

Fig. 28.2 B Metastatic adenocarcinoma from prostate.

usually found on the trunk as an indurated plaque or nodule in women, generally is an adenocarcinoma (28.2). Many cases called "metastatic", are actually direct extension of the cancer into the skin, and not truly metastatic.

- Tumor nodules or single-filing strands (1.128) with pleomorphic, hyperchromatic nuclei, increased numbers of mitoses in the dermis or in the lymphatics or blood vessels. Nuclei sometimes appear somewhat square or rectangular
- Epidermotropism may occur as in Paget's disease (18.13)
- *Glandular formations* or "signet rings" sometimes present, may contain *mucin*
- Positive staining for pankeratin, CK7, GCDFP (gross cystic disease fluid protein) common
- Her-2/neu (c-erbB-2): positive staining in breast cancer correlates with negative staining for estrogen and progesterone receptors and a poor prognosis. Estrogen receptor or progesterone receptor staining usually indicates better prognosis, with better response to hormonal therapy

P

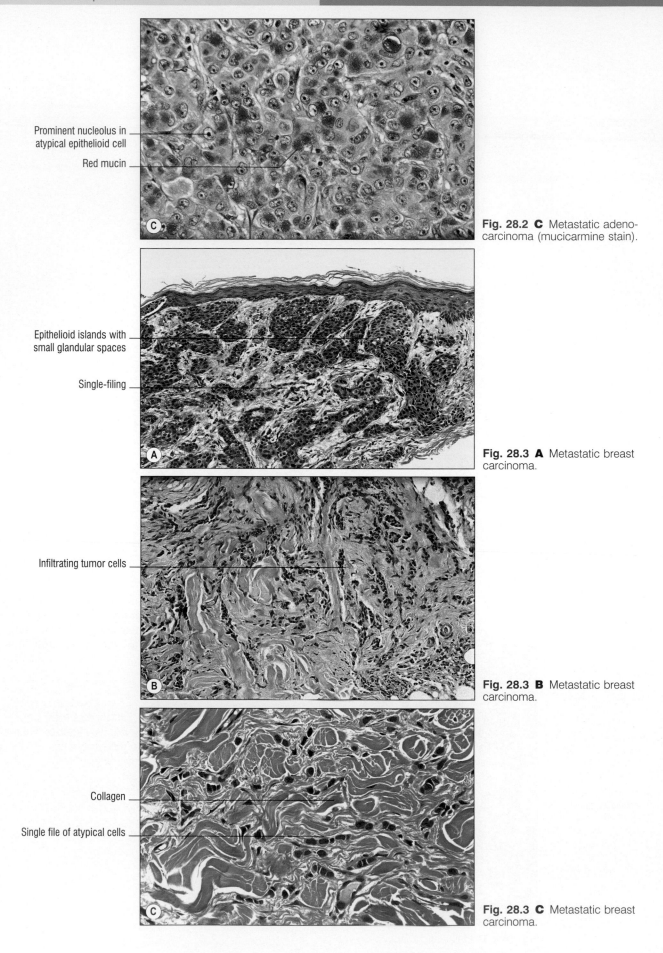

Prominent nucleolus in atypical epithelioid cell

Red mucin

Fig. 28.2 C Metastatic adeno-carcinoma (mucicarmine stain).

Epithelioid islands with small glandular spaces

Single-filing

Fig. 28.3 A Metastatic breast carcinoma.

Infiltrating tumor cells

Fig. 28.3 B Metastatic breast carcinoma.

Collagen

Single file of atypical cells

Fig. 28.3 C Metastatic breast carcinoma.

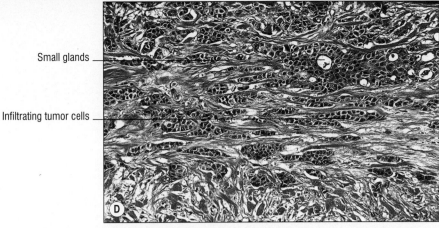

Fig. 28.3 D Metastatic breast carcinoma.

Small glands

Infiltrating tumor cells

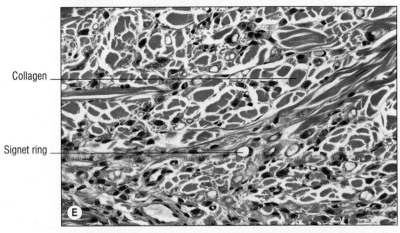

Collagen

Signet ring

Fig. 28.3 E Metastatic breast carcinoma (signet-ring type).

Variations

1. Scirrhous carcinoma (carcinoma en cuirasse): cuirasse is a leather armor suit. Morphea-like induration, subtle single-filing (1.128) of tumor cells in sclerotic dermis (1.125), often with hyperchromatic angulated nuclei.
2. Inflammatory (telangiectatic) carcinoma (carcinoma erysipelatoides): red patches that may resemble a rash, cellulitis, or radiation site, but blood vessels or lymphatics contain tumor cells.
3. Paget's disease of the breast (18.13).

Differential diagnosis

1. Other adenocarcinomas (28.2), sweat gland neoplasms (Chapter 23), basaloid neoplasms (1.11).

28.4 Metastatic renal cell carcinoma

(see Fig. 28.4A,B)
Despite being an uncommon adenocarcinoma, this tumor has an affinity for skin metastases (7% of patients), which often present as *red, friable nodules* resembling a pyogenic granuloma (25.3).

P

- Tumor lobules in the dermis, often surrounded by epidermal collarette
- Large *clear cells* (containing glycogen and lipid, so they are PAS positive, diastase labile, and oil-red-O positive) with central nuclei that usually are only mildly atypical
- *Vascular stroma*, often with *extravasation of erythrocytes* (1.40) and hemosiderin (1.58)
- Positive staining for both pankeratin and vimentin, RCC, CD10, and EMA, negative with CEA and mucin stains

Differential diagnosis

1. Other clear cell tumors (1.22).

28.5 Metastatic small cell carcinoma

(see Fig. 28.5A,B)
Several different rare small cell tumors may metastasize to the skin, usually producing nodules, especially on the trunk and scalp.

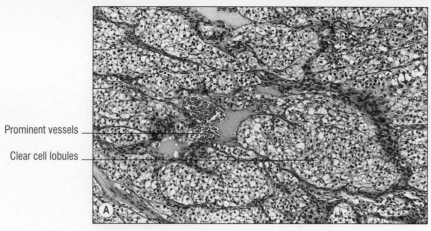

Fig. 28.4 **A** Metastatic renal cell carcinoma (low mag.).

Prominent vessels

Clear cell lobules

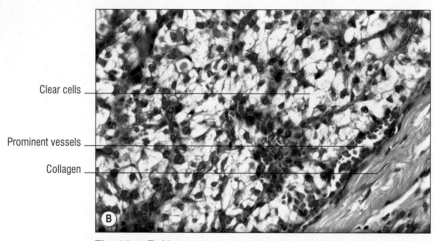

Fig. 28.4 **B** Metastatic renal cell carcinoma (high mag.).

Clear cells

Prominent vessels

Collagen

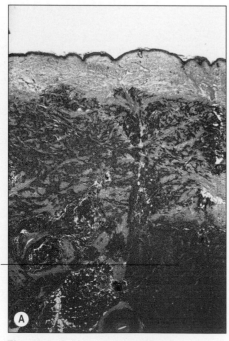

Dense small cell infiltration

Fig. 28.5 **A** Metastatic small cell carcinoma from lung (low mag.).

- *Diffuse* infiltration of the dermis by nodules or cords of cells with atypical *small round nuclei* and little cytoplasm, often increased number of mitoses

P

Variations

1. Metastatic neuroendocrine carcinomas may have neurosecretory granules by electron microscopy, but this is seldom used now that we have immunostains. "Oat cell" small cell carcinoma of the lung is one of the more important neuroendocrine tumors that may be found in skin. Mostly adults, NSE+, chromogranin+ in 30%. Small cell carcinoma of lung is usually CK7+, TTF-1+, neurofilament+, CK20neg, CEA+ in 50%. CK20 is usually negative, but if positive there often is a perinuclear diffuse granular pattern instead of the globular paranuclear dot of Merkel cell carcinoma.

2. Thyroid neuroendocrine carcinomas are rarely found in skin. Follicular thyroid carcinoma often positive for thyroglobulin and thyroid transcription factor-1 (TTF-1). Medullary thyroid carcinoma often positive for calcitonin.

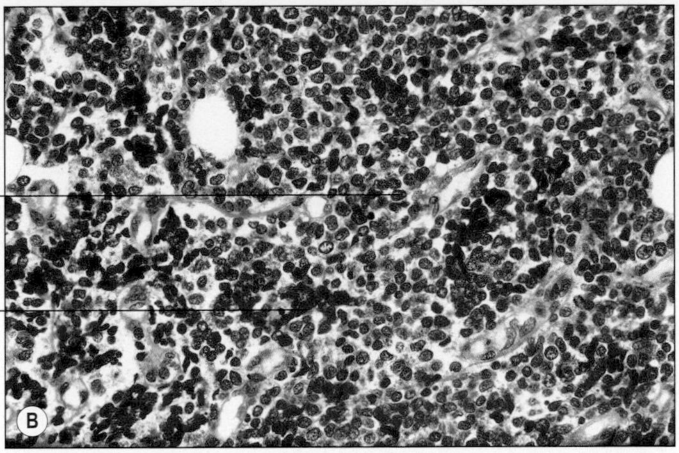

Fig. 28.5 **B** Metastatic small cell carcinoma from lung (high mag.).

3. Carcinoid: mostly adults, type 1 from bronchus or "foregut" which is argyrophil stain positive, and type 2 "midgut" small intestine and appendix which is argentaffin stain positive. May contain eosinophilic cytoplasmic granules. Immunostaining similar to other neuroendocrine tumors, positive for NSE and neurofilament. Neurosecretory granules by electron microscopy.

4. Extraskeletal Ewing's sarcoma (a primitive neuroectodermal tumor, also known as peripheral neuroectodermal tumor, PNET, "peanut"): mostly children, abundant vascularity, pale cytoplasm may contain PAS-positive glycogen, positive for FLI-1 and CD99 (but Merkel cell carcinoma, rhabdomyosarcoma, and lymphoblastic leukemia are also CD99 positive), positive for vimentin, neurofilaments, and chromogranin, negative for desmin, NSE, chromogranin, S 100, myogenin, and pankeratin.

5. Neuroblastoma (another primitive neuroectodermal tumor, PNET): mostly children at birth, adrenal origin, may form Homer–Wright rosettes. Positive for NSE and neurofilament. Other rare PNET tumors in the skin include cutaneous ganglioneuroma (26.1), peripheral neuroepithelioma, and pigmented neuroectodermal tumor (keratin and HMB-45 positive). Myogenin is negative.

6. Embryonal rhabdomyosarcoma: mostly children, occasional strap-shaped rhabdomyoblasts, positive for PTAH, desmin, muscle-specific actin, CD99, myogenin, myoglobin, and Z-bands by electron microscopy. FLI-1 is negative, unlike Ewing's sarcoma.

Differential diagnosis

1. Other small cell tumors (1.22). All of these may be difficult to distinguish without clinical correlation, special stains, or electron microscopy. Merkel cell carcinoma (26.8) and lymphomas are far more common in skin than any of these. TTF-1 is positive in small cell carcinomas of the lung and thyroid carcinomas, but negative in Merkel cell carcinoma.

28.6 Metastatic sarcoma

A wide variety of sarcomas (mesenchymal origin) can rarely metastasize to the skin, but they are far less common than the carcinomas (epithelial origin). They can originate from internal sites, or from cutaneous sarcomas (Chapters 25, 26, 27, and 29).

- *Spindle cell infiltration* of the dermis in most cases, although sometimes can be epithelioid
- Positive staining for *vimentin*, with negative staining for pankeratin, in most cases. Other more specific stains depend upon the specific type of sarcoma

P

Variation

1. Metastatic alveolar soft part sarcoma: uncommon soft tissue sarcoma, children or young adults, most common origin on buttock, distinct organoid or nested pattern, variable expression of vimentin, S100, CD68, NSE, SMA, desmin. It has a specific translocation der(17)t(X;17)(p11.2;q25) which fuses the TFE3 transcription factor gene to the APSL gene. An antibody against the carboxy-terminal portion of TFE3 is highly specific and sensitive for this tumor, except sometimes it can be positive in renal cell carcinoma, some granular cell tumors, and perivascular epithelioid neoplasms.

Differential diagnosis

1. Other spindle cell neoplasms (1.131).
2. Less commonly, other small cell neoplasms (1.130), or epithelioid cell neoplasms (1.38).

CHAPTER 29

Miscellaneous Remnants and Neoplasms

29.1 Nevus lipomatosus

(see Fig. 29.1)
Rare clustered papules or nodules of the buttock with onset at birth or childhood.

- Adipose present in superficial dermis
- Increased dermal blood vessels often

Differential diagnosis

1. Lipofibroma variant of acrochordon (27.4): much more common, adult onset, usually solitary, pedunculated nodule with a narrower base. Many doctors misname these large tags "nevus lipomatosus" by mistake.
2. Goltz syndrome (11.8): nearly no dermis, clinical features much different.
3. Piezogenic pedal papules (29.1): papules on the *heels*, occasionally painful (1.96), thought to be pressure-induced herniations of adipose through an atrophic or secondarily thickened dermis.
4. Adipose may also be found superficially in the dermis in Proteus syndrome, Michelin tire baby, lipedematous alopecia (10.13), some lipomas (29.2), some melanocytic nevi (20.5), and healed old wounds.

29.2 Lipoma

(see Fig. 29.2A–E)
Very common soft subcutaneous (1.135) nodules.

- Proliferation of *normal-appearing adipose* in the subcutaneous fat
- Sometimes sharp demarcation (rarely a capsule) from normal adipose

Variations

1. Angiolipoma: *many small blood vessels*, often *thrombi* (1.137), more likely to be well circumscribed and painful (1.96).
2. Fibrolipoma: increased *fibrous* tissue.
3. Spindle cell lipoma: usually on posterior neck (1.86) or upper back, more in males, CD34+ *spindle cells* (1.131) in *mucinous stroma* (1.83), increased collagen and mast cells (1.78).
4. Pleomorphic lipoma: usually on posterior neck (1.86), hyperchromatic adipocytes, bizarre *floret giant cells* (1.84) that have overlapping nuclei, a pseudomalignancy (1.118), resembles liposarcoma but only has rare lipoblasts and has no necrosis.
5. Infiltrating lipoma (intramuscular lipoma): *skeletal muscle trapped* between mature adipocytes.
6. Chondroid lipoma: rare, encapsulated, chondroblasts and lipoblast-like cells, myxoid stroma, S-100+ in cartilaginous areas, may resemble hibernoma (29.4), myxoid liposarcoma (29.5), or extraskeletal chondrosarcoma.
7. Myolipoma: well-circumscribed subcutaneous nodule, mostly smooth muscle positive for actin and desmin, with about one-third adipose.
8. Angiomyolipoma: probably is a variant of angioleiomyoma (29.6) with fatty metaplasia. The angiomyolipoma of the kidney is associated with tuberous sclerosis (27.3), but is somewhat different and probably not related to the subcutaneous lesions.
9. Dercum's disease (adiposis dolorosa): *multiple painful lipomas* (1.96), usually with ordinary histology or angiolipoma.
10. Multiple symmetric lipomatosis (Madelung's disease): multiple diffuse lipomas, mostly in males, often in a horse collar distribution.

Differential diagnosis

1. Liposarcoma (29.5): large size, *lipoblasts*, and cytologic atypia.

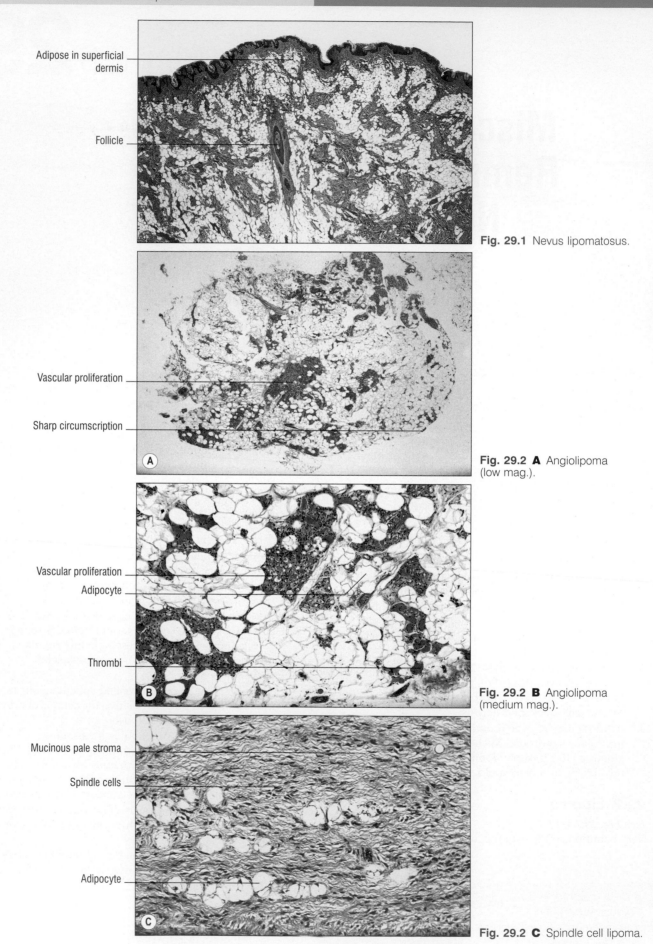

Adipose in superficial dermis

Follicle

Fig. 29.1 Nevus lipomatosus.

Vascular proliferation

Sharp circumscription

Fig. 29.2 A Angiolipoma (low mag.).

Vascular proliferation

Adipocyte

Thrombi

Fig. 29.2 B Angiolipoma (medium mag.).

Mucinous pale stroma

Spindle cells

Adipocyte

Fig. 29.2 C Spindle cell lipoma.

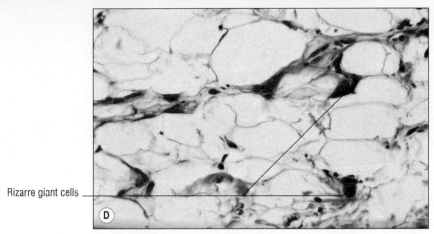

Bizarre giant cells

Fig. 29.2 D Pleomorphic lipoma.

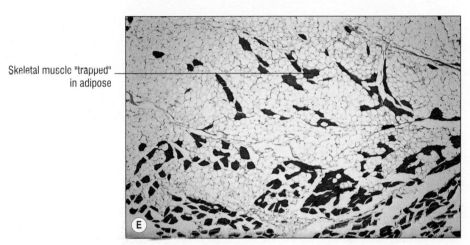

Skeletal muscle "trapped" in adipose

Fig. 29.2 E Infiltrating lipoma.

29.3 Benign lipoblastoma

Rare *subcutaneous nodule or mass in young children*, more common in males. Lesions may recur after excision, but do not metastasize.

P
- Subcutaneous tumor (poorly circumscribed or encapsulated) of immature fat cells with *lipoblasts* (lipid vacuoles displace the nuclei)
- Mucinous stroma (1.83)

Differential diagnosis

1. Liposarcoma (29.5): histologically almost identical, but occurs in adults, with more cytologic atypia.

29.4 Hibernoma

(see Fig. 29.4)
Very rare benign lipoma of immature brown fat in adults. It grows slowly, and is most common on the *neck* (1.86), *upper back*, and axilla (1.10).

P
- Subcutaneous encapsulated tumor of *mulberry cells* (large cells with a central nucleus and multivacuolated granular cytoplasm), sometimes mixed with mature adipocytes

Differential diagnosis

1. Lesions with foam cells (1.46) or clear cells (1.22), such as foamy macrophages related to fat necrosis in panniculitis (1.101) are rarely confused with a hibernoma.

29.5 Liposarcoma

(see Fig. 29.5)
Uncommon deep subcutaneous mass in adults. Superficial lesions have a better prognosis, and have been called *atypical lipomatous tumors*. More common on thighs and buttocks.

P
- Tumor in subcutaneous fat or soft tissue consisting of cells containing lipid with variable differentiation toward adipose tissue
- *Lipoblasts* (cells with several lipid vacuoles displacing the nuclei) or signet-ring cells (single lipid vacuole displacing the nucleus)
- *S-100 protein* may be positive in some liposarcomas

Variations

1. Well-differentiated liposarcoma: *resembles benign lipoma* except lipoblasts present, often diagnosed only after a supposed benign lipoma recurs. Spindle cell liposarcoma (1.131) is also well-differentiated and resembles benign spindle cell lipoma.

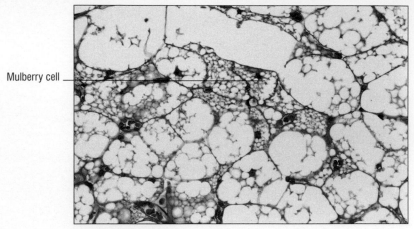

Mulberry cell —

Fig. 29.4 Hibernoma.

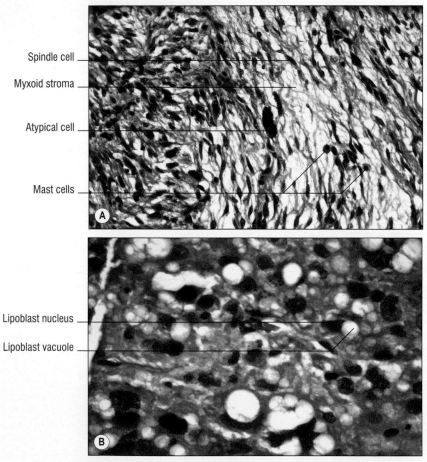

Spindle cell —

Myxoid stroma —

Atypical cell —

Mast cells —

A

Lipoblast nucleus —

Lipoblast vacuole —

B

Fig. 29.5 Liposarcoma (pleomorphic).

2. Myxoid liposarcoma: *myxoid stroma* (1.83) with stellate cells, many "chicken-wire" capillaries, and sometimes focal positive desmin and smooth muscle actin.
3. Round cell liposarcoma: *densely cellular* with numerous *small*, *round*, *hyperchromatic nuclei*, very few lipoblasts
4. Pleomorphic liposarcoma: *extremely bizarre giant cells*, many mitoses

Differential diagnosis

1. Benign lipoblastoma (29.3): liposarcomas almost never exist in children, and usually turn out to be a lipoblastoma instead.

2. Lipoma, especially pleomorphic lipoma (29.1).
3. Most other sarcomas, especially malignant fibrous histiocytomas (27.11), usually do not have lipoblasts and are S-100neg.

29.6 Leiomyoma

(see Fig. 29.6A–F)

Uncommon benign solitary or multiple *red nodules*, often *painful* (1.96), most common on the *shoulder* (1.140) or *upper arm* (1.6).

P

- Proliferation of benign smooth muscle bundles, with *blunt ended cigar-shaped spindle cell nuclei* and abundant pink cytoplasm on longitudinal section, and round nuclei with vacuoles around them on cross-section
- Positive red staining with *trichrome*, and immunostaining with *desmin*, muscle-specific actin, or smooth muscle *actin*

Variations

1. Piloleiomyoma and genital leiomyoma: poorly circumscribed smooth muscle bundles in the dermis. These originate from arrector pili muscles or sexual smooth muscle.
2. Angioleiomyoma: *well-demarcated deep dermal or subcutaneous nodule* (1.135) that *"shells out"* when excised, most common on lower leg, with smooth muscle proliferation originating from the smooth muscle in the walls of *dilated blood vessels*, sometimes with mucinous areas (1.83).

3. Smooth muscle hamartoma: congenital plaque that may be large, sometimes with gooseflesh papules within it, usually on trunk or extremities, sometimes with prominent hairs, may occur with Becker's nevus (20.3).
4. Angiomyolipoma and myolipoma (29.2): more adipose tissue present in subcutaneous nodule.
5. Pleomorphic leiomyoma: some benign leiomyomas can have atypical nuclei, but lack the features of leiomyosarcoma below. Also known as atypical leiomyoma, bizarre leiomyoma, symplastic leiomyoma (meaning "lacking cellular structure", referring to degenerative changes), or apoplectic leiomyoma (referring to degenerative areas "like a stroke").
6. Reed syndrome (leiomyomatosis cutis et uteri): hereditary cutaneous leiomyomas (autosomal dominant with incomplete penetrance), uterine fibroids (leiomyomas), fumarate hydratase mutation, renal cell carcinoma (10%).
7. Dermatomyofibroma (myoid fibroma): see 27.1.

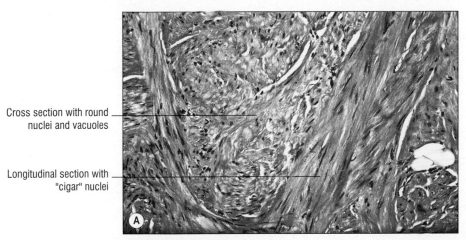

Cross section with round nuclei and vacuoles

Longitudinal section with "cigar" nuclei

Fig. 29.6 A Piloleiomyoma.

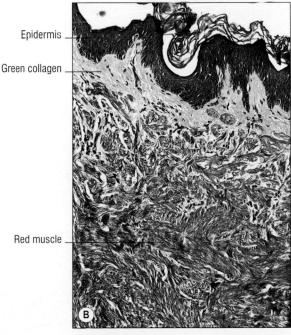

Epidermis

Green collagen

Red muscle

Fig. 29.6 B Piloleiomyoma (trichrome stain).

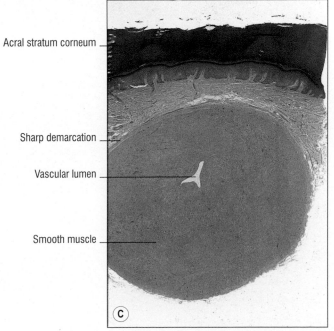

Acral stratum corneum

Sharp demarcation

Vascular lumen

Smooth muscle

Fig. 29.6 C Angioleiomyoma (low mag.).

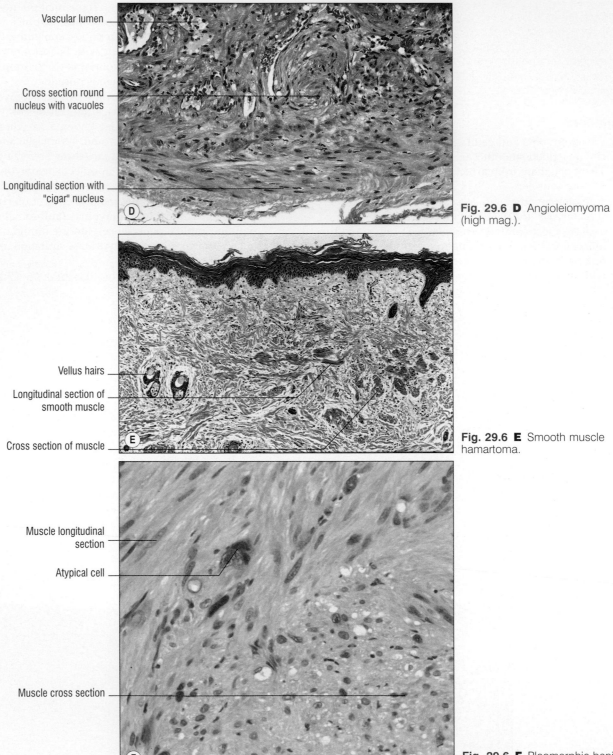

Vascular lumen

Cross section round
nucleus with vacuoles

Longitudinal section with
"cigar" nucleus

Fig. 29.6 **D** Angioleiomyoma
(high mag.).

Vellus hairs

Longitudinal section of
smooth muscle

Cross section of muscle

Fig. 29.6 **E** Smooth muscle
hamartoma.

Muscle longitudinal
section

Atypical cell

Muscle cross section

Fig. 29.6 **F** Pleomorphic benign
leiomyoma.

8. Myoepithelioma: not related to leiomyoma, but placed here because it can be SMA+ and has the stem myo- in the name. Subcutaneous myoepitheliomas are reminiscent of those of salivary glands, but present as a subcutaneous mass, with a spindle cell whorling pattern, and a hyalinized or chondromyxoid stroma. They are Sox10+, S100+, pankeratin+. EMA variable. Don't confuse with myofibroma (27.19).

Differential diagnosis

1. Dermatofibroma (27.1): epidermal hyperplasia, nuclei less blunt-ended, different staining with trichrome, desmin, and actin-neg.
2. Neurofibroma (26.1): nuclei less blunt-ended, wavy appearance, S-100+, desmin and actin negative.
3. Accessory nipple (29.12) and normal nipple: has increased smooth muscle, but breast tissue sometimes present.
4. Normal scrotum and vulva: normally has increased smooth muscle.
5. Leiomyosarcoma (26.7): solitary, larger, more cellular, more atypical, more infiltrating pattern, more than one or two atypical mitosis per ten high-power fields, necrosis sometimes.
6. Other spindle cell tumors (1.131): rarely cause difficulty.

29.7 Leiomyosarcoma

(see Fig. 29.7A,B)
Rare dermal or subcutaneous nodule or plaque, most common on the extremities, may metastasize. Dermal leiomyosarcomas have a much better prognosis than deep subcutaneous ones.

- Smooth muscle proliferation as in leiomyoma (29.6)
- *Atypical pleomorphic nuclei* with hyperchromatism, increased numbers of *mitoses* (usually more than one per ten high-power fields), necrosis sometimes
- *Desmin, muscle-specific actin* usually positive, S-100 rarely positive
- Myofibrils may be identified by PTAH stains

Differential diagnosis

1. Atypical leiomyoma (29.7): has atypical nuclei, but no mitoses, no necrosis, is benign.
2. Other spindle cell neoplasms (1.131).

29.8 Osteoma cutis

(see Fig. 29.8A–C)
Uncommon dermal or subcutaneous papule or nodule, often *white* (1.150) if close to skin surface. Often arises as *secondary metaplastic ossification* from injured tissue, such as sites of previous injection, surgery, trauma or infection, or neoplasm degeneration, especially in *pilomatricoma* (22.3) or basal cell carcinoma (18.14).

- *Eosinophilic bony tissue* in the dermis or subcutaneous fat; *osteocytes* (within lacunae) usually present, *osteoclasts* (multinucleated cells) sometimes present, osteoblasts sometimes present, and distinct *trabeculae* often present
- Calcification may be present (1.19, 8.15)
- Hematopoiesis is rarely present within the bone

Variations

1. Miliary osteomas of the face: more common type of osteoma cutis, multiple whitish or skin-colored (1.129) papules of the face (1.44), usually related to *acne scarring*.
2. Albright's hereditary osteodystrophy: hereditary cutaneous ossification of dermis, fat, and fascia, beginning in childhood, related to abnormal tissue response to parathyroid hormone. Do not confuse with Albright's syndrome (McCune–Albright's syndrome, 20.2).
3. Nevus of Nanta: melanocytic nevus with osteoma (20.5).
4. Gardner's syndrome (19.1).

29.9 Cutaneous endometriosis

(see Fig. 29.9)
Rare *skin-colored, red, or blue nodules*, most commonly surgically *implanted in gynecologic surgery scars*, and sometimes as a remnant on the *umbilicus* (1.143). Signs and symptoms may fluctuate with menses.

- *Endometrial glands*, straight or tortuous, lined by a pseudostratified columnar epithelium with active secretion resembling apocrine glands
- CD10+, *typical fibrovascular myxoid stroma* (1.131)
- *Extravasated erythrocytes* (1.40) and hemosiderin (1.58) common

Differential diagnosis

1. Sweat gland neoplasms (Chapter 23) and adenocarcinomas (28.2) usually do not have CD10+ stroma and the glands look different.

29.10 Accessory tragus

(see Fig. 29.10A,B)
Somewhat common *congenital papule or nodule*, usually *congenital* in the *preauricular area*, rarely on the cheek or neck.

- Pedunculated (1.106) papule or nodule containing numerous vellus hair follicles and often cartilage

Variation

1. Wattle: location on anterior neck, like the wattle of a turkey.

Differential diagnosis

1. Acrochordon (27.4).

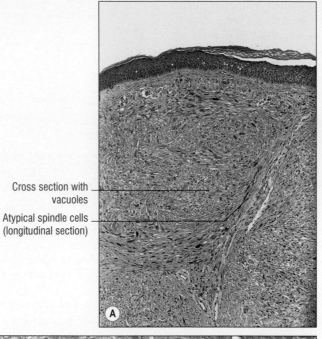

Cross section with vacuoles

Atypical spindle cells (longitudinal section)

Fig. 29.7 A Leiomyosarcoma (low mag.).

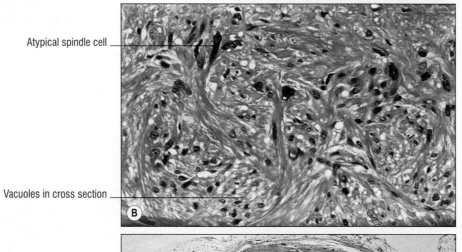

Atypical spindle cell

Vacuoles in cross section

Fig. 29.7 B Leiomyosarcoma (high mag.).

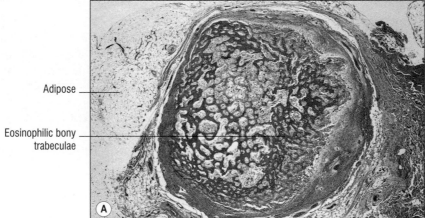

Adipose

Eosinophilic bony trabeculae

Fig. 29.8 A Osteoma cutis (low mag.).

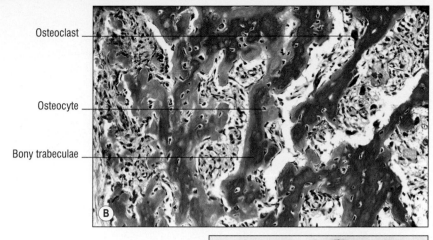

Osteoclast

Osteocyte

Bony trabeculae

Fig. 29.8 B Osteoma cutis (high mag.).

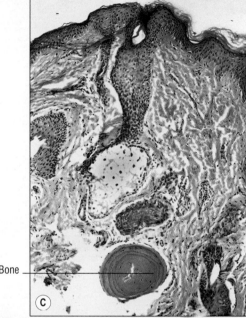

Bone

Fig. 29.8 C Facial osteoma.

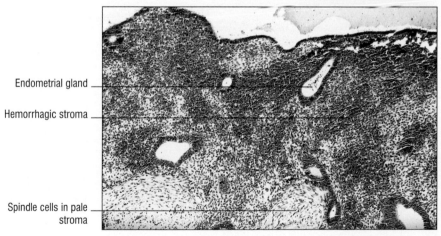

Endometrial gland

Hemorrhagic stroma

Spindle cells in pale stroma

Fig. 29.9 Cutaneous endometriosis (medium mag.).

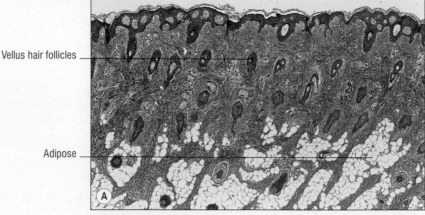

Vellus hair follicles

Adipose

Fig. 29.10 A Accessory tragus.

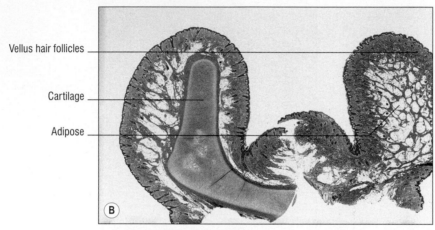

Vellus hair follicles

Cartilage

Adipose

Fig. 29.10 B Congenital wattle.

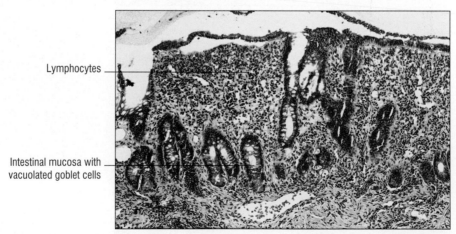

Lymphocytes

Intestinal mucosa with
vacuolated goblet cells

Fig. 29.11 Omphalomesenteric duct polyp.

29.11 **Omphalomesenteric duct polyp**

(see Fig. 29.11)

Rare *pedunculated* (1.106) *red papule*, usually *congenital* in *umbilical* area (1.143), may clinically resemble a pyogenic granuloma (25.3). It is important to consider a connecting fistula or concurrent intestinal malformation.

- Ectopic gastric, small intestinal, or colonic *intestinal epithelium with goblet cells* present within eroded periumbilical skin
- Diffuse lymphocytes common in the stroma

Differential diagnosis

1. Metastatic adenocarcinoma (28.2): cytologic atypia.
2. Gastrostomy, ileostomy, or colostomy site.

29.12 Accessory nipple (supernumerary nipple, polythelia)

Common, *congenital*, sometimes pedunculated (1.143), *brownish* (1.18) macule *or papule* or nodule on anterior chest or abdomen *along milk line*, often mistaken for a melanocytic nevus (20.5) clinically.

- Epidermis with mild papillomatosis and hyperpigmentation
- Increased smooth muscle bundles
- Mammary glands and ducts present in dermis and subcutaneous fat

Differential diagnosis

1. Leiomyoma (29.6).
2. Sweat gland tumors (Chapter 23).
3. Seborrheic keratosis (18.2), if biopsy is too superficial.

CHAPTER 30

Special Stains

It has been said that special stains merely color what you don't know a different color.[51] The Olympic dermatopathologist can diagnose most lesions with routine hematoxylin and eosin (H&E) staining. The very best special stain in dermatopathology is deeper levels sectioned through the block! It is unwise to rely excessively upon special stains, without regard to the overall routine staining features and the clinical setting. Exceptions to the rules are common, and the stereotypical staining results do not always hold true, so beware! A favorite pastime is publishing results that are exceptions. It is enough to make some of us go back to becoming Neanderthal H&E aficionados. In the OJ Simpson trial, I learned that if the glove does not fit, you must acquit. In dermatopathology, this means that if the pathologic diagnosis does not fit with the clinical situation, you must go back and reconcile. For difficult neoplasms, it is often better to perform a battery of several stains so that the pathologist is not dependent upon just one as providing the definitive answer. Some of these stains have technical pitfalls, and staining results (such as sensitivity, specificity, exact color of the stain) vary when methods are modified. For example, the immunoenzyme staining methods result is a brown color when peroxidase and diaminobenzidine (DAB) are used, while the use of a different chromogen, such as aminoethylcarbazol (AEC) may produce a red color. This can be especially helpful when brown melanin is prevalent and you are trying to identify melanocytes with an immunostain. Except where indicated, most of these stains can be performed on formalin fixed, routinely processed tissue.

Acid fast bacillus (AFB): (see Ziehl–Neelsen, Fite, Kinyoun's)

Actin (muscle-specific actin, MSA) and smooth muscle actin (SMA): myofibroblasts, myoepithelial cells are positive (see Muscle). Positive in leiomyosarcoma, glomus cell tumor, inclusion bodies of recurrent digital fibromatosis, half of cellular neurothekeomas

Adenosine triphosphatase (ATPase): blood vessels, nerve fibers, Langerhans cells, monocytes, some B lymphocytes are brown–black (not used routinely)

Adipophilin: monoclonal antibody that stains a protein on the surface of intracellular lipid droplets Membranous staining pattern in sebaceous neoplasms and granular cytoplasmic staining in xanthomatous lesions. Positive in 60% of metastatic renal cell carcinomas, but negative in other clear cell neoplasms of the skin

Alcian blue: acid mucopolysaccharides are light blue at pH 2.5; only sulfated acid mucopolysaccharides such as heparin and chondroitin sulfate are positive at pH 0.5

Alcian blue–PAS: often useful in cryptococcosis, where the gelatinous capsule stains blue with Alcian blue, and the fungal wall stains red with PAS

Aldehyde fuchsin (Gomori): acid mucopolysaccharides and elastic tissue are blue; collagen is red

Alizarin red: calcium salts are reddish–orange, more specific for calcium than von Kossa

ALK1 (anaplastic lymphoma kinase, CD246): positive in 50% of systemic anaplastic large cell lymphomas (ALCL), less likely positive in primary cutaneous ALCL (24.5), usually negative in lymphomatoid papulosis and Hodgkin disease

ALKc: similar to ALK1, said to stain more intensely

Alpha-1-antichymotrypsin (AACT) and alpha-1 antitrypsin: macrophages have brown or red immunostaining, positive in fibrohistiocytic neoplasms, including some examples of atypical fibroxanthoma, but sometimes positive in carcinomas and melanomas

Amyloid: stains with Congo red, crystal violet, thioflavin T, pagoda red 9 (Dylon), Scarlet red (RIT), PAS, and immunostains directed against amyloid are available (8.4)

Aniline blue (Mallory trichrome): collagen is blue; muscle is red

Apolipoprotein D (Apo D): positive in dermatofibrosarcoma protuberans (DFSP) and neural tumors, negative in dermatofibroma and most other soft tissue tumors

Argentaffin (Fontana Masson ammoniated silver nitrate): melanin and granules in type 2 midgut carcinoids are black (28.5)

Argyrophil (silver nitrate impregnation, Grimelius): melanin, reticulum fibers, nerves, Langerhans cells, type 1 foregut carcinoids (28.5), Merkel cell carcinomas are black (26.8)

Auramine O: acid-fast bacilli have yellow fluorescence when viewed with fluorescent microscope; slide should be kept in the dark and read within 48 hours

Bax: a protein promoting apoptosis, positive in breast carcinoma, Hodgkin lymphoma, Merkel cell carcinoma

bcl-1 (cyclin D1): a regulatory subunit of protein kinases involved in the G1 phase of the cell cycle, positive in mantle cell lymphoma, invasive breast cancer, some hairy cell leukemias, some plasma cell myelomas

bcl-2 (b-cell lymphoma/leukemia-2): expression of this oncogene inhibits apoptosis, present only in the basal layer of trichoepithelioma, as opposed to more extensive expression in basal cell carcinoma. Negative in squamous cell carcinoma. Positive in the germinal centers of lymph nodes of follicular center cell lymphoma (not in *primary cutaneous* follicular center cell lymphoma unless there is nodal involvement). Positive in large b-cell lymphoma of the leg, primary cutaneous marginal zone lymphoma, and mantle zone lymphoma.

©2012 Elsevier Ltd, Inc, BV
DOI: 10.1016/B978-0-323-06658-7.00030-0

Negative in normal or reactive germinal centers, and Burkitt lymphoma

bcl-6: nuclear staining in B cells in normal germinal centers, positive in B cells outside germinal centers in follicular center cell lymphoma, positive in most cases of cutaneous diffuse large B-cell lymphoma of leg, negative in mantle cell and marginal zone lymphoma

BDCA2 (blood dendritic cell antigen 2, CD303): expressed by plasmacytoid dendritic cells

Ber-EP4 (EpCam, CD326): stains many types of non-keratinized epithelial cells, positive in pulmonary adenocarcinoma and basal cell carcinoma, negative in mesothelioma and squamous cell carcinoma. Will stain some examples of extramammary Paget's disease, microcystic adnexal carcinoma and desmoplastic trichoepithelioma, but less often than basal cell carcinoma

Ber-H2: (see CD30)

Best's carmine: frozen sections needed, glycogen is red

Bismarck brown: mast cell granules brown

Bodian: nerve filaments (axons) are black

Bombesin: a neuropeptide sometimes found in Merkel cell carcinoma, but some studies found it more likely to be positive in metastatic neuroendocrine carcinoma in the skin than in Merkel cell carcinoma. Rarely used except on antiquated test questions

Brown–Brenn: (see Gram)

Brown–Hopps: (see Gram)

CA-125: positive in metastatic ovarian carcinoma and tumors of the fallopian tube, endometrium, endocervix, and mesothelioma, but negative in breast and colon carcinoma

Calcitonin: medullary carcinoma of the thyroid is usually positive, while papillary and follicular thyroid cancers are usually negative

Calcium: (see Alizarin red, von Kossa)

Calponin: an actin-binding protein that interacts with tropomyosin and calmodulin. Positive as marker for myoepithelial cells, so helps to distinguish microinvasion from in situ ductal breast carcinomas. Positive in pleomorphic adenoma of the salivary gland. Postitive in some atypical fibroxanthomas

Calretin: a calcium-binding protein that buffers intracellular calcium. Positive in follicular infundibulum, eccrine glands, adipocytes. Stains 80% of mesotheliomas, positive in ameloblastoma, granular cell tumor, 14% of adenocarcinomas

Cam5.2: an antibody directed toward CK8–CK18 (see CK8)

Carcinoembryonic antigen (CEA): sweat glands (especially eccrine) and sweat gland neoplasms, adenocarcinomas, Paget's disease, and epithelioid sarcoma. Prostate carcinoma, bladder carcinoma, hepatoma, melanoma, sarcoma, and sebaceous neoplasms are usually negative

CD stains (clusters of differentiation): with some exceptions, many of these are used as leukocyte markers; only some of those commonly used in dermatopathology are listed

CD1a (leu 6): Langerhans cells, precursor T lymphocytes. Langerhans cell histiocytosis, but sometimes positive in myeloid leukemia and mycosis fungoides. Positive in intraepidermal Langerhans microgranulomas of eczema, contact dermatitis, and other inflammatory conditions

CD2 (leu 5, Til): T lymphocytes (not used as much as CD3)

CD3 (leu 4): T lymphocytes. Monoclonal CD3 antibody is the most specific T-cell marker, and most commonly used. The polyclonal CD3 sometimes reacts with B cells. Positive in T-cell lymphoma, lymphomatoid papulosis, natural killer cell lymphoma, negative in B-cell lymphoma

CD4 (leu 3): helper-inducer T lymphocytes (class II major histocompatibility complex restricted). The ratio of CD4:CD8 in mycosis fungoides is usually greater than 3:1. Zanolimumab is an antibody against CD4 used in some malignancies

CD5 (leu 1): mainly T lymphocytes, some B cells in mantle zone. Positive in B-cell chronic lymphocytic leukemia (B-CLL) and mantle cell lymphoma, occasionally positive in intravascular large B-cell lymphoma, and anaplastic large cell lymphoma. Negative in cutaneous marginal zone lymphoma and follicular center lymphoma. Staining may be depleted in mycosis fungoides, like CD7

CD7 (leu 9): T lymphocytes and natural killer cells, the first T-cell-specific antigen to be expressed as T cells mature, and the first marker to be lost (deleted) in mycosis fungoides

CD8 (leu 2): cytotoxic-suppressor T lymphocytes, subset of natural killer cells. CD8 is expressed to a lesser degree than CD4 in mycosis fungoides (except for an aggressive CD8+ variant), but CD8 is predominant in pagetoid reticulosis and subcutaneous T-cell lymphoma

CD10 (common acute lymphoblastic leukemia antigen (CALLA)): B cells in mantle cell lymphoma, follicular center cell lymphoma when there is a follicular pattern, cutaneous diffuse large B-cell lymphoma of leg type, acute lymphoblastic leukemia–lymphoma, and Burkitt's lymphoma. Also positive in renal cell carcinoma, endometriosis stroma, and atypical fibroxanthoma. Negative in marginal zone lymphoma and chronic lymphocytic leukemia/lymphoma

CD11a: stains most normal leukocytes. Positive in some intravascular large B-cell lymphomas (24.13). Anti-CD11a antibody therapy (efalizumab) is a psoriasis treatment

CD14: it is proposed that CD34 progenitor cells in the bone marrow differentiate into either CD14+ cells (most macrophages in skin, most histiocytoses, most diseases in Chapter 7, extramedullary hematopoiesis), or CD14neg cells, which become Langerhans cells that express CD1a (24.18)

CD15 (LeuM1): granulocytes, monocytes, often positive in Hodgkin's disease (24.15), sometimes positive in peripheral T-cell lymphoma and adenocarcinoma

CD19: B cells. Positive in chronic lymphocytic leukemia/small lymphocytic lymphoma (24.16)

CD20 (L26, Bl): B cells in germinal centers and peripheral blood, positive in most B-cell lymphomas (Chapter 24), negative in plasma cells. Target of the drug rituximab

CD21: positive in normal B-cell marginal and mantle cells, and follicular dendritic cells. Used to assess localization of bcl-2, bcl-6, and CD10 within follicular center cell lymphoma (24.8) and marginal zone lymphoma (24.9)

CD22: mature B cells, hairy cell leukemia, negative in plasma cells

CD23: some B cells, follicular dendritic cells, receptor for IgE, positive in B-cell chronic lymphocytic leukemia (B-CLL), sometimes positive in marginal zone lymphoma, usually negative in mantle cell lymphoma

CD25 (IL-2 receptor, TAC): activated T cells and B cells, and activated macrophages, positive in adult T-cell leukemia–lymphoma, more often positive in advanced mycosis fungoides, evaluated to predict better response of mycosis fungoides to denileukin diftitox (Ontak) chemotherapy

CD30 (Ki-1, BerH2): activated T cells and B cells, large atypical cells of large cell anaplastic lymphoma, lymphomatoid papulosis type A, Hodgkin cells, Reed–Sternberg cells, occasionally found in large lymphocytes reacting to scabies, molluscum, and tick bites

CD31 (PECAM-1): monocytes, granulocytes, B cells, T cells, endothelial cells, most commonly used sensitive vascular neoplasm marker (better than CD34 and factor VIII-related antigen for this)

CD33: early myeloid cells, myelogenous leukemia

CD34 (QBEnd 10, human progenitor cell antigen): hematopoietic cell precursors, endothelial cells, some dermal dendrocytes, nerves. Most commonly used to stain dermatofibrosarcoma protuberans (27.10), giant cell fibroblastoma, nephrogenic fibrosing dermopathy and scleromyxedema (also positive in young fibrosing wounds, but negative in morphea and scleroderma), hemangiopericytoma, spindle cell lipoma, solitary fibrous tumor, and sclerotic fibroma. Also positive in neurofibroma, and most examples of leukemia cutis. Stains 50% of epithelioid sarcomas. Not as sensitive for vascular neoplasms as CD 31 and *Ulex europaeus*, but works well for Kaposi sarcoma. Stains connective tissue around normal follicles and is more likely to stain stroma immediately adjacent to epithelium of trichoepithelioma, whereas basal cell carcinoma more likely to have a zone of non-staining around the basaloid aggregates

CD35: granulocytes, monocytes, erythrocytes, B cells, follicular dendritic cells. Used to demonstrate dendritic meshwork in lymphoid follicles

CD38: plasma cells, mainly used for myeloma (24.12). Also positive in some cases of chronic lymphocytic leukemia and other lymphomas

CD43 (leu 22): granulocytes, monocytes, mast cells, T cells, positive in most leukemias, and granulocytic sarcoma (24.16). Positive with CD5 in chronic lymphocytic leukemia and chronic lymphocytic lymphoma. Positive in some B-cell lymphomas along with CD20, such as mantle cell lymphoma, but negative in follicular center cell lymphoma and marginal zone lymphoma

CD45 (leukocyte common antigen (LCA)): when the designation CD45 is used without the restricted designation (R subtypes, or isoforms, such as RA, RB, RC, RAB, RAC, RBC, RO, RABC), LCA stains most leukocytes (benign or malignant), negative in neutrophils, useful in identifying lymphoid lineage in some undifferentiated tumors such as most lymphomas or leukemias, as opposed to other malignancies

(Chapter 28, especially 28.5). Negative in some Hodgkin lymphomas, and often negative in myeloma, myelogenous leukemia, and acute lymphoblastic leukemia. Naïve lymphocytes have high mass and have all three exons RA, RB, and RC. Activated or mature memory lymphocytes have low mass because RA, RB, and RC are spliced out and are called RO

CD45R (4KB5, CD45RABC, contains all three RA, RB, RC exons): T lymphocytes, and some B lymphocytes

CD45RA (MT-2): naive T lymphocytes and B lymphocytes (mantle cell)

CD45RB: B cells, some T cells, macrophages, negative in Langerhans cells. Negative in epidermotropic T cells of mycosis fungoides in frozen sections. In paraffin sections, CD45RB is strangely positive in epidermotropic T cells of mycosis fungoides, negative in contact dermatitis (opposite of CD45RO)

CD45RO (UCHL-1, this shortest null form of CD45 lacks RA,RB,RC exons): memory T lymphocytes (mature activated T lymphocytes), granulocytes, monocytes, negative in B cells and natural killer cells, positive in some T-cell lymphomas. Positive in mycosis fungoides lymphocytes in frozen sections and flow cytometry, but negative in epidermotropic lymphocytes of mycosis fungoides in paraffin sections

CD52 (Campath-1): T cells, B cells, monocytes, macrophages, eosinophils, and mast cells. Negative in neutrophils. Positive in most lymphoid malignancies, including advanced mycosis fungoides, negative in Hodgkin lymphoma. Positive in Langerhans histiocytosis, but negative in normal Langerhans cells. This antigen is the target for alemtuzumab (anti-CD52)

CD54 (intercellular adhesion molecule 1 (ICAM-1), a ligand for LFA-1 (CD50)): positive in many activated T cells and B cells, monocytes

CD56 (leu 19, NCAM): best known for staining natural killer T lymphocytes such as natural killer cell lymphoma, but also positive in Schwann cells and neural neoplasms, neuroblastoma, many neuroendocrine tumors such as Merkel cell carcinoma, myeloma, many leukemias, some melanomas, can be somewhat non-specific

CD57 (leu 7, NK1): natural killer and other T lymphocytes, Schwann cells and myelinated areas of neuroma and neurofibroma, neuroendocrine cells, some cells within follicles of follicular center cell lymphoma

CD63: (see NKI-C3)

CD68 (KP1): stains lysosomes of monocytes, macrophages (true histiocytes), mast cells; often used as a fibrohistiocytic neoplasm marker (most tumors in Chapter 27), but it is not very specific, since any tumor with lysosomes can be positive, and sometimes stains melanoma, more specific than CD20 (not present in myelogenous leukemia or T-cell lymphoma), positive in B-cell malignancies, extramedullary hematopoiesis, plasmacytoma, some myelomas

CD74 (LN2): B cells, activated T cells, macrophages. Positive in many B-cell lymphomas, myeloma, myeloid leukemia, Langerhans cell histiocytosis. More likely to stain malignant fibrous histiocytoma than atypical fibroxanthoma. Rarely used for anything

CD99: positive in endothelial cells, some lymphocytes, negative in neutrophils. Positive in metastatic Ewing's sarcoma (28.5) and peripheral neuroectodermal tumors in the skin (28.5), some Merkel cell carcinomas (26.8), rhabdomyosarcoma (28.5), lymphoblastic lymphoma (24.16), some other lymphomas and leukemias, and melanoma (not used for that). It has been criticized as a non-specific marker for cell "smallness", since it is positive in many "small cell tumors" (1.22) except neuroblastoma

CD117 (c-kit): positive in mast cells (24.17), hematopoietic stem cells (including extramedullary hematopoiesis, 24.19), melanocytes, gastrointestinal stromal tumor, small cell carcinomas (28.5), myelogenous leukemia, granulocytic sarcoma, clear cell sarcoma, and some other carcinomas (breast, lung, stomach). Positive in adenoid cystic carcinoma but not in basal cell carcinoma

CD123: expressed by plasmacytoid dendritic cells type II (formerly called plasmacytoid monocytes). Mainly used for blastic plasmacytoid dendritic cell neoplasm (24.7). Positive in clusters in primary cutaneous marginal zone lymphomas (24.9) and some other B-cell lymphomas, but negative in most follicular center cell lymphomas (24.8) and large B-cell lymphomas of leg type (24.10). CD123+ cells are more common around blood vessels of lupus erythematosus than dermatomyositis, claimed to be a useful finding

CD138 (syndecan-1): plasma cells, endothelial cells, fibroblasts, melanocytes, and keratinocytes. Mainly used for multiple myeloma (24.12), but positive in squamous cell carcinomas and melanomas

CD163: more specific for monocytes and macrophages (histiocytes) than CD68 and other macrophage markers. Positive in most fibrohistiocytic proliferations. Positive in 80% of atypical fibroxanthomas. Positive in some immature myeloid cells

CD207 (langerin): specifically expressed by Langerhans cells

CD246: (see ALK-1)

CD271: (see p75)

CD281 (Toll-like receptor 1)

CD282 (Toll-like receptor 2)

CD283 (Toll-like receptor 3)

CD284 (Toll-like receptor 4)

CD289 (Toll-like receptor 9)

CD303 (blood dendritic cell antigen 2 (BDCA2)): expressed by plasmacytoid dendritic cells type II

CD326: (see Ber-EP4)

Chloroacetate esterase (naphthol ASD, NASD, NASDCl, CAE, Leder stain): mast cells and myelocytic cells (except myeloblasts) have red granules in cytoplasm, negative in monocytes and lymphocytes, often used in mastocytosis (24.17) and myelogenous leukemia (24.16)

Cholesterol: (see Schultz)

Chondroitin sulfate: (see Mucopolysaccharides, acid)

Chromogranin: stains neuroendocrine neoplasms such as carcinoid and Merkel cell carcinoma. Negative in melanocytic nevi and melanoma

CK5/6: positive in non-keratinizing epithelium, mesothelioma, metastatic squamous cell carcinoma of the lung, negative in adenocarcinoma of the lung. More commonly positive in primary malignancies of skin than in metastases to skin

CK7: positive in glandular epithelium. Positive in metastatic carcinomas of the ovary, lung, bladder, pancreas, and breast. Positive in mesothelioma, Paget and extramammary Paget disease. Stains some cases of Merkel cell carcinoma and basal cell carcinoma. Negative in most colon, hepatocellular, neuroendocrine, and prostate carcinoma, squamous cell carcinoma, Bowen disease, and desmoplastic trichoepithelioma

CK8: Cam5.2 is a common example of an antibody directed mainly toward CK8 and CK18, a low molecular weight keratin. Positive in almost all non-squamous epithelium, negative in squamous epithelium. Positive in Paget disease, extramammary Paget disease, many adenocarcinomas, breast ductal carcinoma, eccrine glands, and neoplasms. Variable in apocrine and sebaceous glands and neoplasms

CK10: increased CK10 staining in inflammatory linear verrucous epidermal nevus (ILVEN) compared with linear psoriasis was found by Vissers et al, but not widely performed

CK15: positive in microcystic adnexal carcinoma and desmoplastic trichoepithelioma, negative in basal cell carcinoma and squamous cell carcinoma. Positive in primary skin adnexal carcinomas and mostly negative in metastatic adenocarcinomas from internal organs

CK18: usually positive in adenocarcinoma, negative in squamous cell carcinoma

CK20: positive in adenocarcinomas of the colon, stomach, pancreas, and bile system, mucinous ovarian tumors, transitional cell carcinomas of the urinary tract. Merkel cell carcinoma has classic perinuclear dot pattern. Merkel cells sometimes present in trichoepithelioma are CK20+, usually absent in basal cell carcinoma. In general, tends to stain metastases to the skin from primary sites below the diaphragm, whereas CK7 tends to stain those from above the diaphragm, though this is an oversimplification. Renal cell carcinoma and prostate carcinoma tend to be negative for both CK7 and CK20. Negative in squamous cell carcinoma, non-mucinous ovarian tumors, and adenocarcinomas of the breast, lung, endometrium. Negative in non-Merkel cell small cell carcinomas and mesothelioma. When positive in extramammary Paget's disease, then underlying visceral malignancy is more likely

CM2B4: stains the large T-antigen of the polyoma virus, found in 60% of Merkel cell carcinomas (26.8), sometimes found in other skin cancers

CMV (cytomegalovirus): can be demonstrated by a commercially available immunostain

Collagen: (see Aniline blue, Movat's pentachrome, Trichrome, Verhoeff–van Gieson)

Collagen IV: the collagen found in basement membranes, used to map subtypes of epidermolysis bullosa

Colloid: staining similar to amyloid

Colloidal iron (Hale): this is a two-step stain wherein the colloidal iron binds to acid mucopolysaccharide, and then Prussian blue is used to stain the iron blue; hyaluronidase can be used with this stain to remove the hyaluronic acid form of acid mucopolysaccharide

Complement: (see Immunofluorescence)

Congo red: amyloid is pink–red, green birefringence when polarized; unfixed frozen sections may give better results but are not absolutely necessary

Crystal violet: acid mucopolysaccharides and amyloid are metachromatically purple with blue background

CXCL-13: follicular T-helper lymphocytes, angioimmunoblastic T-cell lymphoma

Cyclin D1: (see bcl-1)

Cytokeratin (keratin): cytoplasm of epithelial cells (squamous cell carcinoma, adenocarcinoma) are positive. Lymphomas, sarcomas, and melanomas are negative. There are at least 20 keratins, which usually appear in pairs: *type I* (acidic, low molecular weight, numbered from 10–20) and *type II* (basic, high molecular weight, numbered from 1–9). CK5 and CK14 are paired in the basal layer, CK1 and CK10 in the suprabasal layer, CK6, CK16, and CK17 in palmar/plantar skin, and CK4 and CK13 in suprabasal mucous membranes. Mutation of K-5 and K-14 occurs in epidermolysis bullosa simplex (6.6), mutation in CKl and CK10 occurs in epidermolytic hyperkeratosis (11.1), and mutation of CK4 or CK13 occurs in white sponge nevus (17.11). Several different keratin stains are commercially available. AE1 is a low molecular weight keratin, more commonly positive in the basal portion of the epidermis and in adnexa. Other popular low molecular weight keratins are cam5.2 and PKK-1, often used for Paget's disease. AE3 is a high molecular weight keratin, more commonly positive in the middle and superficial portion of the epidermis, negative in basal layer and adnexa. Often a "keratin cocktail" or "pankeratin" stain is used (such as a mixture of AE1 and AE3), or MNF-116, which is used to help to assure that most undifferentiated carcinomas will stain positively

D2-40 (podoplanin): relatively specific for lymphatics, but like all lymphatic markers, sometimes blood vessels are positive. Positive in basal cells of adnexal structures. Used for lymphangiosarcoma, lymphangioma, and for staining lymphatics to demonstrate that metastases are within lymphatics. Sometimes positive in Kaposi sarcoma and angiosarcoma. D2-40 is positive in dermatofibroma, negative in dermatofibrosarcoma protuberans. D2-40 is positive in primary benign and malignant adnexal tumors, negative in tumor cells of metastatic carcinomas

DeGalantha: tissue should be fixed in absolute ethyl alcohol, and not processed routinely; urates are black with yellow background

Desmin: skeletal and smooth muscle (leiomyoma, leiomyosarcoma, embryonal rhabdomyosarcoma) positive; less specific for muscle than actin stains. Vascular smooth muscle and glomus tumors stain in a minority of cases

Dieterle: spirochetes and certain other organisms are black

Dihydroxyphenylalanine oxidase (DOPA oxidase): not used routinely, special processing needed, melanocytes are black

EBER: Epstein–Barr virus encoded RNA, by in situ hybridization. Positive in some lymphomas (Chapter 24), especially natural killer cell lymphoma (24.6), lymphomatoid granulomatosis (24.11), and Hodgkin lymphoma (24.15)

Elastic tissue: (see Verhoeff, Weigert's, Orcein, Movat's, 1.31): immunostain for elastin available and said to be superior to Verhoeff

Endothelial cells: (see Factor VIII-related antigen, *Ulex europaeus* lectin, CD31, CD34, vascular neoplasms in Chapter 25) with electron microscopy, the typical organelles are Weibel–Palade bodies, and they contain von Willebrand factor

Epithelial membrane antigen (EMA): positive in normal skin adnexa and adnexal neoplasms (eccrine, apocrine, sebaceous). Positive in Paget's disease, many adenocarcinomas, Merkel cell carcinoma, epithelioid sarcoma, and meningioma. Usually negative in basal cell carcinoma, sarcoma, lymphoma, melanoma. squamous cell carcinoma is variable. Like ALK-1, more likely to be expressed in systemic large cell CD30+ lymphoma than by primary cutaneous anaplastic CD30+ lymphoma (24.5)

Factor VIII-related antigen: endothelial cells, useful in identifying vascular tumors (Chapter 25) that are differentiated enough to express the antigen, not as sensitive as CD31; see also Endothelial cells in this chapter

Factor XIIIa: macrophages and dermal dendrocytes (antigen presenting cells related to Langerhans cells). Often used to stain dermatofibroma, but also positive in fibrous papule, atypical fibroxanthoma, multinucleate cell angiohistiocytoma, juvenile xanthogranuloma, other xanthomas, neurofibroma, and cellular neurothekeoma. Negative in dermatofibrosarcoma protuberans (used with CD34 which is positive in dermatofibrosarcoma protuberans and negative in dermatofibroma). Sometimes positive in nephrogenic systemic fibrosis. Unfortunately antibody clone AC-1A1 (mouse monoclonal) will sometimes stain keratinocytes, whereas rabbit monoclonal antibody (EP3372) is said not to have that problem

Fat: (see Oil-red-O, Sudan black B, Scarlet red)

Feulgen: DNA has red to purple with green background

Fibrin: (see Phosphotungstic acid–hematoxylin, Periodic acid-Schiff, Movat's pentachrome, and Immunofluorescence)

Fite: *Mycobacterium leprae* and other acid-fast bacilli are red (*M. leprae* and atypical acid-fast bacilli may be over-decolorized by other acid-fast bacilli stains such as the Ziehl–Neelsen stain)

FLI-1: nuclear staining of endothelial cells (in contrast to CD31 and CD34 which are cytoplasmic stains). Postive in vascular neoplasms, normal breast epithelium, Ewing's sarcoma, peripheral neuroectodermal tumors, lymphocytes and lymphoblastic lymphoma, Kaposi sarcoma, angiosarcoma, lung adenocarcinoma, Merkel cell carcinoma. Negative in rhabdomyosarcoma and other non-vascular sarcomas, carcinomas, melanoma, and colon adenocarcinoma

Fontana–Masson: (see Argentaffin)

FOX-P1 (Forkhead box protein 1): large B-cell lymphoma

FOX-P3 (Forkhead box protein 3): T-regulatory lymphocytes

Giemsa: nuclei are blue; cytoplasm is pink; erythrocytes are red; inclusion bodies, plasma cell cytoplasm, mast cell granules, *Histoplasma*, *Rickettsia*, some bacteria, Donovan bodies, and *Leishmania* are purple or blue

Glial fibrillary acidic protein (GFAP): glial cells, astrocytes, Schwann cells, positive immunostaining

GLUT-1 (glucose transporter-1): positive in erythrocyte membranes, placentas, proliferating and involuting infantile hemangiomas. Negative in normal blood vessels, pyogenic granuloma, and other vascular neoplasms, vascular malformations, and non-involuting congenital hemangiomas (NICH) and rapidly-involuting congenital hemangiomas (RICH)

Glycogen: (see Best's carmine, Periodic acid-Schiff): prevalent in many clear cell tumors (1.22)

Gold chloride: Langerhans cells; black

Gomori aldehyde fuchsin: (see Aldehyde fuchsin)

Gram's (Brown–Brenn, Brown–Hopps): Gram-positive bacteria are blue; Gram-negative bacteria are red (Gram negatives do not tend to stain well on tissue sections with these stains)

Grimelius: (see Argyrophil)

Granzyme A and B: protein (like TIA-1) found next to perforin in cytoplasm of cytotoxic lymphocytes and natural killer cells. A high percentage of granzyme in Hodgkin lymphoma, natural killer cell lymphoma, and mycosis fungoides is associated with worse prognosis

Grocott–Gomori methenamine silver (GMS): fungi are black with green background counterstain

Gross cystic disease fluid protein (GCDFP): positive in apocrine glands, useful in the staining of Paget's disease (18.13), some metastatic breast cancers, and apocrine sweat gland tumors (Chapter 23)

Hale: (see Colloidal iron)

HAM-56 (human alveolar macrophage-56): macrophages and endothelial cells positive. Negative in lymphocytes and neutrophils. Positive in fibrohistiocytic neoplasms such as xanthogranuloma and dermatofibroma

Hemosiderin: (see Perl's, Prussian blue, Turnbull blue, 1.58)

Her-2/neu (c-erbB-2): positive staining in breast cancer, correlates with negative staining for estrogen and progesterone receptors and a poor prognosis

Herpes virus antigens: various immunoperoxidase or immunofluorescence kits are commercially available (14.2)

Histiocyte: (see Macrophage)

HMB-45 (human melanin black, gp100): a glycoprotein on melanosomes. It is less sensitive but more specific for melanocytes than S-100 (like MART-1). It is more likely to be positive in the superficial aspect (negative in deeper dermal portion) of benign nevus ("stratification" of staining), and more diffuse or patchy in the dermis in melanoma. Unfortunately, it tends to be negative in desmoplastic melanoma. It will stain some dysplastic nevi, Spitz nevi, liposarcomas, and breast cancers

HPV (human papillomavirus, 14.1): can be demonstrated by a commercially available immunostain, by in situ hybridization, or polymerase chain reaction (PCR)

Hyaline: (see 1.35 and Periodic acid-Schiff)

Hyaluronidase: often used with Alcian blue or colloidal iron stains; removes hyaluronic acid from the tissue; sections stained with or without it may help identify an acid mucopolysaccharide

ICOS (inducible co-stimulator protein): angioimmunoblastic T-cell lymphoma

Immunofluorescence, direct method: frozen sections are prepared after transport of the specimen in special media such as phosphate-buffered normal saline, Michel's media, or Zeuss media; then they are most commonly stained with fluorescein isothiocyanate (FITC)-labeled anti-IgG, IgM, IgA, C3, and fibrin; this is important in the diagnosis of autoimmune blistering disorders such as pemphigus, pemphigoid, pemphigoid gestationis, dermatitis herpetiformis, linear IgA bullous dermatosis, chronic bullous disease of childhood, epidermolysis bullosa acquisita, and also lupus erythematosus, and vasculitis

Immunofluorescence, indirect method: serum is used instead of tissue used in the direct method. In dermatopathology, this is commonly used for some of the blistering disorders mentioned under direct immunofluorescence

Immunoglobulin light chains (κ or λ): B lymphocytes have positive immunostaining. B-cell lymphoma and plasma cell myeloma may show predominant monoclonal staining of one light chain more than the other (24.11 and 24.12)

Immunoglobulins: (see Immunofluorescence)

Iron: (see Prussian blue, Perl's, Turnbull blue)

Kappa: an immunoglobulin light chain found on B lymphocytes. Kappa:lambda ratio usually 2:1. If ratio is far off from this, then clonality is present, suggesting malignancy (lymphoma or multiple myeloma)

Keratin: (see Cytokeratin)

Ki-1: (see CD30)

Ki-67 (MIB-1): nuclear antigen associated with proliferation, and is expressed more in malignant lesions than in benign ones. Staining in less than 5% of the dermal melanocytes suggests nevus, whereas staining more than 10% of the cells favors melanoma (these numbers vary depending upon the study). Also used with lymphomas: Ki-67 stains more than 90% of the cells in reactive germinal centers, but less than 50% of cells in the follicular centers of follicular center lymphoma of the non-diffuse type

Kinyoun's carbol fuchsin: acid-fast bacilli are red

L-26: (see CD20)

Lambda: a light chain found on B lymphocytes (see Kappa)

Langerhans cells: (see Adenosine triphosphatase, Gold chloride, CD1a, CD207, Argyrophil, Peanut agglutinin, S-100 protein), Birbeck granules are seen by electron microscopy

Langerin: (see CD207)

Leder stain: (see Chloroacetate esterase)

Lendrum phloxine–tartrazine: acidophilic inclusion bodies of orf, milker's nodule, and herpes viruses are red on a yellow background. Nuclei stain blue. Negri bodies are negative

Leukocyte common antigen: (see CD45)

Leu stains: (see CD stains)

Lipids: (see Oil-red-O, Sudan black B, Scarlet red)

Lymphocytes: (see CD stains)

Lysozyme (muramidase): myeloid cells (including myeloblasts, myelocytes, and neutrophils), histiocytes, monocytes are positive. Has been used for fibrohistiocytic proliferation, but sometimes will stain melanoma and carcinoma

LYVE-1 (lymphatic vessel endothelial receptor 1): lymphatic endothelial cells, negative in blood vessel endothelial cells

Macrophage (true histiocyte): stains with alpha-1 antitrypsin, lysozyme, HAM-56, CD68, Mac-387

MART-1 (*m*elanoma *a*ntigen *r*ecognized by *T*-cells, Melan-A, MLANA): Melan-A is a different antibody recognizing the same antigen. Positive in melanocytes, somewhat comparable in its staining to HMB-45. Expression is regulated by Mitf. It will stain most examples of nevus, (including blue nevus and desmoplastic nevus), and melanoma, but tends to be negative in desmoplastic melanoma. Highly specific for melanocytes (but less sensitive than S-100). Negative in tumors of epithelial, mesenchymal, or lymphoproliferative derivation. Brown or red immunostaining

Masson trichrome: (see Trichrome)

Mast cells: (see Giemsa, Toluidine blue, Bismarck brown, Chloroacetate esterase, Tryptase, CD117)

MB1: (see CD79a)

MB2: B lymphocytes on paraffin-embedded tissue

Mel5 (tyrosinase-related protein-1, TRP-1): stage III and IV melanosomes. Positive in melanocytes, and epidermal component of melanocytic nevi and melanoma. Often negative in desmoplastic melanoma, amelanotic melanoma, and dermal components of nevi and melanomas. It has been used for Mohs surgery of lentigo maligna

Melan-A: (see MART-1)

Melanin: (see Argyrophil, Argentaffin, and other silver stains)

Melanin bleach: uses peroxide, potassium permanganate, or ferric chloride to remove melanin from cases in which it obscures nuclear characteristics

Melanocytes: stain with S-100, HMB-45, or MART-1; melanin stains will be positive if melanin is present; electron microscopy will show organelles known as melanosomes

Melanoma cocktail (pan-mel): sometimes various combinations of HMB-45, MART-1, and tyrosinase are used to enhance staining of suspected melanomas, when they must be distinguished from other metastatic tumors

Mel-CAM: an adhesion molecule that may play a role in communication between keratinocytes and melanocytes, which may play a role in lentigo maligna and melanoma development. Mainly used in research at this time

Methenamine silver: (see Gomori)

Methylene blue: pigment in ochronosis stains black; acid mucopolysaccharides stain metachromatically purple

Methyl green–pyronin (MGP): frozen sections needed, methyl green stains DNA in nucleus green; pyronin stains RNA in nucleoli and plasma cell cytoplasm red; useful in myeloma and angioimmunoblastic lymphadenopathy

MIB-1: (see Ki-67)

MiTF (microphthalmia transcription factor): heterozygous loss of MiTF leads to Waardenberg syndrome type II (white forelock and deafness). MiTF is positive in most cellular neurothekeomas, angiomyolipoma, PEComa, some melanocytic neoplasms, mast cells. Negative in malignant schwannomas, positive in 3–30% of desmoplastic melanomas. Like SOX-10, nuclear immunostaining of melanocytes with MiTF is supposed to be better than the cytoplasmic staining found with MART-1 and HMC-45

MLH3, MSH1, MSH2, MSH6, PMS-2: the proteins from these five mismatch repair genes often fail to immunostain in sebaceous neoplasms of Muir–Torre syndrome and colorectal carcinoma

MNF-116: a pankeratin stain that is positive in most epithelial elements and carcinomas

Movat's pentachrome: collagen and reticular fibers are yellow; muscle and fibrin are red; mucin is blue; nuclei and elastic fibers are black

MSA: (see Actin)

Mucicarmine: epithelial mucin (acid or neutral mucopolysaccharide) is red; usually used for sialomucin, adenocarcinoma, Paget's disease, capsule of *Cryptococcus*; not a good stain for dermal mucins

Mucopolysaccharides, acidic: found in ground substance of connective tissue and in diseases with mucinous or myxomatous areas (1.83), and in sialomucin; stained with Alcian blue, colloidal iron, crystal violet, toluidine blue, aldehyde fuchsin, Giemsa, and mucicarmine

Mucopolysaccharides, neutral: found in basement membranes, fibrinoid areas, and colloid or hyaline (1.35); stained with periodic acid-Schiff (PAS) and mucicarmine

MUM-1 (multiple myeloma oncogene-1): positive in myeloma, melanoma, primary cutaneous diffuse large B-cell lymphoma of leg type. Positive in some cases of large cell anaplastic lymphoma, lymphomatoid papulosis, and Sezary syndrome. Negative in diffuse form of follicular center cell lymphoma and mycosis fungoides

Muscle: (see Trichrome, Aniline blue, Verhoeff–van Gieson, Phosphotungstic acid hematoxylin, Movat's pentachrome, actin, desmin)

Myelin basic protein (MBP): myelin sheath tissue, Schwann cells, oligodendrocytes. Positive in neurofibroma, neuroma, schwannoma and granular cell tumors, but negative in neural nevi

Myeloperoxidase: positive in myelogenous and monomyelocytic leukemia

Myogenin: positive in immature myoblasts in fetal limbs, negative in adult skeletal muscle. Positive immunostaining in rhabdomyosarcoma and Wilms' tumor. Negative in Ewing's sarcoma, neuroblastoma, and other PNET tumors (28.5)

Myoglobin: positive in skeletal muscle, negative in smooth muscle. Positive in rhabdomyosarcoma

MyoD1 (myogenic differentiation 1): positive in nuclei of immature myoblasts in developing muscle, rhabdomyosarcoma, PEComa, and angiomyolipoma, but negative in normal adult skeletal muscle

Nerves: (see Bodian, Adenosine triphosphatase, Myelin basic protein, S-100 protein)

Neurofilament: an intermediate filament found in neurons and axons and neural tumors that contain axons, such as neuroma and neurofibroma, but negative in schwannoma (Chapter 26). Positive in neuroblastoma and some other peripheral neuroectodermal tumors (28.5), carcinoid, Merkel cell carcinoma

Neuron-specific enolase (NSE): neural tissue, granular cell tumor, Merkel cell carcinoma and other neuroendocrine tumors, some melanocytes and melanocytic tumors; it is sometimes joked that it should be called non-specific enolase, because it sometimes stains other things, such as smooth muscle, some melanomas, some lymphomas, renal cell carcinoma, and sweat ducts

NGFR (nerve growth factor receptor, see p75): useful to stain desmoplastic melanomas that are S-100 negative[155]

NKI-C3 (CD63): positive in cellular neurothekeoma, juvenile xanthogranuloma, some melanocytic neoplasms, angiomyolipoma, breast cancer, PEComa (27.21)

Non-specific esterase (α-naphthol acetate esterase or α-naphthol butyrate esterase): granular cell layer, sweat glands, monocytes, histiocytes are positive; negative in neutrophils

Oil-red-O (ORO): need frozen sections of fresh or formalin-fixed, but otherwise unprocessed tissue; neutral lipids are red; most commonly used for sebaceous carcinoma

Orcein–Giemsa (O and G): mast cell granules are purple; elastic fibers and melanin are brown–black; nuclei are dark blue; collagen is pink; amyloid and most cytoplasms are light blue; most useful in identifying elastic fibers

Osteopontin: weak staining in Spitz nevus, strong staining in invasive melanoma, but this stain is not in widespread use

p16 (CDKN2A, a cyclin-dependent kinase inhibitor): a mutation found in some familial melanomas and dysplastic nevi, and many other malignancies. Positive staining in Spitz nevus

p53: a suppressor gene product found to be mutated in many malignancies

p63: a homologue of p53. Positive in more than 90% of benign and primary malignant adnexal tumors, and negative in most metastatic adenocarcinomas in the skin. Positive in benign prostate glands, negative in prostate cancer. Positive in some carcinomas at their primary sites other than skin. Negative in primary mucinous carcinoma, unlike other primary adnexal tumors

p75: nerve growth factor receptor (NGFR, CD271), apoptosis-promoting protein in the tumor necrosis factor superfamily, strongly expressed in epidermis, fibroblasts, endothelial cells, nerves, adipocytes, sebaceous glands, sweat glands, and catagen and telogen follicles. Useful positivity in some S-100neg desmoplastic melanomas, but is also positive in dermatofibrosarcoma protuberans, Schwann cell tumors, neurotized nevi, synovial sarcomas, rhabdomyosarcomas, granular cell tumor, hemangiopericytoma, and peripheral nerve sheath tumors

Papillomavirus antigens: various immunoperoxidase antibodies are commercially available that stain papillomavirus (14.1)

PAX-5 (paired box gene-5): a B-cell-specific activator protein found in immature and mature B cells, negative in T cells. More sensitive and specific than CD20 for B-cell lymphoma. Positive in some Merkel cell carcinomas

PCNA (proliferating cell nuclear antigen): an indicator of cell cycling; more likely to be positive in malignancies

PD-1: immunoregulatory lymphoid cells

Peanut agglutinin: Langerhans cell histiocytosis stains positively, but not as specific as CD1a

Pentachrome: (see Movat)

Perforin: cytotoxic T-cells

Periodic acid-Schiff (PAS): glycogen, neutral mucopolysaccharides, fibrin, hyaline, fungi, and basement membranes are pink or red; diastase can be used with PAS (PAS-D) to remove glycogen and thus render a negative result when staining glycogen-laden cells (the other substances listed are PAS+, diastase resistant, while glycogen is PAS+, diastase labile)

Perl's potassium ferrocyanide: iron (hemosiderin) is blue

PGP9.5 (neuroectodermal protein gene product 9.5): positive in neuroendocrine tumors, neurofibroma, cellular neurothekeoma

Phosphotungstic acid hematoxylin (PTAH): muscle and fibrin are blue; collagen is red; demonstrates granules of granular cell tumor, myofibrils of leiomyosarcoma, muscle striations in rhabdomyosarcoma, red to purple inclusion bodies of recurrent digital fibromatosis

Plasma cells: (see Methyl green–pyronin, Immunoglobulin light chains)

Podoplanin: (see D2-40)

Procollagen-1: procollagen is synthesized by fibroblasts, then cleaved to make collagen. Positive immunostaining in atypical fibroxanthoma, nephrogenic systemic fibrosis, scleromyxedema. Positive in a minority of desmoplastic melanomas and spindle cell squamous cell carcinomas. Negative in desmoplastic trichoepithelioma and sclerosing basal cell carcinoma

Prussian blue: iron (hemosiderin) is blue

PSA (prostate-specific antigen): prostate cancer positive

PTAH: (see Phosphotungstic acid hematoxylin)

PTEN: a tumor suppressor gene coding for a protein for which immunostaining is available

RCC (renal cell carcinoma): this protein is expressed in both normal kidney and renal cell carcinoma, immunostain available

Reticulum: (see Argyrophil, Wilder)

S-100 protein: when used without modifier, S-100 usually refers to the "B" subset, as opposed to "A" below. Melanocytes and melanocytic tumors, glial and Schwann cell tumors, granular cell tumor, eccrine and some apocrine glands, Langerhans cells, Langerhans cell histiocytosis, chondrocytes, smooth and skeletal muscle, leiomyosarcoma stain positively. The name S-100 derives from its solubility in 100% saturated ammonium sulfate at neutral pH. It is sometimes joked that it is called S-100 protein because it stains 100 different things (it does not have high specificity), but nevertheless it is a commonly used workhorse for melanocytic and neural neoplasms because of its availability and sensitivity (more than 90% of melanomas and benign neural tumors, 30% of malignant nerve sheath tumors). Be aware that it occasionally stains unexpected things such as histiocytic proliferations, liposarcomas, and breast adenocarcinoma

S-100A6: positive in cellular neurothekeoma, atypical fibroxanthoma, other fibrohistiocytic neoplasms. More positive in neurotized portion of melanocytic nevi. More diffuse in Spitz nevus, while patchy in melanoma

Scarlet red: frozen sections of fresh or formalin-fixed, but otherwise unprocessed tissue, are needed; lipids are red–brown

Scarlet red (RIT): amyloid is red

Schultz: frozen sections needed, cholesterol and cholesterol esters are blue–green; positive in xanthomas (except eruptive type) and Tangier's disease

Sialomucin: epithelial mucin found in Paget's disease, adenocarcinoma, and mucocele are positive with both neutral mucopolysaccharide stains (such as periodic acid-Schiff) and with acid mucopolysaccharide stains

Silver stains: (see Argentaffin, Argyrophil, Gomori methenamine silver, Bodian, Warthin–Starry, Dieterle, Steiner, von Kossa, Wilder)

SMA: (see Actin, smooth muscle)

Sox10: a neural crest transcription factor found in Schwann cells, melanocytes, and myoepithelial cells. Positive in almost all melanomas, myoepitheliomas, and half of malignant peripheral nerve sheath tumors (more than S-100). It is particularly helpful for staining desmoplastic melanomas where S-100 fails to stain the melanocytes, or when S-100 stains background stromal cells. Like MiTF, nuclear immunostaining of melanocytes is supposed to be better than the cytoplasmic staining found with MART-1 and HMB-45

Steiner: a silver stain, spirochetes, bacillary angiomatosis, granuloma inguinale organisms stain black

Stromelysin-3: strong staining correlates with more aggressive subtype of breast cancer. Positive in dermatofibroma and stroma of trichoepithelioma, negative in dermatofibrosarcoma protuberans and stroma of basal cell carcinoma

Sudan black B: frozen sections of fresh or formalin-fixed, but otherwise unprocessed tissue are needed; lipids are black, positive in Niemann Pick disease, Gaucher's disease, and Fabry's disease

Synaptophysin: positive in Merkel cell carcinoma and other neuroendocrine neoplasms, similar to chromogranin. Negative in normal Merkel cells, melanocytic nevi and melanoma

TCL-1: T cells, plasmacytoid dendritic cells type II

TdT (terminal deoxynucleotidyl transferase): a nuclear DNA polymerase found in immature B cells and thymic T cells (precursor cells), most often used for lymphoblastic lymphoma (24.16). Sometimes positive in Merkel cell carcinoma, acute myeloid leukemia, Ewing's sarcoma, and pediatric rhabdomyosarcoma. Negative in Burkitt's lymphoma.

TFE3: highly specific and sensitive for alveolar soft part sarcoma (28.6), except sometimes it can be positive in renal cell carcinoma, some granular cell tumors, and perivascular epithelioid neoplasms

Thioflavin T: amyloid has yellow fluorescence when examined with fluorescent microscope

Thyroglobulin: papillary and follicular thyroid carcinoma, negative in non-thyroid adenocarcinomas

TIA-1 (T-cell intracytoplasmic antigen): positive in lymphocytes having cytotoxic granules and cytolytic potential (see also Granzyme). Positive in natural killer cell lymphomas, subcutaneous T-cell lymphomas and most anaplastic large cell lymphomas. Worse prognosis when highly expressed in mycosis fungoides. Negative in B-cell lymphomas, Hodgkin lymphoma, and lymphoblastic leukemia

Toluidine blue: acid mucopolysaccharides and mast cell granules are purple

Trichrome, Mallory: (see Aniline blue)

Trichrome, Masson: muscle and keratin are red; collagen is green; nuclei are black; useful for distinguishing some leiomyomas from dermatofibromas. Most labs omit the black nuclear stain and actually provide a "bichrome" of green and red. Postive staining in inclusion bodies of recurrent digital fibromatosis

TRP-1 (tyrosinase-related protein-1): (see Mel5)

Tryptase: mast cells; brown or red immunostaining

TTF-1 (thyroid transcription factor-1): positive in thyroid carcinoma, small cell carcinoma of lung, and 75% of lung adenocarcinomas. Usually negative in Merkel cell carcinoma

Turnbull blue: iron and hemosiderin are blue

Tyrosinase: enzyme in melanocytes, it will stain most melanocytic nevi and melanomas and probably is highly specific. Less sensitive than S-100 but more sensitive than HMB-45. Positive only in a minority of desmoplastic melanomas

UCHL-1: (see CD45RO) a pan-T-lymphocyte marker

Ulex europaeus lectin: (see also Endothelial cells) endothelial cells and vascular neoplasms are positive. It has good sensitivity with strong staining, but lower specificity than CD31, so not used so much anymore. Stains keratinocytes also

Urates: (see DeGalantha, von Kossa)

Verhoeff–van Gieson (VVG, elastic Verhoeff–van Gieson, EVG): Verhoeff stains elastic tissue black; van Gieson stains collagen red and muscle and nerves yellow

Vimentin: mesenchymal cells (including fibroblasts, muscle, endothelial cells, lymphocytes, histiocytes, melanocytes, and Schwann cells). Negative in most epithelial tumors and adenocarcinomas; positive in most sarcomas and lymphomas. Since it is so non-specific, and stains at least some component of most tissues strongly, it is often used mainly to prove good tissue preservation and antigenicity

von Kossa: carbonates, phosphates, oxalates, sulfates, urates, chloride and other anion salts are brown–black; usually used to stain calcium salts

Warthin–Starry: (see also Silver stains) spirochetes, granuloma inguinale, rhinoscleroma, bacteria in bacillary angiomatosis, and melanin are black with yellowish–brown background

Weigert's resorcin–fuchsin: elastic fibers are purple to black

Wilder: reticulum fibers are black; collagen is red

Ziehl–Neelsen: acid-fast bacilli are red; Fite stain is preferred for leprosy and *Nocardia*

References and Further Reading

We have not provided a voluminous list of references because nowadays most information is easily found electronically on the Internet, and any such compilation is quickly outdated.

A. Standard textbooks of dermatopathology

1. Barnhill RL, Crowson AN, eds. Textbook of dermatopathology. 3rd edn. New York: McGraw-Hill; 2010.
2. Elder DE, Elenitsas R, Johnson BL, et al. Lever's histopathology of the skin. 10th edn. Philadelphia: Lippincott-Williams & Wilkins; 2009.
3. Weedon D. Weedon's skin pathology. 3rd edn. Edinburgh: Churchill Livingstone; 2009.

B. "Oldies but goodies" dermpath books out of print

4. Farmer ER, Hood AF, eds. Pathology of the skin. 2nd edn. New York: McGraw-Hill; 2000.
5. Graham JH, Johnson WC, Helwig EB. Dermal pathology. Hagerstown, MD: Harper & Row; 1972.
6. Maize JC, LeBoit PE, Burgdorf WH, et al. Cutaneous pathology. Philadelphia: WB Saunders; 1998.
7. Mehregan AH, Hashimoto K, Mehregan DA, Mehregan DR. Pinkus' guide to dermatohistopathology. 6th edn. New York: McGraw-Hill; 2001.
8. Montgomery H. Dermatopathology. New York: Harper & Row; 1967.
9. Rapini RP, Jordon RE. Atlas of dermatopathology. Chicago: YearBook Medical Publishers; 1988.

C. Dermatopathology atlases and synopses

10. Ackerman AB, Ragaz A. The lives of lesions: Chronology in dermatopathology. New York: Masson; 1984.
11. Ackerman AB, Mendonca A. Differential diagnosis in dermatopathology I. 2nd edn. Philadelphia: Lippincott Williams & Wilkins; 1992.
12. Ackerman AB, Guo Y, Lazova R, Kaddu S. Differential diagnosis in dermatopathology II. 2nd edn. Philadelphia: Lippincott Williams & Wilkins; 1999.
13. Ackerman AB, Briggs PL, Bravo F. Differential diagnosis in dermatopathology III. Philadelphia: Lippincott Williams & Wilkins; 1993.
14. Ackerman AB, White WL, Guo Y, Umbert I. Differential diagnosis in dermatopathology IV. Philadelphia: Lippincott Williams & Wilkins; 1994.
15. Ackerman AB, Jacobson M, Vitale PA. Clues to diagnosis in dermatopathology. Chicago: ASCP Press; 1991.
16. Ackerman AB, Guo Y, Vitale PA. Clues to diagnosis in dermatopathology II. Chicago: ASCP Press; 1992.
17. Brinster NK, Liu V, Diwan AH, McKee PH. Dermatopathology: High-yield pathology. Philadelphia: Saunders; 2011.
18. Busam KJ, ed. Dermatopathology. Philadelphia: Saunders; 2010.
19. Elder D, Elenitsas R, Johnson B, et al. Atlas and synopsis of Lever's histopathology of the skin. 2nd edn. Philadelphia: Lippincott Williams & Wilkins; 2007.
20. Elston DM, Ferringer T, et al. Requisites in dermatopathology. Edinburgh: Saunders-Elsevier; 2009.
21. Grant–Kels JM, ed. Color atlas of dermatopathology. New York: Informa; 2007.
22. Hood AF, Kwan TH, Mihm MC, et al. Primer of dermatopathology. 3rd edn. Philadelphia: Lippincott Williams & Wilkins; 2002.
23. Ko CJ, Barr RJ. Dermatopathology: Diagnosis by first impression. Edinburgh: Saunders; 2009.
24. McKee PH, Calonje E, Granter SR. Pathology of the skin with clinical correlations. 3rd edn. Philadelphia: Mosby; 2005.
25. Okun MR, Edelstein LM, Fisher BK. Gross and microscopic pathology of the skin. 2nd edn. Canton, MA: Dermatopathology Foundation Press; 1988.
26. Schaumburg–Lever G, Lever WF. Color atlas of histopathology of the skin. Philadelphia: JB Lippincott; 1988.
27. Shum DT, Guenther LC. An atlas of histopathology of skin diseases. Pearl River, NY: Parthenon; 1999.

D. Standard clinical dermatology textbooks

28. Bolognia JL, Jorizzo JL, Rapini RP, eds. Dermatology. 2nd edn. London: Mosby; 2008.
29. Burns T, Breathnach S, Cox N, Griffiths C. Rook's textbook of dermatology. 8th edn. Oxford, England: Wiley-Blackwell, 2010.
30. Wolff K, Goldsmith LA, Katz SI, et al. Fitzpatrick's dermatology in general medicine. 7th edn. New York: McGraw-Hill; 2007.
31. Elston D, ed. eMedicine dermatology (online at emedicine.com). St. Petersburg: eMedicine Corporation; 2010.
32. James WD, Berger TG, Elston DM. Andrews' diseases of the skin. 11th edn. Philadelphia: WB Saunders; 2011.

E. Clinical dermatology

33. Callen JP, Greer KE, Paller AS, Swinyer LJ. Color atlas of dermatology. 2nd edn. Philadelphia: WB Saunders; 2000.
34. Cohen BA. Pediatric dermatology. 3rd edn. London: Mosby; 2005.
35. du Vivier A. Atlas of clinical dermatology. 3rd edn. Edinburgh: Churchill Livingstone; 2002.
36. Wolff K, Johnson RA. Fitzpatrick's color atlas and synopsis of clinical dermatology. 6th edn. New York: McGraw-Hill; 2009.
37. Ghatan HEY. Dermatological differential diagnosis and pearls. 2nd edn. New York: Parthenon; 2002.
38. Habif TP. Clinical dermatology: A color guide to diagnosis and therapy. 5th edn. St. Louis: Mosby; 2010.
39. Hall BJ, Hall JC. Sauer's manual of skin diseases. 10th edn. Philadelphia: Lippincott Williams & Wilkins; 2010.
40. Harper J, Oranje A, Prose N. Textbook of pediatric dermatology. 2nd edn. Oxford: Blackwell Science; 2006.
41. Marks JG Jr, Miller JJ. Lookingbill and Marks' principles of dermatology. 4th edn. Philadelphia: WB Saunders; 2006.
42. Mallory SB. An illustrated dictionary of dermatologic syndromes. 2nd edn. New York: Parthenon; 2006.
43. Paller AS, Mancini AJ. Hurwitz clinical pediatric dermatology. 3rd edn. Philadelphia: Saunders; 2005.
44. Schachner LA, Hansen RC, eds. Pediatric dermatology. 4th edn. Philadelphia: Mosby; 2010.
45. Spitz JL. Genodermatoses. 2nd edn. New York: Lippincott Williams & Wilkins; 2004.
46. Weston WL, Lane AT, Morelli JG. Color textbook of pediatric dermatology. 4th edn. St Louis: Mosby; 2007.

F. Normal skin histology

47. Freinkel RK, Woodley DT. The biology of the skin. New York: Parthenon; 2001.
48. Montagna W, Kligman AM, Carlisle KS. Atlas of normal human skin. New York: Springer; 2010.

G. Specific topics in dermatopathology

49. Ackerman AB, Boer A, Bennin B, Gottlieb GJ. Histologic diagnosis of inflammatory skin diseases. 3rd edn. New York: Ardor Scribendi; 2005.
50. Ackerman AB, Cavegn BM, Casintahan MF, Robinson MJ. Resolving quandaries in dermatology, pathology, and dermatopathology. Philadelphia: Promethean Medical Press; 1995.
51. Billings SD, Cotton J. Inflammatory dermatopathology: A pathologist's survival guide. New York: Springer; 2011.
52. Caputo R, Gelmetti C. Pediatric dermatology and dermatopathology. London: Taylor and Francis; 2002.

H. Hair

53. Dawber R, Van Neste D. Hair and scalp disorders. 2nd edn. London: Taylor and Francis; 2004.
54. McMichael AJ, Hordinsky MK, eds. Hair and scalp diseases. New York: Informa; 2008.
55. Olsen EA, ed. Disorders of hair growth. 2nd edn. New York: McGraw-Hill; 2003.
56. Powell J, Stone N, Dawber RPR. An atlas of hair and scalp diseases. New York: Informa; 2001.
57. Sperling LC. An atlas of hair pathology with clinical correlations. New York: Parthenon; 2003.
58. Whiting DA, Howsden FL. Color atlas of differential diagnosis of hair loss. Canfield, NJ: Canfield; 1996.

I. Nails

59. Baran R, Dawber RPR, de Berker DAR, et al, eds. Baran and Dawber's diseases of the nails and their management. 3rd edn. Oxford: Blackwell Science; 2001.
60. Baran R, Dawber RPR, Haneke E, et al. A text atlas of nail disorders: Techniques in investigation and diagnosis. 3rd edn. London: Taylor and Francis; 2003.
61. Scher RK, Daniel CR III, eds. Nails: Therapy, diagnosis, surgery. 3rd edn. Philadelphia: WB Saunders; 2005.

J. Oral pathology

62. Neville BW, Damm DD, Allen CM, Bouquot JE. Oral and maxillofacial pathology. 3rd edn. St Louis: Saunders; 2009.
63. Regezi JA, Sciubba JJ, Jordan RCK. Oral pathology: Clinical and pathologic correlations. 5th edn. St Louis: Saunders; 2007.

K. Immunofluorescence

64. Kalaaji AN, Nicolas MEO. Mayo clinic atlas of immunofluorescence in dermatology. Rochester, MN: Mayo Clinic Scientific Press; 2006.
65. Jordon RE. Atlas of bullous disease. Edinburgh: Churchill Livingstone; 2000.
66. Valenzuela R, Bergfeld WF. Immunofluorescent patterns in skin diseases. Chicago: American Society of Clinical Pathologists Press; 1984.

L. Electron microscopy

67. Hashimoto K. Skin pathology by light and electron microscopy. New York: Igaku–Shoin; 1983.
68. Lever WF, Schaumburg–Lever G. Histopathology of the skin. 7th edn. Philadelphia: JB Lippincott; 1990.
69. Zelickson AS. The clinical use of electron microscopy in dermatology. 5th edn. Buffalo, NY: Westwood-Squibb Pharmaceuticals; 1991.

M. Histotechnology and special stains

70. Bancroft JD, Gamble M. Theory and practice of histological techniques. 6th edn. Edinburgh: Churchill Livingstone; 2007.
71. Carson FL, Hladik C. Histotechnology: A self-instructional text. 3rd edn. Chicago: ASCP Press; 2009.
72. Chu PG, Weiss LM. Modern immunohistochemistry. Cambridge: Cambridge University Press; 2009.
73. Dabbs DJ. Diagnostic immunohistochemistry: Theranostic and genomic applications. Philadelphia: Saunders; 2010.
74. Horobin RW, Bancroft JD. Troubleshooting histology stains. Edinburgh: Churchill Livingstone; 1997.
75. Kiernan JA. Histological and histochemical methods: Theory and practice. 4th edn. Oxfordshire: Scion; 2008.
76. Prophet EB, Mills B, Arrington JB, Sobin LH, eds. Armed Forces Institute of Pathology: Laboratory methods in histotechnology. Washington: American Registry of Pathology; 1992.
77. Schach CP, Smoller BR, Hudson AR, Horn TD. Immunohistochemical stains in dermatopathology. J Am Acad Dermatol 2000; 43:1094–1100.
78. Wick MR, ed. Diagnostic histochemistry. Cambridge: Cambridge University Press; 2008.

N. Surgery and skin cancer

79. Gross KG, Steinman HK, Rapini RP, eds. Mohs surgery: Fundamentals and techniques. St Louis: Mosby-YearBook; 1999.
80. Gross KG, Steinman HK, eds. Mohs surgery and histopathology: Beyond the fundamentals. New York: Cambridge University Press; 2009.
81. Maloney ME, Torres A, Hoffmann TJ, eds. Surgical dermatopathology. Oxford: Blackwell; 1999.
82. Morgan MB, Hamill JR Jr, Spencer JM, eds. Atlas of Mohs and frozen section cutaneous pathology. New York: Springer, 2009.
83. Roenigk RK, Ratz JL, Roenigk HH Jr. Roenigk's dermatologic surgery: Current techniques in procedural dermatology. 3rd edn. New York: Informa; 2007.
84. Robinson JK, Hanke CW, Siegel DM, Fratila A. Surgery of the skin. 2nd edn. Procedural dermatology. London: Mosby; 2010.
85. Vidimos AT, Ammirati CT, Poblete–Lopez C. Dermatologic surgery: Requisites in dermatology. Edinburgh: Saunders; 2009.

O. Skin neoplasms

86. Abenoza P, Ackerman AB. Neoplasms with eccrine differentiation. Philadelphia: Lea & Febiger; 1990.
87. Ackerman AB, Cerroni L, Kerl H. Pitfalls in histopathologic diagnosis of malignant melanoma. Philadelphia: Lea & Febiger; 1994.
88. Ackerman AB, Reddy VB, Soyer HP. Neoplasms with follicular differentiation. 2nd edn. New York: Ardor Scribendi; 2001.
89. Ackerman AB, Massi D, Nielsen TA. Dysplastic nevus: Atypical mole or typical myth? New York: Ardor Scribendi; 1999.
90. Balch CM, Houghton AN, Sober AJ, Soong S-J, et al. Cutaneous melanoma. 5th edn. St Louis: Quality Medical; 2009.
91. Cerroni L, Gatter K, Kerl H. Skin lymphoma: The illustrated guide. 3rd edn. Hoboken, NJ: Wiley-Blackwell; 2009.
92. Gottlieb GJ, Ackerman AB, eds. Kaposi's sarcoma: A text and atlas. Philadelphia: Lea & Febiger; 1988.
93. Magro CM, Crowson NA, Mihm MC. The cutaneous lymphoid proliferations: A comprehensive textbook of lymphocytic infiltrates of the skin. Hoboken, NJ: Wiley; 2007.
94. Mooi WJ, Krausz T. Pathology of melanocytic disorders. 2nd edn. New York: Oxford University Press; 2007.
95. Nouri K, ed. Skin cancer. New York: McGraw Hill; 2008.
96. Piepkorn M, Busam KJ, Barnhill RL. Pathology of melanocytic nevi and malignant melanoma. 2nd edn. New York: Springer; 2010.
97. Requena L, Kiryu H, Ackerman AB. Neoplasms with apocrine differentiation. Philadelphia: Lippincott Williams & Wilkins; 1998.
98. Rigel DS, Robinson JK, Ross MI, et al. Cancer of the skin. 2nd edn. Philadelphia: WB Saunders; 2011.
99. Steffen C, Ackerman AB. Neoplasms with sebaceous differentiation. Philadelphia: Lea & Febiger; 1994.
100. Wick MR, Swanson PE. Cutaneous adnexal tumors. Chicago: ASCP Press; 1991.

P. Soft tissue neoplasms

101. Fisher C, Mentzel T, Montgomery EA, et al. Diagnostic pathology: Soft tissue tumors. Manitoba: Amirsys; 2011.
102. Fletcher CDM, ed. Diagnostic histopathology of tumors. 3rd edn. Edinburgh: Churchill Livingstone; 2007.
103. Weiss SW, Goldblum JR. Enzinger and Weiss's soft tissue tumors. 5th edn. St. Louis: Mosby; 2007.

Q. Dermatopathology journals

104. American Journal of Dermatopathology. New York: Lippincott Williams & Wilkins.
105. Dermatopathology: Practical & Conceptual. New York: Ardor Scribendi.
106. Journal of Cutaneous Pathology. Oxford: Blackwell.

R. Journal references

107. Ackerman AB, Nussen Lee S. Neoplasms in all organs of Muir–Torre syndrome are carcinomas. Dermatopathol: Practical & Conceptual 1999; 5:312–318.
108. Ackerman AB, Penneys NS. Formalin pigment in skin. Arch Dermatol 1970; 102:318–321.
109. Ackerman AB, Magana-Garcia M, DiLeonardo M. Naming acquired melanocytic nevi: Unna's, Miescher's, Spitz's, Clark's. Am J Dermatopathol 1990; 12:193–209.
110. Ackerman AB, Walton NW III, Jones RE, Charissi C. "Hot comb alopecia"/"follicular degeneration syndrome" in African-American women is traction alopecia. Dermatopathol: Practical & Conceptual 2000; 6:320–336.
111. Andrade DM, Ackerley CA, Minett TS, et al. Skin biopsy in Lafora disease. Neurology 2003; 61:1611–1614.
112. Balch CM, Gershenwald JE, Soong SJ, et al. Final version of 2009 AJCC melanoma staging and classification. J Clin Oncol 2009; 27:6199–6206.

113. Ball NJ, Golitz LE. Melanocytic nevi with focal atypical epithelioid cell components: A review of seventy-three cases. J Am Acad Dermatol 1994; 30:724–729.

114. Bergman R. Immunohistopathologic diagnosis of epidermolysis bullosa. Am J Dermatopathol 1999; 21:185–192.

115. Bhawan J, Cao SL. Amelanotic blue nevus: A variant of blue nevus. Am J Dermatopathol 1999; 21:225–228.

116. Boer A, Hoene K. Transverse sections for diagnosis of alopecia? Am J Dermatopathol 2005; 27:348–352.

117. Boyd AS, Rapini RP. Acral melanocytic neoplasms: A histologic analysis of 158 lesions. J Am Acad Dermatol 1994; 31:740–745.

118. Candiago E, Marocolo D, Manganoni MA, et al. Nonlymphoid intraepidermal mononuclear cell collections (pseudo-Pautrier abscesses): A morphologic and immunophenotypical characterization. Am J Dermatopathol 2000; 22:1–6.

119. Chang A, Wharton J, Tam S, et al. A modified approach to the histologic diagnosis of onychomycosis. J Am Acad Dermatol 2007; 57:849–853.

120. Chen KR, Su WP, Pittelkow MR, et al. Eosinophilic vasculitis in connective tissue disease. J Am Acad Dermatol 1996; 35:173–182.

121. Clarke PGH. Book review: A critical review of apoptosis in historical perspective. Am J Dermatopathol 2000; 22:288–290.

122. Connelly MG, Winkelmann RK. Solid facial edema as a complication of acne vulgaris. Arch Dermatol 1985; 121:87–90.

123. Cowper SE, Kilpatrick T, Proper S, et al. Solitary fibrous tumor of the skin. Am J Dermatopathol 1999; 21:213–219.

124. Magro CM, Crowson AN, Mihm MC, et al. The dermal-based borderline melanocytic tumor: A categorical approach. J Am Acad Dermatol 2010; 62:469–479.

125. Doud MS, Lust JA, Kyle RA, Pittelkow MR. Monoclonal gammopathies and associated skin disorders. J Am Acad Dermatol 1999; 40:507–535.

126. Duncan WC, Tschen JA, Knox JM. Terra firma-forme dermatosis (letter). Arch Dermatol 1987; 123:567–569.

127. Garcia J, Cohen PR, Herzberg AJ, et al. Pleomorphic basal cell carcinoma. J Am Acad Dermatol 1995; 32:740–746.

128. Ferrara G, Argenziano G, Zgavec B, et al. "Compound blue nevus": A reappraisal of "superficial blue nevus with prominent intraepidermal dendritic melanocytes" with emphasis on dermoscopic and histopathologic features. J Am Acad Dermatol 2002; 46:85–89.

129. Fine J-D, Eady RAJ, Bauer EA, et al. Revised classification system for inherited epidermolysis bullosa: report of the second international consensus meeting on diagnosis and classification of epidermolysis bullosa. J Am Acad Dermatol 2000; 42:1051–1066.

130. Hall JR, Holder W, Know JM, et al. Familial dyskeratotic comedones. J Am Acad Dermatol 1987; 17:808–814.

131. Headington JT. Tumors of the hair follicle. Am J Pathol 1976; 85:480–505.

132. Higby DJ. A practical classification of lymphomas (letter). N Engl J Med 1979; 300:1283.

133. Horenstein MG, Jacob JS. Follicular streamers (stelae) in scarring and non-scarring alopecia. J Cutan Pathol 2008; 35:1115–1120.

134. Ivan D, Diwan AH, Lazar AJ, Prieto VG. The usefulness of p63 detection for differentiating primary from metastatic skin adenocarcinomas. J Cutan Pathol 2008; 35:880–881.

135. Kalra L, Treloar A, Price R, et al. Blue sclerae and iron deficiency in general practice. Lancet 1987; 1:335.

136. Kerl H, Soyer HP, Cerroni L, et al. Ancient melanocytic nevus. Semin Diagn Pathol 1998; 15:210–215.

137. Ko CJ, McNiff JM, Glusac EJ. Melanocytic nevi with features of Spitz nevi and Clark's/dysplastic nevi ("Spark's" nevi). J Cutan Pathol 2009; 36:1063–1068.

138. Li N, Bajoghli A, Kubba A, Bhawan J. Identification of mycobacterial DNA in cutaneous lesions of sarcoidosis. J Cutan Pathol 1999; 26:271–278.

139. Liang H, Wu H, Giorgadze TA, et al. Podoplanin is a highly sensitive and specific marker to distinguish primary skin adnexal carcinomas from adenocarcinomas metastatic to skin. Am J Surg Pathol 2007; 31:304–310.

140. Lokich JJ, Moore C. Chemotherapy-associated palmar–plantar erythrodysesthesia syndrome. Ann Intern Med 1984; 101:798–799.

141. Lowe L, Rapini RP. Polarizable foreign material in granulomas of sarcoidosis. J Cutan Pathol 1990; 17:305.

142. Lowe L, Rapini RP. Newer variants and simulants of basal cell carcinoma. J Dermatol Surg Oncol 1991; 17:641–648.

143. Magro CM, Crowson AN, Shapiro BL. The interstitial granulomatous drug reaction: A distinctive clinical and pathological entity. J Cutan Pathol 1998; 25:72–78.

144. Mahaisavariya P, Cohen PR, Rapini RP. Incidental epidermolytic hyperkeratosis. Am J Dermatopathol 1995; 17:23–28.

145. McCalmont TH, Brinsko R, LeBoit PE. Melanocytic acral nevi with intraepidermal ascent of cells (MANIAC S): A reappraisal of melanocytic nevi from acral sites (abstract). J Cutan Pathol 1991; 18:378.

146. McNeely MC, Jorizzo JL, Solomon AR, et al. Primary idiopathic cutaneous pustular vasculitis. J Am Acad Dermatol 1986; 14:939–944.

147. Metry DW, Hebert AA. Benign cutaneous vascular tumors of infancy. Arch Dermatol 2000; 136:905–914.

148. Metze D, Rutten A. Granular parakeratosis, a unique acquired disorder of keratinization. J Cutan Pathol 1999; 26:339–352.

149. Mones JM, Ackerman AB. Proliferating trichilemmal cyst is squamous cell carcinoma. Dermatopathol: Practical & Conceptual 1998; 4:295–310.

150. Mutasim DF, Bridges AG. Patch granuloma annulare: Clinicopathologic study of 6 patients. J Am Acad Dermatol 2000; 42:417–421.

151. Nagasak T, Lai R, Medeiros LJ, et al. Cyclin D1 overexpression in Spitz nevi: An immunohistochemical study. J Cutan Pathol 1999; 21:115–120.

152. Nonaka D, Chiriboga L, Rubin BP. Sox10: A pan-schwannian and melanocytic marker. Am J Surg Pathol 2008; 32:1291–1298.

153. Peterson JL, Read SI, Rodman OG. Familial myxovascular fibromas. J Am Acad Dermatol 1982; 6:470–472.

154. Prieto VG, Sadick NS, McNutt NS. Quantitative immunohistochemical differences in Langerhans cells in dermatitis due to internal versus external antigen sources. J Cutan Pathol 1998; 25:301–310.

155. Radfar A, Stefanato CM, Ghosn S, Bhawan J. NGFR-positive desmoplastic melanomas with focal or absent S-100 staining: Further evidence supporting the use of both NGFR and S-100 as a primary immunohistochemical panel for the diagnosis of desmoplastic melanomas. Am J Dermatopathol 2006; 28:162–167.

156. Rapini RP. Obtaining a skin biopsy and interpreting the results. Dermatol Clin 1994; 12:83–91.

157. Rapini RP. "New" diseases in dermatopathology. Adv Dermatol 1997; 12:213–236.

158. Rapini RP. Spitz nevus or melanoma? Sem Cutan Med Surg 1999; 18:56–63.

159. Sariya D, Ruth K, Adams-McDonnell R, et al. Clinicopathologic correlation of cutaneous metastases: Experience from a cancer center. Arch Dermatol 2007; 143:613–620.

160. Signoretti S, Annessi G, Faraggiana T. Melanocytic nevi on palms and soles: an histologic study according to the plane of section (abstract). J Cutan Pathol 1996; 23:62.

161. Smith ES, Hallman JR, DeLuca AM, et al. Dermatomyositis: A clinicopathological study of 40 patients. Am J Dermatopathol 2009; 31:61–67.

162. Subrt P, Jorizzo JL, Apistharnthanarax P, et al. Spreading pigmented actinic keratosis. J Am Acad Dermatol 1983; 8:63–67.

163. Swerdlow SH, Campo E, Harris NL, et al. WHO classification of tumours of haematopoietic and lymphoid tissues. Lyon: IOARC Press; 2008.

164. Tschen JA. Pagetoid dyskeratosis. J Am Acad Dermatol 1988; 19:891–894.

165. Werchniak AE, Perry AE, Dinulos JG. Eosinophilic, polymorphic, and pruritic eruption associated with radiotherapy (EPPER) in a patient with breast cancer. J Am Acad Dermatol 2006; 54:728–729.

166. Wheeler CE Jr, Carroll MA, Groben PA, et al. Autosomal dominantly inherited generalized basaloid follicular hamartoma syndrome. J Am Acad Dermatol 2000; 43:189–206.

Index

Page numbers followed by "f" indicate figures, "t" indicate tables, and "b" indicate boxes.